American Romanian Academy of Arts and Sciences

A. Ardelean, Andreea-Daniela Antochi, C. Aurian-Blăjeni, O. Buda, P. Deme, P. Firu, Norina Forna, Corina Frandeş, Z. Györi, O. Haţegan, M. Ifrim, G. Litarczek, A. Majuru, Liana Moş, C. Precup, V. Preda, V. Săhleanu, Casiana Stănescu, C. Toth, N. Ursea

TREATISE
OF MEDICAL, MORPHO-FUNCTIONAL, MOTRICITY, CULTURAL AND META-PSYCHOLOGICAL ANTHROPOLOGY

Under the editorial supervision of
Acad. Prof. Mircea Ifrim, MD
Secretary General of the Academy of Medical Sciences

Acad. Prof. Mircea Ifrim, MD and collaborators
TREATISE OF MEDICAL, MORPHO-FUNCTIONAL, MOTRICITY, CULTURAL AND META-PSYCHOLOGICAL ANTHROPOLOGY

Authors: A. Ardelean, Andreea-Daniela Antochi, C. Aurian-Blăjeni, O. Buda, P. Deme, P. Firu, Norina Forna, Corina Frandeş, Z. Györi, O. Haţegan, M. Ifrim, G. Litarczek, A. Majuru, Liana Moș, C. Precup, V. Preda, V. Săhleanu, Casiana Stănescu, C. Toth, N. Ursea
COVER: Iulian Gherstoaga
ARA Editors: Ioana Onica, Ruxandra Vidu
PUBLISHER: ARA Publishing House
COVER ILLUSTRATION: *The Creation of Adam*, Michelangelo, Sistine Chapel ceiling
COVER: Iulian Gherstoaga
TRANSLATOR: Andreea - Daniela Antochi

ISBN: 978-1-935924-27-2

Under the editorial supervision of
Acad. Prof. Mircea Ifrim, MD
Secretary General of the Academy of Medical Sciences

ARA Publisher: http://www.AmericanRomanianAcademy.org

I dedicated this work as homage to my teachers

Assoc. Prof. Dr. Eugen Floru, MD

Acad. Prof. Dr. Şt. Marius Milcu, MD

Prof. I. Th. Riga

Acad. Prof.Dr B. Menckes, MD

Acad. Prof.Dr Victor Preda, MD

Outstanding personalities of Romanian and international medicine, who passed away and to whom I owe my training in the field of anthropology.

Special thanks to the management of the "Vasile Goldiş" Western University of Arad, who helped me with the work and research facilities required for the issuing of this treatise.

AUTHORS

Aurel Ardelean – Academician Professor Univ. Dr., MD, The "Vasile Goldiş" the University of Arad

Antochi Andreea - Daniela - MA in East- Asian Studies, University of Bucharest

Aurian-Blăjeni Corneliu – Doctor in Medical Sciences;

Buda Octavian – Professor, MD, the "Carol Davila" University, Bucharest;

Deme Paul – Assistant Professor, the "Vasile Goldiş" University of Arad;

Firu Pătru – Professor, MD, the "Carol Davila" University, Bucharest;

Forna Norina – Professor, the University of Medicine of Iaşi, Dean, corresponding member of the Academy of Medical Sciences;

Frandeş Corina-Daniela – Lecturer, MD, the "Vasile Goldiş" University of Arad;

Györi Zsolt – Assistant Professor, the "Vasile Goldiş" University of Arad;

Haţegan Ovidiu – Doctor in Medical Sciences, lecturer, the "Vasile Goldiş" University of Arad;

Ifrim Mircea – Acad. Prof. Dr. The "Vasile Goldiş" the University of Arad, Secretary General of the Academy of Medical Sciences, Awarded with the National Order of the "Star of Romania" in rank of Knight;

Litarczek George – Academician Professor Doctor in Medical Sciences, the "Carol Davila" University, Bucharest;

Majuru Adrian – Historian;

Moş Liana Mioara – Professor Doctor Dean at the Faculty of Medicine, the "Vasile Goldiş" University of Arad;

Precup Cris-Virgiliu – Assoc. Prof., MD, the "Vasile Goldiş" the University of Arad, specialist physician in forensic medicine;

Preda Victor – Academician Professor, the "Iuliu Haţieganu" University of Cluj;

Săhleanu Victor – Academician Professor doc. MD, Director of the Centre for Anthropologic Research of the Romanian Academy, Bucharest (during 1990-1998);

Stănescu Casiana – Lecturer, MD, the "Vasile Goldiş" the University of Arad, specialist physician in gynecology;

Toth Csongor– Assistant Professor, the "Vasile Goldiş" University, Arad;

Ursea Nicolae – Academician Professor MD, the "Carol Davila" University, Bucharest.

Table of Content

PREFACE
TO THE SECOND EDITION

The Treatise of Medical, Morpho-functional, Motricity, Cultural and Meta-psychological Anthropology gives an original and extremely complex view regarding the creation of the "human" phenomenon, which is the subject of anthropology and it can prove any passing day the great philosopher Socrates's axiom '*I know that nothing is known!*'

Creationism-evolutionism, science-religion, opposition or complementarity, these are the great questions to which the anthropology is looking for answers on its turn. Anthropology may be accounted for an inter-disciplinary science where multiple other areas interfere, like medicine, both fundamental and practical, the motricity without which the human being cannot be thought of, with direct applicability in health and sports, in the cultural phenomenon emanated by the human being, and recently, the metapsychology as the paranormal human aspects are a reality.

The current work outstands by the originality of dealing with such complex issues, which also explain the presence among the authors of some personalities from various fields approaching this topic. In the same time, there can be noticed the presence of some valuable young persons, trained in the vivid school established by the *Acad. M. Ifrim.*

Acad. M. Ifrim trained himself with masters who were direct disciples of the *Prof. Francisc Iosif Rainer*, the founder of this anthropological science in Romania, worldwide acknowledged, the first International Congress of Anthropology being held in Bucharest under his presidency.

The great academician *Ştefan Marius Milcu, Rainer's* student, called *Mircea Ifrim* as *Rainer*'s "grandson"; this "grandson" continuing the anthropological research under his guidance and some other distinguished students of Prof. Rainer, among which we name *Eugen Floru, Theodor Riga, Neagu Natalia* and others.

This treatise has both philosophical and practical value. Philosophically, it brings to-date data on the place where the phenomenon "human"stands, in essence, pleading with current data that "*there is the spirit above the substance.*"

Practically, the data of medical, motricity, and morpho-functional anthropology, conditioned both genetically (genotypic) and by the environmental action (para-typical), are of practical use: – for medicine where, for instance, the bioenergy which represented an enigma in the past (telepathy, telekinetic, etc.) can be certified today with extremely complex equipment, the alternative medicine with its various fields being acknowledged by the World Health Organisation. The individualised therapy relying upon the anthropological typologies is imperiously required, *Paracelsus* stating that it is more important to know "*what kind of patient has a certain disease than to know what kind of disease has a certain patient*" – the same standing for the physical education, an important element of prophylaxis in the competition sports, where the constitutional typology selection is of essence; – as for the culture which is nothing else but the emanation of the human being's complexity – and, not lately, for each human being who, knowing better him/ herself if possessing some notions of anthropology may develop harmoniously, achieving a better correlation between aspiration, vocation and possibilities which may provide him/ her an optimal evolution.

As a conclusion of this treatise, I express my entire consideration to the authors and, not in the last, to the work coordinator, Acad. Prof. Dr. *M. Ifrim*, who proves himself a valuable researcher and a worthy "grandson" of the Professor *Francisc Rainer*, being educated in the vivid school of this great coryphaeus of the Romanian and international school of this science who said that "*a teacher is great if his students go higher than him.*"

Acad. Prof. Cristiana Glavce, M.D.
Director of the National Institute of Anthropology of the Romanian Academy

PREFACE
TO THE FIRST EDITION

A preface can be useful to a work only if it avoids the "benevolent" formalism in its appreciation. According to this standpoint, we shall present a commented analysis of the complex anthropologic interrelations considered under the motricity aspect in the vision of this monograph.

Adopting the concept of anthropology as a complex multi-band interdisciplinary science, the work presents the essential parameters of the human organism in dynamics. The critical role of the psycho neuro muscular ability as a basic factor in sanogenetic and performance physical training is pointed out.

By considering anthropology in the complexity of the interrelated components, which have defined it from its very beginning in the nineteenth century, a reductionist presentation of the problems has been avoided. In this perspective, the author shows in the first chapters the main stages of human ontogenesis, very necessary to the understanding of the mechanism of Motricity, generally and in sport especially.

A whole chapter, dealing with the "*hereditary determination of the human organism, genotypic and para-typical interrelations of importance in sports activity*," is substantiated by the investigation of the relation between the neuro motricity capacity of the parents and their offspring, extended up to the endowment for a certain sports category. An exemplification of the veracity of this hereditary relation is completed with a similar analysis biopsychic and biochemical mechanisms of genetics, able to explain this potential capacity favoring sports performances.

In the anthropologic assessment of the factors which define the psychoneuromotricity capacity in sport, the necessity of also utilizing the constitutional typology should be emphasised. The complex problems of these interrelations are set forth clearly, in a logical sequence. The examples of sports performances analyzed using modern technology in the anthropologic perspective are conclusive for the problems of the treatise and for its utility in practice. The description of biorhythms as complex anthropologic parameters is meritorious.

The morphological chapters of sport anthropology are presented in the light of the unity between form and function, a characteristic feature of the Romanian school of anatomy, promoted in our country by *Fr. I. Rainer*, who also held the function of Head of the Department of Anatomy – Biomechanics and Anthropology of the National Academy of Physical Training and rector of the latter. This conception permitted to approach new aspects of the organism of a performance sportsman. Particularly instructive from this point of view are the psychological parameters and the elements that characterize movement: speed, force, resistance, and skill.

Skill as a bio-psychomotricity quality is described in its complexity, with aspects related to the mechanisms which determine it and some elements of high applicability, representing an original and valuable contribution of the author. These chapters as a whole are of the utmost interest and utility for the organizer, the coach, and the sportsman. The constitutional type presented from the somato-physiological, motricity and psychic point of view and determined genotypically and para-typically is a new element both on the conceptual and applied plane.

Likewise, the integration of the biological forms in their dynamics with the various factors of the natural and educative environment should also be emphasised. In this way, a complete anthropologic representation, which considers the social and cultural complexity, characteristic of man and human populations, is obtained. The author's opinion, according to which the factors play a part in the achievement of performances and generally in sports efficiency, is just. It is shown by conclusive arguments that the genetic potential may be brought into being through education and sports training.

An outstanding merit of the author consists in the fact that he reviewed the problems of sport and implicitly of physical training in the perspective of an anthropology applied in the forms of movement of the human organism. The originality of this approach is also pointed out by the fact that the traditional anthropology is a predominantly static discipline, with few attempts to define a man by dynamic parameters. It is obvious that sport is a science only as far as it includes data of anthropology, genetics, physiology, biomechanics, mathematics, etc., remaining otherwise a simple limitative practice which, under the conditions of the current advances, can no more meet the requirements of performance. The only working tool of the specialist in the field of physical training and sport is the human organism, a fact which fully justifies the absolute necessity of knowledge, in their complexity, of the anthropologic aspects defining the phenomenon man.

The sports anthropology is, undoubtedly, an editorial event of a high originality, offering a rich, informative material also in the medicine of the healthy man, in which physical training under its various form represents a sanogenetic requirement. In addition, on the conceptual anthropologic plane, the work brings a meritorious contribution to the development of anthropology in a dialectical materialistic, functional vision, passing beyond the descriptive stage, limited only to morphological aspects, and illustrating once more the actuality of the ideas of Professor Fr. I. Rainer, who pointed out that "*the form shows at the same time the function*".

This treatise represents a valuable contribution to the theoretical and practical foundation for both anthropology and sport and physical training in general. We appreciate the book should be available in the library of every specialist in the field of anthropology, medicine, and physical training, as well as of those who have in their Profession a tangency with the biological complexity of the human body.

Academician ȘTEFAN M. MILCU

FOREWORD

The *Treatise of Medical, Morpho-functional, Motricity, Cultural and Meta-psychological Anthropology* which represents the second revised and completed edition of the monograph published in 1988, tries to present a series of new data occurred lately in the science of the anthropology, processed through the prism of the authors' personal experience and their original research.

The monograph's purpose is both conceptual and philosophical, giving a cosmic vision to the "human" phenomenon, pleading for Platon's philosophy, for whom the real world is the shadow of the fire existing in the celestial world, and a practical, anthropological one, as it results from the work, which, by knowing and deepening the constitution, physical and cultural typology, can bring concrete solutions in medicine, physical education, sports, culture, etc. Being aware on the fact stated by the great neurologist Ashby that, in the field of cognitive and thinking capacities, the "*unknown is much higher than the known fact.*" The authors understand that the process of knowledge is extremely difficult and complex and that the current monograph does nothing else but to prove the Chinese saying '*the higher you are, and you look, the valleys seems deeper and darker*' or as the philosopher *Fr. Bacon* said '*partial knowledge leads to unfaith, and knowledge, as deeper as it gets, leads to faith*'.

We leave it up to the experts and readers to evaluate the work and to suggest us everything which might improve it in a future edition.

We give a special thanks to the "Vasile Goldiş" Western University of Arad, to the Acad. Aurel Ardelean, its president who generously granted us access to the Institute of Life Sciences, which resides on the Platform of the Academy of Medical Sciences, so that we could perform such research in this area, and that this work could be published.

Acad. Prof. Dr. Mircea Ifrim
Secretary General of the Academy of Medical Sciences

CHAPTER I.
MEDICAL FUNDAMENTALS OF THE ROMANIAN ANTHROPOLOGY

Francisc Iosif Rainer (1874-1944): medicine, anthropology, culture

Member of the Scientific Department of the Romanian Athenaeum (1933)
Titular member of the Academy of Medicine (1935)
Honorary Member of the Romanian Academy (1943)

"There is a synthesis of the knowledge which may throw a bridge between man and goodness by art and science!"
Francisc Iosif Rainer

"Rainer is the most erudite person I know!"
Ion Cantacuzino

The Romanian modern scientific and cultural world owes the scientist *Francisc Rainer* an absolute unique creation in the field of anatomy and anthropology, thanks to his works and to the schools he established in Iaşi (1920-1944) and Bucharest (1920-1942). Besides the great neurologist *Gheorghe Marinescu*, *Rainer* was one of the most distinguished students of *Victor Babeş*, a regular participant in the works of the "Society of Anatomy," head of the laboratory of the Medical Clinic at the Colţea Hospital, a "spiritus rector" of the anatomy in Romania. *Francisc Rainer* is the founder of the medical anthropology in our country and, at the same time, the founder of the School of Anthropology in the capital of the country. *Rainer* had an integrating conception of the anthropology, being fully persuaded by the "*tight ratio between the biology and the culture.*"

However, let's make first a leap in time...

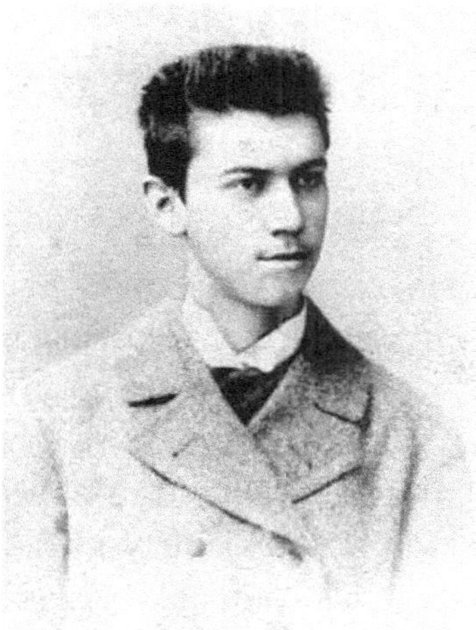

Student in the First year of Medicine. Image from 1892, at 18 years old.

"Over 125 years ago, in the current University Square, there was still for another few years, a garden where one could lose oneself for some moments at any time of the day. A young high school pupil used to come in this garden at noon to spend his break quietly. The Saint Sava College was nearby, and that retreat was for our young man only a passage in between two walks. He was sitting on one bench and eating his homemade lunch. A frugal snack and, while eating, he was looking far, at the rumor on the street. Then, he went to the University`s Library, using the entrance from the Faculty of Science, entrance which is currently blocked. This high school pupil's name was *Francisc Iosif Rainer*. And, this was the beginning of his concerns to get closer to the knowledge, and his reading at the University`s Library placed him entirely in the neighborhood of the sciences, of the concrete from the immediate worldliness. Here and under such circumstances, the high school pupil *Rainer* decided to study medicine. And so, in this story, he entered in the year of grace, 1892." 52 years later, in 1944, still on a summer day, he was lying down on his bed and very weakened, he found himself at the end of a road which he felt arriving without anything being able to stop it. He asked for paper and pencil to write down, but he gave up, saying people around that, at eight o'clock, `his way was about to end.' "*I have two things inside me, one is what becomes spirit when I die, the other is the soul of the body, which dies at the same time with it,*" said the scientist during his last year of life. Moreover, while on his way of departure, he still felt a grasping hand and to comfort those around him, he was whispering "still... still...", but then he wept as the last words had been spoken. And crying, head turned towards the windows; he slept into eternity... While that high school pupil was getting ready to enter the Faculty of Sciences and go upstairs to the library in search of the human perfection..." (*The Biography of a Universal Personality* by Adrian Majuru, in Francisc Iosif Rainer, *Daily Notes. Conferences. Travel Diaries*, edition cared by Adrian Majuru, Oscar Print Publishing House, Bucharest, 2012, page 9)

Francisc Rainer's concerns are difficult to be framed into distinct areas, as he had a confession to make for each hour of the day. And this scientist's confession was the synthesis of some elaborate concerns and research, coming from medicine and passed through the filters of the universal culture or cut from the literature, art, or philosophy and adjacent added to his medical excurse. That surprised the most, and his faculty colleagues said that he "was a phenomenon." Actually, the ability of the answer triggered from particular and developed to general was built only by personal effort. Very simply, *Rainer* said that to his students: "*The personality develops by solving issues raised by reality. The choice of the favorite solutions in this solving sets the type of the personality. The clashes with reality are important, and not the ghosts of the things. We may be sure that the only way given to us to evolve is that of the personal effort. We cannot evolve, but by our intuition, therefore, each of us must find the personal way to grow his/ her qualities*".

Benchmarks for an Exceptional Career

Born in 1874 in a family of Austrian intellectual in Bukovina, Austrian citizen, *Francisc Iosif (Josef) Rainer* gets a certificate of naturalization as Romanian only in 1904, at 30 years old. He studies in Iaşi and Bucharest, where he enrolled at the Faculty of Medicine in 1892. Ever since the faculty, the Professor of psychiatry *Alexandru Obreja* receives him as preparatory at the laboratory of the Chair of Histology (1894). In 1920, he was transferred as Professor and, then, as head of the Department of Anatomy and Embryology at the Faculty of Medicine of Bucharest. It is the time when another stage of the Professor's life begins: his encyclopaedic concerns of modern anthropology. From that moment, *Rainer* will define the anthropology as *the science of the Human phenomenon*.

The cooperation between *Francisc Rainer* and the great sociologist and ethnographer *Dimitrie Gusti* and the institutionalization of the Romanian anthropology concretizes via the complex campaigns of research of the rural Romanian population from the mountain area and by the publishing of the monograph *Anthropological Surveys in Three Romanian Villages in the Carpathians*, fundamental work in the Romanian Anthropology. In 1939, the volume received the *Oroveanu Award* of the Romanian Academy whose Honorary member he became in 1943.

The anthropological school that he established carries the seal of his original, innovative and interdisciplinary thinking in the knowledge of the human being in its bio-cultural integrity and in the dynamics achieved with the environment. This integrated vision for the human being, shaped by the European scientific world by the end of the 20th century, was introduced in our country by Professor *Rainer*. To him as well, we owe the establishment of the only Institute of Anthropology bearing his name, in 1937, at Bucharest, Institute which he conceived from construction details to the research directions which are still current and which placed the Romanian anthropology among the most modern schools at international level. The major topic to which he dedicated his entire career was that of the correlation substance – life. Ever since the beginning of the education and research in the field of anatomy, embryology, and anthropology, he imprinted a fecund direction to the synthesis between morphologic and functional, admirably synthesized in the sentence engraved on the frontispiece of his laboratory: "*Anatomy is the science of the living matter.*"

This orientation mainly influenced the Romanian school of morphology. His research, though low in number due to the scientist's excessive scrupulosity and probity, represented highly valuable contributions in the universal morphological science. They have been published in the medical press of the country ("The Hospital," "The Journal of Medical Sciences") and abroad (in the French and German media) or communicated to various societies (the Anatomic Society, the Society of Medical Sciences, the Society of Biology, etc.). Otherwise, with much modesty, Rainer wrote that: *Without a doubt, the person dealing with science often has the occasion to have more or less unusual findings, but usually, they do not have this quality... Basically, this is the reason why the number of publications synthesized in the following pages is narrow compared to the quite long number of years since I have been working.*

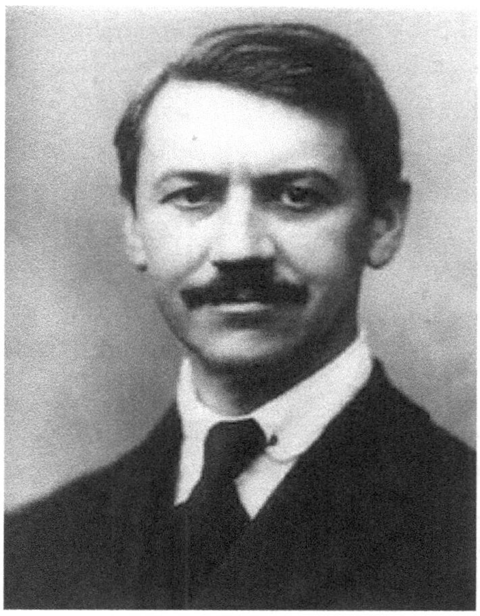

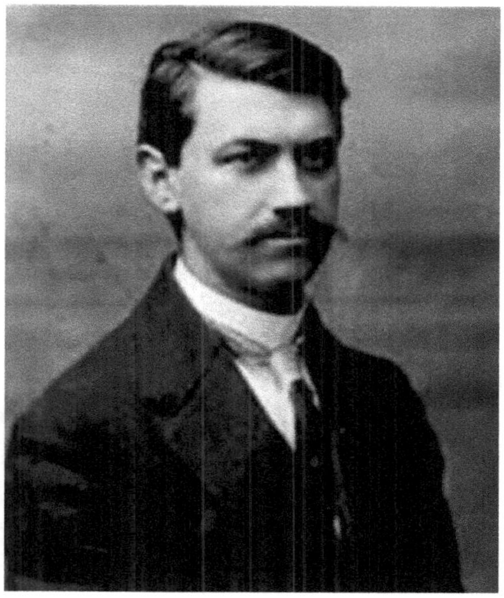

Portrait images, years 1910-1920

In 1945, under the aegis of the *Society Romanian Athenaeum* and the *Romanian Academy,* four posthumous volumes in Romanian and French had been published, the volumes comprising just a part of this scientific works. Of the numerous observations and morphologic research, we must mention: the referential description of the sub-epicardium lymph nodes in humans, of some anatomic impairment of the *Willis'* arterial polygon; the structural particularities of the epididymis, the coexistence of the duodenum-jejunum pits with the upper and lower duodenal pits, the anatomy of the lymph vessels of the heart and skin etc. The heart lymphatic system may be regarded as *Francisc Rainer*'s main scientific contribution in anatomy. Using the new techniques of repeated inoculation, completed with studies of microscopy and compared anatomy, he brings entirely new data both in their description and morpho-functional interpretation. Another work of high value, with finalized character, is that on the dura mater functional structure. Prof. *Rainer* deducted the existence of the pituitary portal system which his student, *Grigore T. Popa,* will describe magisterially and he predicted the existence of the cardiac fascia – which today bears the name *His* – long before its discovery by *His*.

Also, *Fr. Rainer* carried on a significant organizational and methodological activity in the field of the anatomic education. He organized the Department of Anatomy by a modern conception, expanding the area and arranging the annex laboratories, turning it into a modern institute of morphology and embryology. The anatomic Museum is completed and organized by his care, processing the anatomic preparations of the most instructive and valuable ones. In order to prepare the material of dissection, Prof. *Rainer* set up the prosectorium – the corpses service – at the Faculty of Medicine, as well as the Institute of Anthropology, a unique institute in our country, one of the fewest of Europe. *Fr. Rainer* contributed in the organization of the Institute of Physical Education (being the holder of the Anatomy Department of the Institute mentioned earlier), and he organized the education of the artistic anatomy at the Academy of Belle Arts.

Francisc Rainer: the Professor

His wife said about him that, up to 40 years old, until 1913-1914, he had lived in a "prolonged adolescence," which he went out unexpectedly with a tremendous responsibility: the course of anatomy at the Faculty of Medicine of Iaşi. In the opening of this course, *Rainer* had stated a principle of life and a pedagogical method built in silence and full privacy during the 17 years of clinician at the Colţea Hospital: "*I have always had the persuasion that there was no higher feeling, not so vast and Profound thinking that one could not share to some young minds and hearts. It is the most beautiful meaning of the teacher to find the ways for it. How far I am from this ideal, no one else could know but me! However, the value I put on your beings, I think that you already have felt it. Without hesitating, I may say that I have seen in you all Your future*".

Rainer entered the pedagogical life with the faith in the solidarity of the human souls, trying to acquire "*a soul and intellectual wealth with the thought to pass it to the others",* though *"the borders of the soul one cannot find this way, walking, and, as long as you would wander on all the paths, so deep would be its meanings*". He felt so tight to the human soul that it seemed a *murder* to him to mock the *youth*.

He worked thoroughly and with great delicacy with the young souls, both in the course room and in the dissection areas. One day in *Rainer's* life was not only an early debut, but it also varied as a program, all these variations serving to just one purpose: the knowledge of the human soul. The working day started in the morning at two or three o'clock, and he read in the morning what was harder to read. He read from two to eight o 'clock and then he entered in the healthcare service. At five o'clock in the afternoon, he was on the Kisseleff Road, in the second round, telling his close one: "*not only the walk but also to sit on the grass and then to answer after a quarter of an hour.*" Riding the bike was either every day or twice, thrice a week. One of the things he put was turning the energies. He proposed that *Iosif, Bruckner,* and *Buşilă* get united, that each takes one book to which each to make a reference. The most important things he wrote calligraphically and placed them on walls, on boards, saying he needs to see what we wrote when passing by. He said there was no meaning to live if one could not do anything...

This happened in 1897. Years later, *the physician Negreanu* noted this fact and its results achieved through a continuous individual effort of improvement: *Who had not suffered from insomnia in his/ her life, troubled by great cosmic matters, this one is not worthy to be called human or to live. This is a human the one who can die for an idea. At the [the monographic campaign] the monograph in Fundul Moldovei (Bukovina), Rainer went with the students in the evening, looked to the sky and gave astronomic explanations and recited from the second part of Faust. He made large steps. He climbed the mountain with an unseen fastness. He made fencing with Pipart, Bădescu, and Pancu all the time. Rainer* built on the same background of knowledge of general culture and strict specialty an applied endeavor on the specific form of the anatomy course. In the same time, he taught to students at medicine, plastic arts and at the National Institute of Physical Education. For the latest, his course explanations looked as: *The walk is formed by a succession of positions where all the body parts are engaged; it is a personal act, depending on the ratio of levers of the body segments and it also depends on the person's temper. The state of soul is also reflected by this basic element of ours. The shape our shoes takes while using them gives us certain clues on the way how the chain of forces in our body act against the gravity (...) In the chromatic mass comprising "genes" carrying the abilities which we are endowed with from our ancestors, the body shape, the temper, the soul qualities and even the human destiny are imprinted.* Then, he emphasized that *all physical qualities must be acquired by endeavors and sweat by each generation apart, as in our being, only the phenotype may be influenced by environment and education in a certain amount.*

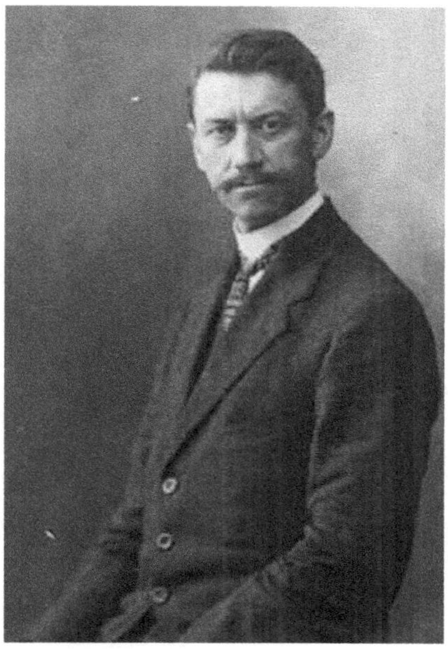

Francisc Rainer in 1914, at 40 years old.

There was another approach for the students at plastic arts, *Rainer* saying that *we must educate the student's eye for perceiving various subtleties and shades, we must sharpen the faculty of differentiation.*

On this Professor's projection on the final result of an academic lecture, one of his ex-students at Belle Arts, Ms. *Aurora Pavelescu* remembered after almost two decades, in 1945, how the Prof. *Rainer*'s course of artistic anatomy had been developed: *Examining the living model, our attention was drawn on the ratios. The Professor explained us a ratio scheme by Fritsch's method. It was simple and easy to calculate. The length of the backbone was measured, that dividing into four areas (modules). With the help of these modules, the ratios scheme is combined. As we had been familiar with finding on the living model the spots representing the centers of the joints, we could take the measures to apply them in the scheme. On one part, the limbs lengths as it should have been by ratio rules was enlisted, and on the other, there was what we really found out. Most of the times, the disproportion was impressive.*

Measuring a larger number of models, we got familiar with such a procedure and, in time, we could figure out at first sight if a human body was proportionate or not. (...) We could notice the deposits of adipose tissue on the female models. The Professor explained us the changes occurring while getting older. The male models gave us the opportunity to examine the musculature, to figure out what is the muscular tonus. We were informed on the superficial sanguine vessels. Each class allowed us to find new details. One by the other, we were described: the ear, the nose, the eye, anatomically presented and then compared to models and in various works of art, by age and authors. We noted the color of the iris, and we were told how its various colors could be explained. We interpret the special particularities of the face, either as fetal characteristics, or as pathological elements, or as racial difference. (...) Sometimes, in front of a model, the student called to examine him, does not notice all details. Then, the Professor helps him/ her. For instance, he asked if he had seen somewhere else the lines on the neck, seen at a young woman. The Professor reminded us that they could be seen at Venus of Milo and so, they are a sign of beauty. It is the so-called "Venus's necklace." He gave us a lot of examples of esthetical details: the fat cushion located by the axilla on the great pectoral or the lateral inferior lumbar dimples. All were details carefully figured on the antic statues.

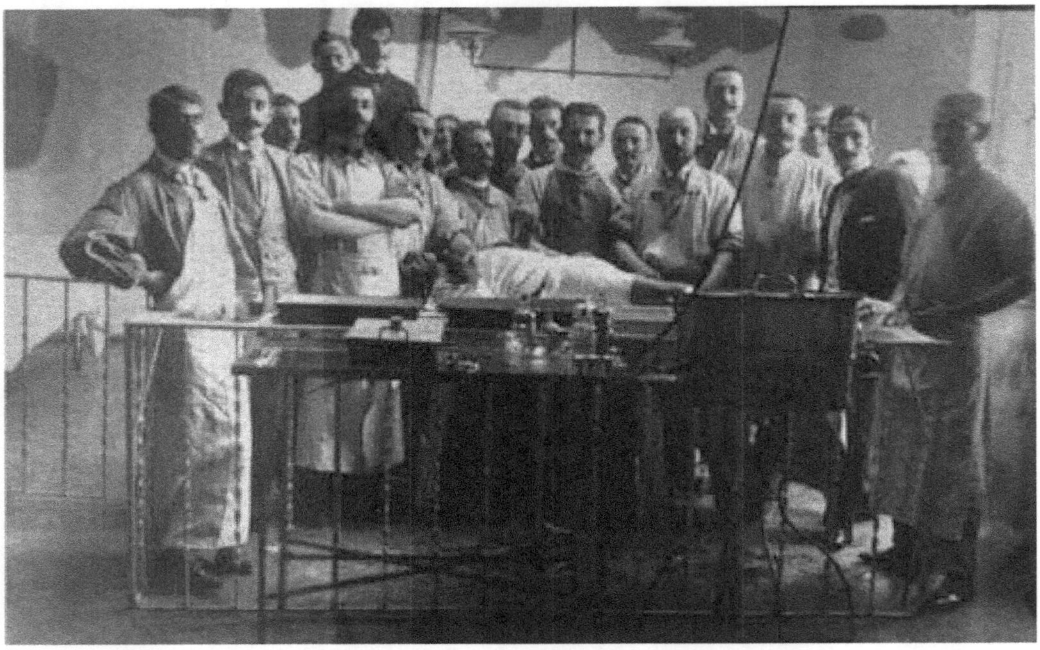

Fr. Rainer, trainee at Colţea, by 1900. In the image, he is in the upper line, in a black suit. In the middle of the group, Thoma Ionescu; the second at right, Victor Gomoiu.

As for the lectures held by *Fr. Rainer* at the Academy of Belle Arts, the Professor *Gheorghe Ghiţescu* – Professor's student and follower – considered that the anatomy as "*science of the living matter met naturally at Rainer with the science of the external shapes of the living body, with the artistic anatomy. (...) Beyond the field of anatomy and the discussion on de muscular modeling in rest and movement, at special classes or during plain incursions related to the anatomic problems, the vast area of the differentiated external morphology and the expression opened up*". For his students at Medicine, *Rainer* had a scientific endeavor oriented towards the immediate intervention, not without comprising the creative intuition. He said that there are required "*not much knowledge, but and few organic, reality-connected, adequate knowledge without which one is lost at patient's bedside.*" *Rainer* was one of the most valuable Professors in the Romanian medical education, his lectures and conferences being of an outstanding clarity and erudition. Over the years, his students at the Faculty of Medicine said "with admiration" to *Mircea Vulcănescu*, how the intuition led *Rainer to the discovery of a functional correlation between the organs without apparent connections between them, but even to some important anatomic characters which the study of the corpses did not allow for, as they were not obvious but in the structure and functioning of the living body.* For *Rainer*, the body unity was *a method requirement, a perspective of the spirit, a hidden element which has to order out the development of the intelligence operations when it is tried to clarify a concrete fact, a shape.*

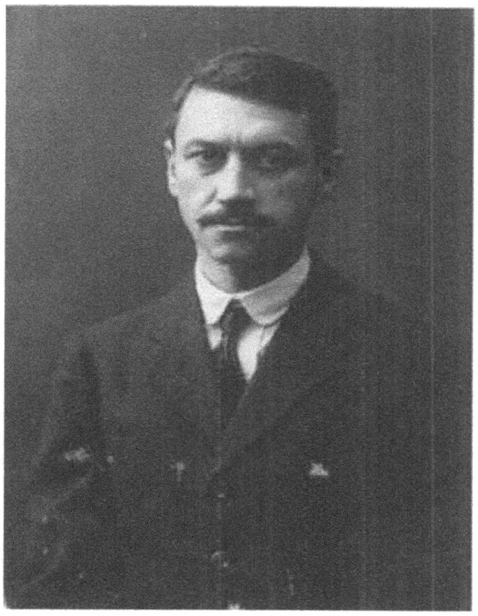

Photograph made in November - December 1916.

Rainer also addressed to the broad audience in a public conference held at "Dalles" Hall for ten years, somewhere between 1932 and 1942. The clarity of his observations and the clear language, the simple and exact wording persuaded each time. There were at least two situations: once during the field research, with *Dimitrie Gusti*, where, each time, *Rainer* succeeded to persuade the peasants from isolated villages to come and cooperate with the sociologists and physicians who came in their village, and, on the other hand, he succeeded to persuade a very diverse audience, consumer of culture, on this niche concerns linking the philosophy to the biology, to the anthropology and the universal literature and most of all of the common, yet sensible and hardly noticeable connection between such diverse areas. The two inseparable sides, the biological and the cultural, created the *Phenomenon Human Being. Rainer* used to say that *any conception of life resulting only from the biological is subhuman, but no conception of life should oppose to the biology. Francisc Rainer* always highlighted the social and cultural importance of population's education.

Pioneering in teaching anatomy

The hardly built erudition ever since the high school years helped *Rainer* in achieving the first remarkable discovery, and this discovery was not made only as results of his works in the Colţea wards, but, especially, to the association of the medical practice to the original reading of *Goethe's* poetic and scientific works, as well as that of the works of the great British naturalist *Charles Darwin*.

Rainer developed his work and research method by developing the comparisons between varied fields of concern, proving how tight is the connection between science and culture. Thus, *Goethe's* line "*Geprägte Form, die lebend sichentwick elt,*" i.e., *the pattern of the shape, which develops alive,* helped him give the most innovative definition of the human anatomy: *the Anatomy is the science of the living matter. Rainer* considered the anatomy as *science, as a branch of the biology; he presented the anatomic forms in their mechanical and functional causality.* In the same time, *Rainer* had the *spirit of observation and biological judgment. Rainer* was the founder of the functional and biological school of anatomy, *the scientific anatomy in our country,* which was not descriptive, nor it relied on the fragmentary description of the organic parts, *as it did not represent an inventory, but a functional, evolutionist anatomy. The scientific culture*, said *Rainer, is not equal to information or orientation.* At *Francisc Rainer*'s method of research in the anatomy, it *becomes a science of the movement, of the development, of the causal chaining in time and space of the forms, which so appear as phenomena whose origin is historically conditioned during the* phylogenetic.

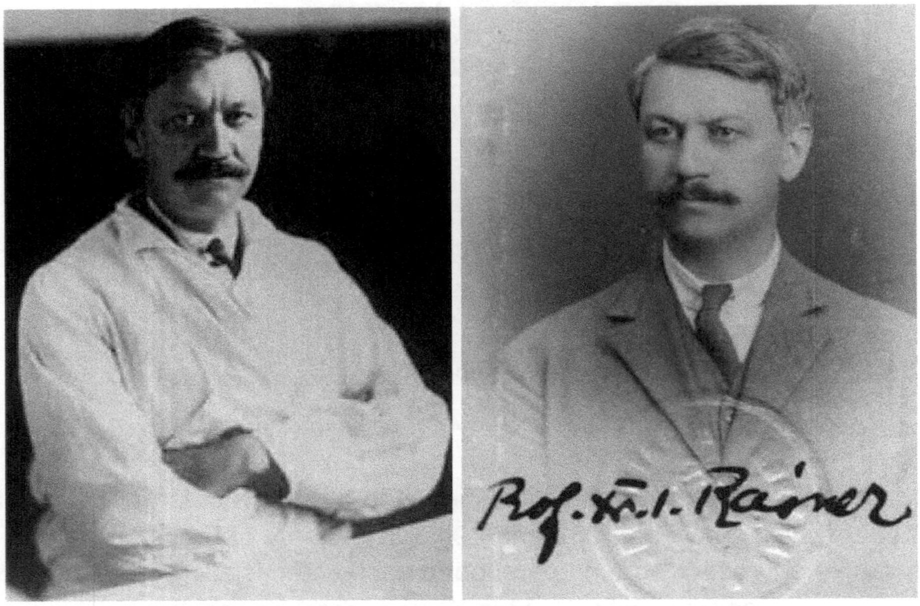

Fr. Rainer in a portrait photo of 1926 and a photo with signature.

For *Rainer,* it was very important to have a *clear speech, adjusted to the work, not as an actor.* He told his students during one of his lectures on anatomy in 1920: *Any form of the living matter, being stimulated, always responds by the reactions inherent to its structure. The energy power applied on the optical nerve gives light sensation, on the acoustic nerve – hearing sensations, on the tongue – tasting sensations.* Or on another occasion: *Let's not imagine that the centers in the brains governing the words articulation are identical with centers of the ideas. Thus, in order to express more accurate an idea, it is required to excite these centers. This cannot be made better but by articulating in our speech with tight teeth. May someone conceives a more beautiful idea without being expressed in words if these centers are not exercised*?

He was a visual person, remembering his ex-students of the anatomy course. *He described the things as if the vision was a muscular action. He put the images from the books in three dimensions at once. Constantin I. Parhon*, ex-colleague of the department with Prof. *Rainer* ever since Iaşi, said in the middle of the 40's: (...) *we can state that Rainer is the one who put the grounds for the scientific anatomy at our faculty, so conceived as we found written on the frontispiece of the institute he ran: "The Anatomy is the science of the living form".(...) Rainer introduced the real scientific education of the Anatomy which is the study of the body and the organs, tissues, etc. as phenomena whose determinism must be investigated by all means. (...) I mention in particular the fact of constantly highlighting the role which the traction exerted by the muscular constrictions has in the architecture of tendons, aponeurosis, and bones.* Consequently, *Rainer* created in the anatomy "a new method of thinking and work. He is the first who gave a new direction to the study of the anatomy, (...) where the living matter is tightly linked to the structure, and this one to the function; so, it is the expression of the functional structure. *Rainer* was among the first who dwelt with the functional structures and, in our country, the first who gave impetus to that research".

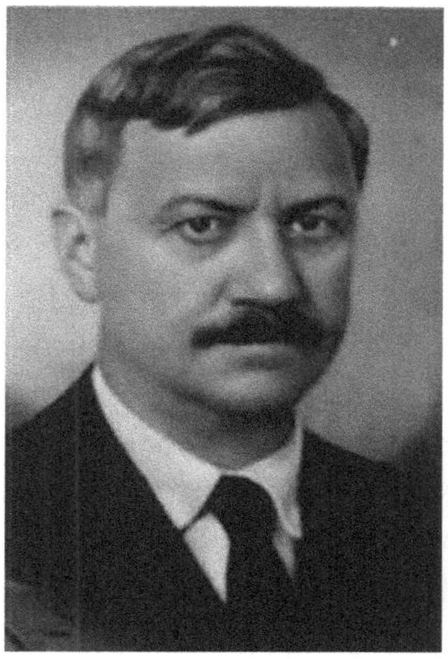

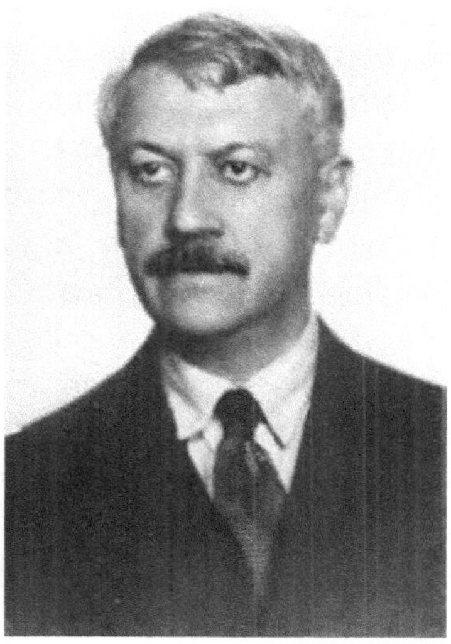

Fr. Rainer – two late photos, the one at right is in 1942, at 68 years old.

The founding of the School of Anthropology of Bucharest

Since his arrival as Professor of anatomy at the Faculty of Medicine of Bucharest, *Francisc Rainer* has introduced elements of anthropology. The first Ph.D. dissertation based on anthropological research, and supervised by him, is defended by *Valentina Roşca, MD,* in 1926 (from a somatological investigation in a Normal School for Girls).

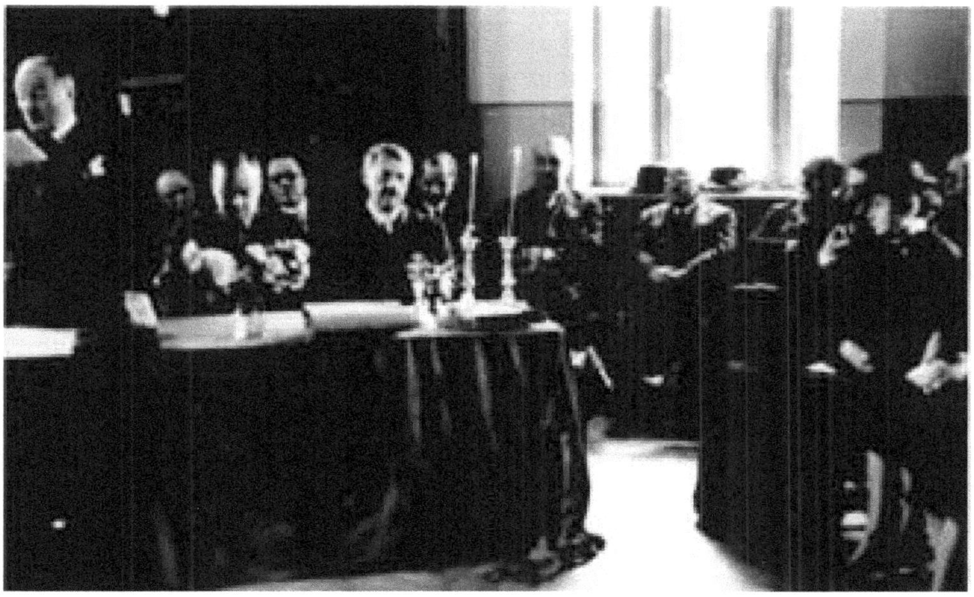

D. Mezincescu, C. Stoicescu and Fr. Rainer (at the Presidium) at the inauguration of the Institute of Anthropology, 1940. In the back row on the left, C. I. Parhon, and in front of the window, in the middle, Grigore Antipa.

Francisc Rainer had lectures of anthropology ever since 1923 at the Institute of Physical Education where there was the Department of Anatomy and Anthropology. They were the oldest lectures on the subject in our country. The final point of this concern is the foundation of the Institute of Anthropology in 1940. Practically, he is the founder of the scientific anthropology in our country and, at the same time, he is the creator of the school of anthropology of Bucharest. Rainer was a holist, being convinced on the vital ratio between biology and culture. In the same time, in Rainer's view, the disease was considered as a *mass phenomenon*, also having *an anthropological significance* and, as such being able to clarify *not only the conditions of life of a population by offering us clarification on its level of vitality, but also indications to discern the direction to which the selective process tends.*

Rainer made popular several fields of anthropological research which were made known both inside the academic system, and outside of it, through public conferences. Among the bravest topics approached in front of a large audience, there is the conference *Issue of the Human Races* and *The Origin of the Egyptian People*. In the matter related to the concept of "race", *Rainer* proved that "there cannot exist a pure race, and whether it once existed, it could not be kept as such because of the populations' exoduses from one side of the continents to the another, movements caused by the need for food or by the cataclysms occurred on Earth. He could not accept the theory of the hegemony of the Aric (Arian Editor's note) race in the European culture, and especially in the culture of the ancient Greeks who developed, according to him, from an older Aegean culture, which, at its turn, was under the influence of the culture of the peoples from the Eastern Mediterranean basin: Egyptians and Chaldeans".

The history of the Romanian people finds itself also in the details of the biodiversity studied with the instruments specific for the medical anthropology, biology, and sociology, applied by the Professor *Dimitrie Gusti* for the last ones, and, in the first cases by the Professor of anatomy *Francisc Iosif Rainer*. The collaboration between the two of them gave an added value to the intern-disciplinary research in our country and showed what can be achieved by joining together the applied sciences, in understanding the phenomenon HUMAN, through the prism of its biological and cultural bipolarity and, from this perspective, to reveal a synthetic image of the Romanian people's history and evolution. We can go down in time with the help of the biology, of the laboratory analyses or of the various categories of measurement which the medical anthropologic often subsumes the cultural anthropology. All these details are determining in the classical study of history. The general conception of the anthropological research coincided, in its essential features, with the one carried on almost at the same time in Europe. We can talk here of a genuine scientific and European cultural synchronism. He also added the complex research on the Sanguine type. Besides his anthropological concerns, he also performed the serologic diagnosis of syphilis and performed a large number of medical consultations which were very required as soon as the peasants felt that they were not performed in vain.

The organization of the research was the following:

I. The probative first passed to the nurse in charge with the blood samples and the processing of the reactions for establishing the sanguine group and the séro-diagnostic of syphilis.

II. Then, they came to me, and I was performing the anthropological work, gathering the metric and descriptive data.

III. Afterward, another assistant took the sheets.

IV. It was now the turn of the assistant who took photos.

V. If necessary, in the end, there was the consultation performed by two clinical assistants.

The so-gathered scientific material is formed of over one thousand anthropologic sheets, of the results of more than 2,500 serologic reactions for establishing the blood groups, of about 500 photographic clichés, each having three views of the same person. The anthropological photograph was made by respecting the technique of *Frankfurt Horizontal*, face, Profile and three-quarters. The assistant who took photos in the three *Gusti-Rainer* campaigns was the later academician *Ştefan Marius Milcu*, by then Professor *Rainer's* assistant. In the Auditorium of the Romanian Academy, Professor *Dimitrie Gusti* made a "warm and touching characterization of the Professor *Francisc I. Rainer`s* personality. *Rarely there were reunited in such a happy way, as we have met with him, in one bundle, skills such as the scientific reasoning, the organizing mastery, and the soul noblesse. Professor* Rainer *was a true philosopher, practicing, without showing up, the wisdom – unlike so many other who show it without practicing it. Professor* Rainer *was a pioneer in opening new pathways and with regard to anthropology of the Romanian people, creating the scientific grounds through the research he performed on the field for the first time, in three Romanian villages, which are also the first anthropological peasants' monographs in the world science! The Academy thoughts of recognition return to the one who created the anatomy of the living being the place which he rightfully has among the first world's scientists.*

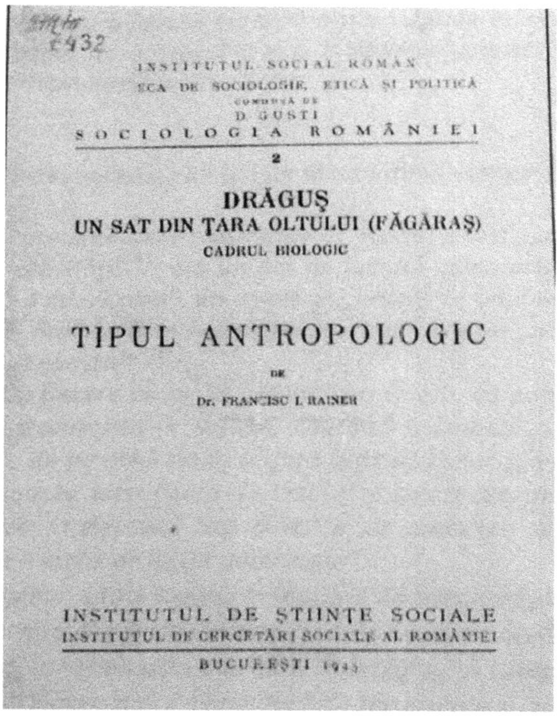
INSTITUTUL SOCIAL ROMAN
ECA DE SOCIOLOGIE, ETICĂ ŞI POLITICĂ
CONDUSĂ DE
D. GUSTI
SOCIOLOGIA ROMÂNIEI
2
DRĂGUŞ
UN SAT DIN ŢARA OLTULUI (FĂGĂRAŞ)
CADRUL BIOLOGIC
TIPUL ANTROPOLOGIC
DE
Dr. FRANCISC I. RAINER
INSTITUTUL DE ŞTIINŢE SOCIALE
INSTITUTUL DE CERCETĂRI SOCIALE AL ROMÂNIEI
BUCUREŞTI 194[illegible]

The results of the three campaigns in Nereju, Drăguş, and Fundul Moldovei were published in the *Enquêtes Anthropologiques dans trois villages roumains des Carpathes – Anthropological Surveys in Three Romanian Villages in the Carpathians* (Official Journal and the State Publishing Houses, the Central Publishing House, Bucharest, 1937), work awarded by the Romanian Academy, and after which *Rainer* was elected as honorary member of the Romanian Academy. In addition, *Rainer* created a very rich and unique collection of skulls (over 6.000 studied and cataloged pieces) together with a large number of casts of exotic skulls, a rich collection of pathological bones; all these were the grounds for the establishment of the Institute of Anthropology, which bears his name nowadays. The Museum of Anthropology was opened to the public on the ground floor of the Institute of Anthropology on the occasion of the 17th *International Congress of Anthropology and Pre-Historical Archaeology*, hosted in Bucharest in September 1937. The museum was closed in 1952, as the building ground floor, specially designed for being a museum, was taken over by the Faculty of Medicine and turned into laboratories for students.

Rainer's Personality in the Contemporaries' Memory

For those who knew him, *Rainer* was *an exemplary of race, as rarely shows up in the middle of a community;* he was a person of *Cinquecento humanist facture, with a classical culture, with a pathetic vision of the truth, a true humanist Polyhistor of encyclopedic nature. The most astonishing fact in his nature is the anxiety of search; he was a tireless researcher, belonging to the Faustian type of our civilization.* On each occasion of meeting the young ones, the audience, his close persons or foreign personalities, *Rainer was searching in the souls looking for the gold grain seen everywhere by Dostoievski. He raised the curtains from the young eyes in the grandiose shows of nature. He unlocked the disciples' mind from the stone carcass of the traditions, and he opened unsuspected perspectives to the eyes eager for learning science. The Wiseman's learning was a lesson of character, of dignity, of the fulfillment of his duty towards the society – lesson of great humanity.*

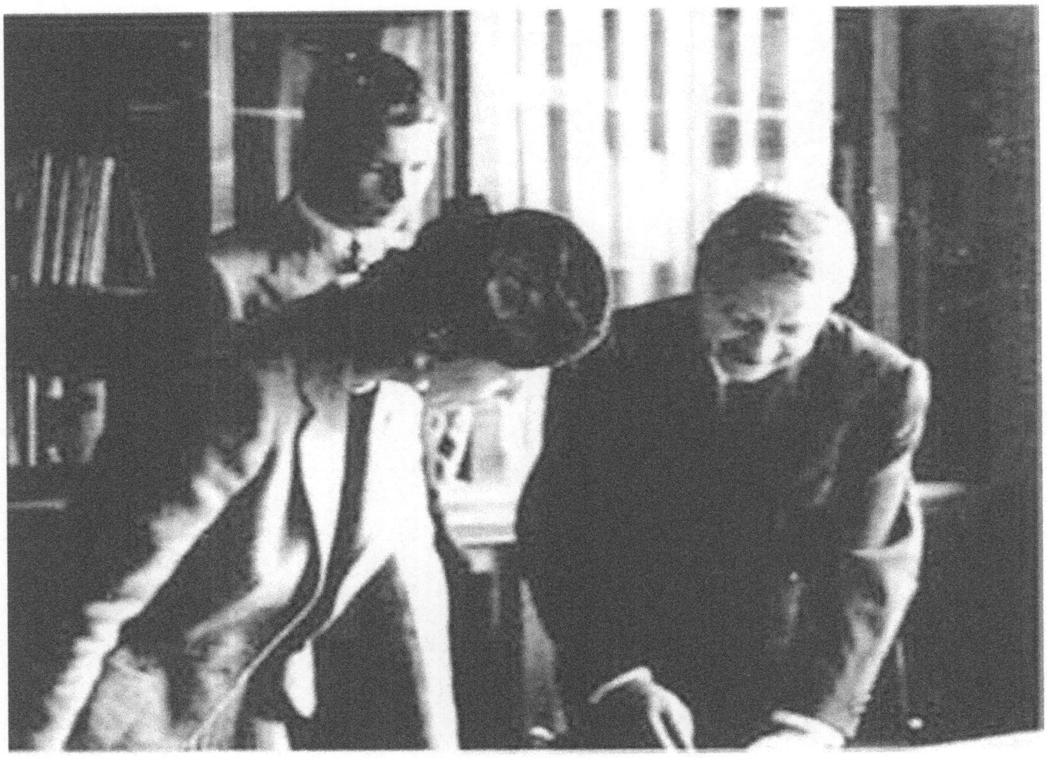

Queen Mother Elena and King Mihai I visiting the Institute of Anthropology in the fall of 1940.

Rainer was always concerned by the issue of the dynamic intuition and not only once he was heard by his assistants and students speaking with enthusiasm of *Goethe's* studies of chromatics. At *Rainer,* the intuition *was not a passive contemplation of the object, but the Bergson's pattern – the result of a long and thorough preparation of the thought by observation and continuous reflection on it.* Influenced by *Johann Goethe, Charles Darwin, Rudolf Virchow* and *Claude Bernard, Rainer* created a scientific model of research which, in the view of his contemporary, *did not find up today either imitators or adepts. Rainer* era *impregnated by the Greek culture, speaking the language, he was a disciple and thorough connoisseur of Goethe's works who had a deciding influence on him. Connoisseur of the painting schools from various ages, he pleased himself with setting up links between the characters' anatomy and the way they were plastically, artistically performed.*

For many of his students, Professor *Rainer* was *an outstanding creation, endowed with the most selected qualities of teacher, organizer, and person of humanity, honesty and justice, of noblesse and wisdom.* Professor *Ion Zamfirescu* remembers that *Rainer saw in words not only a conventional or accidental coat for the idea but also the way of functioning of this idea, a materialization of its essence. He said, "Not only the sound but the thinking itself must live in the word." I understood from* Rainer", continued Professor *Zamfirescu*, *what is the function and what striving force may have the idea of functioning in the processes generated by minds observation and knowledge.* Rainer was able to *call on any detail from Balzac's* The Human Comedy*, the entire intellectual gestation of Beethoven's quartets or even a funny event from the* Baron of Münchhausen's Stories. *Rainer* had a spiritual connection with the youth; he told his friends: *With all my being, I feel connected to the human soul, I think it is a crime to mock the youth.* His ex-student, Dr. *G.T. Dinischiotu* remembered the classes of anatomy from the first year of faculty when Professor *Rainer* tried *to develop our power of observation on multiple sensitive ways, being persuaded that a phenomenon is not well-known unless it can be evoked plastically. For that, we made hours of bone casts, hours of drawing on the anatomy notebook, hours of live palpation. (...) Nothing seemed banal any longer under the light projected by such a comprehension. And, sometimes, the horizon which the Professor opened for us was so wide that, at the same time with the thrill of understanding, we also felt that emotion always triggered by the direct contact with the huge phenomena of life.*

The later physician, *E. Floru*, remembers the trips made with the Professor in the group of students at the first year of medicine, trips made around Bucharest. *I remember*, writes *E. Floru of the classes of fencing in one afternoon, nearby the Comana Monastery. I remember the readings from Claude Bernard, on the Lake Snagov banks when the lake was not drained, and it was covered by water lilies. How deep entered in us the words of the great researcher, combined with the teacher's explanations!*

The way of research and scientific elaboration wished by *Rainer* was an ideal one: *The spirits searching while resting and thoroughly formulating, only under the stimulus of the topic induced pleasure.* Under this projection of ideas, Rainer *intensely stimulated generations of youth to the benefactor effort of the intellect growth. (...) This is all that matters in our world: the high goal.*

Professor *Rainer*: A State of Mind. His Students and Successors

Rainer had very clear life principles. Of morality and internal struggle. Of solidarity with the souls wanting to rise by science and sustained work. Rainer stated: I could not be interested in a person who does not agitate an idea for the general welfare. I feel deep gratitude to the society that entrusted me with a department as there are means for the progress of your being. Moreover, I must show it my gratitude by defending its interests. The life urge is integrated to the activity in the society: We owe to give society as much as we can, and we do not have the right to be resentful for the injustice, as each of us owes more to society than society owes us. Rainer worked for the love of full achievement of things. The life and the surroundings are a trip which needs to be carefully analyzed. He recommended 'do not read like you are driving a fast car, like an American who wants to see Rome, but read like you are walking in a carriage, fully admiring the views.

Rainer built his ideal of life being marked by three personalities: *Virchow*, who, by his research on the cellular pathology, made him rely on concrete, *Claude Bernard*, who, by the criticism of the experimental methods, completed his method, and *Goethe, by his critical studies and philosophical poetry*. The intimacy of the thoroughly study topic and delivered to the others after long years of verification made *Rainer* state that *you have the right of talking to the other only when you see the county of knowledge and ideas as such a height; and when you are able to raise the others at the same height, so that they have the feeling that they breathe freely and feel the winds of the heights.* To succeed in such a strength of clarity in speech, in substantiation, one must first face the own weaknesses and defeat them one after the other. One must reach there where you alone can count yourself worthy of any speech and action compliant with nature. *Don't let yourself turned back by some criticisms or by the resulting whispers... However, if it is good to work or to speak, do not see yourself unworthy. They have their own inner guide and listen to your own instincts. Do not worry, but follow straight your path, guided by your own nature and by the universal nature: Regardless, both follow a unique path.* Ever since 1919, *Rainer* recommended that *we must not do to anyone the honor of revealing the offenses brought to our sensitivity.*

Starting from *Plutarch's* urge in the ancient times: *Know yourself and by that you will know the meaning of your existence and the entire Universe, Rainer* goes further saying that *it is an amputated limb of the citadel, the one who splits his private soul from that of the rational beings, as the soul is the core.* This truth is similar to the urge left by the chemist *Ştefan Minovici* before his premature death in 1935: *Listen to your conscience, for it is the soul and the soul is divine!*

Rainer gave voice to the conscience, by listening to his soul. He succeeded indeed to make school, but also to set up new institutions. The Institute of Anatomy and Embryology of Bucharest, and then the Institute of Anthropology are his creation. The School of Anatomy was innovated by his way of thinking and research. *Rainer* was the first to give a *new direction to the study of the anatomy. He shows that the anatomy is no longer the science of the corpse. The corpse anatomy data are required only as departure points for developing the anatomic thinking.. (...) The living shape is tightly connected to the structure, and this to the function; therefore, it is the expression of the functional structure. Rainer* is considered to be the creator of the new orientation in medicine, and, briefly, his method meant *developing broadly and sort of cinematographically the body, from the cell to its full achievement; the functional interpretation of the systems building the human and their interdependence are issues which predominantly concern the course of anatomy and decide the frame for presenting the details which form the material of the anatomical science.*

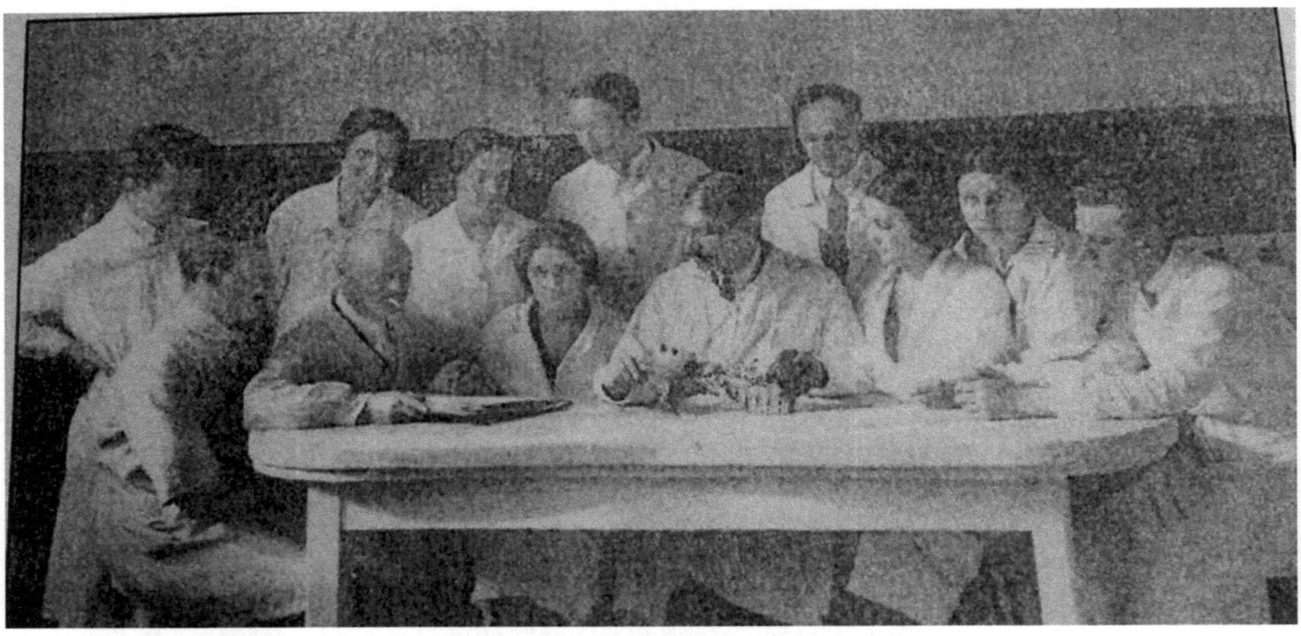

Professor Rainer with his assistants, 1926. Eugen Floru, in the back, at right Natalia Neagu, placed on Professor's left.

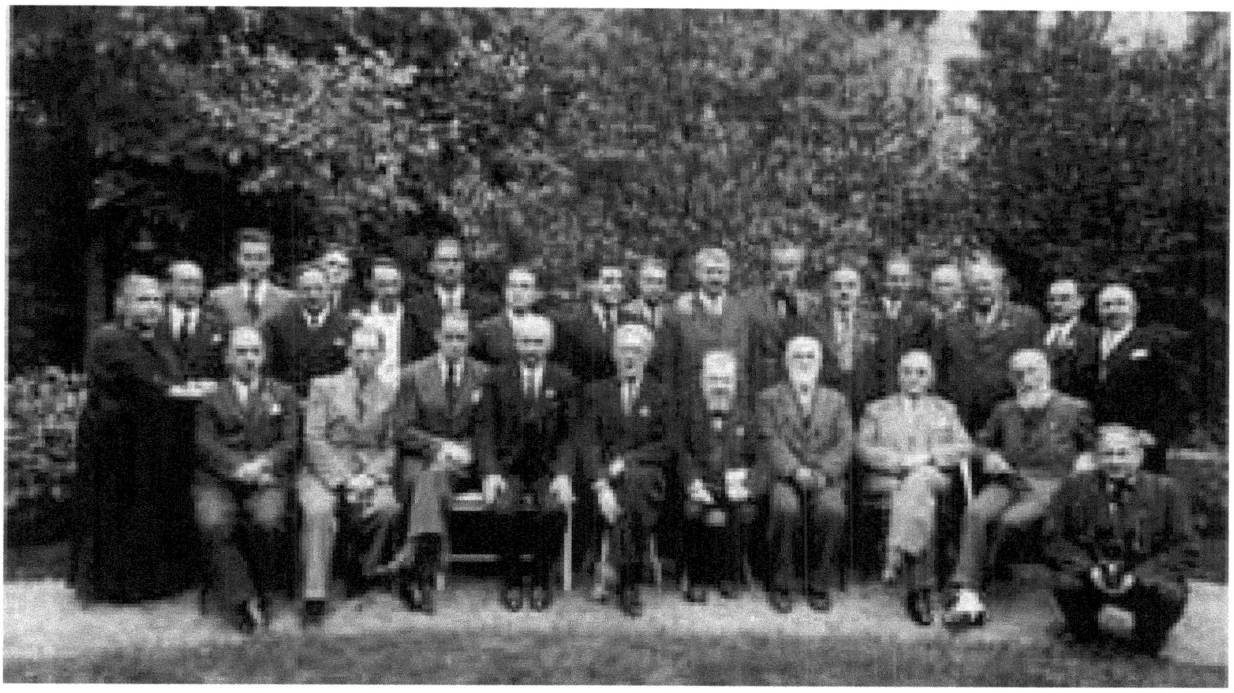

Photograph taken in the yard of the Rainer family on the occasion of the First International Congress of Anthropology and Prehistoric Archaeology, hosted at Bucharest in the fall of 1937, under the presidency of Professor Rainer. First row, from left to right: Prof. Niţescu, Lhuer, Lopez-Rez (minister of Spain), Prof. Sćerbakinski (Prague), Prof. Stolykwo (Krakow), Prof. Babor, A. de Villemereuil, G. Paul Boncour, Henri Berr (director of the International Centre for Synthesis), Ivo Franić (Zagreb). The second row, starting from left to right: Mrs. Dr. Rainer, Dr. Floru, Costin Kiriţescu, Z. Iagnov, Dr. C. Ciurea, Dr. O. Vlăduţiu, Dr. A. Tudor, Dr. B. Menkes, Dr. Ioaniţescu, Dr. Stănescu, Prof. Rainer, Ştefan Popescu, Prof. Bălan, Bartocz Lajos, Ing. Baiulescu.

Dimitrie Gusti said about *Rainer* and his work that "it was a real preach by the experience of his life" of *culture Benedictine*. The physiological direction in the morphology created by *Fr. Rainer* was developed both in Iaşi (1928-1942) and in Bucharest (1942-1947) by his student, *Grigore T. Popa*, Rockefeller scholar (at *Rainer's proposal*) in 1925. Doctor in medicine and surgery of the Faculty of Iaşi, Professor Rainer's assistant ever since his student years, he follows his master at the Department in Bucharest, where he is a lecturer, being in the same time teacher of anthropology at the Institute of Physical Education of Bucharest (1923-1927). In 1928 he was appointed a tenured Professor in the Department of Compared Anatomy and Embryology at the Faculty of Medicine in Iaşi, a position held until 1941 when he transfers to Bucharest.

However, *Rainer's* most famous student is the Nobel Laureate *George Emil Palade* (1912-2008). *Palade* enrolled at the Faculty of Medicine of Bucharest which he successfully graduated in 1936. He discovered his call and passion for research still in the faculty, being appointed assistant during the student years at the Institute of Anatomy run by Professor *Francisc Rainer*. In 1940 he was awarded the title of Doctor in Medicine with the dissertation *The nephron of the cetacean Delphinus Delphi. Study of compared morphology and physiology*, under *Rainer's* coordination. Already associate Professor in Bucharest, *Palade* left in 1946 to the United States as a researcher in *Robert Chambers's Laboratory* at the Department of Biology of the University of New York. *Palade* accepts the Belgian biologist's, *Albert Claude*, an invitation to work at the Rockefeller Institution, a position held for 27 years. Between 1973 and 1990, he was head of the Department of Cellular Biology of the Yale University. On December 10, 1974, he received the Nobel Prize in Physiology and Medicine together with *Albert Claude* and *Christian de Duve* for "their findings on the cell structural and functional organization."

Ştefan Marius Milcu (1903-1997), the personality of reference of the Romanian Endocrinology, *Rainer's student* and *C. I. Parhon's* successor defended his doctoral dissertation at the Faculty of Medicine of Bucharest in 1928 – *Is the carotid corpuscle a paraganglioma?* –, being awarded the title of Doctor in Medicine, under *Rainer's* supervision. He was preparator (1924-1927), and, then, assistant (1924-1935) at the Institute of Anatomy and Embryology of the Faculty of Medicine of Bucharest, led by Prof. *Rainer*. Tenured Professor (1948-1973) at the Clinics of Endocrinology of the Institute of Medicine and Pharmacy of Bucharest where he was rector between 1953-1955. Between 1957-1977, he ran the Institute of Endocrinology C. I. Parhon of Bucharest. Vice-president of the Romanian Academy (1963-1964), *Milcu* studied all sectors of endocrinology regarding the pathogenic of the endocrine imbalances and the biochemistry of the endocrine syndromes. He thoroughly studies several aspects of the inter-relations of the nervous system with the endocrine glands, highlighting the change in the tissue reactivity to hormones in relation to the integrity of the nervous system. He is considered to be a pioneer in applying the radioactive isotopes into the Endocrinology. He also performed research on vegetal and animal biology concerning the stimulating effect of the hormones on some culture plants and animals. He led complex anthropological surveys on the population from various areas of the country (Bicaz, Porţile de Fier, etc.). Also concerned with the history of medical science, *Milcu* wrote about anthropology in the context of culture. *Rainer* had always been concerned by the issue of the dynamic intuition and not only once his assistants and students heard him talking with enthusiasm of *Goethe's* chromatic studies. For *Rainer,* the intuition "*was not a passive contemplation of the object, but the Bergson's block – the result of a long and thorough preparation of the thought by observation and continuous reflection on it.*"

Rainer discovers the pituitary port system, demonstrated afterward, at *Rainer's* impetus by his student *Popa* whom *Rainer* sent to England with a state scholarship. *Popa* publishes in the medical literature together with Prof. *Una Fielding* totally "forgetting" that the real discoverer was Professor *Rainer*. Thanks to this omission, the pituitary port system gets to be known as the Popa-Fielding system which is not according to the reality. He was the most fervent supporter of the anthropology in our country and the one who saved the Bucharest anthropology from cancellation, after 1950. Practically, the Schools of Anthropology of Iaşi and Cluj had been cancelled, the anthropologists from those schools being politically imprisoned or marginalized. After 1955, famous personalities of these schools have been brought by the Acad. *Ştefan Milcu* in the staff from Bucharest, despite the restrictions of political order.

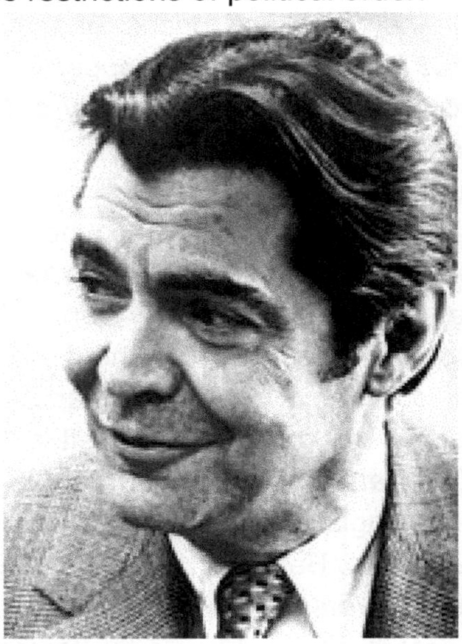

George Emil Palade (1912-2008)

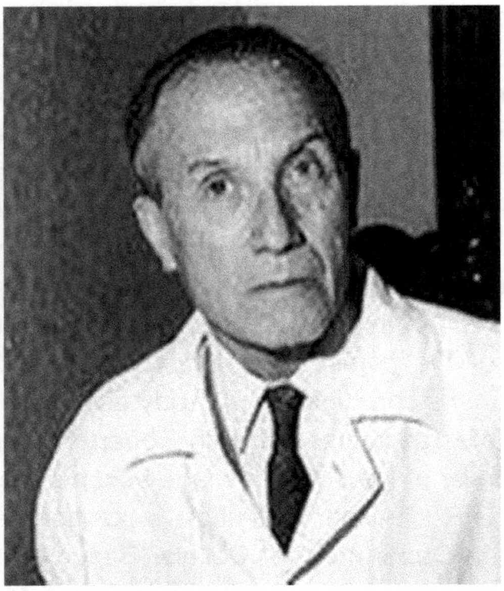

Ştefan Marius Milcu (1903-1997)

Ştefan Milcu succeeds to keep the institute of anthropology in the building specially erected by *Rainer* (where it still carries on its activities in our times), turning it into the Centre for Anthropological Research, initially in the Institute of Endocrinology (1952-1955) and, then, under the direct patronage of the Romanian Academy. Acad. *Ştefan Milcu* kept his promise made to his magister to develop and continue Rainer's school of anthropology. He helped his colleagues and defended the anthropology in times of sorrow, taking the leadership of the Centre for Anthropological Research from 1952 to 1964.

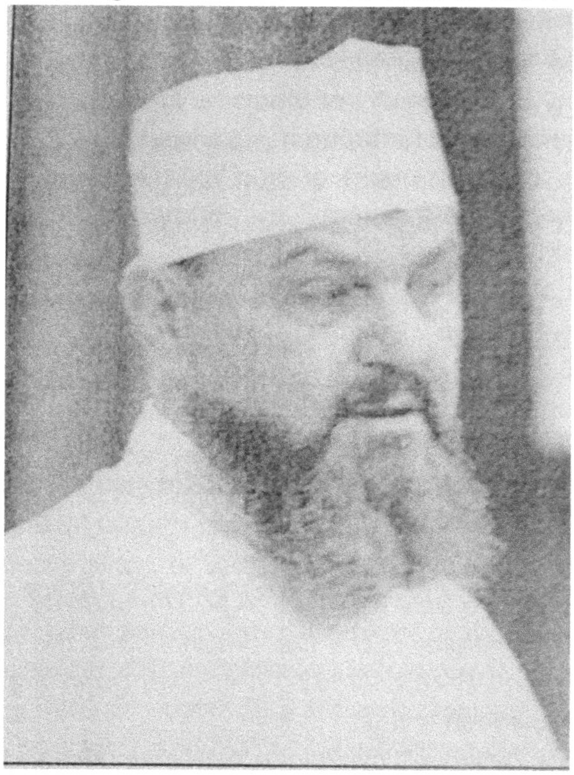

Ilie. Th. Riga (1908-1977)

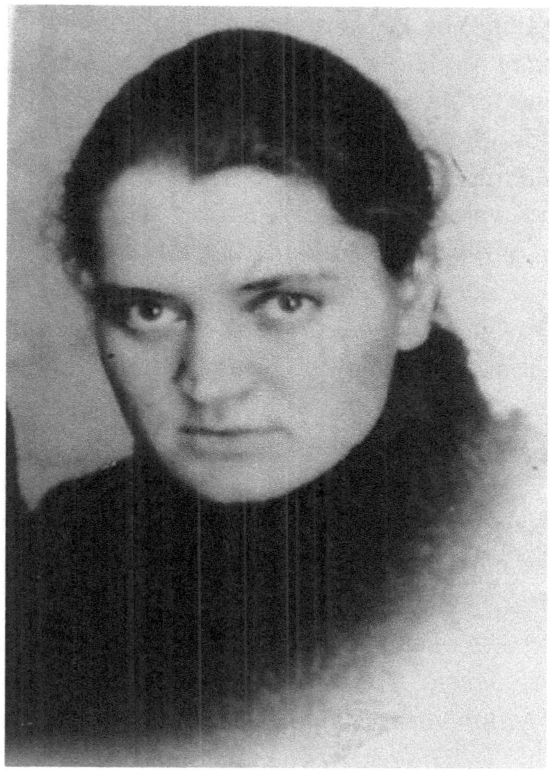

Natalia Neagu (1912-1999)

After the political opening in 1964, even if not leading the anthropology officially, until his last days of life, the academician *Milcu* supervised and coordinated the activities of the Centre for Anthropologic Research and fought for turning it again in an institute named after his creator, *Francisc I. Rainer*. Another *Rainer's* successor, *Ilie Th. Riga* (1908-1977) developed the academic education of anatomy and surgery at the Faculties of General Medicine and Paediatrics of the Medical-Pharmaceutical Institute of Bucharest. During 1957-1960, he published in premiere a massive *Course of Human Topographic Anatomy with clinical applications and operatory and experimental surgery*. In parallel, *Riga* has developed the academic education of zoology at the Faculty of Veterinary Medicine of Bucharest by fundamental works of compared anatomy, in cooperation with *Vasile Gheţie* and *Eugeniu Paştea*.

Convinced evolutionist and encyclopaedic spirit, *Ilie Th. Riga* developed and enriched the biological and medical anthropology by the technical innovation of *anthropometrical compass* for body measurement, by elaborating and substantiating the concepts of *anthropomorphosis and bio-morphological constructive type*, he laid the basis for the characterisation of the anthropological size of the individuality and variability in connection, of the integration by anthropomorphosis and of the continuous cerebral evolution (by encephalisation, cerebralisation, frontalization, occipitalization, lateralization, suprastructuring, development and evolutionary scaling from archi- and paleo-structures to neoformations). During 1945-1947, *Riga* was the initiator of the publishing of the *Complete Works (scientific, medical and academic)* of his magister *Rainer*, under the auspices of the Romanian Academy, of the University of Bucharest and the Romanian Athenaeum. He is also the author of an essential biography on *Francisc Rainer's* life. In March 1942, supervised by *Rainer, Natalia Neagu* (1912-1999) defends her doctoral thesis on the topic *The Role of the Nasal Sept in the Mechanical Construction of the Face.* Following her master's footsteps, she studied the embryogenesis of the heart, where she has a series of priorities in elucidating the heart septation. She studied the skull development, and, in particular, the masticatory apparatus; she cooperated with *Pătru Firu* in the study of the embryogenesis of the masticatory apparatus. The basis of research in embryology of the Romanian Academy was at Timişoara, at *Benedict Menckes*, with whom she was colleague as an assistant with *Rainer*. She had been working for decades at the Department of Anatomy of the Faculty of Medicine in Bucharest and she cooperated with personalities of the Romanian school of morphology, as well as with *Lucia Bareliuc*, together with whom she published three classical books of embryology, one of them being awarded the *Victor Babeş* Award of the Romanian Academy. It is proper to mention a series of Professor *Rainer*'s outstanding Ph.D. candidates:

Eugen I. Floru: *Contributions to the status of the iliotibial tract*, June 1925; *Valentina Roşca: On the teenagers' growth and development*, 1926; *Benedict Menckes: On the innervation of the superficial arch of the palm*, April 1930; *Ion Juvara, Morphological analyse of the diaphragmatic hernias in adults*, October 1938; *Ion Cotăescu: Contributions to the stage of the fibrous apparatus*, June 1940, *Raul Robacki* and others.

Mihai Neagu Basarab surprised with sophistication the art of the doctorate at *Francisc Rainer*. *Who sees a doctoral dissertation issued under Rainer's guidance is surprised by the low size of such an important academic endeavor. That is why it is appropriate to provide details. Professor Rainer claimed that an original work is valuable only when it can be summarized. One of Rainer's essential contributions in developing the anatomy is the first description of the heart lymph vessels. The great German anatomist Hermann Brauss (1868-1924) when reaching the heart lymph vessels in his treatise* Anatomie des Menschen *writes:*

> *"The lymph vessels of the heart had been described by Rainer. As the work cannot be synthesized, we reproduce it in extenso."*

And, then, there are the two pages of Rainer's work of Anatomischer Anzeiger *of 1907, between quotation sign. Thus, we should not be surprised that, among Rainer's assistants, there resulted in almost twenty, first-hand Professors, and a Nobel Prize laureate who, supervised by* Prof. *Rainer, studies the nephron of the cetacean Delphinus Delphi*, opening the horizon for the *contemplative anthropology* which the Prof. *I. Th. Riga, MD* and the Professors *Gheţie* and *Paştea* develop, at the Faculty of Veterinary Medicine.

Animated by the passion for truth, evolutionist, a Darwinist and rationalist in the scientific thinking, a person with firm Democratic beliefs, *Fr. Rainer* places himself in an honorary place in the gallery of the coryphaei of the Romanian medical-biological thinking. During his times, he was a shiny example of scientist – citizen. Outstanding scientists such as *Francisc Rainer* have lived with the conscience that they have the mission to create a modern Romania, with solid institutional culture and an occidental system of values, living under the moral imperative of the civilizing role of the science, and, in this case, of the medicine as a privileged area. Their stringent concern was to overcome in an accelerated rhythm the scientific and cultural gap between the occidental world and to turn the Romanian society into a benchmark for the Western civilization at the gates of the Orient. The diversity of documented testimonies presented here prove the tight connection between the personality of the Professor *Francisc Rainer* and the European culture. He succeeded to comprise in one view and to express with simple words, truths on the biological phenomenon called Human, linking the antic art and philosophy to

Goethe's poetic and scientific works in order to stop on the details in the development of the living form whose primordial element, the living matter is in balanced interdependency between the genotype and the phenotype. Between what is hidden inside and what comes from far by successive inheritance and what is outside and suffers changes due to the environment and the surroundings.

Bringing back in the memory *Fr. Rainer's* personality, honorary member of the Romanian Academy, is a duty of homage and gratitude towards the referential figure of the Romanian Anthropology. The anthropological school he founded wears the seal of his original, innovative and interdisciplinary thinking in the knowledge of the human being in its bio-cultural integrity and the dynamics achieved with the environment. This integrating vision on the human, shaped in the European scientific world by the end of the 20th century, was introduced in our country by Professor *Rainer*. With these iatro-historical landmarks on Professor *Francisc Rainer's* life and scientific work, on this occasion, we also wish to bring homage to his universal personality and his indulgent soul, stoic in relation with the posterity. Stoicism gave by the Professor by a question he asked himself by the end of his life, like looking in a mirror:

"*I wonder if your destiny was real?*"

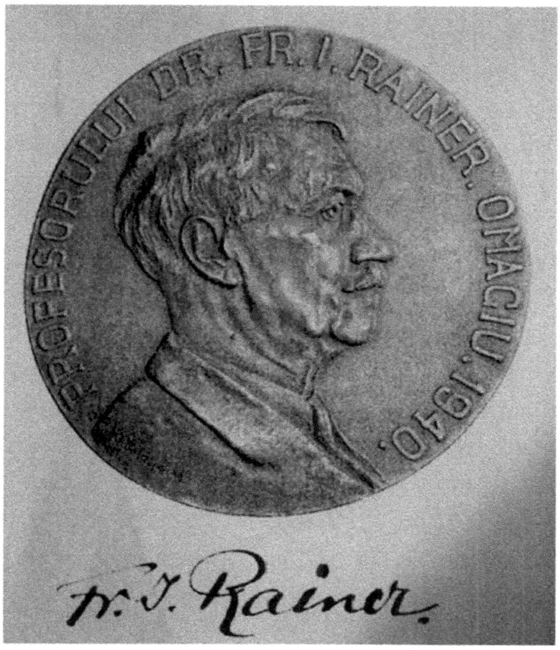

THE HISTORY OF ANTHROPOLOGY IN ROMANIA

"It is more important to know what person has a certain disease, than what disease has a certain person."
***Theophrastus Bombastus von* Hohenheim**

The anthropology studies the person and its material and spiritual production. In Romania, the first notions of anthropology as a science, we find in the first half of the 19th century, when the first book in Romania, unsigned, written in Cyrillic, is presenting notions of human anatomy and physiology with elements of psychology, concluded by the description of the "types of temper". These data being probably taken from the first course of anthropology at the University of Paris, where Prof. *A. de Quatrefages* starts with the human's anatomy and physiology, compared to that of the animals, and continues with elements of psychology framed according to the conditions of the external environment. In the end, there are also shown the beliefs, and the customs of the populations reported to their working tools in their evolution.

The first Romanian historical writing mentions the physical features, the characteristics of the psychical and socio-cultural life of the native populations, and of the populations who crossed or stopped in the territory of our country. Thus, the first anthropologic information is very early, and we can talk about notions of anthropology once with the publishing of the *Treatise of Anthropology* by *Vasici Ungureanu* (1830). Afterward, a series of doctoral dissertations of some Romanian physicians publicly defended in Paris, Berlin, Vienna and Budapest approach anthropological issues, and so affiliate Romania to the countries with tradition in anthropology.

The first lecture with anthropological elements is held in Iaşi by Prof. *Cizak* (1850). During the same period, there begin the first anthropological research, their results being published in specialty foreign journals. By the end of the 19th century, the great Romanian cultural and scientific journals *Convorbiri literare*, directed by *Titu Maiorescu* and *Dobrogeanu-Gherea's Contemporanul* published articles of anthropology on the origin of man, of the human races, as well as original theoretical and conceptual contributions such as *Ghibănescu's* study, *Evolution and Education*, dealing the matter "movement" from inorganic to organic up to the human being. By the end of the 19th century, in full Europeans' colonial expansion, the main concerns of the scientist in biological sciences focuses on the natural origin of the human species, making a direct connection to *Darwin's* theory of the human evolution. Thus, it shows up the conflict with the monotheist religions which support the man's creationist theory. Most of the aspects concerning the "human phenomenon", starting with the biological notions and continuing with the psychical, socioeconomic, cultural, religious ones, and so on, are issued empirically, by simple comparative observations, acknowledging that the human is a bio-psycho-social being, a topic developed afterwards, scientifically, by anthropology.

The beginning of the 20th century marks a well-defined development and direction of the anthropological research both on historical populations (in cooperation with the archaeologists), and on current ones. The worldwide famous anthropologist *Eugène Pittard* not only trains a series of Romanian specialist but, for years (1900-1937) he participates with them in field studies in the most representative areas of Romania: both on cores of native population and in regions with a real population mosaic, such as Dobrogea. As a result, there are published in foreign publishing houses monographs on the Romanian populations and a large number of articles in famous journals of anthropology.

In the first decades of the 20th century, data, and the first mappings of the metric characteristics of Romanian populations start being gathered systematically. During the same time, the measurements for recruitment are set (after the French School of Anthropology) setting up a referential database for the evolution of the population in time.

In Iaşi, Prof. *Botez* introduces elements of anthropology in the academic courses of the Faculty of Natural Sciences and, in the same time, substantiates the School of Iasi which has a particular weight in the development of the Romanian Anthropology.In parallel, the schools of anthropology of Cluj and Bucharest take shape and develop, each with a particular specificity. The School of Cluj, run by the Prof. *Papilian*, with a strong medical and social imprint, in the period between the world wars. Famous personalities of the Romanian anthropology from this school are removed from the circuit of the specific life after 1944, and so developing this anthropologic center. The remaining research is actual even nowadays, by their multi-disciplinary character of approaching the issues, and by the broad scope of approached areas: from paleoanthropology to the anthropology of the contemporary populations, developing research of medical, demographic, auxological, racial and sociocultural anthropology. The disappearance of the School of Cluj did not prevent though the entry in the national and international circuit of the anthropological issues approached by the experts from Cluj.

The Objectives of Anthropology

The Society of Anthropology is established in 1862 having *Paul Broca*, the famous discoverer of the first human fossils in the Inferior Pleistocene *Pitecantropus Yawanensis,* as director. This society opens a school of anthropology where the observation and the metrics are systematically taught as working methods and the mathematical statistic processing as method for data analyses; on this occasion, it is introduced the system for codified observation with registration on special, standardised sheets and with proper tools, of high precision; on the same occasion, the topics of study are also presented, topics which extended their area up to our days; the following topics outstands for the same first stage:

1. The physical (anatomical) anthropology also introduces the methodology based on observation and metrics established and adopted by the German *Martin-Saller* School. This methodology was also adopted in our country, *Rainer* installing at the Institute of Anthropology, recently established in Bucharest, the entire German equipment, including the highly performing Leica type photographic device, assisted by *Eugen Floru*, who continues his works.

2. The biological anthropology has been developed at the Institute of Anthropology of Brussels and introduced in Iasi by the Prof. *Botez* and the Prof. *Olga Necrasov*, and in Craiova by the Prof. *Nicolaescu Plopşor* and *Firu Ion*, at the Museum of Oltenia.

3. The etiology and the cultural anthropology are developed by the schools in the USA; these topics were developed in our country by the Institute of Ethnology of Bucharest, run by Prof. *Vulcănescu*.

4. The prehistoric anthropology (Paleontology) – palaeoanthropology – is also developed in Romania, in Bucharest, Iaşi, and Craiova, introduced by the Assoc. Prof. Eugen Floru, MD Prof. *Olga Necrasov*, Prof. *Nicolaescu Plopşor* and *Ion Firu*.

5. Linguistic anthropology.

6. Demography and medical geography developed at us by the Acad *Şt. Milcu*, show up simultaneously in various schools in the world, among which Romania, approaching three main topics: the morphology of the body and the head in the philo-ontogenetic evolution of the human being; the human physio-psychological features; the socioeconomic aspects, considering the human as a bio-psycho-social being.

7. The comparative anthropology, developed by *I. Th. Riga*, Prof. *Gheţie* and *Paştea* from the Faculty of Veterinary Medicine.

At the beginning of the 20th century, there is an anthropological “movement” in the world, driven by each country`s desire to “anthropologically” investigate the population from their countries and colonies, to present them in anthropological journals diverse by Profile. An extensive ethnographic and craniological material is gathered and stored in institutes with museums, like casts, masks, photograms, etc, as study material for the young anthropologists. After the anthropological publications, there were the battles for ideas, the colonists being particularly interested as they wanted to claim the superiority of their country`s race to that of the colonies` races. Racism takes a national appearance in Hitler's Germany where one of the biggest genocide in history happened, in full century of industrial civilization. In opposition to Hitler's trend, another extremist empire, Soviet Russia, triggers a likely genocide against those opposing to the Marxist – Leninist conception, relying on the essential "guided" role of the environment, of the socialist way of life which creates a "superior human being." These extreme Nazi trends were criticized by *Fr. Rainer*, on the occasion of conferences on human genetics, presented at the University of Bucharest. In the presence of the German Nazi authorities, in 1940, *Rainer* said, proving that there is no relation between the size and the shape of the skull and the intelligence: biologically all people are the same. The Soviet extremist trends had been blamed by Prof. *Gr. T. Popa*, in a conference in Dallas, in 1945, the reason for which he suffered a lot, accelerating his death in full creative activity. In our country, beginning with 1933, *Gusti* and *Rainer* organize the well-known medico-anthropological analyses, concluded with three volumes where the first anthropological research in three villages from Romania are presented: Nereju, Fundul Moldovei and Drăguş (Făgăraş). *Rainer* and his assistants from the Institute of Anatomy and Human Embryology make observations, metrics, and photographs by the age standard and establish the diagnostic of the regional types of our country, in percentages, most of them being a mix. In these areas, predominant are the three fundamental types in Romania: Alpine, Dinaric, and Mediterranean to which the Carpatho-Danubian Northerners are added, the Faelic and the Osteuropids of our country which are mentioned as "elements."

These volumes were presented at the International Congress of Anthropology and Archaeology, held in Bucharest, on September 1-8, 1937, occasion to visit and work at the Institute of Anthropology, established by *Rainer* and endowed with a collection of 6300 human skulls, measured and labelled by *Rainer* himself, with the registration of the data concerning their names and surnames, year of birth and the disease that caused the death. In addition, there have been registered in the institute another 200 children skulls, from birth to 16 years old, a collection unique in the world, also labeled by *Rainer* himself, and further studied by *Pătru Firu*.

Another over 10 000 pathological osseous parts have been prepared and systematically placed in special exhibits, bones representing the osseous pathology of the population in Romania during the interwar period. *Pătru Firu* has described many craniofacial pathology pieces in several works. Osseous tuberculosis with the extraordinary collection of "hunchbacks," tertiary syphilis, the osseous tumors, including the cranial ones and the rheumatoid lesions are only a part of this extraordinary collection, partially presented by his students. At the Congress, Prof. *Pittard*, who performed the first anthropological studies on the population in Dobrogea together with Dr. *Suzana Pop* asked Prof. *Rainer*:

- *Who is going to use this extraordinary collection of skulls and osseous pathology?*

Rainer answered:

- *Everyone according to its power of understanding.*

On the same occasion, *Rainer* confesses telling:

- *The dominant feeling of my entire existence is the deeper comprehension of life in its human shape.* Rainer admits that the human is a biological being, but if one applies to human the laws of biological, it becomes inhuman.

Socio-economic aspects of anthropology

In the contemporary age, Europeanization by a federation of free associated states is designed. It is intended to unite all European populations, regardless of their nationality, ethnicity, race or religion. The federation can be established by respecting the human rights, the democratic principles and the products exchange on a free market. The nationalist extremist ideas are rejected in a States Federation. During this time, it is still studied in Anthropology the morpho-physiological and behavioral variability of the humans as individuals, as precisely this variability unites the people in a federal State, choosing different Professions which allow for the technological and cultural advances. This way the productivity of work increases, the number of products on the free market, the populations standard of life increases. The individual variability is determined by a unitary population genic foundation which is to stabilize itself by the reorganization of the federalized populations and is to give a new creative and energetic impetus to the descendants.

Genetic anthropology

The population genic foundation programs the somatic development (biological), the psychological (spiritual) and behavioral (social) ones with certain limits of variability which can be established anthropologically depending on the age, gender and the time of research. The deviations from these "normal limits" are considered pathological. In here the medical anthropology is to intervene, with its specifications, the dentistry, the gastroenterology, the nephrology, etc. The European Union has already assumed the idea of elaborating a *Charta pathological*, which was partially drafted by dentists, in Romania by *Firu* and *Rusu*, using the étiopathogénie methodology by the WHO. Based on this *Charter,* population programs for prevention of the constant (pathological) impairments may be developed. A detailed report on the strategy for prevention of the oral-dental-maxillary conditions in relation to the noxious factors of external environment was presented by *Firu* and *Rusu* at the Balkan Medical Days of October 1999, in the presence of the WHO leadership.

According to *Rainer*, *Milcu,* and *Firu*, the "exotic" populations known as "colonial" have a biological evolution almost at the same level, the differences being only in percentage, their behavior and tools being different because of the particular socio-cultural conditions. Even today there are people in the world who have tools from the Neolithic age, others on the stage of the individual, familial agriculture, without mechanized tools. The "industrial" man of today intends to produce more and cheaper to increase all people of the Earth life standard, to prevent the famine and the epidemic chronic diseases and to increase people's life expectancy. Thus, the anthropology intends to cooperate with all humanist, technological, cultural, social, ethnological, historical, biological, medical sciences in order to know the noxious factors from the internal and external environment, to accomplish a physical and spiritual health by proper education.

Medical Anthropology

The medical and anthropological investigations carried on by *Milcu*, *Dumitrescu* and *Firu* continue the socio-anthropological investigations performed by *Gusti* and *Rainer*.

Rainer developed a physical anthropology of study of the regional types in our country, after the standardized model of the International Society of Anthropology. Professor *Rainer* created an anthropology of the osseous pathology, by the extraordinary collection of skulls and pathological bones belonging to the interwar period population of Romania. *Milcu* continues the medical-anthropological investigations, initiated by *Gusti* and *Rainer*, creating a medical anthropology, currently acknowledged at international level.

Dental anthropology

Under Prof. *Milcu's* guidance, Prof. *Firu* created a dental anthropology by approaching the phylogenesis and the ontogenesis of the dental-maxillary apparatus. With this occasion, he proved that the phylogenesis and the ontogenesis might be regarded as pathological factors in the hereditary conditions of the dental-maxillary apparatus, such as the mandibular prognathous, the pro- or retro alveolar positions which benefit from surgical treatment. Many phylogenetic dental anomalies considered as "syphilis" skeletons are now rejected. Thus, we consider that the mandibular prognathous is a phylogenetic hereditary condition, unlike other hereditary conditions which can be chromosomal.

Studying the limits of craniofacial variability in groups of children and adults (about 10 000 subjects from the medical-anthropological investigated area during 1950-1960) *Firu* performs somatograms, photograms, and Xray-encephalograms. Based on them, a diagnostic can be made of a dental-alveolar-maxillary anomaly. The orthognathic surgical techniques which *Firu* has initiated and developed in Romania, rely precisely on these anthropological methods of investigation. Applying the same anthropological methods to the operated patients, the efficiency and the value of the surgical technique could be evaluated.

Today the modern contemporary person emphasizes the socioeconomic life, the "historical" character of the humanity, its creative skills in technology, literature, biology, medicine, morals, religion, etc. The human being represents an "unique" original being, it is essentially an "ontological" being, as *V. Săhleanu* said, another *Milcu's* brilliant student: accidentally, biologically, the person can be sick, suffering. The theological experts say that the disease can be of body and soul, and at its healing participate the physicians and the church servants, gifted by God to heal the soul conditions.

Thus, in the current days, the biological diagnostic of the disease may become necessary, and we need to add sometimes the psychosomatic medicine or the priest's counseling for the soul condition. The biological rehabilitation must also be followed by the behavioral rehabilitation of the person in the society, being favorable to the creativity and the social work. The occlusal rehabilitation at an edentulous patient with functional prosthetics restores not only the patient's biological functions, mastication, and deglutition but also the psychosocial ones, speaking, physiognomy, receptivity, affectivity, etc.

The philosophical, predictive anthropology

How does an anthropologist study "the human" today? The philosophical anthropology recommends a methodology of knowledge on the "concrete" human using a five ratio relationship, according to *V. Săhleanu*:

1. The connection between the biological person and the socio-cultural human, by developing the old formula: the human is a bio-psycho-social being.

2. The connection between the population group, the mesological factor – factors from the external environment – biogenesis, climate, nutrition, pollution factors, etc. – and the socioeconomic factors – the sociogenesis, the stress, the noise, the pollutant gas, etc.

3. Establishing the biological "normal" (the health within some limits of normal variability) and the social normal – behavioral, ethological, comparative with the psychosocial deviations within limits admitted by the legislation of the respective population group.

4. Establishing these limits of normal biological and social variability is accomplished by medical-anthropological investigations, with the participation of all medical, sociological, psychological specialties, using the current office technique.

5. The analyze of all these data in the past, present and future conclude with a strategy for prevention of the biopsychosocial deviations from the population, community investigated group. The

strategy may be adjusted for other population types from a certain geographic area to achieve the standardization of the methods of investigation, recording, analyzing, and evaluating.

The beneficent interventions for the person's bio-psycho-social health, from child to old person, have not been easily accepted by some population groups, due to some inefficient educations. The training of the civilized "person" with proper culture, educated in the family and at school, is performed slowly, patiently; when such a person is a teenager and may fit in the society with a particular Profession, the society advances, establishes cooperation and the life become beautiful, with high standards.

The four socioeconomic world crises along the centuries

At the International Congress of Anthropology held in October 1988, *Firu* presents the report the *Worldwide economic and social crises.*

Analysing the humans' life from the superior Pleistocene (30 000-10 500 years B.C.) when our shared ancestor *Homo sapiens* showed up and until the contemporary person, we find an extensive morphological and behavioural diversification which starts with the three races (leuco-, melano- and flavoderm) differentiated from the *Homo sapiens*, between 30 000-10 500 years B.C. In Holocene (10 500-5000 years B.C.) *Homo sapiens* showed up, from whom, in order, there showed up the Alpines (Sumerians, Carpi, Etruscans, Basks), Armenoides (Caucasians), Mediterranean types (Indites, Semites, Italo-Balkans), Northern Dynaric (Carpatho-Danubian and Osteuropides, Faelics) and mongoloid elements. At these forms, the three morphological constitutional types and the ectomorphs, the mesomorphs, the endomorphs and other psychical, endocrine types, etc.

From the beginning, all these series of *Homo sapiens* descending humans presented four characteristic trends which are:

– aggressiveness, even towards the congeners, confirmed by the dictum *Homo homini lupus*;

– opulence: eat a lot, gather fortune, fight for power and subordination;

– imitability: fashion clothing, tendency to have more than the neighbours;

– creativity, this is the best quality, leading the humans to the current culture and civilisation.

This last quality allowed the humanity to pass over the three economic and social crises which took place in Neolithic (5000-2000 B.C.), in the Bronze Age (2000-750 B.C.), in the feudal age (750 B.C.-2000 A.C.) and the current informatics age after 2000 years.

In the Neolithic-Eneolithic (5000-2000 B.C.), the labor division is accomplished into:

– agriculture workers (Sumerians)

– hunters (Acadians).

Each of them had their faiths and customs and wished to stay independent. The conflict between them concretised with the solving of the first economic-social crisis by organising the states with totalitarian management (kings, emperors, with aristocrats, priests and slaves), with the adoption of the Taurus cult from the agriculture workers and of the Hemiobol (hunters). The conflict groups were the Sumerians (Alpines) and the Acadians (Armenoids). This stage corresponds to the Sign of Taurus (4500-2000 years B.C.) in astrology.

In the Bronze Age (2000-750 B.C.) the Mediterranean differentiate with the three groups (Indites, Semites, Italo-Balkanics), which have a different evolution: the Indites emigrate in India, continuing the agriculture and the cult of Taurus. Some Semites entered into conflict with the Assiro-Babylonians forming, after reconciliation, by affinity, the Assiro-Caldeean state. The Hittites and the Egyptians built and developed an agriculture empire with an impressive development of the architectural art and the religion, anticipating the monotheism. The Greeks develop the agriculture, the manufacture, the trade oversees, the sheep raise and promotes the peaceful cooperation and the democratic principles. The Sign of Aries during this time span corresponds to the cult of the Aries, adopted by the shepherds in the area. The second socioeconomic crisis develops by the expansion of the Imperial Roman State, imposing the peace in the Mediterranean area, with the army formed by the Mediterranean (Romans) related to the Northerners Carpathians-Danubians (the she-wolf legend).

Between the years of 300-2000 A.C. begins the religious crisis concluded with the victory of the Christianity and the development of the theocracy. This stage corresponds astrologically with the Sign of Pisces, favourable for the development of the religion. The agriculture is the economic basis of time, which allows the formation of some small led by feudalists. After the victory in Valmy of the French revolutionaries, the national states develop with the integration of some ethnical, religious or of different typologies groups. This idea led to the formation of some large, hegemonic nations with expansionist tendencies, with wars leading to the loss of 60 million persons during the last 100 years when the premises for the fourth crisis occur. Astrologically, we enter the Sign of Aquarius which favors the development of the technology (the technocracy). The industry replaced the agriculture. We are now talking of the industrial human, with a particular technical culture, with the development of the technological and biological sciences, with the generalisation of the informatics, the time and space being no longer a barrier in the economic, technical, biological, medical information, etc. Instead of the libraries, the speciality journals, the tapes and floppy disks showed up, allowing for the experts' information and for the data processing in record time. The crisis occurs between the population groups with primitive agriculture, poor and sick, and the industrial countries with populations with much higher life standards, with low child mortality and a life expectancy index of over 70 years old.

How is this fourth economic world crisis going to be solved? The idea of the national states and the totalitarian empires is gone. The peace can no longer be imposed by force, for the state leaders' welfare. It goes back to the democratic principles and the free market, initiated by Greeks in the area of the Greek citadels. The national states union is imposed as a federation, and not as a hegemonic state, applied in Greece. The human rights initiated by Christianity, become the religion of this age, respecting the beliefs of some persons yet. Normally, globalisation is to be reached, to the establishment of some technological, medical standards (in investigations, in medical treatments, etc.) and, in general, in all the sciences which could advance freely and could stimulate the endowed persons' creative activity, of those gifted in various economic-social areas. A better life is intended for all population groups in the world, without limiting the persons' habits and customs. The technocracy is to save the humanity in the following decade from the famine and the inter-human wars leaving space for the human creativity, inhibiting the tendencies of aggressiveness and opulence.

All these principles, applied in the industrialised countries led to the rise of the life standards and the increase in the life expectancy. The developing countries, such as Romania, and even the poor countries want to reach decent life standards. All this could be achieved only by education and by the work of the people in the respective communities, with the democratic support of the industrialised countries.

Other personalities of the Romanian anthropology

Victor Papilian

D. Gerota's disciple and the first Romanian Professor of anatomy in Cluj, *V. Papilian* was the founder of a great Romanian school of human anatomy, embryology and anthropology in this city. *V. Papilian* performed a large number of anthropological researches and he established the Cluj Society of Anthropology.

Constantin Maximilian

Constantin Maximilian (1928-1997, born in Bucharest) performed high school and academic studies. (the Faculty of Medicine, 1947-1953, in Bucharest). He continued his specialisation in anthropology at Moscow (1957) and in the USA in medical genetics (1968-1969). Between 1950-1953, he was a scholar of the Romanian Academy at the Centre for Anthropological Research, and between 1953-1957, he became a researcher at this centre, at the Section of Paleoanthropology, participating in the study of several caves and of some Neolithic settlements (Ohaba-Ponor, Sărata Monteoru, Peştera Muierii). He drafted several works of anthropology among which: *Sărata Monteoru. Anthropological Study* (1962), the first monograph of this kind in the Romanian medical literature, distinguished with the *Victor Babeş* Award of the *Romanian Academy*. He was a member of the *French Society of Anthropology* and member of the *Romanian Academy*.

Eugen Floru

He was a lecturer in the Department of Anatomy run by *Francisc I. Rainer*. He made world famous findings such as the *Ilio-tibia tract in anatomy and, outside the paleoanthropology, elements on the "perforated calcaneus at Schitişor"*.

Olga Necrasov

Olga Necrasov (born 1910, Sankt Petersburg) performed high school and academic studies (the Faculty of Sciences, the Department of Sciences of Nature) at Iasi. She continued her specialisation in serology at the Laboratory of Bacteriology and Experimental Medicine of the Institute of Hygiene in Poland, in compared anatomy at the Institute of Anatomy of Lvov, in contemporary anthropology at the Institute of Anthropology of Cracow, in anthropometry and classical anthropology at the Institute of Anthropology in München. In 1940, she defended her doctoral dissertation on *Anthropological Researches in the North of Romania - Recherches anthropologiques dans le nord de la Roumanie*.

She was a Professor of compared anatomy, anthropology and embryology-histology; director of the Centre for Anthropologic Research of Bucharest; head of the Department of Anthropology of the Iaşi Branch of the Romanian Academy. She studied the compared and functional anatomy of the nervous system in fish, the morphology of the skeleton of the mammals from the Quaternary paleo-fauna, the contemporary anthropology and paleoanthropology, etc. She was also interested in the development of the Biology in Romania, as well as on the contribution of some Romanian scientists (*I. Borcea, P. Bujor*).

She was member of the Commission of Anthropology and Ethnology of Romania (since 1960), in the National Committee for the International Biological Program, hosted by UNESCO, member of the *Biological Society of Romania, of the Society of Anthropology* by the *Slovakian Academy of Science, of the Royal Institute of Anthropology of Great Britain and Ireland, of the Society of Anthropology* of Vienna; she was awarded the Order of *Scientific Merit* (1974), with the Commemorative Medal *Ales Hrdlicka* (1962), with the *Paul Broca* Award and Medal (Paris, 1980). She was corresponding (1948) and full (1990) member of the *Romanian Academy*.

Cantemir-Moise Rişcuţia

Cantemir-Moise Rişcuţia (1923, born Cetatea Albă, Bessarabia) graduated the Faculty of General Medicine of Bucharest (1949). His doctoral thesis in the speciality of anthropology was carried on at the *Francisc Rainer Institute,* and it was named *Study on the malar bipartition at Romanians*. He also followed courses in biological and cybernetic statistics and independent studies of painting. After functioning initially in the clinics of endocrinology and internal medicine, he became a scientific researcher in anthropology, activating at the *Cantacuzino Institute* (1956), *the Medico-Legal Institute* (1960; he founded the first laboratory of forensic anthropology) and the

Victor Babeş Institute (1970; he founded the Laboratory of anthropo-biology) as a main scientific researcher, with the speciality of physical anthropology, paleoanthropology and judicial expertise. Until retirement (1993), he has been active there, a time when the laboratory of *Victor Babeş Institute* has been cancelled. He specialised in physiognomic reconstitutions, developing a new method of stereo-morphologic study – photo-stereometric – which allows for an exact, mathematical interpretation of the living form, by analysing the bright level curves, projected on the human body or the skeleton. He studied series of skulls in the cemeteries of Histria, Târpeşti and Orlea. He reconstituted the physiognomy of several fossils, being considered as one of the most important worldwide experts: Pithecanthropus *Sangiran II* (1965-1967), Pithecanthropus *Modjokertensis* (1967), *Homo Sapiens Praesapiens Steinheimensis-Berckhemer* (1972).

Other prestigious works consisted of: the reconstitution of *Ludwig van Beethoven*'s physiognomy; investigation, at *Palermo*, of the circumstance of *Nicolae Bălcescu*'s death and burial; anthropological research on the people of the *Apuseni Mountains*, performed with a complex methodology (classical and original somatometry, of the evolutionary morphology, somatoscopy on historical taxonomic criteria – phyletic –, genealogical databank, photo-stereometric investigation in taxonomic purpose on large series, population informatics processing). Despite a large number of contributions in a less explored area, probably Dr *Rişcuţia* becomes publicly known only in 1970 when after the imprint of a psychopath bite, left on the victim's skin, he drew four possible portraits of the dental archway owner. One of these portraits was identical to that of the famous criminal *Râmaru* and, finally, led to his identification.

Mircea Ifrim has an activity of research approaching among others the anthropological constitutional typology, completing it with the motricity typology (1988). He published 32 monographs among which: *The motricity anthropology*, where he presents his research in the field of the constitutional typology, considered for the first time in its complexity – morphologically, physiologically, psychically, motricity, and genetically. He is a student of the academician *Şt. Milcu*, Assoc. Prof. *Eugen Floru*, Prof. *I. Th. Riga*, MD, and others. He is concerned with cultural anthropology, as seen in the publised monography *Sailing through the Storm*. He was a first assistant and close collaborator for the above mentioned. This brief presentation of the personalities marking the Romanian anthropology would not be complete without naming other physicians who dedicated themselves to this fascinating branch of the medical sciences: *Horia Dumitrescu* (1893-1988), *C.S. Nicolaescu-Plopşor* (1900-1968), *Traian Herseni* (1907-1980), *Suzana Grinţescu-Pop* (1908-1977), *V.V. Caramelea* (1915-1994), *Vladimir Georgescu* (1929-1992), *Maria Cristescu* (1929-2000), *Alexandra Bolomey-Georgescu* (1935-1995).

Conclusions

The anthropology has developed as a science of socio-economic knowledge and tendencies in the world. There have been in Romania valuable scientists who actively participated in the introduction of the anthropological subjects and methods, so developing the medical aspects of this science. *Fr. Rainer* remains the creator of the anthropology in our country, founding an Institute which is bearing his name, an extraordinary collection of skulls and pathological bones, selected, labelled and presented invaluable scientific works.

The Institute of Anthropology, today *the National Institute of Anthropological Research Fr. Rainer* survived during the communist times due to the "elastic" intelligence of Prof. *Milcu*, such as he was characterised by *Rainer,* surprisingly introducing as main subject "the origin and the formation of the Romanian people", researches that showed in 10 years, from 1950-1960, while *Milcu* was the director of this institute, that the population in Romania is a people's mosaic, with particular somatopsychical qualities, our country having as treasure people's intelligence and capacity for adjustment to the new international socio-economic evolutions. In fact, one of the first researches of population genetics in the world is that of Acad. *Drăghicescu* who publishes in 1932 the monograph *Genetics of the Romanian people*. His ideas are acknowledged by the academician *M. Maliţa* in the monograph *Homo fraudes*. *Milcu* creatively develops medical anthropology, stimulating his favourite students, by proposing one of them, *Firu*, as the institute director in 1960, and the latest creative developement being the dentistry anthropology and performing the national program of research for the prevention of the oral-dental-maxillary conditions depending on the external and internal environments.

After 1960, the new director, Prof. *Olga Necrasov*, MD, develops a biological anthropology, continued by the current director *Cristiana Glavce,* MD. After the Revolution, Prof. *V. Săhleanu*, MD, became director of the Institute and developed in particular the philosophical anthropology with works of great value in this field. After 1990, the Institute gets back its institutional personality, allowing the achievement of an objective topic in the research program, i.e. *the Anthropological Structure of the Current Historical and Prehistorical Populations on the Territory of Romania, in the perspective of the last decade of the 20th century.*

The topics frame in the fundamental research on the biomedical and sociocultural aspects of the phenomenon human, in its current complexity and its individual and populations evolution. The human individual is approached in its unitary complex as a living body. The biological aspects (normality and pathology) and the sociocultural ones dwell in the synchronic and diachronic perspectives. The componence of the researchers' team of the Centre reflects the specificity of the Romanian school of anthropology. Each expert, representatives either of the positive sciences (physicians, biologists, IT experts, biophysicists), either of the humanist sciences (philologists, sociologists, psychologists, historians) tends to cover a broader thematic spectrum, in the contemporary anthropological research. The distribution of topics intends to bring up new aspects in the knowledge on the contemporary and historical humans.

The research thematic of the center starts from the paleoanthropology going to the contemporary anthropology and from the biological anthropology to the sociocultural one. This reflects both preserving the tradition of the institutionalized anthropology of our country since 1937, and our researchers' current concerns are belonging to the concerns at a worldwide level. The proofs of the high level of the scientific research within the Institute are the six awards and the diploma "Academy Merit" awarded by the Romanian Academy. We mention the seven zonal anthropological atlases with the multi-disciplinary approach of some regions with importance in the Romanian people's formation and continuity. Also, there is the publishing of ten volumes of authors or collective works in various anthropological fields, as well as the two volumes of the *Anthropological Atlas of Romania* which is a panorama on the entire country considering the population typological structure. The most important objective of the Centre researchers is to elaborate an anthropological atlas for the whole country. The first volume referring to Wallachia was published in 1999. The "Francisc I. Rainer" Institute of Anthropology (the ex-Centre of Anthropological Researches), under the aegis of the Romanian Academy, has been publishing annually without interruption ever since 1950 the journal in Romanian *Studii de cercetări antropologice – Studies of Anthropological Research* and since 1964, the *Annuaire roumain d´Anthropologie – Romanian Yearbook of Anthropology*. In addition, several materials have been published in national and international prestigious journals. From 1952 to 1999, it was published in here the journal in Hungarian *Studies and Researches of Anthropology* (suspended due to lack of funds in 1999). We consider that the Romanian anthropology by everything it represents and has been achieving may be attached to the prestigious schools worldwide while preserving its specificity of inter-disciplinary research and institutional priority. Today, the *Centre for Anthropological Research Fr. Rainer* represents an institution known worldwide, appreciated for its works and each year included in the European anthropological movements, as each year, this Centre organises debates, congresses, symposiums of international interest.

CHAPTER II.
THE OBJECTIVES OF THE MEDICAL, MORPHO-FUNCTIONAL, MOTRICITY, CULTURAL AND META-PSYCHOLOGICAL ANTHROPOLOGY

As defined by *Blumenbach*, anthropology is a science of synthesis studying the human as a biological phenomenon, with two important directions of investigation: physical anthropology and cultural anthropology *(Keiter)*. *Physical anthropology* is actually a branch of the morpho-physiology studying the origin, the evolution and the morpho-physiological density of the human being. Within it, we can differentiate the paleoanthropology (approaches the evolution of the human being, having tangencies with the compared anatomy, the embryology, the genetics, the archaeology, etc.), the morpho-anthropology (formed by neurology, which studies tissues and organs and the somatology which approaches the body as unitary entity, under somatic constitutional typological proportion), the physio-anthropology (consider the physiological characters both considering their adaptability to various environmental conditions, and their physiological constitutional typology), the heredo-anthropology (monitors the hereditary determinism of the human constitutional typology, the genetics of the populations by the prism of the unit in the diversity of the human being, the evolution of the human being conditioned by the interaction between the hereditary fund of the environmental factors), the anthropo-demography (which approaches the aspects connected to the demographic trends of the populations, by the particularities of age of the bodies conditioned by the processes of growth and development, by the correlations between the sexual determinism of the human being and the evolution of the demographic phenomena).

Cultural anthropology approaches aspects from the sphere of the supra-structure of the human being, considered as social phenomenon, the man being the only biological being which, beyond its biological environment, also has a social environment and at whom besides transmitting the hereditary information via the genes, there is also a transmittal from one generation to another of the intellectual information by the articulated language and the writing. The cultural anthropology mainly comprises the archaeology (the history of the old cultures), the ethnology (the theory of culture), the linguistics (the study of speech and language), etc.

Acad. *Ştefan Milcu* considers that "anthropology is a branch of the sciences of the nature, located at the border between the biology and the social sciences, which, considering the inter-relations with the environmental, geographical and historical factors, deals with the study of the human variability, of its origin and races".

Historically, anthropology has an old evolution, developed in tight connection with genetics (which, in fact in some researchers' view, is a part of anthropology), which defines the hereditary side of both somatic-constitutional and psychological typology of the human, and the complex processes of human individual's growth and development and of the multiple phenomena which condition the populations' characteristics and dynamics, ethno- and phylogenetically. The beginnings of anthropology and genetics date since *Aristotle.* In the *History of Animals, Aristotle* places the human being among the animals, considering it as the being superior organised, it introduces the term of anthropology and makes the first references to genetics, showing that from malformed persons the children are also malformed, and that malformations may be hereditary or caused by the factors of the environment. *Aristotle* highlights that "the soul is above the matter". Also, in the Indian books dating from the second millennium before our era, there are notes on the unfavourable consequences of the consanguine marriages. Some horses' pedigree was marked down on the Babylonian plates of Ninive.

In his works, *Herodotus* describes differentiated anthropological characters of the Mediterranean, Caucasian and Scythian populations. *Isidorus* shows that the person's look differs from the geographic area of origin. *Hippocrates* – the Father of medicine – makes several references of genetics, showing that children with blues eyes are born from parents having blue eyes, and gives so the first reference on the transmittal of the recessive homozygote characters. For the first time, *Albertus Magnus* shows that the human being is formed by a heredity side and from a part determined by the factors of external environment and describes the possibility for hereditary transmittal of the acquired characters. He highlights the existence of some hereditarily transmitted malformations such as polydactyly, hermaphrodism, situs inversus, and reveals that the nutrition may alter the heredity.

After this period, there follows a long stagnation in the field of anthropological and genetic findings, and also in the field of anatomy, and then, in the times of Renaissance, it is recorded a new qualitative leap in these areas. So, *Leonardo da Vinci* shows the existence of the resemblances between humans and animals; *Bernier* (1620) makes the first classification of the human races, and *Galen* reveals the link between the constitutional type and state of disease.

Later on, *Linné* places the man among the primates, showing the existence of some constitutional types, such as the gothic – tall, unpigmented, the Finnish – blond and Lapponian. In addition, he considers the current species as *Homo sapiens sapiens* (wise person), with the variants *Europeus, Americanus, Asiaticus* and *Africanus,* by the geographical area of location.

Lamarck claimed that the evolution of the animal world is the result of the adjustment to the environment and the transmittal of the acquired characters, while *Darwin*, based on the natural selection and variability, substantiates the origin of species, humans' included. Later, *Regnier de Graaf* discovers the ovarian follicle, and *L. Hamm,* the spermatozoids. Actually, between evolutionism and creationism is an acerb dispute, but the creationism and the meta-psychology gain field.Ulterior, *Gregor Mendel* emphasises the fundamental processes of the heredity by experimental research on plant bringing as corollary explanations on the hereditary substrate of the anthropological typology. Thus, he crosses types of plants and mathematically analysed the achieved results, substantiating the notions of dominance, recessive, homozygous, and heterozygotes. We add to this the conquests of *Flemming, Strasburger, Waldeyer* (1875), *McClung* (1902) on the gender chromosomes, followed by those of *Morgan* in 1910, who substantiates the chromosome theory of heredity. These findings take a peak in 1953 with *Watson* and *Crick* researches which prove the existence of the DNA and of the genetic code, as biochemical material substrate of the genes and, respectively, of the heredity, followed by the studies of anthropology and genetics of the populations, of molecular, medical, radio-biological, immunity, cytological medicine, of dermatoglyphic pharmacology, etc., which took a particular impetus lately. In our country, the beginnings of the anthropology can be found in *Dimitrie Cantemir's* work, *Descriptio Moldaviae,* where it is mentioned the influence of the geographical location and the socioeconomic conditions of the populations. Later on, *Nicolae* and *Mina Minovici,* worldwide personalities, organise the first forensic institute in Europe, at Bucharest, introducing the anthropological methods in the forensic medicine for the first time in the world.

Afterwards, *C. I. Parhon,* the author of the first treatise of endocrinology in the world (1909), performs pioneering studies in bio-typology, bringing original contributions, of worldwide value in the endocrine interpretation of the constitution, proving the role of the endocrine glands in the occurrence and the evolution of the races and in the determinism of the individual constitutional type. *Fr. I. Rainer* performs the first medico-anthropological investigations, starting the elaboration of the *Anthropological Atlas of Romania,* organises the first Institute of Anthropology in the South-Eastern Europe, one of the first in the world, which is inaugurated on the occasion of the 17th International Congress of Anthropology and Archaeology, held in Bucharest in 1937. He performs the first researches of anthropological sportive bio-typology in the first laboratory of such a Profile in Europe, which he found as the first rector of the National Academy of Physical Education, he initiates and lectures the course of sportive anthropology for the students in the third year of the National Academy of Physical Education. His contributions in the field of anthropology place *Fr. I. Rainer* among the most outstanding personalities of anthropology at a worldwide level. *Fr. I. Rainer*'s researches are continued by the Acad. *Ştefan Milcu,* who develops the anthropological studies in our country on the structure of the Romanian people, on the endocrine type and constitution, on the correlations between the constitutional typology and the sports performance, on the somato-physiological qualities of some groups of populations, on the genetic determinism of some biological characters etc., bringing original contributions acknowledged at worldwide level. They bring him international notoriety able to take to highest peaks the prestige of the Romanian anthropology and genetics.

In this context, the *sportive anthropology* detached itself from the anthropology. In our country, it was substantiated by scientists such as *Fr. I. Rainer* and the Acad. *Ştefan Milcu.* Professor *Rainer* taught at the National Academy of Physical Education in the third year of studies the course of anthropology, after the course of anatomy at Year I and of biomechanics at year II. *The sportive anthropology* whose content we consider it is better expressed by the wording *Motricity anthropology,* belonging to the Acad. Prof. Dr *Mircea Ifrim* (1988) has as an object a complexity of elements involved in the entire sports activity and, especially, in the process of selection and training, conditioning more and more the achievement of the sportive performance.

The anthropological findings based on computerised programs start being more and more efficient in acquiring the performance. The simple law of Physics explains how forces are sent from one point to another. For each athlete, an ideal anthropological diaphragm can be established corresponding to his/ her physical characteristics. Comparing this model-trajectory with sports person's real movements in action is possible to detect the useless gestures, the inappropriate movement, the false impulses and the attitudes dispersing the force or reducing the strength. Besides all the above, the computer, programmed with anthropology parameters allows establishing the value of the angles of each joint during a performance, as well as the positions of the gravitational centre, elements which can be found in the monograph *Antropologia motrică – Motricity Anthropology* written by Acad. *Mircea Ifrim* (1988).

We tell few elements of the global concern on motricity anthropology. The high jumper, the Dutch *Ruud Wielart* has been anthropologically analysed by *Gideon Ariel.* Examining his jumping schemes, one can state that he can reach easily five extra cm; the position of his gravity centre is excellent, but when crossing over the bar, he stretches his leg too soon. In order to raise well his leg, he is forced to bend his back and reaches the bar. If he waits for one more fraction of a second to raise his lower limbs, all his body would be beyond the bar, and he could lean easily. Instead, he possesses a good technique: he stops his acceleration right before detaching from the soil, which is excellent as he recovers a maximum of strength to raise himself.

On the other hand, it was noticed that *Ruud Wielart* slightly lacks strength and that he has to develop certain muscles: the strength using to lean on the soil right before the jump should be able to be equal to approximately eight times higher than his weight, like at the best jumper. However, it is much lower. Proper training can easily rectify the flaw.

The case of the American disc shooter *Mac Wilkins,* who won the gold medal at the Olympic Games in Montreal in 1976, is also an example of anthropological analyse. Few months before the games, *Gideon Ariel* has analysed the champion's technique. At that time, *Mac Wilkins* was throwing the disc at 66 meters, which represented a good performance, but he was far from the 69 meters of the world record. Calculating the forces of the sportsman limbs related to the anthropological constitutional type and studying the schemes of his throws, Dr *Ariel* has noticed that the American athlete right before throwing the disc was moving his knee like a spring, instead of blocking it. By doing this, he was losing a part of the strength which should have been sent to the disc." As such" – comments Gideon *Ariel* – "it was simulated on the computer, the throw performed by a fictional *Mac Wilkins*, who would not move his knee. The prediction was spectacular: he might get three extra more meters". Three days later, after blocking his knee with an orthopaedic device, *Mac Wilkins* was getting over the world record, reaching 70.86 m. Another American athlete made a similar mistake: the weights thrower *Terry Albritton.* After analysing his moves anthropologically, *Gideon Ariel* advised him *not to bend anymore the knee before projecting the weight,* so that the arm receives a maximum force. He even predicted that, if he rectified this flaw, he would become world champion. A month later, this prediction turned real.

The anthropological analyse of the javelin thrower, *Bill Schmidt, the* technique also gave considerable results. Physician *Ariel* discovered that the sportsman was losing strength by "letting his hip fell" at the time of the throw. *Schmidt* quickly rectified his standing and threw the javelin beyond 92 meters, thus two meters far from the world record. Coupling the computer programmed on anthropological parameters serves not only to improving the performances, but it also allows for the elimination of the useless efforts and the technical mistakes. For instance: since ancient times, long jumpers were convinced that must have knurled steel to press to jump up on the plan. However, *Gideon Ariel* discovered that, at the jump time, the foot, in contact with the ground, pushes less than it is achieved by accelerating the other lower limb launched before and, by that, of the torso.

In theory, *Gideon Ariel* considers that we can analyse any sports performance. Yet, some disciplines are harder to "dissect". For instance, this is for the natation, as we must take into consideration a supplementary element: the water. We are about to build an aquarium swimming pool so we can record the swimmers during the training. Pole vault also raises problems, to the extent that you cannot neglect the characteristics of the pole used. Generally, the approach is delicate for all disciplines where the aesthetics plays an important part. We can improve a gymnastics movement, but it is not sure that the aesthetics might gain from that. For the artistic ice-skating, it has been tried to find out how the judges analysed the mandatory figures, why did they favour a certain skater and not the other. Is it that the hand's movement caused their choice or the movement of the leg, of the head, of the arms? We ended up by establishing that, in reality, the trunk position caused the decision: it has always been very straight, regardless of the legs and arms movements. If the team sports resist to such analyses – as the strategy takes a vital place – is it still possible to improve the way how each rugby or football player hits the ball? In reality, *Dr Ariel*'s anthropological method is applicable wherever there is movement.

What happens when no flaw, no movement error is discovered in an athlete? Do you tell him/ her that he/ she has reached the maximum and no progress can be expected? It is quite rare to meet flawless sportspersons. Often, when the moves close to the perfection, the athlete still might lack strength. The anthropological analyse detects such deficiencies and, in such a case, it is possible to elaborate an appropriate training program. When this element is also accomplished, we found ourselves regarding the ceiling phenomenon, characterised by reaching the upper limit of genetic adaptability. For *Gideon Ariel,* for instance, the ideal sprinter must have an ultra-quick movement of the legs firstly. However, the fastness of this movement is tied to the neuromuscular system. In order to select the best runner for 100 or 200 meters, the coaches are though interested in measuring the legs reflex of extension. At an equal timing, the runner with the longest lower limbs and the shortest torso will have the all the odd to defeat his/ her opponents.

For certain sports, the American anthropology expert has tried to calculate the human limits, these absolute records which the sportsperson cannot defeat without jeopardising his/ her life. At 100 meters, the limits for possible must be around 9.6 seconds; beyond this limit, there is the risk that the muscles break and of certain bones fracture. At long jump, the world record of the American *Bob Beamon* (8.90 m) is not far from the ultimate limit, which has to be of 8.96 m. However, *Beamon* is quite close to the ideal athlete: his running is extremely fast, and his movements are perfectly synchronised, his anthropological type reaches the optimum for this test. At the time of the jump, he develops a force of 770 kg in the hip joint which is at the limit of the muscular rupture. At high jump, one day, possible, the 2.70 m are going to be reached while the world record is 2.38 m. In the same way, doctor *Ariel* compared *Dick Fosbury*'s jump (Gold Medal at the Olympic Games in Mexico in 1968, where he inaugurated the so-called method of "dorsal rolling") with *Valeri Brumel*'s jump when he defeated the world record by "ventral rolling". He simulated on the computer the height which *Brumel* might have used the *Fosbury flop*, which has a higher vertical component. The Soviet would have defeated the world record: in theory, he was able to reach 2.41 meters!

There are only certain coaches who are still reticent: they fear that the anthropology and the biomechanics jeopardise their Profession! "No way", replies doctor *Ariel*: *the motricity anthropology is nothing but a new tool meant to improve our knowledge of the sportsperson effort and the athletes' performances. The psychological relations between coaches and sportspersons play a primordial part in the competition, and there is no way I could replace them.*

In the same line, we mention that the *motricity anthropology* approaches:

– the relation between the ideal and the real shapes;

– the way to use the physical exercise for the competition, respectively, the topics of the motricity anthropology for getting maximum efficiency;

– the relation between the constitutional bio-typology and the performance;

– the concept of health considering the sportive activity; both mass sports and competition one compels to the reconsideration of the concept of anthropological normality (eg.: degree of gigantism of basketball players, the weightlifters' weight, etc.);

– the morpho-physiological and cultural effects of the physical education and sport on the population;

– the ethnological aspects of the physical education and sport;

– an aspect of very broad inter-disciplinary complexity (sports imply physical, cultural, social models);

– scientific investigation of the concrete motricity situations and individualised anthropological studies on highly-performant athletes;

– the incidence of the new sciences in the sport's investigation: the theory of the systems, the cybernetics, the semiotics, the structural analyse, the axiology, the praxeology, the futurology, the auxology, the bio-typology, the bio-statistics, the bio-rhythmology, the psycho-somatic, the ergonomics, etc.;

– the perspectives opened by sport for the philosophical anthropology;

– the relation between the genetic determination and sport.

Motricity anthropology is a global discipline, a science of the nomo-sphere which is not identical to the noosphere but is comprised in it. The anthropology presents major implications in forming the students' dialectical philosophical conception, of the concept of biological advance in the light of determinism and indeterminism, of the innovator spirit in thinking, being one of the subjects with powerful medico-social and philosophical character, both materialist and idealist.

Essentially, this multitude of aspects forms the subject of the motricity anthropology, which can be synthesised in some basic landmarks, as it follows:

– The processes of growth and development with their implications on the motricity movement;

– The constitutional somato-physiological, motricity and psychical typology, conditions by the genetically determined biological rhythms and the correlations between the constitutional type in its ensemble and the requirements of the sportive competition activity; the interrelations between the genotype and the para-type in building the constitutional type (the phenotype);

– Genetic and anthropological determination of some characters with major significance in achieving the sportive performance;

– The anthropologic and genetic methodology of evaluation of the sportive potential and efficiency.

Lately, *motric anthropology* gets involved in the sportive competition activity in two essential parts, respectively in:

– sportive selection which, performed anthropologically and genetically, has a considerably superior efficiency to that which does not take account on these criteria, the only ones able to scientifically predict the evolution of the biotype and of the measure where this becomes an optimal anthropological type in the sports area he/ she was selected for;

– guidance of the training based on the knowledge of the individual anthropological particularities of each subject, which allows that the sportive efficiency is considerably increased, being known that the conditioning for reaching the upper limit of genetic adaptability of the Motricityity relies on an optimal individualized dosage of the effort which the body could take.

In addition, *motric anthropology,* by deciphering the processes of growth and development, the body particularities of age, and of the dosage of the physical effort considered as environmental factor, in relation to these morpho-physiological characteristics of the body – genotypically and para-typically determined –, gets majorly involved in directing the entire activity of physical education and sport during the entire ontogeny of the human being, since birth to adulthood and senescence, so that the physical effort, performed scientifically, on anthropological and genetic grounds, actually constitutes a factor for harmonious growth and development of the body in its building stage, and then in a factor of promotion and maintaining the state of health during the entire human existence.

Thus, it results that motricity anthropology, the inter-disciplinary science detached a few decades ago from the anthropology and having a rich tradition in our country by the great scientists *Fr. I Rainer* works and continued by *Şt. M. Milcu*, *Iuliu Haţeganu* and *Mircea Ifrim*, has a particular value for the competition sport, and for the guidance of the physical education and sport consistently to the imposed requirements, of being one of the essential factors of the harmonious development and of preserving the population's state of health, essential goals for the progress of our nation. *Cultural anthropology* aims for phenomena in correlation with everything that the culture stands for, a result of the nervous system activity in its complexity, on which we are going to detail later on. The culture is distinct for each population group, being connected to the population and individual genetics, sides of the morpho-functionality of the anthropology. *Meta-psychological anthropology* concerns the "human" phenomenon, considering its behaviours of physical, ethereal, astral, mental, and spiritual body, aspects which we are going to detail in the chapter presenting each of them thoroughly. Our approach is an element of certain novelty in the universe of the anthropology conferring an unapproached up to now a vision in the field of this science, the current work approaching this aspect in the premiere.

CHAPTER III.
THE HUMAN ONTOGENESIS

The human body ontogenesis, respectively the viability since the conception to the exit, acknowledges three important periods:

– the period of growth and development;
– the period of maturity and reproduction;
– the period of involution (the senescence) (the term of senility indicates an early involution).

Considering the normal duration of these stages, we mention that the growth and development stage covers 22-23 years, and, as proven by the American school via researches performed on a multitude of species from the animal world that the total life duration, normally, must be five times higher than the period of growth and development. Thus, for the humans, around 120-125 years. However, due to some artificial factors of the environment, factors largely created willingly or forced by the human being, this average life duration decreased considerably. Among these noxious factors, we mention the excessive nutrition (especially after 45 years old, when the metabolism reduces to 70% of its initial value), the sedentary, the nervous stress, factors which are placed on the first plan.

We are going to approach especially the period of growth and development, without mentioning the period of maturity and reproduction which is subject of the anatomy and physiology and to the period of senescence (according to the American school classification it begins at 75 years old), which is the subject of the gerontology.

In addition, we are going to correlate the constitute periods of growth and development with the influence of the sportive effort which represents one of the essential environmental factors both for achieving a stronger body, and for preserving the state of health, and for building a stronger body, apt to the highest morpho-physiological parameters for the further periods of maturity and senescence. It is a scientifically proven fact that the senescence begins with the conception and it is conditioned – just like the maturity – under all aspects to the period of growth and development, essential for the entire ulterior evolution of the body. We also shall refer to the correlation and the dosage of the effort with the anthropological particularities of age, related to the requirements of the highly performant sport.

Growth and development – laws and periods

We understand by growth and development a dynamic complex of biological processes which the human body suffers in its evolution until the maturity.

The growth is a quantitative process of cell multiplication concerning the gain of weight, volume and dimensions of the body, while the development is a qualitative process of cell differentiation translated by functional changes and qualitative improvement marking the improvement and the adaptation of the body apparatuses and systems, their complex evolution and coordinated integration in a unitary whole (fig. 1).

Rainer voiced his conscience by listening to his soul. He indeed succeeded in teaching but also in founding new institutions. The Institute of Anatomy and Embryology of Bucharest are his creation. The school of anatomy was innovated by his method of thinking and research. *Rainer* was the first who "*gave a new direction to the study of the anatomy. He shows that the anatomy is no longer the science of the corpse. The data of the corpses anatomy are needed only as starting points for the development of the anatomical thinking. (...) The living form is tightly connected to the structure, and this one to the function; thus, it is the expression of the functional structure*". *Rainer* is considered to be a creator of the new direction in medicine, and, briefly, his method consisted of developing in great lines and sort of cinematographically of the body from cell to its full achievement, the functional interpretation of the systems building the humans and their interdependence, they are issues predominantly concerning the class of anatomy and decide the framework to present the details forming the subject of the anatomical science. On *Rainer* and his work, *Dimitrie Gusti* said that it was a "real preach by the experience of his life" of "*Benedictine of the culture*".

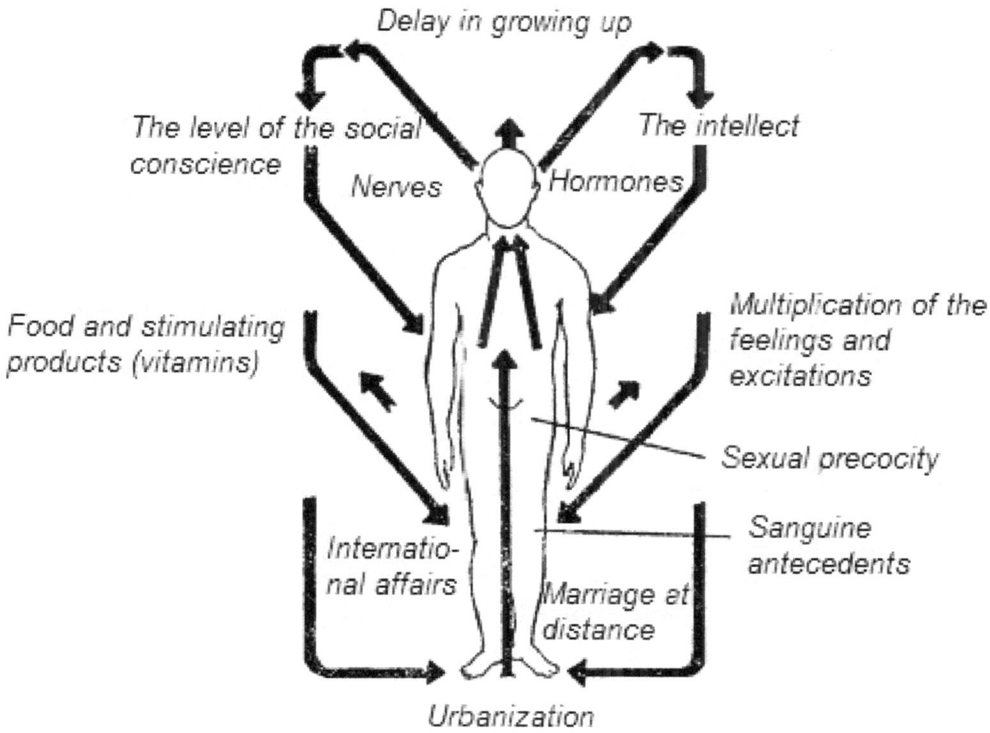

Fig. 1. Intricate of the endogenous and exogenous factors and their consequences on the constitution and acceleration. (by R. Nold).

These processes are conditioned by the action of some internal factors, represented by heredity, by the neuroendocrine genetic determined mechanisms and by some series of external factors from which we quote: during the intrauterine period – mother's state of health, and the pregnancy normal evolution, then geo-climatic factors, the alimentation, the environmental pollutants, etc. Among the external factors, the motor activity, the physical exercise, the physical and psychical efforts (as these two type of solicitation in sports cannot be dissociated), by phenomena of adjustment, compensation and overcompensation which trigger, stimulate, and, in some circumstances, even guide the growth and the development.

The physical exercise and any motricity activity develop obviously the elements of the locomotricity apparatus. By them, there are employed at a high level of solicitation, the breathing and the circulation, the nutritive exchanges and the processes of regeneration, the neuroendocrine regulation systems. Their exercising accomplished the functional structure of the tissues, stimulate the growth and leads to a better integration of the elements forming the body.

Training the apparatuses, systems and functions of the body, their use beyond the moderated level of current requirements cause response reactions with the character of over-adjustment and over-compensation, phenomena explaining the beneficial effects of the physical exercise on the whole individual evolution. The processes of growth and development recognize complex neuroendocrine regulations.

Regulating the process of growth. A large complexity of structures and nervous circuits intervene in this regulation, as it follows:

1. The extra-hypothalamic existence of some secretions of somatostatin (STH):

– At the central level, in the tonsils, in the periventricular organs and mesencephalon;

– At the periphery, at the stomach base, of the pyloric centre and of the pancreas, where it is secreted by the delta cells. It seems like somatostatin is also involved in the digestive regulations.

2. At hypothalamus level:

– conditioning the secretion of somatostatin is achieved by the ventromedial and arched nuclei of the hypothalamus and by the intervention of the noradrenergic, dopaminergic and serotoninergic neurones;

– a multitude of neurohormones with the neurotransmitting role are triggered; their final action on the growth hormone release varies; among these neurohormones we mention:

- The hormone of the arched nucleus, leading to the somatostatin secretion which inhibits, by feedback mechanisms, the arched nucleus in this action if it is in high peripheral concentration;
- The hypothalamic dopaminergic neurones, located in the tuberoinfundibular area, which have both positive and negative action on the somatostatin secretion, depending on the level of their concentration;
- The hypothalamic serotoninergic neurones have an exclusively positive action on the secretion of STH.

It is considered that the increase in the STH secretion during the physical exercises reduces the glycaemia and increases the concentration of arginine, performed via the serotoninergic hypothalamic bodies. The glucoreceptors of the ventromedial thalamic nucleus which are sensitive to the disorders of use of the intracellular glucose also intervene: the acetylcholine inhibits the secretion of STH, the beta-endorphins have of positive action on the secretion of STH. They act both by stimulating the noradrenergic neurones and by reducing the vegetative action of the dopaminergic neurones upon the increase of the STH concentration.

3. The receptors of the adrenergic hormones stimulate the increase of STH and, the noradrenergic ones inhibit it.

4. Through the ventromedial nucleus, the free fatty acids have a negative action on the secretion of STH.

5. The pyrogenic substances have a positive action through the thermo-regulating hypothalamic nuclei.

Laws

The processes of growth and development develop themselves by certain strict norms which can be systematised in the following five laws (by *Adrian Ionescu*, in the paper *Creşterea şi dezvoltarea- Growth and Development*).

1. The Law of unequal and asymmetric growth of the tissues and organs

The tissues and constitutive organs of the body grow and develop unequally and in various periods of time during the evolution of the human body. For instance, from birth to maturity, the brains grows four times, the liver grows nine times, the spleen 13 times, the kidneys 14 times, the heart 20 times, and the intestine 30 times.

The tissues and organs may grow faster or slower; some develop continuously, other known periods of stagnation or ever may devolve. Among those increasing rapidly, we may count some components of the nervous system. During the first year of life, the central nervous system, and especially the eye and the internal ear, reaches to sizes and proportions close to the final ones. The sexual organs have almost explosive development up to the puberty. Still then, the thymus and the lymphoid organs start devolving. Though developing unequally, the tissues and organs keep a certain degree and certain limits of proportionality, which do not trouble too much the harmony of the shapes, and the balance of functions.

Also, asymmetries occur between the two vertical halves of the body in the shape and placement of the organ or the length and thickness of the segment, particularly in the level of the upper and lower limbs *(Kucera).*

This asymmetry is characterised by:

a) Between the pair organs there is a functional asymmetry; for instance, at right-handed, the upper limb is longer, thicker, the shoulder more lowered and the opposite is for the left-handed;
b) The normal asymmetry of the pair organs and the trunk evolves progressively with the age, opposite to the growth and in the same way as the function;

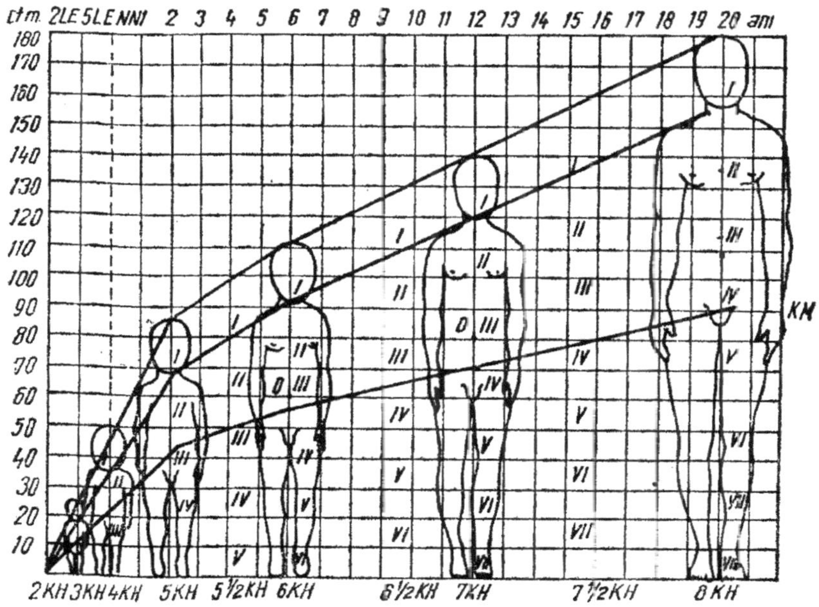

Fig. 2. Proportion changes of the body limbs during the growth (according to Stratz).

c) At right-handed, the superiority of length and thickness of the right upper limb, compared to the left one is, most of the time, accompanied by a crossed functional superiority.

The above elements have particular importance in sports, as it was proven that there is a symmetrical and asymmetrical sport, in the meaning that the sportsperson with a higher level of right-left symmetry has resulted in the symmetrical sports, while in the asymmetrical ones, the subjects with marked right-left asymmetry are more performant.

2. The law of different rhythm of growth and development

There is a certain system of growth and development at the level of each organ and tissue, conditioned by the hereditary factors. Most of the somatic elements follow the rhythm of growth of the stature and of body weight, which becomes for us benchmarks or terms of comparison. Generally, the organs keep their own rhythm of growth and structural differentiation and functional perfection. (fig. 2, 3) Important variations of rhythm are also found in the growth of the various parts or regions of the body. Thus, while the head doubles its height since growth to the maturity, during the same timeframe, the trunk grows approximately three times, the upper limbs four times, and at 12 years old – seven times.

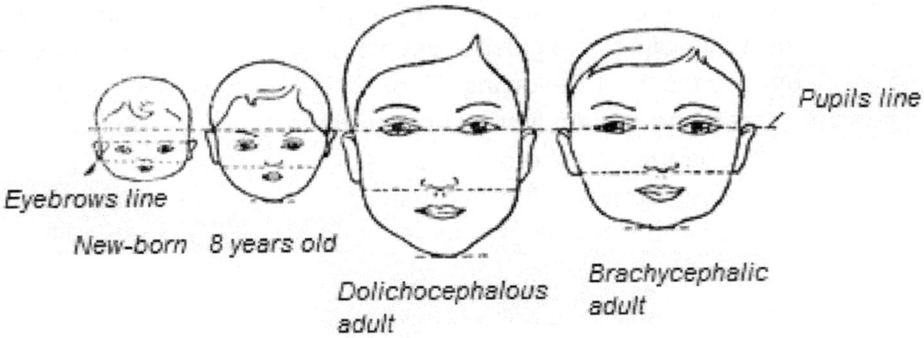

Fig. 3. Particularities of the massive facial growth and the proportions between the face levels at dolichocephalous and brachycephalic

As result of the different rhythm of growth and development, physiological discordances and even dissociations may occur between the different parts of the body *(Variot).*

3. The law of proportions

The different rhythm of growth and development also attracts permanent changes in the proportions between the various constitutive parts of the body. Thus the child is not an adult in miniature. The change of proportions between the parties begins from the intrauterine life and continues after puberty. During the body evolution, monitoring the change in the ratios between the height of the head and the stature, we notice that, at the two months old embryo, the height of the head is half of the length of the entire body. According to *Stratz,* at birth, the length of the body is four times the height of the head; at one year old, four times and a half; at two years, five times; at three years old, five times and a quarter; at four years, five times and a half; at five years old – five times and three quarters; at six years old – six times; at eight years old – six times and a quarter; at ten years old, six times and a half; at eleven years old, six times and three quarter; at twelve years old, seven times.

Regarding the ratio between the upper and the lower limbs, it is noticed that during the intrauterine life, the upper limbs are longer than the lower ones; slightly after birth, their length becomes equal; in 10 years, the lower limbs become longer than the upper limbs.

Also, the centre of gravity moves down as long as the child grows. Systematising, we notice the following:

a) There are three periods in the evolution of the variations proportion between the body width and length: from four to six years old, from six to 15 years old, and from 15 years up;
b) Since birth to the adult age, each segment of the body has its own way of behaving related to the height. In anthropology and the judiciary medicine, this law gives the possibility of exactly appreciating the stature of an individual by the size of one of the limbs bones.
c) If one segment of the body has a proportional growth superior to the statural one, the immediate segments, superior or inferior to the considered one, will have a proportional growth inferior to the statural one.

4. The law of the alternation

Regarding the time succession, between the period of growth and development, a series of alternations between the processes of growth and development, between the increase in height and that in weight, between the growths of the various neighbouring body segments. There is an alternation between the active increase of the body size and the development of the organ. In the stages of very intense qualitative growth, particularly during the development of the stature and the increase in weight, the organs development and the improvement of the functions is slowed down. After these long times of quantitative accumulation, there is stagnation or a regression of the growth. During the short break periods, real qualitative leaps occur, leading to a superior organic development.

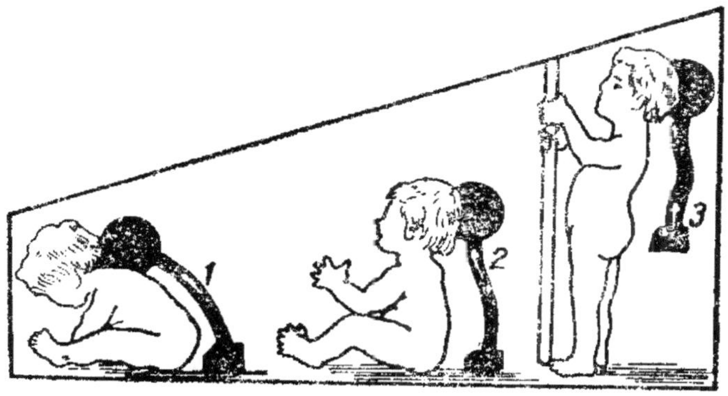

Fig. 4. The occurrence of the backbone curves in children

An obvious alternation often occurs between the rapid and intense increase in height and the reduced growth of the body weight. *Bartels* şi *Stratz* divided the age from one year to 20 years old into alternating periods of "accomplishment" or increase in weight and of "stretching" (elongation) or increase in height. The times of the first accomplishment lasts from one to four years old, and of the first elongation from five to seven years old. The times for the second accomplishment last from eight to ten years old, of the second elongation from 11 to 15 years old. The period of the third accomplishment and stretching last from 15 to 20 years old.

The increase in height alternates with the increase in width or the body thickness. The bones alternate their growth in length with their thickening. At the upper limbs, the increase in the length of the arm (the humerus) alternates with that of the forearm (radius and ulna); at the lower limbs, the increase of the thigh (the femur) alternate with that of the leg (tibia and peroneus).

The most important alternation occurs between the increase in the length of the lower limbs and the increase in the height of the bust (the Godin's great alternation) at puberty.

5. *The law of the puberty maturation.* According to this law, the puberty, by which we understand the totality of the morpho-functional changes occurring in the body once with the beginning of the gonads actions, causes the gender-differentiated growth and development. We are going to present this aspect once with the description of the puberty period.

The criteria for appreciating the growth rely, mainly, on the biometrical examination. The biometrical basic examinations consist in measuring the stature (the distance between the vertex and the soles), of the weight of the thoracic perimeter and the vital capacity. These data are correlated, materialising themselves into the *Brcca, Pignet, Gourtner, Speel* and cardiac indexes which show us the degree of development.

Periods

Regarding the periods of the growth, the data in the literature provide us with a great variety of opinions. The fact is justified as there cannot be a net delimitation of the various stages of growth, seeing as they are tightly connected. Moreover, teaching type reasons claim the existence of such divisions into distinct stages of the growth process.

We are going to present the physiological anatomy particularities of the human body based on the following classification of chronological periods in which the human being lives during its ontogenetic evolution:

1. The embryo-foetal period, from conception to birth.
2. The first childhood, from birth to three years old, when the emergence of the first dentition is completed. It comprises:
    a) The new-born stage (first 30 days);
    b) The nursling stage (30 days – one year);
    c) Little child (ante-preschool, one – three years).
3. Preschool stage (three – six years old). It begins simultaneously with the time when the first dentition has emerged and concludes once with the emergence of the first permanent teeth.
4. School period (six – 16 years). Depending on the occurrence of the puberty (12-14 years old at girls, 14-16 years old at boys), this period is divided into:
    d) Primary school period (ante-puberty): six – 11 years old;
    e) Secondary school period (puberty): 11-13 years old at girls; 12–14 years old at boys;
    f) High school period (post-puberty): 14-18 years old.

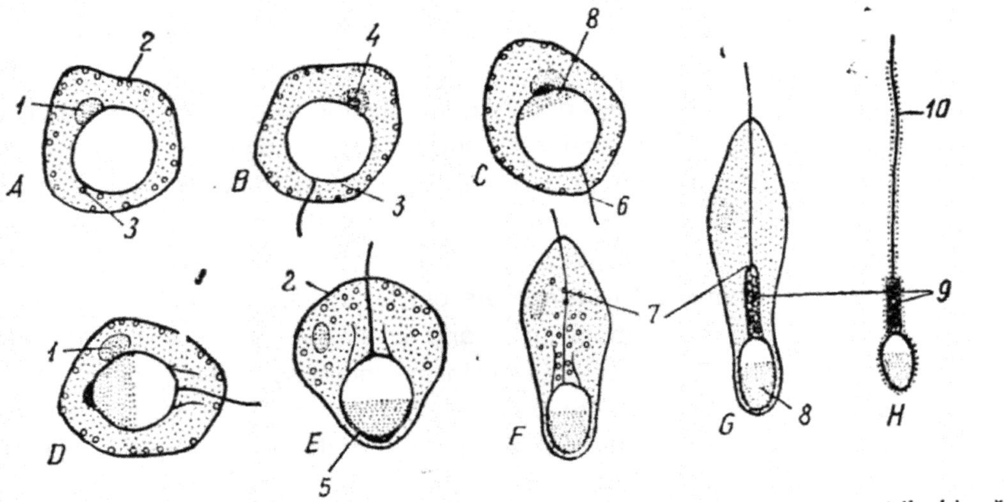

Fig. 5. Spermiogenesis at humans (transformation of the spermatid into spermatozoid) 1- Golgi Apparatus; 2-Mithocondrial; 3-Centriole; 4-Acrosome; 5-Cephalic caps; 6-Axial filament; 7-Innelar structure; 8-Nucleus and cephalic cap; 9-Mid (connecting) piece; 10-Spermatozoid tail. (according to J. Langman)

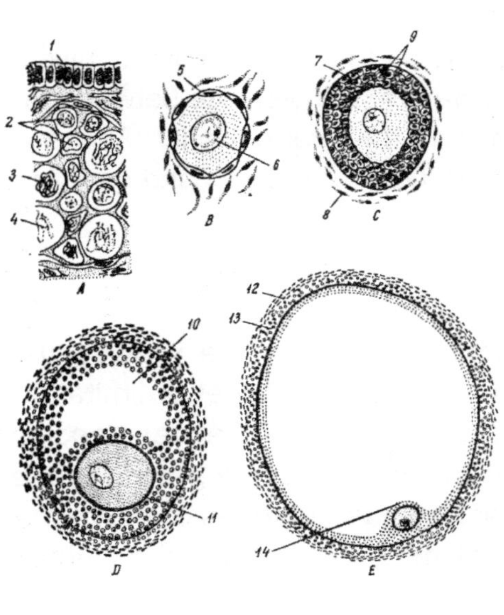

Fig. 6. Oogenesis (according toJ. Langman): A-Section through the ovarian tissue of the embryo after three months: 1- Ovarian epithelium; 2-Oogonia; 3-Oocite of 1 rank (leptotene stage); 4-Oocytes of rank 1 (zygote stage); B-Primordial follicle; 5- The Flattened epithelial cells; 6-the nucleus of the oocyte of rank 1; C- the oocyte of rank 1 in an advanced stage of development; 7-Basal membrane; 8- Ovarian connective tissue; 9-The pellucida membrane about to be formed; D-Oocyte of rank 1 with developed follicular cavity; 10- The follicular cavity; 11-Membrana pellucida; E- de Graaf follicle; 12-External sheath; 13-Internal sheath; 14-Cumulus ooforus.

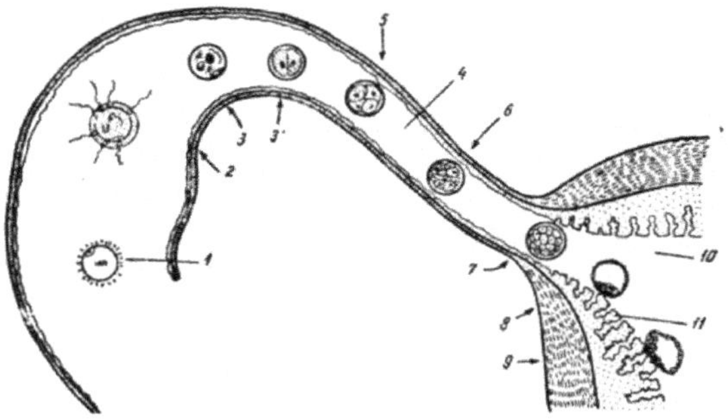

Fig. 7. The evolution of the egg during the first week of development:

1-The ovule surrounded by spermatozoids; 2-Fecundation; 3- The zygote in the stage of two blastomeres (after 30 hours since the fecundation); 4-The fallopian tube; 5- The zygote in stage of four blastomeres (40-50 hours since the fecundation); 6-Stage of eight blastomeres (after 60 hours); 7-Stage of 16 blastomeres (the IV-th by day); 8- Free blastocyst (V-th day); 9-Implantation (between 6 and 20 days since the beginning of the last menses); 10- The uterine cavity; 11-The uterine mucosa..

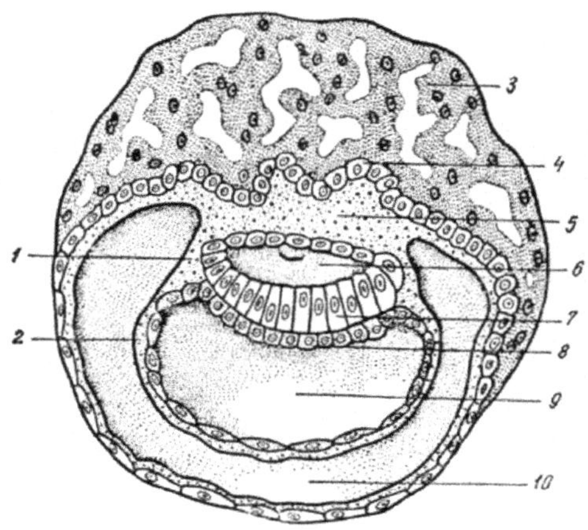

Fig. 8. The blastocyst by the end of the second week:

1-Somatopleure (mesenchyme which doubles the amnion); 2-Splanchnopleura (mesenchyme which doubles the lecytocell epiblast); 3-Syncytiotrophoblast; 4-Cytotrophoblast; 5- The embryo pedicle; 6- the Amniotic cavity; 7-Ectoblast; 8-Entoblaste; 9-Lecitocel; 10-Celom.

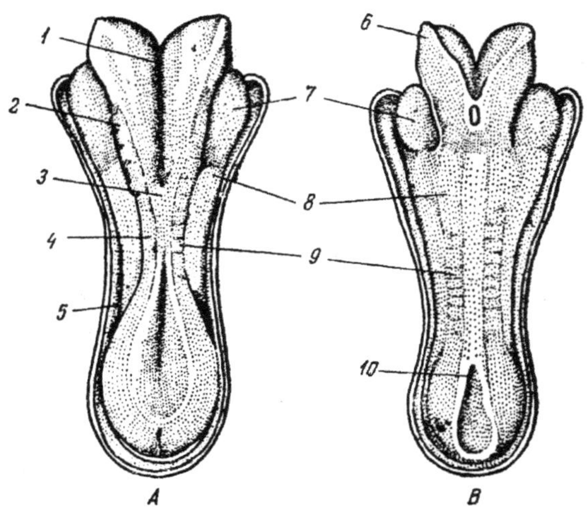

Fig. 9. Dorsal view of the embryo disk (according to J. Langman):

A-Human embryo of 22 days old; B-Human embryo of 23 days old; 1-Natural ditch; 2-Otic placodes; 3-the Ceiling of the neural tubule; 4-Somite about to be formed; 5- The sectioned edge of the amnion; 6-the edge of the neural ditch; 7-The pericardial area; 8-First somite; 9- the 7th somite; 10-The posterior neuropore.

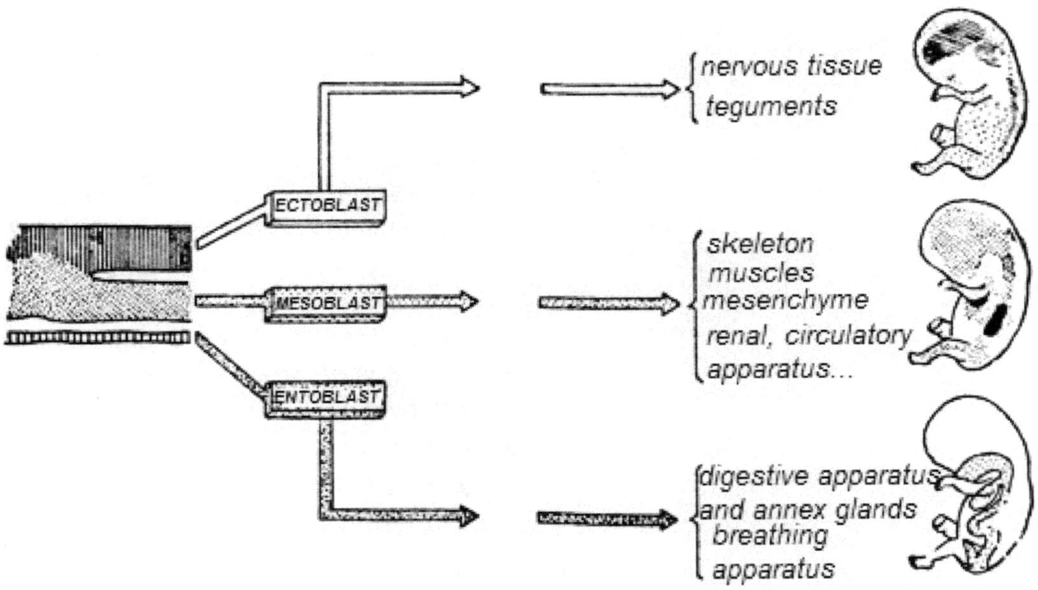

Fig. 10. Derivatives of the embryo layers (according to Tuchman-Duplesis)

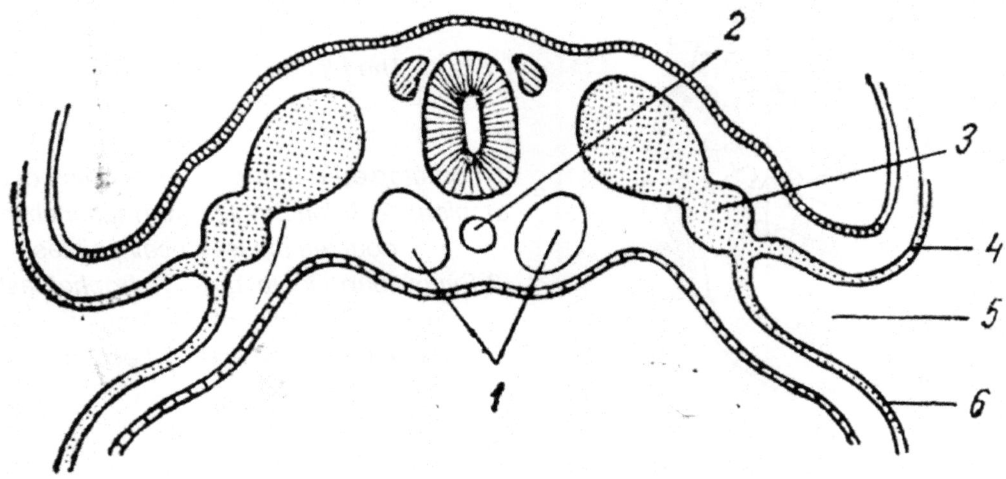

Fig. 11. 21 days old human embryo.
1-Dorsal aortas; 2-Dorsal cord; 3-Nephrotome; 4-Somatopleura; 5-Colon; 6-Splanhnopleura..

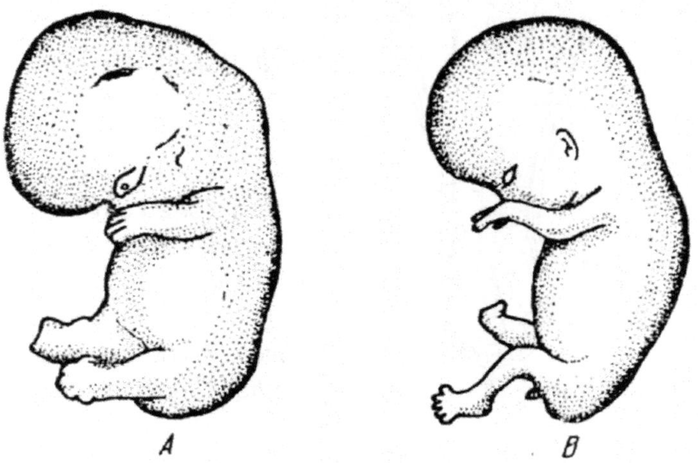

Fig. 12. A. – The aspect of a seven weeks old embryo;
B. – The aspect of an eight weeks old embryo.

We are going to present only the ante-puberty, puberty and post-puberty periods as only these are of particular interest for the motricity anthropology, illustrating only the embryo-foetal stage. The embryo-foetal stage (fig. 4-14; for detailed explanations see The Malformation Risk in the Human Reproduction, M. Ifrim, *Ed. Medicală).*

- *The new-born stage* (first 30 days after birth):

– quick growth in stature;
– weak development of the nervous system with the predominance of the sub-cortical centres;
– rectilinear spine.

- *Nurseling stage* (30 days– one year):

– quick growth in stature and weight;
– the emergence of the dentition;
– at three months the cervical lordosis occurs, at six months the dorsal cyphosis, at nine-12 months lumbar lordosis;
– the thorax presents the anteroposterior diameter smaller than the cross one;
Low muscular mass;
– weakly developed nervous system.

- *Period of a little child (*ante-preschool*, one-three years):*

– the rhythm of growth is slowing down;
– change in the proportions between the head, the trunk and the limbs;
– completion of the first dentition;
– the bones present Haversian irregular systems, thick periosteum;
– wide articular areas between the constitutive osseous segments;
– circumvolutions and cerebral furrows slightly accentuated, undifferentiated cortical cells, nervous fibres incompletely myelinated.

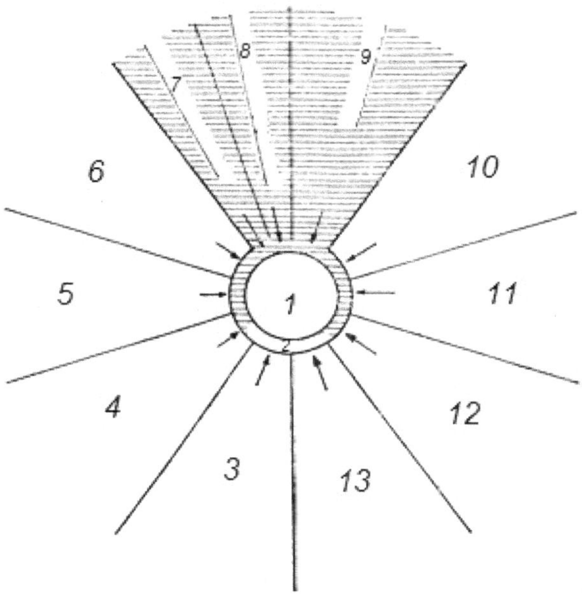

Fig. 13. The teratogens potential factors (according to W. Hirsch). Legend: 1 – congenital malformations of the product of conception, 2 – genotype, 3 – infections, viruses, bacteria, protozoa; 4 – endocrine factors, insulin, cortical-suprarenal hormones, sexual hormones, thyroidal hormones; 5 – nutritional factors, hypovitaminosis, hypervitaminosis; 6 – pregnant's age, deficit of sexual maturation, supra-maturation, 7 – chromosomal aberrations, 8 – genetic incompatibilities; 9 – pathological genes; 10 – noxious due to the radiations, all ionising radiations, X-rays, electronic radium rays, protons and neutrons rays; 11 – chemical factors, hypoxia, anticonception means, drugs; 12 – mechanical factors, abortions and uterus curettage, attempts for abortion, nidation impairment, strangulations, inflammations; 13– unknown causes.

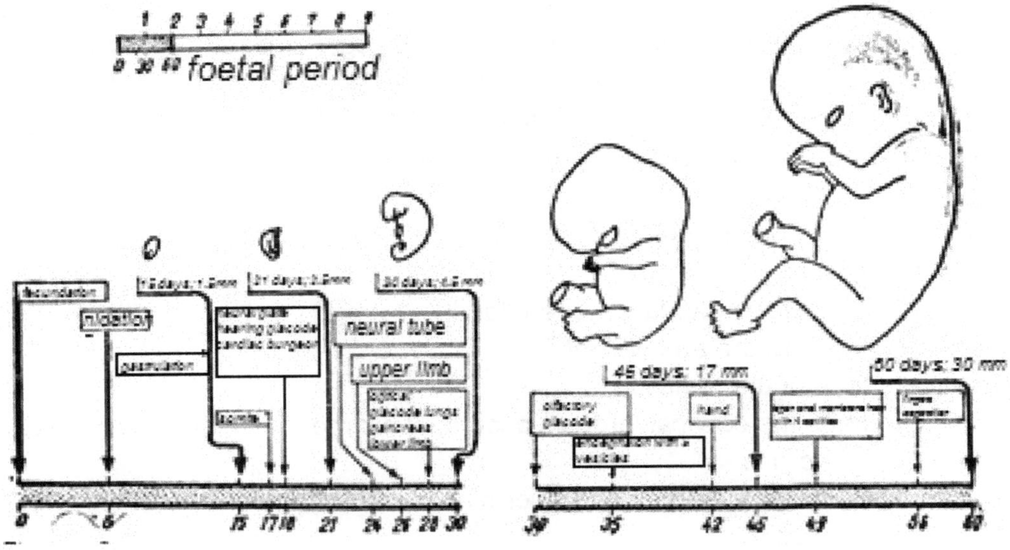

Fig. 14. Stages of development of the products of conception (according to Tuchman Duplesis)

- *The preschool period* (three-six years old)

– *The nervous system:* the brains, as volume, is developed, but the motricity area is still far from the maturation.

– *The locomotor apparatus.* The bones can easily deform after long and extended requirements. The muscles are slightly developed; the muscular fibre is rich in sarcoplasm, it contains more water and fewer proteins, more interstitial connective tissue and less elastic tissue.

– *The breathing apparatus.* The lungs are very wide compared to the thoracic cage; the heart, the mediastinal organs also occupy an area proportionally larger than at the adults.

– The metabolism is very active; the consuming of energy on kilo/body is larger than at the adults.

– The gonads are weakly developed.

- *The school period*

A. *The period of primary school* (six-11 years old girls and six-12 years old boy) – *ante-puberty*

The growth is generally uniform, accelerating by the end of the period, it is mostly made by the elongation of the lower limbs, which causes an accentuated gracilization of the child' body. Up to ten years old, the differences of growth of the children of opposite gender are not high; at this age, it shows up at the girls an acceleration of the growth due to the occurrence of the puberty.

– *The nervous system.* The brains have almost the weight like that of the adult, but functionally, the development is not complete; it is noticed a better development of the first signalising system; the cortical motricity area reaches the maturation (it is complete only at 13-14 years).

The neurones from the anterior ridge of the spine are large and unpigmented until the age of eight years old when the pigmentation starts. At the intumescent level, the voluminous neurones particularly group themselves, but at this age, the nuclei specific for the adult cannot be distinguished at this age. The reticulate formation and the black substance are well differentiated, and until puberty, they do not contain the characteristic pigment.

Regarding the histological structure, the pre-puberty pupil's cerebral hemispheres are alike to those of the adult, but between the cortical fields, the limits are not yet clearly defined and exact. Up to the age of ten years old there can be found in the white substance of hemispheres the lymphoid isolated cells, and their number is increasing after this age. The large pyramidal cells (the *Betz* gigantic cells) present variations regarding the sizes of the basal dendrites, as well as the dimensions of the cell bodies. The differentiation of the cortex is made

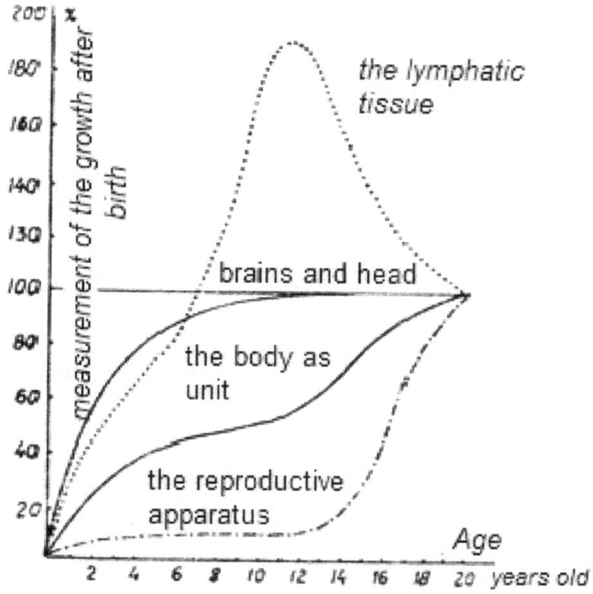

from inside of the surface, by the occurrence of some myelinated areas, from where the process stretches in all directions.

Fig. 15. The dynamic of growth and development of some components of the body.

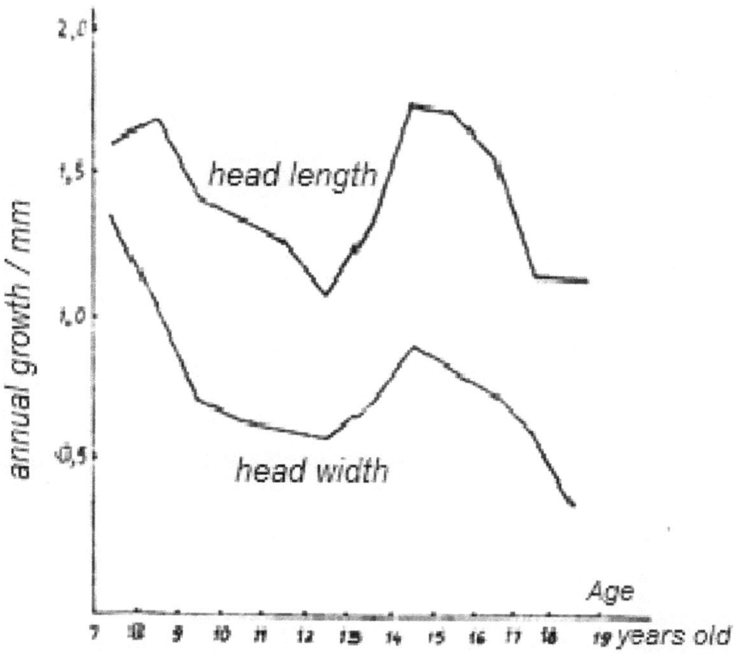

Fig. 16. The dynamics of growth of the cephalic extremity

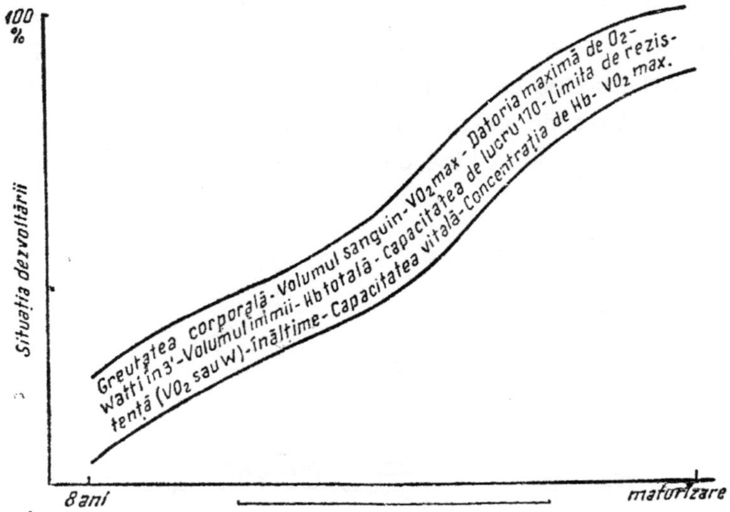

Fig. 17. The curve of the evolution of some functional and morphologic parameters at boys of eight- 18 years old (Bouchard, 1972)
Legend: the situation of the development, 8 ani = 8 years old, maturizare = maturation, greutate corporala = body weight, volumul sanguine = blood volume, datoria maxima de O_2 = maximum O_2 uptake, volumul inimii = heart volume, capacitatea de lucru = work capacity, limita de rezistenta = resistance limit, inaltime = height, capacitatea vitala = vital capacity, concentratia de Hb-VO_2 max. = maximum concentration of Hb-VO_2

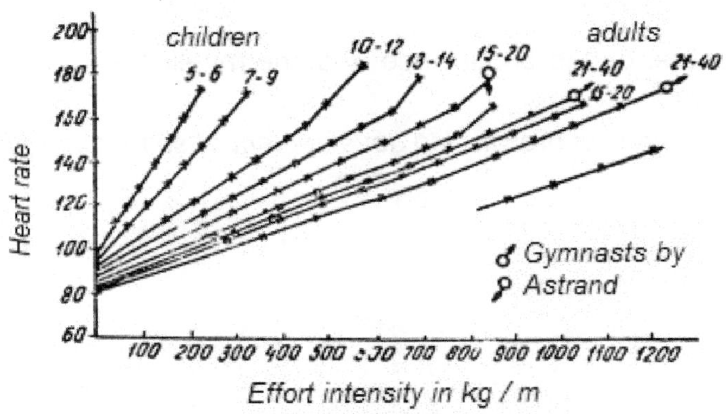

Fig.18. The cardiac frequency dependence on the effort`s intensity, at different ages.(by Hebberlinck)

Functionally, the most striking phenomenon is the lack of balance among the fundamental cortical processes, observing a net predominance of the excitation. Among the various forms of inhibition, mostly the inhibition of differentiation (one of the main forms of internal, conditional inhibition) is weakly developed and slows down the cortical fixation of the newly received elements (words, notions, movements).

The accentuated plasticity of the central nervous system at this age ensures a particular receptivity, but the weak development of the inhibition of differentiation slows down the solid fixation of the new notions. The superior nervous activity perfects itself in the way that, by the end of the respective period, the capacity of cortical inhibition develops, without balancing the excitation. The activity of the glands with internal secretion is, for now, insufficient during this time. The gonadotropic pituitary gland lacks activity while the basophile side of the adenohypophysis produces abundantly the somatotrope hormone *(Şt. M. Milcu)*. The thyroid gland has a low number of follicles. The adrenocortical has the fasciculated and reticulated areas less developed. The thymus is developed, with a large number of fully active *Hassall* corpuscle, its involution beginning right at the half of the period. The gonad has very low secretory activity. The peripheral side of the kinesthetic analyser, in the same time with the vestibular and visual analysers, perfects itself, the movements become more accurate, the coordination is better; the useless, non-economic contraction exclude themselves gradually. The time and space are better estimated.

– *The locomotor apparatus.* The bones are tougher by the consolidation of the lamellar functional systems which causes a slight increase in their resistance to the traction, pressure and rotation requirements.

At the beginning of the period (6-7 years old), the rhythm general of growth is faster then up to that age, following that, afterwards (8-11 years old) to assist to its marked slowing down particularly in the somatic sphere (the growth of the stature) *(Andronescu, A.)*.

Between 7-9 years old, for girls, and 7-11 years old for boys, and compared to the previous stage, the rhythm of ossification and growth reduces; concretely, no longer new centres of ossification appear during this stage.

Between 9-11 years old, for girls and 11-12 years, for boys, is a stage of active proliferation leading to the emergence of the apophyses, of the sesamoid bones, and at the completion of the medullary cavities, a stage which continues once with the puberty.

Completion of the thoracic kyphosis occurs at six-seven years old.

The musculature ends up representing, at six years old, 21.7% of the body weight (compared to 35%, in adults). The muscular fibres, at children with pre-puberty age, are relatively longer than in adults, and the tendon parts are shorter. At the beginning of the period, they are still thin, have large nuclei and are relatively rich in sarcoplasm and water. A large quantity of connective tissue can be found among them. The muscular tonus is lower at the children with ante-puberty age, compared to the adults, which favours the ampler performance of the movements in joints, but slows down the achievement of some fine, differentiate, precise movements. The neuromuscular excitability is lower at the pupils of this age, compared to the adults, the chronaximeter values being higher. The speed of reaction and execution is better, because of the still low muscular mass.

– *The cardiovascular apparatus.* The heart reacts strongly, but not economically to effort; the coronary irrigation is rich; the regulating mechanisms are still weak until seven years, they are not well developed, they are more adequate to slight requirements.

The transversal diameter of the heart is proportionally higher in adults. The increase of the longitudinal diameter occurs at a slow pace, until the puberty. The circumference of the right ventricle at seven years old is higher with 2 cm than at the left ventricle.

At pupils, the ante-puberty vascular net is relatively well established, and the faster development of the arteries of elastic type facilitate the task of the myocardium.

The cardiac frequency in rest is the average of 100/minute at children of six years old, 90/minute at seven years old, 84/minute at eight years old and 80/minute at 12 years old. This tachycardia in the first years of the school age represents quite a significant burden of the myocardium, being given the relatively important expense for maintaining a cardiac rhythm of rest so high and the weak (metabolic) economic efficiency this kind of sustained work. At effort, the situation is more precarious is also more precarious because the volume of the heart being small, any plus of irrigation with blood of the required muscles claims for a considerable increase of the cardiac frequency, which reflects negatively on the functional efficiency of the myocardium which hardly faces the intense requirements for a longer time *(Demeter A.)*.

At rest, the systolic volume at the pupils of ante-puberty age has values around 20 ml at six years old and 30 ml by the end of the period. The cardiac debit is higher at the pupils of ante-puberty age – 2-2.5 litres per minute at rest, and at effort increases approximately 4-5 times – reaching maximum values of 8-9 litres/ minute at 6-8 years old and of 10-12 litres/ minute at 10-12 years old. The arterial pressure at the pupils of ante-puberty age is low at the beginning of the school years, although presenting a tendency in growth. In his researches, *Demeter* found an average value of the systolic arterial pressure of 71.3 mm Hg, the diastolic pressure having as average value 39.6 mm Hg. At eight years old, the values raised up to 75.4/43,8 mm Hg, at nine years old 79.2/47 mm Hg, and at 10 years old at 83.4/49.8 mm Hg.

– *The breathing apparatus.* The nasal cavities are smaller and narrower than at the adults.

The larynx is situated three vertebrae higher than at the adult, and only at 13 years old takes the final position. The elastic fibers of the bronchi are rare at the beginning and, only at 12 years old, they develop more quickly. The breathing bronchi are few in number at the beginning, and the feebly developed interstitial tissue contains less elastic fibers.

The thorax becomes likely to that of the adult in shape but not in size; the transverse diameter is higher, as the anterior-posterior one; the thoracic aperture becomes skewed, the ribs take a downward direction, no longer so leveled. However, thorax stays behind the development of limbs. The lungs begin to be similar in structure to the adult lung, since seven years old, but the volume is still small; thanks to this effort capacity increases, but insufficiently.

Thorax, taken as a whole, develops slowly in children aged ante-puberty. The index of proportionality, appreciated by the formula of *Erismann* (thoracic perimeter - 1/2 size of the stature) presents positive values up to five years in girls and six in boys, when values fall below zero and become negative throughout the entire ante-puberty and pubertal periods ('age of the narrow thorax") *(A. N. Ionescu,* 1963).

Vital capacity increases almost parallel to the anatomic lung capacity, marking a significant leap between six or eight years old. At the end of the ante-puberty period, the vital capacity reaches the average of 1800-2000 ml to pupils who participate systematically in physical education classes in cycle I and of 2200-2400 ml in those who participate in sports activities in school *(Demeter, A. Gogea, A.* et al., 1973).

During the physical exercise, the possibilities of increasing the volume of the thoracic cage in a wide breath of children are low. Therefore, from the smallest effort, these children appeal to the acceleration of the breathing, even this being a limited possibility.

Accessory respiratory muscles (abdominals, big dentals, scalene, pectorals, sternocleidomastoids, etc.), insufficiently developed, may not provide the appropriate expanding of the thorax volume during the effort, the amplitude of the breathing is, therefore, relatively small. It limits reaching high values of breathing minute volume (flow). Thus, at the age of six, breathing minute volume or flow rate at rest is 2.5-2.8 liters/ minute, and at the effort reaches 18 to 20 liters/ minute, which is only 8-10% of the adult breathing flow of an athlete *(Demeter).*

There is no morpho-functional substrate for long and lasting effort. Ensuring the body balance at rest, but mostly during effort meets difficulties because of the kinesthetic analyzer which is insufficiently developed, as well as due to the fact that the gravity center of the body is slightly higher above the ground.

Efforts will go to achieving a correct movement, to eliminating the balance and of other extra movements in walking and running. We must insist on a proper tenure and in achieving a correct rhythm of the movements, paying considerable attention to the more accentuated development of the dorsal and neck expander muscles, as well as to other muscular expanding muscles, aiming to gradually establish the ensuring of a functional balance between the large antagonist muscular groups. The static endurance of the child at this age is low. Instead, the dynamic activity of successive contractions and relaxations is less tiring. The dynamic effort is also encouraged by the high degree of cortical excitability and provides favorable conditions for circulation and breathing. The efforts of strength requiring large muscle tension and those of resistance are not advisable at this age. High attention is to be paid to the proper position of the pupils at the desks in order to prevent deformations of the spine. The balanced lifestyle, the judicious alternation of the physical, intellectual effort and the rest, the balanced nutrition, rich in proteins and vitamins (A, D2, B complex), the outdoors movement will contribute to the harmonious development of the children's body (fig. 15-18).

B. *The period of secondary school* (11–13 years old, girls; 12–14 years old, boys) – *pubertal*

Boys and girls of different chronological age are comprised in this category. However, there is a main criterion uniting them in one single category, which is: *the puberty,* with the great transformations which occur in the entire child's body.

The puberty central phenomenon is the sexual maturation caused by the increased flow of sexual hormones which causes the occurrence of the secondary sexual characters, in the same time with deep somato-vegetative and psychical changes. If until around the age of 11, the endocrine secretions were abundant in growth hormones, after this age, the endocrine system is characterized by an intense increase the secretory activity of the ovary, respectively of the testicle, which by the sexual hormones causes important morphological and functional changes of the body. The event is more accurately marked at the girls by the occurrence of the first menses, while at boys is the emergence of the ejaculation. The body sexualization occurs, the phenomena of sexual maturation being twinned with those of neuropsychological one (*Şt. Milcu).* Mainly, the primary sexual characters appear, consisting of the maturation and the development of the genitalia which take the anatomic shape of the adult, while becoming a function.

Once with the puberty the secondary sexual characters accentuate in boys, the laryngeal development and the change of voice, the axillary and pubic pilosity (of rhombic type), the increase in the muscular mass etc., and at the girls – the development of the mammary glands, the axillary and pubic pilosity (of rhombic type), the characteristic growth of the adipose panicle etc. The skeleton, especially the basin bones, presents differentiation between the two genders. In women, the diameters are larger, the basin being adapted for parturition. In the same time, the other organs and systems forming the human body present morphological differences in the two genders.

The puberty is marked by two extremely important phenomena: the acceleration and the neoteny. *The acceleration* is the constant biological current phenomenon, according to which the current generation, compared to the past ones, register an increase in height and weight. Thus, in our country, compared with 1930-1940, it notices a mean increase in the boys' height of 12-14 cm, and at girls, about 10–12 cm. The explanation for this phenomenon is still controversial, but most authors admit the involvement of three factors: the higher quality diet richer in protein, the urbanization, with the full context of influences that drawn by and the genetic factors.

Lately, it was proved that the melatonin secreted by the pineal gland and having a role in the growth is produced in higher quantity under the influence of the light for a longer period of time. Correlating this with the active 24 hours time which undeniably has increased compared to the past decades, it results in a possible conditioning of a higher secretion of melatonin under the incidence of the artificial and natural light radiation and, thus corollary, an increase in the height of the current generation. *The neoteny* is the biological phenomenon of accelerated somato-sexual maturation and delay of the psycho-intellectual maturation, at the same time with the delay of the social maturation (later socio-professional integration, due to the increase of the school enrolment, connected to the increase in the informational volume required for the specialization in various fields). The acceleration of the somato-sexual maturation is a fact, the age of puberty going down compared to the past decades. So, for instance, in Norway around

1830, the puberty showed up at 17 years old at girls, and now it occurs around 13-14 years old; in our country, compared to 1930-1940, the puberty in boys and girls occurs 1.5 years sooner. The psycho-intellectual maturation which, a few decades ago, ended about 19-20 years old, currently continues to 22-23 years old. It consists in continuing the process of permeabilisation of the synapses in the central nervous systems which grants increased functionality and plasticity of the nervous structures. We mention that the neurological researches have proven that, once with the conclusion of the psycho-intellectual maturation, it begins a process of neuronal destruction in the CNS (approximately 1000-2000 neurons die every day), which continues until death and which is even lower when the psychological and physical activities are more intense.

The phenomenon of neoteny presents both advantages and disadvantages. The major advantage is the high plasticity of the nervous system from where derives the psycho-intellectual capacity, at much higher parameters, of the current generation. The negative consequence is the creation under such circumstances of a biological conflict between the level of psycho-intellectual maturation in progress and the early completed sexual maturation, conflict translated into a high degree of effervescence of the current generation. In such a context, the activity of physical education and sport gets new and extremely important meanings in achieving the necessary balance for optimal solving this biological conflict.

Both acceleration and neoteny prove that the current human species, *Homo sapiens sapiens,* is in the ongoing evolution towards other more evolved hominine shapes. In this respect, the great anthropologist *Teilhard de Chardin* looms for the future a new human form, *Homo sapientissimus,* with clearly higher qualities, able to prove the dialectics evolution and the materiality of the minus where we are currently.We also mention that the puberty varies in duration from one individual to another.

Beyond the primary and secondary sexual characters which become evident, a multitude of changes occur throughout the body: the bones grow in thickness, the vascular system develops, in boys the larynx grows explosively, the trunk grows larger than the limbs, so that the gonadal secretions and the changes in the genital area are reflected in the entire body *(Roussellet),* and the difference in the two genders grows higher. We also emphasize that the environmental and hereditary factors (food, geoclimat, urbanization, etc.) influence the time of installation and during puberty, so individualization and differentiation of puberty chronological age of the biological elements are paramount in the scientific investigation of this development stages of the organism.

Regarding the morphological characteristics of other devices mentioned importance in practice following sports:

- *Musculoskeletal.* The bones at this age are developing mainly on account of their growth in thickness by depositing minerals (calcium and phosphorus) and strengthening the intimate functional structure. They become more resistant to mechanical factors, pressure, thrust and twist the detriment of their previous elasticity.

Spine, 13-15 years there is the closing of the sacral ducts; at 13 years ending the synostosis of the pedicle of the vertebral bodies. Thorax development, during the first part of the pubertal age, is slow (the age of the narrow thorax), followed by a more pronounced development. The humeral head epiphysis is welded to the rest of the girls between 13-16 and 14-17 years old boys. Humeral trochlea ossifies through a double center, which occurs at age 11 in girls and age 13 in boys. We note the disappearance of cartilage in the hip bone and welding Y final at the acetabulum component of the three bones (ilium, ischium, and pubis), 12-16 years for girls and 13-18 for boys. Joints, however, are underdeveloped and ligaments do not provide sufficiently tensile, torsional.

Muscles develop by stretching the fibers and especially not in thickness. Because of this, their surface is still small and the physiological section, consequently, their strength is low. The length of muscle fibers has an advantage in that it increases the amount of mechanical work, with the requirement that there is no global force overcharged more than muscle. Relative strength (force reported in kg/body), at this stage, not only stagnates, but even shows a considerable decline, both in flexors and extensors. However, the growth of absolute force and the relative extensors is slightly higher than the flexors. This raises the need for a greater degree of strength exercises at this age, especially for flexor muscles, preventing downturn driving overall trend accentuated by the end of puberty in girls. Review of old conceptions, which advised against the use of force exercises at pubertal age students, citing arguments morphological and functional are absolutely necessary.

Efforts are contraindicated the maximum strength and large neuromuscular stretches, showing the danger overloaded, the musculo-ligamentous. Instead, the force exercises well-dosed based on working with small dumbbells and dumbbell with gradually increasing intensity, the principle of gradual increase physiological effort, are not contraindicated.

The speed of response and recurrence is developed, but endurance and strength are far lagging behind the adult. So they are not allowed to obtain performance training efforts force and strength; any unwise use of means which develops strength and endurance have negative consequences on growth.

Increase in long bones and lengthening muscles give the characteristic appearance of puberty: tall and thin with narrow thorax, *Erismann* negative index (minimum to 14 -15 years), lower lung volume (risk of tuberculosis), voice changed because boys the rapid growth of the larynx, low muscle tone predisposing to deformities of the spine, flat feet or increased occurrence, the occurrence of juvenile acne, etc.

- *The nervous system.* It grows fast and ends practically the maturation of motricity cortical area of the analyzer. The analysis function and the synthesis of bark grows, the internal inhibition. On this basis, achieving differentiation increases speed and reflexes conditional formats go out slower. The function of the second system to the first system signal dominates.

We must show that at puberty, still persists, to some extent, insufficient inhibition processes subject to the power excitation processes. Because of this, the movements of children at this age are of a sudden, with low accuracy. Excitability and high mobility of the nervous system during puberty, explains the driving speed of reactions in general, but as nerve processes are unstably balanced, coordination does not benefit from favorable conditions for development.

The trend towards irradiation process of excitation is based on all the relative weakening of cortical inhibition process pubertal age pupils, resulting in uneven character and even sudden movements, motricity activity of these students is generally exaggerated, excessive.

- *Cardiovascular system.* The heart is bulky compared with the thorax; regulatory mechanisms are frequently disturbed circulation (predominantly sympathetic), and they exacerbate during effort. We frequently meet regarding the heart, functional murmurs, arrhythmias and hypertension crises. The cardiovascular apparatus develops slowly in the pubertal stage. The arteries have a diameter of greater proportion than in adults, and the veins and lymph system are well represented. Heart rate recorded at the beginning of puberty, 90-100 beats per minute and drops at the end of puberty at 82-88 beats per minute. Systolic volume increases from 30 ml, reaching 13 years equals 40-45 ml, and at 14 years, 45-60 ml. Cardiac output also increases.

However, the heart inotropic being low, cardio-respiratory efforts of short duration and intense are not suitable, requiring too much the heart. We conclude that the cardiovascular system presents an adaptation more difficult to intensive efforts, evidenced by the fact that oxygen-maximum heart rate obtained in absolute values or per kg/body is lower, and the systolic volume and the maximum cardiac output are far from the values of the adult, boys registering values superior to the girls.

- *Respiratory system.* It develops intense pubertal stage.

The nose takes his final form; the larynx goes down taking the shape of the adult topography, the trachea and bronchi grow, lungs increase remarkably in weight and volume, their anatomical capacity increasing with over 50%, the amount of elastic fibers in the lung increases considerably. The respiratory function improves. An increase in the amplitude of respiratory movements (230 ml current volume to 350 ml, from 11 years to 15 years) decreased respiratory rate (from 22-18 breaths per minute on average), vital capacity increases and breathing tissue - judged by the maximum consumption of oxygen per minute - increases considerably (although they are not reached maximum levels of aerobic capacity, so the resistance efforts cannot achieve maximum results).

Although cardiovascular and pulmonary devices are much required due to the rapid growth of body weight, exercise is not contraindicated unless some organ damage. Experience has shown that functional disorders disappear by rational practicing sport.

- *The endocrine system.* The most striking difference from the small schoollar age is the intensive development of small *endocrine glands* and especially *the gonads,* which are fully operational. The secretion of testosterone by the testis and ovary folliculin and progesterone causes both primary and secondary sexual characters and all other morphological changes in other systems and devices. Sexual maturation leads to libido and reproductive capacity - elements that will influence the behavior of young altogether. Higher nervous activity undergoes significant changes. Pituitary lobe and in particular its previous intensifies its activity, increases the secretion of TSH, ACTH and gonadotropin hormones. Thyroid and adrenal activity increases, causing a hyperreactive nervous system and enhanced autonomic instability or lability.

Clinical and experimental observations distinguish between sex determination and the realization of sexual differentiation, an ontogenetic process lasting many years, with milestones in the embryo-fetal life. In the process of sexual differentiation occur as tools of genetic determinism, hormones or other hormone-like substances *(C. Guja).*

Genetic information, especially allosome, causes the formation of gonads unisexual. This is the stage of gonadal sexualisation process that in humans take until the 60th day of embryonic development. Male sexualisation process is then continued using endogenous hormones developed by the embryonic testis (antimullerian principle and the virilizing), while the women continued sexualisation "passive" without requiring such hormones. An argument that this is so important is the castration of embryos during the genitals are sexually undifferentiated and that - regardless of genetic sex - leads to the sexualization of women.

Male and female genitalia appearance thus constitutes a new stage in the process of sexualisation of bodies, hormonal stage. In the process of sexual differentiation, it is also important to have a good "colonization" of primary gonadal by primitive gonocyte. A "poverty" of them in gonocyte is the source of many problems with development and functioning gonads, of many gonadal dysgeneses. Genital tract development is conditional upon the proper functioning of the gonadal endocrine embryo. The active testicle opposes the evolution of the tract towards feminization. In the normal development of the gonads and the accessory sexual organs, the autosomes also get involved. Their participation in the functioning of organs that depend on gonadal endocrine (pituitary, nerve centers, etc.) explains the apparition of the gonadal dysgenesis in autosomal disorders usually associated with somatic abnormalities.

Establishing the genetic sex and creating the basic sexual structures are only two stages of sexual differentiation. It is followed by "sexualisation" of nerve structures, required by the hypothalamic - hypophyseal-gonadal complex operation and "sexual maturation," then puberty, which carries out the development of secondary exterior sexual characteristics, genesis instinct, procreative capacity, etc. Puberty is induced by androgen and estrogen steroid growth. It is not sufficiently studied whether the occurrence of pubertal characteristics and growth plays an organ response. Estrogen controls the breast development, growth, and maturation of the uterus, vagina, menstruation. In addition, progesterone is also responsible for ovulation cycle.

Androgens promote the growth of external genitalia in boys and clitoris and labia majora, girls. They respond and deepening of the voice in boys and sexual hair in both sexes. Growth spurt during puberty has not yet been fully explained. Both testosterone and STH have anabolic effects which promote growth. STH concentration in blood can be experimentally elevated with testosterone and estrogen after the induction of hypoglycemia with insulin. In fact, in both sexes, at puberty, there are higher values of STH than before puberty. Androgens and estrogens thus appear to cooperate with STH to induce puberty growth spurt. The marked growth spurt in boys may be explained by the higher concentration of testosterone in them. Epiphyseal fusion and thereby completing increase is probably due to the action of testosterone and estrogen. STH deficit does not prevent epiphyseal fusion, while a shortage of sex hormones makes the epiphyseal fusion not to occur.

In order to classify the degree of sexual differentiation, there have been proposed several schemes. The ordinary type, android or gynoid is the average type of the studied population. It is a reality only for a given population. The sexual type differs from one race to another. However, the ordinary type does not mean the perfect type. As it was noted by *Jean Vague* (1953), an ideal sexualised type is only met exceptionally rare. This author also believes that by focusing on the average type there can be differentiated several abnormal types.

The first group includes individuals with low somatic abnormalities in which the sexual differentiation is normal. In this group, *Vague* distinguishes several subgroups. Excessive differentiation of normal sexual characteristics gives birth to hyper-android men and hyper-gynoid women. In men, muscles are strong; adiposity is deposited in the upper body, shoulder girdle is well developed, and there is an abundant hair growth. Hyper-Gynoid woman is characterized by adiposity deposition in the lower regions, weak musculature and *cubitus valgus* emphasized.

Poor sexual differentiation creates a great variety of forms. These types are named by *Vague* gynoid man and android woman. The gynoid man presents adiposity in the lower body, rounded forms, deficient muscles, reduced hairiness, and a slightly *cubitus valgus.* The android woman is characterized by depositing adiposity in the upper body and shoulders are moderately developed. In another subgroup, there are summarized irregular variations, represented by limited deficiencies. Thus, some men show a tendency for depositing the adiposity in the lower region and women develop excessively the shoulder girdle. *Vague* includes in the second and third group, individuals with gonadal malformations or genital tract. The secondary sexual characters are also affected. These groups belong to the pathologic.

Endocrine, nervous and neuropsychological changes emphasise the discrepancy between the physical development and functional capacity of the actual body. This manifests through uncertain, clumsy, cumbersome movements or even vasomotor neuro-vegetative disorders (tendency to sweat, to faintness, redness of the face, etc.), irascibility, excitability, with some states of excessive shyness or rebelliousness, explosive attitudes, a tendency towards noisy and competitive games, etc. However, at the cited age, there is the nervous and locomotor substrate that are required in learning complex motricity skills (aptitude improvement) and for the efforts to speed. Considering that each child makes his own puberty, caution should be used for individualising the effort. Sexual differences are large at this point.

The girls exceed boys in the initial growth rate of height and weight. The pelvis development, specific accumulation of panniculus, breasts develop, etc. Because of somatic and vegetative differences between the two sexes, it is necessary to develop separate programs and to work individually. When this age I reached, in the physical educational program are allowed the following: short distance running, jumps, throwing with appropriate sporting materials (Oină balls, small weights, disc and javelin at juniors), sports games alternated with relatively long rest breaks, gymnastics, swimming, etc. Sports with high demands regarding resistance (average distance running, speed skating, cycling), can be included in the training program, provided that they are introduced gradually under medical control, strictly limiting the effort level consistent with the physical and functional capacity of the organism of children of this age.

It is not recommended maximum efforts with high loads of the musculoskeletal system. In preparing children of this age may also be used a large number of exercises in different movements and varied character of the neuromuscular effort. They contribute to the development of dynamic stereotypes, to obtain a baggage rich and developing the functional capacity of the body.

In conclusion, at the age of puberty, physical training models must be applied differently, depending on the nature of work and the specific demands of each sports branches. The fact that the chronological age is not the same as the biological age also requires the removal of rigid application of the indications and contraindications mentioned above.

An in-depth knowledge of the particularities of morpho-functional and psychological characteristics of each child we work with is the only way in which we can avoid the two mistakes that are commonly found in sports life. They are overloading the body through exaggerated efforts and excessive caution, due to which the preparation is maintained at a lower level than the possibilities that the child can offer.

C. *Period of high school (postpubertal)*

Once puberty is completed, the child is turned into a young person (junior) which, from development and the morpho-functional exercise capacity and psychical characteristics, he/she is getting closer and closer to becoming an adult. Studies have shown that at the age of 16-17 years old, some indices of physical development as height, weight and chest perimeter, is getting close and at 18-19 years old they almost entirely reach a similar level as the morphological indices of adults. The period of growth and development postpubertal is quite long, reaching six to eight years or more, especially if we focus on the criterion of complete growth in height.

In the light of chronological age, the stage of postpubertal growth and development extends up to 20-22 years for girls and boys 23-25 years *(Albu, I.,* 1971) (Fig. 19).

- *Locomotor system.* Regarding the spine, we just note the closure of the sacral canal, between 15-18 years.

Limb bones also show a slow growth and completion of ossification. Skeletal ossification occurs at different body segments, and continue along postpubertal period. In most cases, the bones have acquired their final shape and size at the end of the postpubertal period, and welding of the primary ossification centres with the secondary centres occurs later, between 20-25 years. Bones approach the adult bone structure and strength; the conjugation cartilage thins up, marking the beginning of their ossification and growth cessation in height. The thorax is growing in volume and more than the limbs, making proportionality index to increase *(Erismann).*

Muscles increase in volume. By increasing physiological sectional area, the force grows in proportion to the amount of this surface.

It is known from literature that one square centimetre of surface develops at this age approx. 10 kg/strength. Exceptions from the rule apply to women of the same age, who develop on the same sectional area about 7-8 kg/strength, and to young trained teenagers, to which the value/cm^3 exceeds the average value (depending on the degree of training).

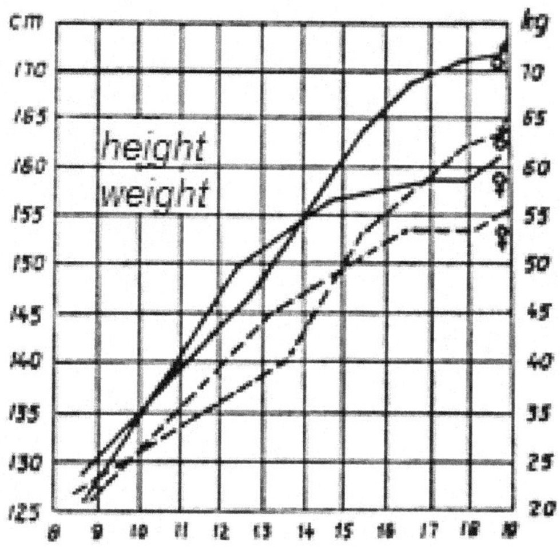

Fig. 19. *Curve height and body weight, the girls during maturation. Postpubertal stage there is a slowdown of somatic development.*

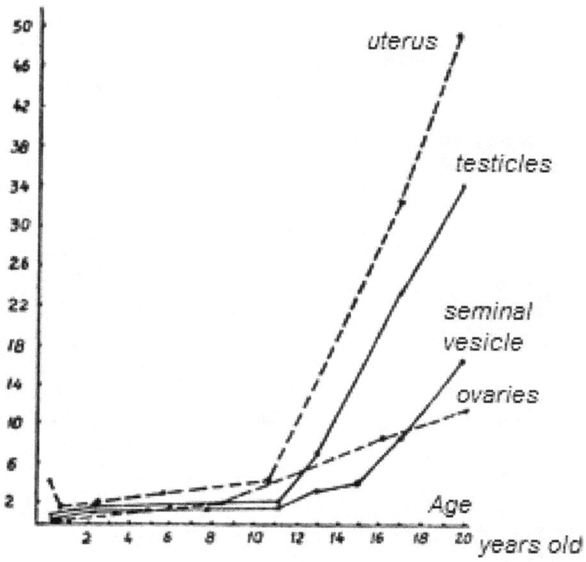

Fig. 20. Weight gain testis, seminal vesicle, ovary and uterus.

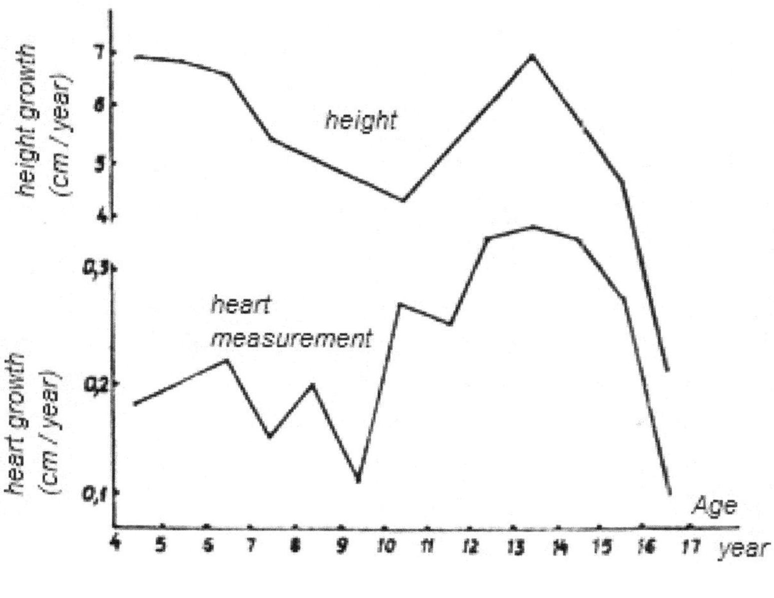

Fig. 21. Dynamics of growth of the heart and body size.

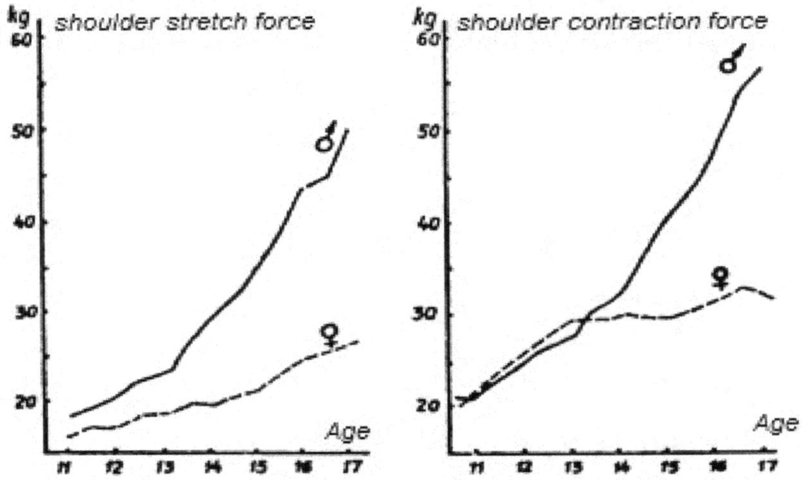

Fig. 22 The dynamics of increasing muscle force with scapular-humeral adduction, retroversion

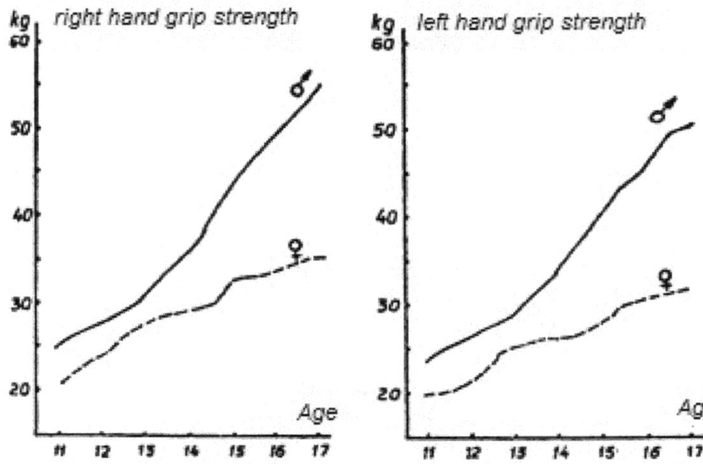

Fig. 23. Dynamics of strength increasements in palmar flexor muscles (right hand and left hand)

However, we must emphasise that in that age period, the force is left behind as value in contrast to the quality of speed and coordination, which is closer to that of an adult. Muscle tone and endurance to static capacity increases (fig. 20 -23).

- *The nervous system* is characterised by the fact that it continues its development, particularly through permeabilization of the synapses. There is a balance between excitation and inhibition, between irradiation and concentration. Plasticity and responsiveness are large, engrams fitting easily, which explains the facility of attributing the motricity skills at this stage. The analysers are close to a degree of maturation close to that of an adult on a morphological level, but lower by a functional level. We note that the functional mobility of the fundamental nervous processes favours the development of speed and skill. However, CNS and analysers resistance is lower, which makes it faster for fatigue to appear, compared to adults where it takes much longer.

- *Cardiovascular apparatus* accelerates its development.

The volume and weight of the myocardium grow, especially the left heart. The surface of the section of the myocardial fibres increases and, consequently, increases the amplitude of contraction. Large arteries and veins reach almost adult size. Systolic volume increases, reaching, at the age of 18, nearly adult values (75 ml boys and 55 ml girls, both at 18 years). Similarly, the cardiac output increases (4.7 litres/minute for boys at 19 years and 3.7 litres/minute for girls). Heart rate and blood pressure have values close to those of an adult. Regarding the economy of the maximum cardiovascular exercise, we note that the maximum pulse-oxygen index recorded a net improvement at this stage *(Demeter).*

- *Respiratory apparatus* approaches regarding morphology, as one of an adult appearance, but it is still far from functional and continues its development.

Now, under a morphological report, there is a widening of the nasal cavity, larynx development, and increasements in the number of the lung elastic fibres. Operational parameters of pulmonary ventilation improve, respiratory rate decreases while the amplitude of respiration increases, vital capacity also increases, maximal oxygen consumption rises considerably. It can be concluded that respiratory function achieves higher standards by both morphological developments and by enhancing functional capacity. The aerobic capacity allows resistance exercises, which have a positive inotropic effect (improvement of capitalization and organs' nutrition). However, the maximum consumption of O_2 per minute/kg body weight, maximum heart rate and oxygen do not reach very high values, other than by training; postpubertal phase being favourable for resistance effort.

Note that, during the present internal secretion, stabilisation, sympathetic and parasympathetic autonomic adjustments occur. At the present age, in addition to efforts based on speed drills, the training program can include efforts gradually of resistance and force. Weight exercises will be determined on a strictly individualised case, based on the morphological and functional development and the actual capacity of effort which the young people reached its physical level by preparing earlier. Efforts which require repeated large muscle strains (functional isometric contractions, lifting weightlifting, etc.) must be very carefully dosed correctly, and those who make such efforts must also perform medical checks, differentiated repeatedly.

* * *

Presenting the main teaching periods of growth and morphologically related particularities, we must emphasise that there is great individual variability of these somato-functional characters and psychological detailed to individuals of the same chronological age. Each of them is unique and genetically determined paratypes, which requires individually marked sports activity. Different exercise capacity of children of the same chronological age (same class) is maintained in the adult, but during childhood, such differences are wider. Moreover, which is very important, exercise capacity in children is unstable and uncertain, which is explained by their significant neuro-vegetative liability, mainly due to puberty, which leaves a mark with high individual variability.

Regarding the individual pace of growth, we should mention that in the last century, especially in recent decades, it is to bee noted in children and young people in most European countries and other continents, an important biological phenomenon, termed by *G. Roberts* (1876) and *E. W. Koch* (1953) "secular trend", characterized by an accelerated growth of some indices of development. Thus, the average height and weight of today`s children and adolescents, are higher than in the last century, and sexual maturity occurs earlier. Although completing the growth process takes place soon, definitive adult sizes are larger. Sexual life was extended not only through an earlier puberty, but also through a later climacteric (menopause); so human longevity became higher. From worldwide obtained data we can conclude that "secular trend" takes place in all economically and socially developed countries of the world, independent of geographical location, climate, ethnic composition, both in towns and villages; in varying degrees, he can achieve all walks of life. In our country, because of the improved living conditions, this phenomenon is particularly pronounced. In this context, we must also mention the phenomenon of neoteny, meaning that of the late psycho-intellectual maturation and accelerated sexual maturity, found recently throughout the globe.

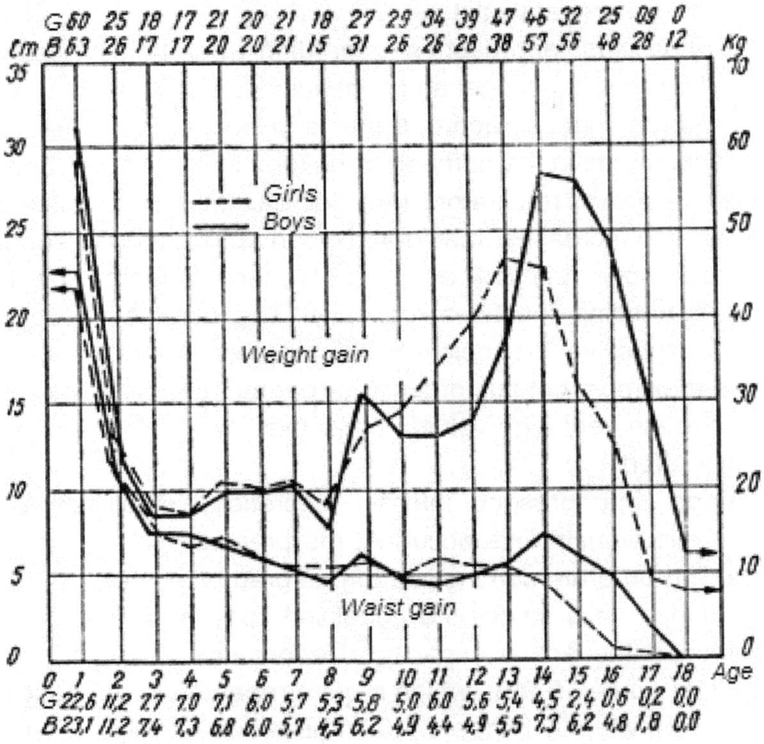

Fig. 24. Annual growth in waist and weight (according to A. Ionescu).

The study of the conditions and factors that determine the phenomena of acceleration and neoteny highlights the influence of civilised life, improved nutrition, advances in prevention and treatment of disease and the benefits of a more rational organisation of work and leisure time of youth. In connection with this latter point of view, it discusses at length the great importance of physical education and sport on growth and development of youth. Research proves the methodical practice effectiveness of physical exercises, both on normal growth and harmonious development of young people and reducing the negative effects of the phenomenon of neoteny.

Summarising, according to data stated by *Adrian Ionescu,* the main somatic and visceral parameters of growth throughout the ontogenetic development of human beings, we emphasise the following: carefully watching developments in body size from birth to 18 years, there is a progressive dispersion in height and weight values. The variation of values is smaller for waist and much greater for weight, for both girls and boys (fig. 24-25). During puberty, 12 -13 years for girls and 14-15 years at boys, the maximum variation and widest dispersion of values are found for both the waist and the weight. After this, the values are coming increasingly closer to the average value. The pace and speed of growth in height and weight, as well as the sequence of more active or slower periods, do not correspond exactly to the two sexes.

Girls have a more accelerated growth in the prepubertal and pubertal periods, when they briefly surpass boys, both in height and weight. Afterwards, the growth slows, stopping before the boys. For them, puberty is later and slower, but on a longer time, which enables further growth in height and weight. After 15 years, boys catch up and surpass girls, sometimes realising severe increases in height.

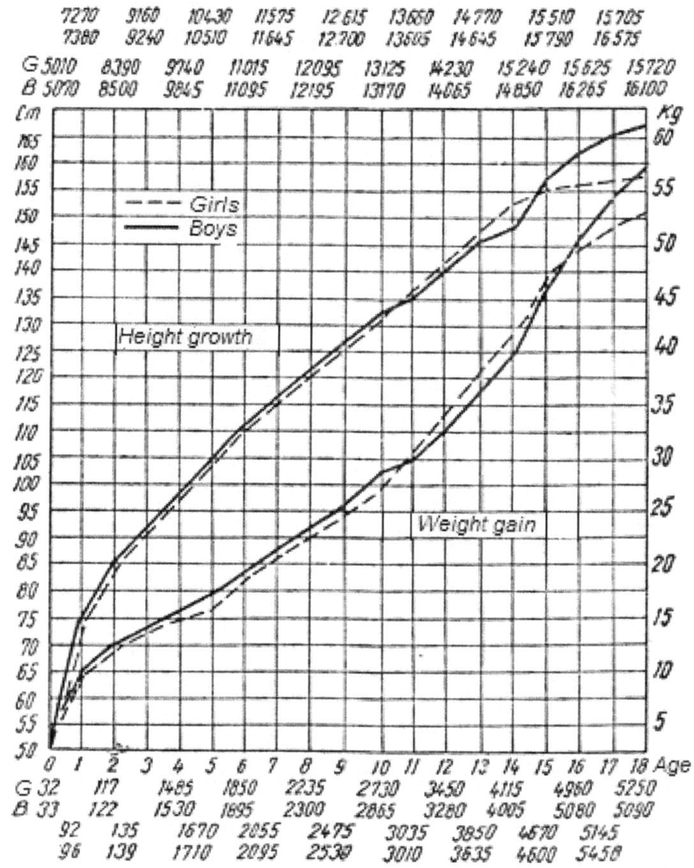

Fig. 25. Increase in height and weight by genders (according to A. Ionescu).

Statistical data show that both the waist and weight continue to grow increasingly less in boys, up to 25-26 years. The overall increase in body height and weight growth is the result of the growth of its component segments: head, neck, trunk, upper and lower limbs. The uneven growth pace of the above-listed segments causes continues changes in body proportions. The most spectacular stages of evolution occur in utero and early life after birth. The second period of great changes is puberty, during which sexual maturation occurs.

The growth of the skull is made in several stages: in the first year, increasing in both sexes is uniform and equal. Between two and six years the occipital and front part predominantly grow, and between six and seven years the base of the skull lengthens; up to ten years the boys head is higher than the girls; between 11 and 16 years the growth is equal. After 16-18 years the size of the boys` heads surpasses the girls` in every sense.

The trunk is the body segment between the neck and lower limbs. The trunk is the most voluminous part of the body. In the intrauterine life, the trunk increases greatly, reaching up to 32-35% of body height. Up to 13 years for girls and 15 years for boys, growth is slow, then becoming increasingly more intense until maturity. The trunk grows nearly three times the length of 18-20 cm, the initial length at birth, and it rises to 50-55 cm in adulthood. Up to 10-14 years, girls have a shorter torso than boys. After puberty, this segment grows faster in girls surpassing boys in the same age at torso length. He gets a final form at women, between 20-25 years when measuring approx. 50 cm, and in men between 30-35 years, when measured on average 54 cm. The biacromial diameter measures about 12 cm at birth; it doubles at six years and nearly triples at maturity. Bihumeral diameter or shoulders width is with a few centimetres higher than the biacromial diameter. At well-developed children and teenagers and shoulders width represents a quarter of the body height. Girls always have narrower shoulders than boys.

The diaphragm divides the trunk into two cavities: chest and abdomen.

The thoracic growth is being looked at by measuring the thoracic perimeter and reporting it to the body height. Analyzing the increase of the thoracic perimeter and body height by age and by making a report between each after *Erismann`s* formula (thoracic perimeter minus half waist), it could draw a number of conclusions about the growth of the thorax from zero to 18 years old(data of the Institute of Hygiene, obtained in 1957 from 310 000 children and young people across the country).

After reaching a maximum equal in both sexes (around the age of six to nine months), the *Erismann* index decreases until puberty. He reaches 0 value at 5 years old girls and six years old boys when it continues to decline, gaining negative values: 4.42 at 12 years old girls and 4.01 at 14 years old boys. Such low values have an important signification regarding the functional capacity of the respiratory apparatus at the ages mentioned above. Once the lower limit is reached, the *Erismann* index begins to rise again, going to positive values at 17 years old girls and 18 years old boys.

The period of 5 - 17 years for girls and 6 - 18 years for boys, in which the *Erismann* index values are negative, is known as the "narrow thorax period" and it represents a long phase of poor evolution of chest dimensions and respiratory function. The pace with which the thoracic perimeter increases at this time is slower than the growth rate in the entire length of the body.

Increased chest perimeter is terminated around the age of 20 years; it reaches on average 85 cm in men and 80 cm in women. It is sometimes observed the slow growth of the chest until almost 50 years, largely due to the development of muscle mass or fat accumulation in the subcutaneous tissues.

The abdomen is the lower floor of the trunk and is divided into the abdomen itself and pelvis. The abdominal perimeter is at birth on an average of 24-25 cm and ranges between 20 and 28 cm. It grows until five years, reaching 47-59cm for boys and 44-57 cm to girls; at ten years is 50-67 cm to boys and 47-64 cm for girls.

The pelvis is, at birth, very small and looks up towards the belly. Its anteroposterior diameter is greater than the transversal. When the child stands up and walks, the pelvis widens and tilts forward and down. The bicristal diameter, which measures about 10 cm at birth, reaches the end of growth at 27 cm. The pelvic diameters double at six years of age and triples at maturity. The hip width at the major trochanter level is at newborn of 7.5 cm, which is lower than the width of the pelvis; it increases quite quickly, doubling at three years, tripling in 11 years and reaching adulthood with a value four times higher.

Starting at seven years, the pelvic dimensions and especially the hips diameter are higher in girls than in boys. There is a direct relationship between torso growth and the whole body height and the increased length of the upper limb. At birth, the upper limbs are equal in length to the torso, which they surpass in two years with 114-116% and six years with 123-124%.

At adults, the ratio of upper limb length and body height ranges after the waist size: at 150 cm high, the upper limb length is 64-71 cm in men and 61-68 cm women. At 160 cm height, 66-76 cm in men and 65-75 cm in women; 170 cm height, 69-83 cm in men and 70-79 cm in women (*Martin*). Legs grow and develop more than the superior limbs, both in thickness and length, especially after childbirth. Legs length doubled up to three years; triples at six years, quadruple at 12 years and it grows five times in adulthood. They get on average at 88 cm in men and 82 cm in women (*Martin*).

Proportionality relationships are established between body segments.

Throwing an overview over the changing proportions of the body, we find that the newborn, the bust and torso are relatively longer than the limbs and upper limbs are longer than the lower ones. At an adult, the bust and torso are relatively shorter than the limbs; upper limbs are shorter than the lower ones.

In girls, body proportions are established earlier than the boys.

Differences between the sexes are not conclusive enough at birth but are increasing progressively until the end of growth. Compared with adult men, women have a longer torso, shorter legs, wider pelvis and hips.

Both boys and girls, body height, determines the overall proportions between segments. To the short people, infantile proportions will prevail, namely long torso and short legs, and at the tall one's, juvenile proportions meaning shorter torso and longer limbs. The proportionality ratio between the upper and lower limbs is subjected to age influences and sexual differentiation. Regarding the ratio between the two halves of the body, we can only talk about a relative symmetry. When we speak of settlement and volume asymmetries of internal organs, we have to mention that with time, some of their functional asymmetries is added.

Thus, the upper limbs are equal to each other only in 18% of cases; right limbs are longer in 75% of the cases, the left side in 7% of cases *(Hasse* and *Dehner).* Differences in length range between 8-10 mm and 20-22 mm. Right upper limbs are thicker and have a greater muscle strength than the left ones because of the predominant use of the right hand. These differences are not detected at birth. In connection with asymmetries of the limbs, chest asymmetries are emphasised, especially the spine, the shoulder girdle, the pelvis. Somatovisceral growth and development also recognises its own dynamics to each apparatus and system in the human body. Muscle growth and development starts right from the intrauterine life and ends after the age of 40 years. At birth, the muscles represent 23.3% of the entire body weight; at nine years is 27.2%; 15-16 years - 32.6%; 17-18 years to 44.8% (*Sovetov*). Distribution of muscle mass and body segments on regions differ by age. In newborns, the muscles of the trunk are 40% of the entire body musculature; t adulthood - only 25-35%; upper limb muscles - 27% in newborn and 28% for the adult; lower limb muscles - 38% for the newborn and 54% the adult.

Quantitative changes in muscle are accompanied by changes in their chemical composition. Thus, while the newborn`s muscles contain much water and few solid substances, the percentage of protein substances and minerals increases with age.

The shape, size, structure and chemical composition of bone varies with age. In newborns, the cartilage weight and the ossified parts represent 15-20% of the child's entire weight. After the completion of ossification, there represent 27.2% of the body weight. At birth, only the diaphyses of long bones and the epiphyses of larger bones of arms and legs are ossified. In infancy, bones contain a large amount of water (up to 69%) and very few minerals (13%). Bones, at this age, have a fibrillar structure, richly vascularized, which ensures bone growth and rapid ossification. Cartilaginous mass, dominant at this age, gives bones a great flexibility and watches the skeleton for fractures.

In childhood, the fibrillary structure of the bones is replaced with a lamellar structure; the water percentage decreases to 45%, on the other hand, mineral salts are increasing to 22%. In the first year of life, lugs grow greatly, increasing with almost four times their volume. However, their growth becomes increasingly slower until puberty then accelerates again gradually to maturity. From birth to 20 years, the heart increases its weight by 12 times. The heart weight, in relation to the weight of the entire body, at birth is higher and varies between 0.44% and 0.52%. Appreciable increases in the absolute weight of the heart is found in the first two years of life and puberty. Heart volume is 19 cm^3 at birth, 50 cm^3 at two years, 93.5 cm^3 to five years, 250 cm^3 at 13 years and 250 -300 cm^3 to the adult.

The digestive segments gradually adapt to functional needs. The liver weighs 125-210 g at birth and is the 23rd part of the body weight; at five years is weighing 500-600 g. The adult liver reaches up to 1400 to 1500 g, representing the 34th part of the body weight *(Sappey)*. Most of the endocrine glands appear from the intrauterine life. Their evolution is conditioned by the role they fulfil in different periods of life.

Pituitary, exercising its multilateral ruling influence on all processes of growth and development, grows slowly, doubling its volume from birth to adulthood. Epiphysis develops up to seven years and then regresses slowly with the development of the sexual glands.

Thyroid shows great individual variation during evolution. In newborns, the gland weighs 1-5 g. After birth, it decreases a little in the first month and then grows intense up to five years. Moreover, it decreases again at six or seven years; it increases intensely to puberty and then slowly to adulthood when it weighs 18-30 grammes.

Parathyroids grow and develop until puberty and slowly decrease until the end of growth.

Thymus grows slowly during childhood, reaching a weight of 5-6 g to seven years, intensely increases up to 14 years, reaching to weight 30-35 grammes, then it gradually atrophies.

The adrenals are well developed at birth, decrease little in the first six months and then grow intensively in the first three years; up to eight years when they reach adult size glands.

Genital glands develop differentially by gender since the third month of intrauterine life.

The testicles descend from the lumbar region of the abdomen; they set about the inguinal channel in the 6th or 7th-month and finishes the descent in the 8th intrauterine month. In pathological cases, one or both testicles may remain in the abdomen (cryptorchidism) or in the inguinal channel (testicular ectopia).

Until puberty, the testicles grow slightly (0.5-2 cm^3), but after puberty their growth accelerates, reaching within a few years 10 times the original size (15-20 cm^3).

The ovaries descent, after birth, from the abdomen into the pelvis, settling permanently in place between one and four years. Ovary weight is of 0.5-0.6 g at birth, reaches 4-5 g at puberty and 6-8 g at adulthood.

The cerebral cortex of the newborn is very underdeveloped regarding its functionality; vital processes being adjusted at this age by the subcortical nerve centres. Higher functions of the cerebral cortex develop under the impulse of analysis. The first conditioned reflexes are formed after the 2nd and 3rd month, along with the development of sight and hearing, and relationship functions to 1-3 years, along with the development of language. The finishing of the cortical functions occurs by the age of 16-18.

Neurovegetative functions develop parallel to the cortical.

The differentiation processes of nerve cells, the fibre myelination and the multiplication of dendritic branches, are conducted intensively up to three years and round off up to eight years. Peripheral nerves, which are very little developed at birth, they increase their weight four times up to 3 years and 15 times until adulthood.

Concluding on all these issues, we point out that a good knowledge of individual characteristics, age, somatic and morphological of the human body, is a prerequisite for obtaining a sporty yield appropriate for scientifically directing all programs of physical education and sport, so that they can fully contribute to the harmonious development of body and to preserve the health of the population.

Correlations between sports activity and the dynamic of maturation and cyclical sexual phenomena

Children and youth sports score the widest circles. The age of starting to exercise entails a permanent decrease (reduction). The early awakened interest in sports for children aims to increase the limits of systematic adaptation of the body to bigger efforts and intensity exercises. With the condition of an early beginning of the training, some children acquire exceptional results. From countless examples can be listed: the 13 years old Australian girl, *Jenny Turrol* – world champion in 800 m freestyle swimming - and *Kornelia Guder* - representative G.D.R. (the fastest competitor in crawl and dolphin, which at 14 years old obtained at München, three silver medals and a year later she had no rival left in Europe, Australia or the USA). There are multiple causes of such phenomena.

Girls, during sexual maturation, lose motivation to exercise. Their construction, as a result of increasing secretion of sexual hormones, changes: there is an increasement in the layer of fat, which prevents the development of physical capacity. Some psychologists interpret the renouncement of girls to practice sport through the difficult period of social adaptation. Increasing the period of training in the sport for children raises the question: what influence have exercises on the physical development of a young body? In connection with this problem, several groups of specialists conducted a series of research (fig. 26-28).

Milianowa showed the beneficial influence of the practice of swimming on the physical development and motricity ability. The best young Hungarian swimmers are characterized by a rapid physical development (assessed by the skeletal age method). *Janowsky* confirmed this following the evolution of 11-14 years old boys who underwent a three-year experiment, performing a program of training in performance gymnastics. There has been achieved a high level of motricity ability and a balanced, proper physical development.

From the above observations, it can be concluded that the body's reaction to training depends on the size of the workout efforts.

Looking at the age when the first menstruation appeared in girls that practice sport, should not be omitted key factors that are influencing the tempo of maturation - the environment and the body construction. Sport, through its influence on the body, as it tells the multitude of issues, is considered an environmental factor.

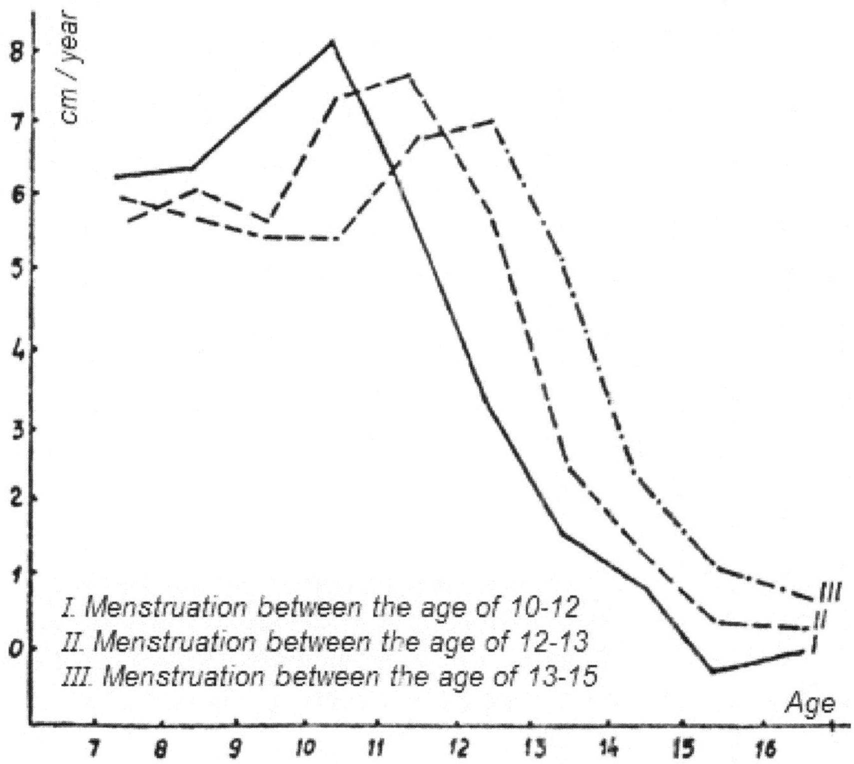

Fig. 26. The height of the growth curve in girls in relation to the menstrual cycle

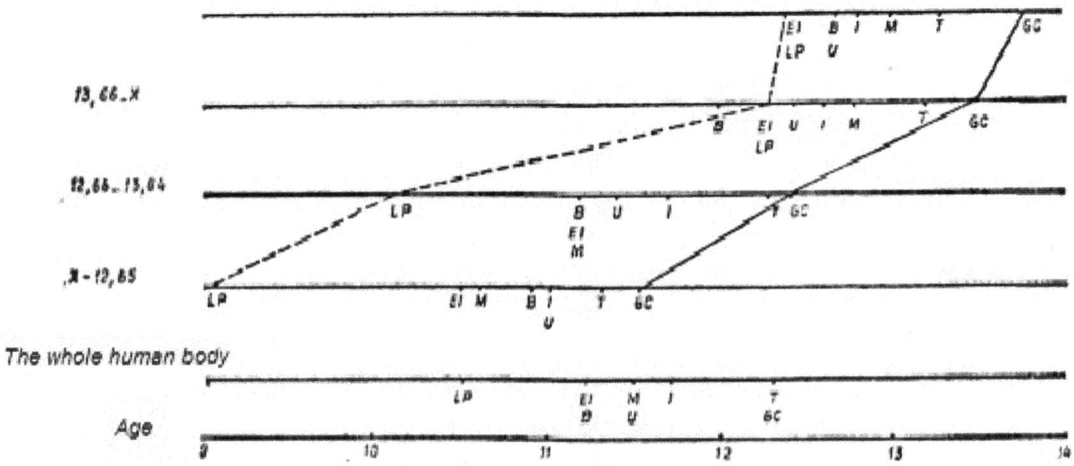

LP - foot
EI - lower extremity
U - shoulders
B – pelvis
I - height
T - trunk
GC - weights
M - hand

Fig. 27. Sequences of puberty leaps of the somatic traits in girls in relation to the menstrual cycle.

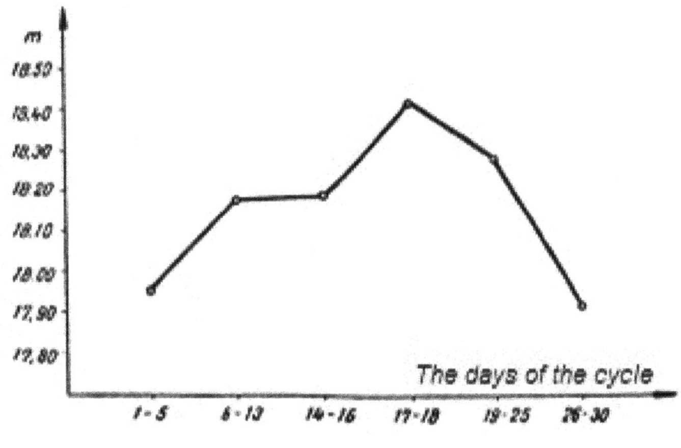

Fig. 28. The results of expressing the arithmetic average in weight throwing during the menstrual cycle.

Specifics of training in various contests amended the athletes` silhouette into a shape suitable for the characteristics of the practised sports discipline. Hereditary factors, on the one hand, and the environment, on the other hand, decide on the course of maturation processes of the body and designating the occurrence of menstruation.

The influence of motion (dynamic) on the occurrence of the first menstruation age is not easy to determine, given the complex nature of the problem in this case. On the one hand, sports training changes the course of maturation, on the other hand, the coaches, making the selection for training groups in various stages of advancement sports, girls are always choosen for the best physical attributes with an accelerated physical development. So they have an ascendancy over other girls of the same age. The listed factors encroach the assessment of the influence of practising sport on sexual maturation. A series of works were dedicated to the mutual ratio of conditioning over the body construction and the first menstruation. It was noted that girls who mature later are characterised by a leptosomatic body building and those that mature earlier have qualities of a picnic body building. In the light of modern research methodology, the occurrence of first menstruation age assessment should be based on accurate clinical history method (asking whether or not started menstruation).

Negative correlations of statistically prove that the higher the maturation begins at a younger age, the increase in body size is smaller (just for other features). An early pubertal jump of the body height indicates the start of a premature maturing. The faster the individuals mature, the greater are the characteristics of the structure of the male and female body. The age of the first menstruation can be considered as a criterion of selection in sports. However, these successes are not always lasting. Masters of the junior's category quite frequently end their athletic career at this stage. Progress is hampered further due to the inefficiency of certain features. There are forecasting methods for body dimensions; however, in the practice of sport, they are less valued.

The greatest difficulty is raised by the tempo evaluation and qualification development of children for one of the sports groups: early developed, normal, or matured late, it is necessary to use the forecast method. Today it may be proposed that the first menstruation`s age should be an additional criterion in selecting girls for schools with basketball profile. From the tall girls, it ought to be selected those that have not yet begun menstruation. This way, many errors are avoided related to the selection of the highest sports girls, which are in a transitional period (puberty jump), and the arising disappointments which are out of the failure of this physical parameter (height). Based on our research results and from data from the literature, it can be stated that the competing high-skill, practising sports games and athletics, girls are selected from among the late appearance of the first menstruation. A delayed maturation process characterises high-performance athletes in Poland. This phenomenon can be interpreted in close connection with the construction of the body and great height a feature of sportswomen and boys silhouette. The average age of first menstruation in Jugoslavian basketball team stands at 14.30 years, and hammer thrower Polish group at 14.43 years.

Regarding the motor activity influence (dynamic) on the course of the menstrual period, we mention the following. It was noted that the changes, which refers to the duration and amount of menstruation under the training`s influence, occurred most frequently in the competitors with the youngest age until 20 years of life. Instead, these changes rarely occur in athletes past 30 years. Without measure physical effort and irrational sportsmanship causes menstrual disorders and impaired genital development. The greatest danger that threatens the health of athletes is cold, accompanying water sports and winter.

In research conducted by gynaecologists on girls highlighted the dependency exists between the occurrence of menstrual disorders, character and intensity of effort. An essential element in analysing women's ability to exercise must be age and physiological maturation. The nervous excitement that appears during menstruation hinders the concentration that is required before start during tournaments. American doctors show a great exercise of tolerance during the menstrual cycle. It is estimated that there are no reasons for interrupting the motor activity in any phase of the menstrual cycle if participation in training and competitions do not cause disturbances during menstruation.

Bulska states that a suitable dosage of exercises do not causes any disturbance in the menstrual cycle, and in 1973 concluded that during childhood (girls) and before puberty there is no prohibition for practising the exercises as gynaecological diseases in girls are very rare at this time. Only mature women should avoid physical efforts during menstruation, in cases where it is very painful, or the amount of blood is too high. *Hoym*, too, considers that there may not be problems in the practice of physical exercises during that period; exceptions are the swimmers during the first days of menstruation. *Astrand* Swedish doctor has conducted research on 114 female swimmers and did not observe in any of them important changes related to the menstrual cycle, although they did not alter the pace of training. No gynaecological complications were reported, and later the tasks were normal. These observations are supported by the results of research conducted on 729 athletes (Lightweight athletics) Hungarian determined that sport has no negative influence on menstruation and future childbirth if the effort dosage is adequate during the cycle. To sports and the birth takes less time and compared to the majority population, the number of caesareans is halved. During the Olympics in Melbourne, it was confirmed that six medals in swimming and sprints were obtained by contestants that were during the menstrual cycle. Pain related to menstrual cycles seldom happens compared to similar disturbances that occur in women who do not practice sports.

A similar point of view it has *Hay,* who, within 20 years with the athletes did not notice any gynaecological disorder caused by physical activity. By this author, it may happen that some competitors to suffer from menstrual pain - then the cause must be found and the disease healed. A similar point of view belongs to *Kiss* who argues that the vast majority of contestants, the intensive physical effort does not influence the course of the menstrual cycle. 90% of women during menstruation train normally: 85% of them have not been changed during the menstrual cycle; 9% were recorded negative changes, and 6% of them - beneficial changes.

Kiss concludes that menstruation and the first three months of pregnancy do not raise any problem for sports training and competitions. *Neal* argues that the various difficult situations related to menstruation, facing coaches in the sport with women in mediately or immediately, have socio-educational causes.

The views presented in works it can be concluded that the rational use of physical exercise does not cause menstrual disorders. Most of the works of different authors that in 60% of women (50-90%) exercise have no influence on menstruation. The favourable impact of exercise can be used to cure the first menstrual disorders and acyclic bleeding. Only 20% of women noted that exercise act unfavourably on menstruation. The menstrual pain was observed more frequently in young women, the students of the first year. Given this, some authors claim that the default of exercise does not cause menstrual disorders, but that the female body is very sensitive to social changes that reflect on changing pattern of the great quantity of blood and the menstrual cycle. The situation of the contemporary research on the influence of sport on the body formulates various multilateral questions that require a deeper study of the problems. Regarding the physical capacity during the menstrual cycle, we note the following. Rich or painful menstrual periods and those of a certain ailment do not always allow contestants to realise in full the training tasks; in many disciplines itself, girls set their workout, avoiding certain exercises during menstruation or opt to participate in training in general (swimmers avoid training in water).

Ziwnowaraja showed that the circulatory system and respiratory functions occur during menstruation, unfavourable changes, revealing unfavourable conditions for sport, and exercise. She demonstrated the occurrence of adverse reactions, psychomotor, so a weakening of nervous system activity by decreasing muscle strength (evident in dynamometric measurements). To assess the influence of physiological changes during the menstrual cycle in the physical capacity the cycle divided into four corresponding periods to the following cycle phases: menstruation (bleeding), phase follicle, ovulation phase and the luteal phase. The highest level of capacity is noted during ovulating and functioning of the corpus luteum. In the coming days entails a slight decrease capacity, to stand up, then, not until the day 22-24 of the cycle. Based on the results obtained during investigations can be considered the dependence of results in sport and the phenomenon of ovulation cycle. We note that research proves a low value on tests of physical capacity in the first and fourth period with a remarkable increase in the III-a period. Subjects with 17-KS values indicated in the urine have achieved a very high physical capacity of the power test, in comparison with the results in the elimination of the low 17-KS. After *Mihail* and collaborators, we should expect the following hormonal fluctuations in the level of substances in the blood: the first three days, a very low level of oestrogen and progesterone. In the 8th – 12th day, a higher amount of oestrogen in the blood. In the 14th – 18th days, a very high level of oestrogen before ovulation, high levels of luteinizing hormone (LH) and oestrogens (FSM), an increase of progesterone; in the XX – XXIII day, a fairly high level of oestrogen, high levels of progesterone. It seems that during ovulation, some interstitial ovarian eliminates more androgens and testosterone than in other periods. Testosterone, like estrogen, is an anabolic hormone and positively influences nitrogen fixation.

It is hard to suggest today how these hormones affect the increasing of the physical ability. They act indirectly by regulating the activity of other glands of internal secretion, and firstly anterior pituitary sometimes can directly influence the intensity of biochemical transformations. During analysis investigations, it was observed that in some sports, there is a noticeable decline in the performance in the last days of the menstrual cycle and before the cycle. Part of sports stated that during menstruation it`s tough and affects their state of elation. Pain often occurs within the circulatory and nervous system. They have confirmed a rhythmic pulse, increased heart rate, increased nervousness, increased the sensitivity of nerve and reflexes, physical and nervous rapidly fatigue. Within this complex pathology is the so-called premenstrual blood pressure, which appears quite strong in some women. It is characterized by a sense of tension, increased excitability, abdominal pain, headache, a painful breast tension, insomnia, visual disturbances and a change in voice. Premenstrual pains are sometimes felt for 1-3 to 5-7 days before menstruation. Based on the data, among the many causes of failure in sport occupies an important role belongs to the cyclicality of hormonal activity of the ovary. Hence the explanation of dependence between sports results and the menstrual cycle.

Having examined the ability of the body stated that, at rest, maximal oxygen consumption is highest in the luteal phase. The highest level of oxygenation in the previous period was recorded at rowers menstruation; it amounts to 14.28 ml, and the lowest level during menstruation was 13.18 ml. The difference between the rate of oxygen during the luteal and menstrual phase and of the folliculin is essential in statistical terms. The research made at the cycle ergometer has shown that all sports induced the greatest effort during the luteal period. The lowest effort was highlighted during ovulation between the 13th and 16th day of the menstrual cycle. To assess physical capacity during the menstrual cycle were used various motricity tests.

Klaus and *Noack* have made force measurements of various muscle groups with 5 tests. In all tests, the highest results were recorded in the period after menstruation. The worst results are reported before and during the cycle. Similar results were obtained in psychomotor research using the *O'Connor*, *Noack, Kretschmer* and *Hindersdorf* test.

In the period, before the menstruation appears obviously depression, nervousness, which can be a cause of the increasing number of accidents in sport. In light of these observations stated that in the period after menstruation, mental condition, cerebral and somatic state in women is the most favourable. The physical ability of the follicle phase is connected to oestrogen. Mixed results were obtained in their research *Witzenrath* and *Hildebrandt.* In research conducted throughout the menstrual cycle, the response time to optical and acoustic signal, 37 girls were noted important differences between the follicle and luteal phase. During menstruation, the results recorded sharp declines and recover only towards the end of phase follicle; simultaneously observed that the reaction time during follicle phase is especially short, the pace slows frequency. In research conducted in the main stages and even in menstrual days, using tests for physical ability, the best results were scored in the second half of the cycle.

Martius, seeking to elucidate many of the exposed problems noted that to athletes, the motor ability could be closely related to the type of construction of the body. *Martius's* opinion, women with a leptosomatic building the highest measure of the motricity pulse and the coordination capacity happens in the first half of the cycle.

Bousenwein studied sports oscillation form. She concluded that the oscillation level of motricity ability in relation to the menstrual cycle should be correlated with the state of training. From research conducted to date have not yet elucidated the physical capacity issues during the menstrual cycle. The processes of growth and development, as well as other periods of life, are conducted differently in every human by genotype and paratypes existing factors. In ilikiologie, a distinction is made between calendar age, measured by astronomical time (years, months, days) since its birth - called chronological age – and biological age, determined by biological criteria. For a given population (and for a specific historical epoch) can be given an average schedule of the bioreutic tempo at which we relate to a particular individual. Age criteria but do not have the precision of physical health standards (such as axillary temperature) or chemical ones (such as blood glucose). Biological age can be reviewed (which are considered as signs of "premature old age" and those of "prolonged or delayed youth") - or take into account certain *synthetic and expressive criteria.* Such an expressive criterion is speed healing. In fact, the biological age of an organism is a result of the biological age of the various parts of the body: tissues, organs, fluids. Changes in age structure and design of tissues and organs define the morphological age, characterised by weakening the activity of organs define physiological age (or functional), those reflected in the chemical composition of tissues and blood - biochemical age. Among age changes are relatively well studied the collagen fibre - the principal substance of connective tissue and is the most common protein in the body.

Not every change with age is a good diagnostic criterion of "age" analysed; are selected those that allow better differentiation between "young" and "old". Some criteria are more convenient, more accurate; some are laboratory tests, others can be determined by medical examination or similar to medical (clinical examination).From applying different criteria and tests can establish a global index which, compared with the standards of the population, the diagnosis of "ageing" of normal time (orthogenesis) or abnormal time ("ageing" accelerated or delayed).

According to research conducted by *F. Verzar* (Basel), the constant changes signalling an involution are: high blood pressure (systolic and diastolic pressure), the low vital capacity of the lung, decreased habituation eye, increasing the perimeter of the chest and abdominal (but last perimeters deducted only after 67 years). According to the data of Geriatric Institute in Bucharest *(Cecilia Enăchescu* and *C. David)*, main involution psychological changes are, in order of frequency: decreased memory, attention and learning ability, decreased libido, increased sensibility slowdown ideation, neuroticism, fatigue, anxiety, irritability and reduced sociability.

The desire to find mathematical expressions (or graphic "mathematisable") for the processes of growth and involution has led to many remarkable results. It is understandable that the simplest representation is based on calendar time (= the calendarist age) as the simplest expression is seen to be a linear function (first-order equation), corresponding to the line (after *V. Găhleanu* "the anthropological dynamic of adulthood").

During calendar is the time clocks adjusted by movements of the stars (or, lately, after carrying out physical processes atomic) is, therefore, physical time, and we can accept as such, possibly with "corrections" to the concept of time uniform and absolute (Newtonian time) by Einsteinian relativity. Alternatively, representation of the biological growth process based on calendar time does not (organisms evolved) curves whose geometric elegance to suggest a suitable analytical expression, simple enough. On the other hand, if after that organic growth is at every moment, live weight proportion reached:

$$\frac{dm}{dt} = km \ ,$$

the descriptive relationship is an exponential law:

$$m_t = m_o e^{kt}$$

Naturally, we must assume the existence of such limiting factors of growth; find that the body growth has a limit characteristic for the species, the more plausible it becomes that the differential equation:

$$\frac{dm}{dt} = k(M - m) \text{ ,}$$

leading to a law of logistic type *(Verhulst, Pearl)*:

$$m_t = \frac{A}{I + e} kt \text{ .}$$

We admit (as *LV Bertalanffy)* that limit the growth resulting from the dialectic of assimilation (proportional to metabolic exchange surface) and disassimilation (commensurate with the living mass volume):

$$\frac{dm}{dt} + k_1 S - k_2 V \text{ ,}$$

which, through integration leads to a different kind of "S curve" than logistics curve. However, it is assumed that the ceiling coincides with the dimensions achieved when "full maturation" relatively confusing concept regarding man, but specified about by the addition - somatic sexual maturation - the cessation of growth in height.

It should be noted that for higher organisms (including man), one logistic type relationship is not able to adequately describe the growth process. To adjust the empirical data needed to "complicate" the analytic relationship, either in the form:

$$m_t = \frac{A}{B + Ce^{f(t)}} \text{ ,}$$

Where f (t) is a polynomial - to superimpose multiple logistic type relationship (adding them possibly terms of a linear relationship), which would correspond the existence of several growth cycles theoretically. In addition, each species (or at least each group of plant species or animals) appears to have a particular analytical expression, not only regarding numerical coefficients, but also the type of equation used. In these circumstances, the mathematical treatment of the particular problems (of weight gain and height growth, etc.) is extremely difficult. It can bypass the difficulty introduced by the use of physical time eliminating the variable "time", for example, applying allometric analysis. In terms of graphic and mathematical representation of involution phenomena, the phenomena of "decline", recorded during ages (after 20 years), the use of physical time is shown to be more appropriate. *Calloway,* who researched (1966) over 100 such processes of decline, finds that there are sufficient three types of representations: linear (the rarest), exponential and power function:

$$y = at^b$$

(found in allometric analysis). As is known, the exponential function can be "linearized" using a logarithmic ordinate and power function can be "linearized" by functional stairs (logarithmic) on the x-axis and the axis of ordinates:

$$y = e^x \text{ , } \ln y = x \text{ ;}$$

$$y = ax^b \text{ , } \text{loy} = \log a + b \log x \text{ .}$$

That physical time is presented as a variable in the description of phenomena of ageing is for *Calloway,* an argument for *physicochemical theories* of ageing. However, *Calloway* does not take into account the "complacent" function power (in fact, it subsumes both the linear and hyperbolic relationship of inverse proportionality), nor that they have linear decreases a less "natural" than decreases (or increases) exponentially. An old investigation of *Lecomte du Nouy's* on wound healing by age revealed a coefficient independent of age, calendar inversely proportional to age. In other words, the law of scarring is *different* at different ages calendar, but can be represented by the same symbols, if is taken into account a "correction" that transforms physical time in a variable, *a hyperbolic function of time.* Everything happens as if for an older man, physical time "moves" faster; as for a man of 50, one-year (representing 1/50 of his life) *time has* another value than for a child of five years (for a year is only 1/5 of his life).

Simplifying terms of the issue, we wonder if *it* is more *appropriate* to represent a biological process over time in *physical units,* or in units of time considered to be "opportunity" that could be called "organic time" or "biological time". The suggestion arising from previous rows is that the biological temporal laws (biological cronorm) might unify if, instead of physical time, it would use a "time organic". The largest (and boldest) try to carry out such a transposition we owe it to *G. Backman* (1942). We will briefly describe his reasoning and results. The basic idea is this: *The organic time is a logarithmic function of physical time.* It is based on the growth rates of organisms, i.e., take the maximum speed of growth (seen as "normal speed") and from the *moment* that is done this speed. The first postulate is denoted by:

$$\log H = k_2 \log^2 T\ ,$$

(where $k_2 < 0$). Time Unit is *tm* and speed unit is *hm; T* and *H* are expressed in these units: $H = h / hm$ and $T = t / tm$. It comes in as a first stage, the expression:

$$\log h = k_0 + k_1 \log t + k_2 \log^2 t$$

linking the rate of growth with the physical time, and the relationship:

$$\log t_m = \frac{k_1}{2k_1}\ .$$

Then the *differential* growth law is of the form:

$$\frac{dy}{dt} = e^{S_0 + S_1 \ln t + S_2 \ln^2 t}\ ,$$

(as opposed to classical *full* growth laws that were exponential law). Through various transformation variable on which we insist, the law is rewritten by using the integral of probability:

$$y = A \frac{\int_{-x}^{x} e\, dx, unde\ x = c_1 \log t + c_2 = c_1 \log t}{t_0 s} = \frac{c_1 \log T}{T_{03}}\ .$$

The value of the constants C_1 is not that easy to obtain. By $T_{0.5}$ denotes the time at which half of the final value is reached. What can be the "final value"? Regarding the human growth, *Backman* prefers to use weight - not height, because height is affected by the curvature of the spine (physiological curvature or "age"). But the average weight grows beyond the end of adolescence, so during youth and adulthood. Thus, *Backman's* growth equation covers the adulthood, "uniting" under the concept of ontogenesis and what, for other authors, is the debut gerontogenesis. Note that for *Calloway* and all authors before him, traced the curve of decline, the "connection" to their growth curves did not represent a sufficiently serious problem.

In its final form using "organic time" and not "physical time," *Backman's* equation adapts satisfactory to the empirical data, is equally valid for many animal and plant species. This advantage may be on account of numerous arbitrary constants intervening in analytical expression (suppleness an analytical expression is the number of such constants), as to the fact that the author, like his predecessors, is forced to admit that the developing of the upper body is the result of several growth cycles. But he could translate as the author believes - the "catching" of a biological meaning. An argument for the last interpretation is to identify, by calculation, the important moments of the life cycle. Thus, sexual maturation occurs when:

$x = c_1 logt + c_2 = 0$,

The symmetry point of the growth function. The squarish structure of this function brought the conclusion that the values:

$$x^2 = \frac{0}{2};\frac{1}{2};\frac{2}{2};\frac{3}{2};\frac{n}{2},$$

Plays an important biological role. The difference between them is constant and has a value which can be regarded as a "quantum critical". Quantum limits $x = \sqrt{0/2}$, $\sqrt{1/2}$, $\sqrt{2/2}$, $\sqrt{3/2}$, may be 'combined' with defined biological events which are identical, - in all organisms. It continues:

$$d(x^2)dt = \frac{2c_1([e(c_1)]log[t + c_2])}{t}$$

It is regarded as an expression of vitality conduct. Then $t_0 = 3 \cdot t_{0,5}$ is the measure of time when life is at its peak and begins ageing rapidly, the $t_a = 4,48 \cdot t_{0,5}$ pass to a slower ageing.

The function:

$$\frac{dx}{dt} = \frac{c_1 \, loge}{t}$$

Represents the realisation in `physical time' of the size of the vital action. *Backman* observed that there is an analogy between `organic time`, as defined by him, and 'dynamic time" in cosmology introduced by *Milne:*

$$\tau = t_0 ln\frac{t}{t_0} + t_0$$

$$x = c_1 \, loge \cdot ln\frac{t}{t_{0,5}}.$$

So, concludes *Backman,* living organisms take place in a "logarithmic world." This development explains why, over the years, we see the calendar time as being "compressed", meaning "accelerated". Calculations show that his "absolute acceleration of physical time" is an increasing function throughout life, with equal slopes:

$$tg\alpha = 0,1/c_1 \cdot loge$$

Thus, after 50 years it is five times higher than when it was at ten years. The relationship is linear:

$$\alpha = 0.1880t.$$

(*Backman* points out that the "true calendar age" of man is not to be reckoned from birth, but from the moment of conception). If "biological length" of the "physical time" unit at the age of ten is taken as a unit in the early embryonic development, it is 13.8 times longer, and at age 65 is 6.5 times shorter." Quanta of organic time" means: a) a structure while the conduct of life; b) the ability to distinguish - beyond the time of sexual maturation, or cessation of growth in length of life stages (adults). (This in contrast to what he says - with satisfaction - *Calloway,* finding the "smooth" character of the curve traced by physical time).

At $x = \sqrt{1/2}$, In the third cycle of growth (fundamental growth cycle), located at the age of 35-40, we find, after *Backman,* the maximum vital capacity of the lungs. It starts the process of slowing down of the relative duration of the systole, decreasement of the accommodating lens and a rapid decline in fertility. The frequency of gallstones increases greatly.

At $x = \sqrt{2/2}$, located at 50 (or 60) years, the climacteric and prostate hypertrophy appear, there is an increasement in the frequency of gastric cancer (and the prognosis worsens)

At $x = \sqrt{3/2}$, the fundamental growth cycle ends (60 or 85 years?) - Which could mean and "end of life".

The 4th cycle (Cycle IV), is stretching from late teens to early puberty. Therefore, the period of youth and the adulthood stage is corresponding to a "post-cycle" (as "primary cycle" ends with the completion of deciduous dentition).

Backman's calculations show us the development process and key moments of the process of "involution" an organic time-dependent, own not only to each species, but also to each individual. An agreement with the curves presented by *Calloway* can be obtained under the assumption that inter-individual variations of the organic involution are distributed randomly, but dependent (within each stage of life, stage shaped by values of the organic time) processes that depend directly on physical time. The reasoning behind the assumptions will appeal to new research (1968) of his *Ph. Burch* related to some diseases - and especially some rare diseases.

Burch also proposes a mathematical model. By hypothesis, he admits that some diseases are arising from the accumulation of somatic mutations. Mutations are random events easily occurring by "chance" through "hazard". If mutations occur in certain cells of immunocompetent clones, a disease can be reached through immunological self-harm. However, it outlines a group of diseases whose distribution after the calendar age, obey an exponential law. The prevalence by age regarding the general population is given by:

$$Pt = S\{1 - \exp(-kt)\}$$

and the rate of occurrence in the general population age *t* is given by expression derived:

$$\frac{dP}{dt} = kS\exp(-kt)\,.$$

A correction must be made for the period of latency. When the model requires at least one mutation in each of n cells, the equation is written:

$$Pt = S\{1 - \exp(-k)\}^n\,.$$

When needed *r* somatic mutations, the equation is written:

$$1 - \exp(kt^r)\,,$$

Where k is defined as Lm^r : *L* is the number of cells at risk of mutation, m is the mutation rate per gene and year. In these models fit remarkably well statistics on diseases: systemic lupus erythematosus, osteoarthritis interphalangeal joints, Dupuytren's contracture, *carpal* tunnel syndrome, Wilson disease, diabetes, urticaria *pigmentosa,* manic-depressive psychosis, schizophrenia, etc. What is strange is that the model is "checked" for tooth loss, the occurrence of canities, involution psychosis, etc. - the typical manifestations "of old age".

In representations, log/log curves that show the dP/dt, depending on age, have a parabolic shape, generally asymmetrical shape with convexity upwards. With the title of example, we give statistical parameters related to diabetes: latency correction =5 year, *r*=5, S=6, 7×10^2 for women, k=109 years^{-5}. We also mention that the comparison of series coming from particular geographical backgrounds, it happens that the statistical parameters differ; it does not differ, however, the type of curve which adjusts these data. All have a maximum at a certain calendar age, which corresponds to the maximum of probability of completing the constellation of pathogenic factors.

CHAPTER IV.
THE HUMAN BODY JUDGED THROUGH AN INTEGRATIVE, SYSTEMIC AND EVOLUTIVE ANALYSE

The adult period of human existence has been researched systematically and analytically less than the extreme periods of the individual life. If the Fundamental and Applied Study of childhood have shaped the scientific fields of puericulture pediatrics and pedagogy - and for "Autumn" and "Winter" of life were established sciences today in full swing - gerontology and geriatrics - the period called "adult", benefitted from unspecified research. We understand by this term that the data on the "man in general" or "middle man" philosophical or statistical abstractions whose practical utility is quite questionable. (First, because the man is presented in two polar variants, the two sexes, further, that the variability of the human within which we focus using racist or constitutional typologies, is not an epiphenomenon, but the root of reacts, adaptive and initiative components - extremely diverse. Human indiv dualization is effective, meaning he has not only a descriptive or identificational signification!). Lately, the period (defined chronologically bad!) of the youth is, in turn, the object of complex research with institutions specially profiled as *the Research Centre for Youth Affairs*, attached to *UTC (The Communist Youth Union)*.

The paradoxical statement after which the adult is an unknown (or, if that adult is a pseudo-known) does not want to be a denial of scientific acquisitions, many on biology, psychology, sociology, etc. of the human (being understood by "man" usually "mature man", in which the processes of growth and organismic differentiation ended and the processes of involution are negligible). Pleading for "adultology" is only an invitation to reconsider and processing of such data in a less used perspective: one that integrates during the "adult" in the vital curve of the body (and more necessary in curve of the individual destiny of personality); one that differs in its content processes, times, stages, crossroads, etc.

Many years ago, *Cl Parhon* showed that to be understood properly, the issue of ageing, it must be classified first in the more general issue of age, *mutatis mutandis*; the same can be said about the adult. Each segment of human life has its biological characteristics (of the assimilation and disassimilation, growth and differentiation, operating bodies, etc.); precisely those characteristics necessitated the emergence of branches of medicine such as paediatrics and geriatrics. To study the biological age differently, *Cl Parhon* proposed as name *ilikibiology*. We can speak as naturally of *ilikipsychology* and *ilikisociology (Al. Chira)* - or, in short, a synthetic *ilikiology*. However, life can and should be studied in connection with the stages of its flow. *Panta rei* - "everything flows" – said *Heraclitus*; therefore, to conduct life phenomenon, as for the study of life in a continuous succession of years - was proposed *(Ehrenberg, Max Burger)* name *bioreutics*. Living systems are evolutionary systems (in a sense given by *V. Conta* for this word): individuals are born, grow up, develop, mature, regress, die. They go through different stages of development and involution, characterised by specific notes; the transition from one stage to another is sometimes smooth, sometimes through crises. In principle, it can be said that the issue of the crisis depends on individual temperament, capacities for social adjustment and self-adjusting. A weak personality, an unreasonable environment can transform seizures (often useful, enriching personality) in disaster for evolution.

One of the adultology problems will be an adequate separation of stages of life (the "age") and the research of any subdivisions of the "adult" stage. Another will be considering the critical, uncritical or potentially critical character of "bioreutical" transformations. Further, these problems (somewhat preliminary) will be connected with the issue of ageing. Abstract: with progressive evolution and involution of the individual. Is it the "adult" period the final segment, continuing the progressive ontogeny is it the beginning of senile decadence or has another scheme (status)?

Human ages and the "adult" period

In humans, as in any repeated typical ongoing process ("phasic" process) growth, maturation and involution of the individual include outstanding quality phases that can be called stages, "ages", etc. In the history of philosophical concerns, medical or scientific about man (as in the history of jurisprudence), the definition of these phases was usually done empirical or even arbitrary. Purely chronological criterion was often a "numerology" criterion, the seven or ten digits playing a greater role in defining the age.

Thus, some Egyptian hieroglyphs, referring to life fully lived that comprise about 60 years notes that it takes ten years to begin to know what life and death is, for another ten years to instruct you for ten years to learn to distinguish good from evil. The philosophy of ancient Chinese *Kung-fu-tze* said that up to 15 years' the child learns by 30 he stands firm, at 40 he begins to overcome the doubts, at 50 he understands the laws of Heavens and at 70, he barely knows what "limit" means! In *Chia-i-Ching* indicates a gradual change in the adult human temperament, from 40 years from decade to decade. At *Hippocrates*, we encounter a division of life into seven periods of seven years; at 49 years would reach true maturity at 56 years the man becomes old.

In Arab tradition "age power" is between 18-30 years. Puberty is located at 13 years and at 40 years old (as in *Talmud*!) – The beginning of the decline.

At *Lorenco (Balthazar) Gracian* (1653), a man of 20 years is the man of will; at 30 years the genius manifests and at 40 years - judgment; Meanwhile, it develops the power to appreciate life in accordance with its true value.

After the rites of the Church of Romanian feudal principalities, "seven ages has a man" cocoon up to four years, child up to 14 years, teenager up to 22, sturdy to 42, male to 56, old up to 69 and mature up to 80!

The *Psalter* of *Dosoftei* (1673) speaks of an age of "greying" that precedes old age. *Cantemir* in his *Divan* distinguished himself seven ages: infancy (up to seven years), childhood (up to 14), teenage (up to 21 years treated with puberty); with the end of this period enters into "real life" which includes joyfulness, manhood, greying and old age.

It is noteworthy that in this staging, criteriology is mixed, bio-psycho-social, taking into account, not only the ectoscopy elements empirical and clinical noticeable (such as the state of the child, or the appearance of secondary sexual characteristics, or gray hair), but also the performance of virtual psychosocial, behavioral traits, affection, resistance. It is noteworthy, too, that this staging only applies to males.

Hufeland divides the first 50 years of life into two equal stages: between 50-60 years ageing occurs, and after 60 years the individual is old. *Schopenhauer* expected a "scheme of life" relatively long; the work includes 40 years, the next 30 being dominated more and more by the contemplative life. *N. Pende*, proposing an ontogenetic or auxological biotypology distinguishes, contrary to the "numerological" tradition, 9 stages in human evolution, along with 9 phases of involution. Three laws dominate the process: a) weight-morphological antagonism (*Viola*): mass varies inversely with differentiation; b) the large and small alternations (*Godin*): There is an alternation between the growth in length, and, respectively, width, of a bone, between the growth of legs and torso, between the growth of two overlapping segments of the body; c) the antithesis of both "hormonal morphogenetic constellations" (*Pende*), after which the catabolic hormones act morphogenetic, in the opposite direction of the anabolic hormones (length/width). Each phase would have an endocrine-type formula that would explain somatic and psychological manifestations. Periods (steps) are, after *Pende:* newborn period (in which there is a "genital crisis")

1. during the first year of life (which highlights the predominance of assimilatory glands: thymus, lymph apparatus, pancreas, the thyroid, parathyroid, pituitary, liver and adrenals

have a lower tone). The characteristic endocrine formula explains growing appetite, the tendency to depositing fat, hydrophilic, but at the same time the susceptibility to exudative skin phenomena to spasmophilia (convulsions), sudden death ("clinical" death). In the second half of the first year of life would occur, however, a hyperthyroid "crisis", hyperparathyroidism hypo hepatica - which might coincide with the occurrence of the first dentition;
2. of *turgor primus* (between 2 and 3 ½ years);
3. of *proceritas prima* ("small puberty"), with first prevalent elongation;
4. of *turgor secundus* (between 9-11 years), acceleration of the weight increase;
5. of pre-puberty *(proceritas secunda)*;
6. of puberty *(turgor tertius)*, where there is predominant the genital hormone constellation formed by pituitary, thyroid and ovary – at women, and by pituitary, adrenocortical and testicles – at men;
7. post-puberty age (or inter-nubile-puberty);
8. adulthood characterised (after *Pende*) by "increasing virility and femininity" and the last increase in width (so *turgor Quartus*);
9. "critical age" (age of life deformation), followed by old age.

Each period (from 1° to 7°) differs from the previous one, as well as the following, by targeting the general vegetative (anabolism/catabolism). Moreover, *Pende's* transition from one to another is done by "crisis", and the whole evolution relies heavily on the resources and environmental influences. It follows, among other things, that the individuals of a more advanced phase (or late) are more likely to distinguish between them; thus adulthood can portray individuals with varied types, and "deformation" (10 °) may occur, in many directions.

In the problem of endocrine constitutional determinism of ages chapter, can be added the idea that the same secretional endocrine gland of several hormones (sometimes partial antagonists between them, such as the pancreas that develop insulin-hypoglycemic and glucagon hyperglycemia) can change the functional dominant from one stage to another. This seems to have been highlighted for the cortico-adrenal, during the beginning and end of ectopic life. An important sentence is an asynchrony evolving and involution, endocrine glands (for old age; thesis was supported *by Șt. Milcu.)*

A special mathematical arguments are contributing their location coordinates rather complex problem. We refer, first, to the relatively recent analyse of growth curves body, carried by *A. Ciureş* and *V. Săhleanu* (1969, 1973) - analysis suggests a <u>quantization</u> weight gain in humans. Namely, the addition of body mass would be done by "micro-quanta" of 16.6 g integrated themselves in "macro-quantum" each about 10 kg. The latest figure is derived from an <u>allometric</u> representation, the relationship between body weight and visceral weight (*Săhleanu* 1952, 1959). In other words, for some organs, is enough only one relation of the type:

$$y = ax^{b} \ ,$$

$$\log y = \log a + \log x \ .$$

(one right line on net of log/log), while the other organs is a need for more (usually two) that, on the graph, are at an angle." Breaking" points coincide around the 10, 20 and 30 kg body weight. As 'critical' points for body growth, since such corresponding "breaking" is observed on the chart represents the height by weight. However - what is still more important for the present discussion - allometric analysis shows that interindividual variations in adults are not based on interindividual variation curves during the growth period. This result would plead for discontinuity between evolutionary period and seemingly stationary age "adult" period. We cannot stop over the evolution stage described by psychoanalysis, a conception that pretends to be <u>biological</u> since it follows the evolution of an "instinct" (<u>libidinal evolution</u>). Gradually, other erogenous zones “crosses” libido (oral, anal, phallic, latency stages, etc.) reaching in the normal cases (“happy”) at an adult erotic type, integrated where the genitality has its well-defined place. The original design of *S. Freud* completed and composed by *K. Abraham, S. Ferenczi, Klein,* etc. is more interesting for psycho-pedagogues and auxologists than 'adultologists”. However, for “adultologists” are fundamental two concepts derived from this perspective: the fixing in a certain stage (fixing due to an accident biographical or relationships within the family, abnormal) and the regression to a hypo-evolved stage.

Psychoanalysis has, among other things, the merit of having helped to found a scientific sexology. But, while the psychoanalysts are concerned with sexual instinct avatars, for the auxologist and “adultologist” of today is more concerning, the measure in which the sexual polarisation of soma occurs (and concomitantly the psyche). Sexual immaturity (with the persistence of infantile characteristics, adolescent, etc.) will be distinguished as such, the polarisation more or less pronounced (between the hyperginic and the hyperandric type) and the presence (open or latent) of heterosexual notes. After a remark once made (*Săhleanu*, 1958), a coefficient of ambisexuality is an organismic balance factor; morbid conditions may be allowed to man by “hypo feminity” (e.g. hypoestrogenism), etc.

The relations between “adultology” and sexualisation anthropology are more complex, the hypothesis of “foetalization” *(L. Bolka)*, of the retardation, or of “pedogenetic” character of the human being, continue to enjoy the attention in science. Not coincidentally man is a primate with an extremely long childhood! “Paedogenesis” human explains *(G. Rohe)* Oedipus complex and infantile notes the co-substantial of the constitution of the female adult infantilising forming, by this author, complement adaptive of elongation of childhood. On the other hand, *G. Maranon* issued a *vue d'esprit* on the classification of human ontogenetic development between male and female poles. The man would go through a “feminoid phase” in puberty, and the woman (through a genuine process of retard, we would say) would present a masculinization barely sketched for climacteric. Incidentally, we would like to note that during the adult life of the woman, there is usually a development of sexual libido, sensitivity genital and ability to orgasm - suggesting a “virilization”, more exactly, a quality of a modus male type.

Delineation and age assessment depend on biological and social factors and their respective cultures ages, as mortality age or average length of life. It was thought for a while that in traditional China there were many “patriarchal”. In reality, apparently, the Chinese married early procreate without delay; Wealthy man around the age of 40-45 years he became an in-law and still lived a quiet life and less active, a life of “old man”. However, it would be simplistic and therefore incorrect to believe that prestige of certain age directly reflects the demographic situation. It was stated (and we have associated this opinion) that the recovery of old age is a human social feature. It would be possible to achieve some degree of development of productive forces; the presence of the elders should be a burden. It was claimed (without abundant documentation ethnographic) that in some primitive tribes, old people are killed or left to die or commit suicide - in order not to burden for the tribe. *Clemens of Alexandria* noted, two millennia ago that “Hyperborean” kill those of them who manage to reach the age of sixty. Such cruel habits were attributed to some Germanic people, who lived at the beginning of our era.

Recent ethnological research shows, however, that hordes of subhuman primates, the valid old has a useful function in relation to the life experience gained. The social value attributed to different ages has an obvious cultural mark - there is a general human standard.” Valuing” social age (note essentially biological in man) is an illustration of the biological and social dialectics, an example of biosocial character.

In ancient Egypt, the same hieroglyph designates old man as the ruler as the head or the “large man” socially important. This suggests that the prestige of old age in civilisation. The ancient Hebrew, elders, have a dominant social role.” Patriarchs”, leaders, authors of laws and holy books, founders of religions are longevity wise. Longevity for some of them recorded in *the Bible* is implausible. Respect for old age has passed in Christianity. The Father is represented in religious icons, as an old man with a white beard.

Homeric Hellas does not identify old age with wisdom and majesty. The ideal man is young; the apotheosis of man is in his person. Age is awkward, unsightly, to *Pindar* at *Sappho*. The hero is glorified, for example, *Achilles*. Subsequently, the credit granted to elders differentiated by type of civilisation developed (commercial, militarist, etc.).

Cicero is forced to take action against discrediting age. Life is a journey; each portion of the road has its peculiarities. *Seneca* condemns the misuse and waste of time at all ages. White hair is the sign of time passing - and not its proper uses. For the Germanic warrior, supreme glory was ideal; death of old age does not bring glory, but glory can bring immortality. As such, old age could not enjoy prestige. The saying: "*Who does not have elders should go and buy them*" expresses high appreciation that some people give to the experience and wisdom of age. However, what is "old"? The label has an overwhelming sociocultural determinism - sometimes autobiographical, and it can be shown that, often, the "old" means "adult".

In the *H. Ibsen`s* dramatic opera, there are some attitudes and significant lines. The *Lady from the Sea*, a girl of eighteen, considered to be strange the idea of marrying one of her former teachers because it is "very old"; in fact, he was 38 years old. *Builder Solness*, still at the age where it can inspire passion erotic, is fiercely opposed affirmation of the young, he acts as if it belongs to the generation of older people. *Erasmus of Rotterdam* saw the need, at 37 years, to address the disadvantages of old age. Much the same age, the ill *Ch. Darwin* spoke in a letter to a friend about "his old bones." He lived his great works on both biologies again and had published fifty years earlier. At 32, *G. Papini* was writing an autobiography *A finished man*: literary work later proved the contrary.

The average length of life was remarkable in the nineteenth century, from 28 to 45 years old. However, until the twentieth century, the growth of the average length was achieved, up to 70 years, thus normally ageing elders - a frequent category. Conveniences brought by civilisation and natural training of older in works of great responsibility in forced reconsideration "labels".

The seminar in Kiev (1963), held under the auspices of the World Health Organization, distinguished, apart from youth and maturity, three age categories:

a) Transition or middle-age, between 45-60 years old;
b) Early old age (from 60 to 75 years old);
c) Old age (after 75 years old).

To change the (contemporary) attitude towards "middle" ages is characteristic the appearance, in 1952, of a successful publicist volume: *Life Begins at Forty*, by *American Walter Pitkin*. By this author, true life could begin at 40 years, a life full of achievements, if we knew how to live it in time. True, says *Pitkin*, that at 40 years old in some way we get old, and "lose" by this ageing but also, and gain the maturity and a better use of resources and expertise can lead to a positive balance. However, only in comfort and civilisation, life would "restart" at such an age. As an argument in favour of his thesis, *Pitkin* brings data which suggests that the lifetime characteristic of species is the degree of civilisation. *Pitkin* is optimistic, and that reviews the biographies of famous people who have stood in his youth (as was *Wordsworth, Ibsen, Curie, Linné*). It was only after 40 years have become "interesting" people like *Titian, J. Conrad, H. Hoover*; triumphs of creators like *Handel, Bach, Haydn, R. Wagner, Michelangelo, Goya* were entered after (or long after) 40 years. It quoted *H. Ford* repeating that "no one has done anything important before forty years" - which, of course, is an exaggeration - even if *Thorndike* calculated that the common age at which people produce their masterpieces value is 47.7 years (statistics on 331 cases). Lately, on the contrary, there is a tendency for the devaluation of adulthood (and, even more, the older age). It has roots in the economy as considerations on (mostly) industrial labour. Scientific-technical dynamism, speed "moral" deterioration of technology raises a serious issue of periodic retraining. The holder of technical cultures older than 20 years, for example, is often overtaken by a new avalanche. Therefore, we sometimes encounter (in Western literature) strange appreciation after an engineer for 40 years, for instance, it is "too old".

In a close relationship, there are involved economic calculations regarding the profit made by using an individual's age X, counting salary expenditures (possibly training) and for retirement. The higher the calendar's age is, the better the chances of a negative balance, and at a certain age, employment seems clearly understaffed.

We are witnessing, also to a decrease in the average age of the performer's athletes. A thorough and adequate training, at a relatively early age, make the victories in the competition to rely increasingly on natural advantages (and psychomotor) of adolescence and early youth. Competitive sports performance status, makes the Olympic land or championships to be abandoned at dwindling "age limits". Conditions for good enhancement of the creative capacities of young people going at the same time, to a decrease in the average age at which Nobel laureate, at least in some sectors (physics).

Regarding the political, international life in the last decades showed that the destiny of countries could be entrusted with the same confidence personalities relatively young (as President *Kennedy*) or old folks (as Chancellor *K. Adenauer*). Not all people carry out their "life run" as fast. Not every man is "showing his/her age" some seem "old before our time." Early ageing is a fact scientifically proven just how youth is admitted to be juvenile, persistent and prolonged. Therefore, in ilikiology there is a distinguishing between calendar age measured by astronomical time (years, months, days) since birth – also called chronological age and biological age, determined by biological criteria. For a given population (and for a specific historical epoch) it can be established an average timetable which relates to the bioreutical tempo of a particular individual.

Age criteria do not have the precision of physical health standards (such as axillary temperature) or chemical ones (such as blood glucose). Biological age can be reviewed (in which are into consideration signs of "premature old age "and "prolonged or delayed youth") - or consider certain synthetic and expressive criteria. Such an expressive criterion is the healing speed. In fact, the biological age of an organism is a result of the biological age of the various parts of the body: tissues, organs, fluids. Changes in age structure and design of tissues and organs define the morphological age, characterised by the weakening of the activity of organs define the physiological age (or functional), those reflected in the chemical composition of tissues and blood - biochemical age. Among age changes relatively well studied we find the collagen fibre - important substance of connective tissue and the most common protein in the body. It speaks of an actuarial age related to the probability of death calculated with the help of mortality tables." Life expectancy" of an individual depend upon the biological state of his own body and not the characteristics of the group to which he/she belongs.

The notion of biological age applies to any living being. For ilikiology, which is specific to man, were proposed terms of psychological age (mental) and social age (sociological). Youth and old age are characterised by certain traits of spiritual life through a particular state of psychic functions - dependent on the state of the nervous system, but also the experience and trials of life. Also, they are characterised by certain social roles by interests and through a more or less intensive social life, etc. For elders, the interest in life is a good index for assessing the psychological age and - especially - social (*Olga Văleanu*). By *J. Galtung, Fr. Mahler* and others, age is presented as a decrease of options for a specific "role". The essential options are made in youth (or even before). Some authors prefer the synthetic term of biosocial age, insisting that it has a "historic character", varying with the development of society stage, geographic region, habits, etc. Psychological criteria in age assessment are something else than mere figures of speech. "*You are still young as long as you admire and to the extent that you admire,*" wrote *Bacon*. In fact, today`s psychologists tend to admit that the stages of life do not replace completely each other, but also provides gains that would require being preserved. "*Childhood never goes away from us, it is a permanent source of deriving all the twists and turns of our lives,*" said *George Călinescu*, and continues: "*Our age is measured after the intensity of life... Brilliant is the youth you have achieved through adulthood.*" Another great contemporary writer *I. Ducici* noted: "*The old age of man begins where ends his liveliness... the man gets older only all his passions age.*" *M. Gramsci* believed that "*you are getting old when you start to fear death.*" We add two significant quotations: <u>the belief that you can accomplish anything</u> would be the mystery of youth (*I.S. Turgheniev*), the spirit remains forever young (*J. Renard*). *Goethe* observed that every human`s decade has his own luck, his hopes, his specific capabilities. As I said on another occasion (1972), by analogy with what we noted for the proper physiological and psychological domain of individual life we could talk about a good "rate of soul wound healing" and a spiritual fecundity characteristic of youth. Unlike the physiological sphere, the mentality`s homoeostasis characterises old age rather than youth. *J.Galtung* argued recently (1972) that "openness" of mind, in the cognitive and axiological domain, diminishes much after the age of 25 years. At this age, the "cosmological" and "axiological" configuration ends, starting with a double process of completing accepted paradigms with notions that are consistent, tending to neglect others, to reject what threatens to unsettle or restructure.

I proposed, in this context, the concept of Axiological age - concept essentially "anthropological" and to be explained on another occasion. Mutations are, however, events that occur at the sub-molecular level of the living matter, regarding its biophysical structure. Ageing is attributed to many authors, to phenomena that occur at the same basic level (cross-linkage, colloidal hysteresis errors of transmission of genetic information, even somatic mutations). For diseases studied by *Burch*, as well as some phenomena of "older age" labelled as involution phenomena, appear thus, founded explanatory, the mathematical dependence to physical time - taken as an independent variable.

Organismic development studied by *Backman* is, on the contrary, a sequence of events to another level of integration, biologically specific. Such progress, genetically programmed and equipped with cyber self-regulation is described clearer and more appropriate regarding the organic time. We can also issue an additional hypothetical interpretation: the number of mutations as mutually independent random events increases (on average) proportionally with the physical time, the "chrono-nomic" dependence being linear. It is possible that some "setbacks" with a straight aspect to physical time to express random storing of biological incidents, a constant risk. In many discussions over organic time (biological) the time of physiological events is approved with psychological time. Still, *Schopenhauer* (1851) noted that estimating the passing calendar time we do it in relation to our age (so he would be "perceived" as being ten times longer at the age of five than the age of 50). The reasoning was resumed *E.Mach* (1903) and then the *Lecomte du Nouy*, in his commentary to speed wound healing study, taken as an indicator of biological age.

Bergson (1910) admits that for inanimate matter there one time, unitary and universal, while each living organism has its own time, which not only arises after individual rules but also in non-uniform flow.

Benussi (1913) speaks about a physical and subjective time; the latter depends on the flow (apparently) of "filling" the bag of events.

Backman (1942), establishing his law of accelerating physical time in living organisms, not heeding, sufficiently, biological productivity of various time intervals of physical time, during vital cycles. Each new cycle introduces an acceleration of the body events, increasing - temporarily - biological productivity of physical time. Analog can be reported the psychological social, cultural "productivity" - the physical time units, or units of biological time. We speak of "fruitful years" or a "sterile adolescence". When "it seems" that time passes quickly or slowly (in situations where we have too many to-dos or when we anxiously wait), that assessment is made in relation to the standards of "productivity". When we appreciate the time that has passed, we add criteria related to achievements and hopes fulfilled or not, the favourable or unfavourable character of situations, etc. An accurate assessment of the variation with age, regarding the psychological flow of time, is difficult. Short intervals tend to be judged in relation to physiological rhythms (i.e., Pulse rate), thus introducing an additional dependency, secondary to organic time. It is assumed that the "inner metronome" does not accelerate with age since there were not reported any difficulties of timing and tempo, at musicians of different ages. An available measure would be, possibly, the amount of information able to be "metabolized" by consciousness, in a given period of physical time, - or the quantity of information actually "metabolized". However, this amount depends on the exogenous and endogenous informational contribution (from memory), the width of the field of consciousness, the "training" as well as the "temperament".

With the progress of phylogenetics, all living beings have gained increased capacity of utilising the physical time. The increase conduction velocity in nerves, shortening reaction time, speed up metabolic processes in warm-blooded - "enrich" (virtually) with events, the time lived by the animal. *C. Wittenberger* also insisted on this aspect. However, the life experience of the species, fixed in genetic programs (including behavioural programs) as well as the individual one in ontogenesis, ensures not only effectiveness (rich reactivity), but also efficacy (goals) and efficiency (high yield). Only in this way, it achieves a high individual use (and subjective) of "objective" time; teaching, in all its forms and qualities - from infusorians to humans - means a virtual acceleration of psychological time versus physical time. Then, contrary to what *Mach* wrote, the 'second': beaten by the pendulum, seems longer now than in childhood, because between two beats of the pendulum, it can intersect and it can be serialised with more information. Thus adulthood is characterised by including it in the "chrono-biological" ontogenetic program which is characteristic for the species, which makes it dependent on the "organic time". In the same time, it is undermined, substantially and energetically, on molecular and sub-molecular level, the thermodynamics and quantum processes directly dependent on "physical time".

Cyber and information peculiarities of the psychic life make the "psychological time" to flow unevenly, whimsical but not random and it can support the organic time easements, but being able to adjust after the timing and physical model. The psyche is able to achieve an acceleration of his own time, for a better resource exploitation permits by the physical and bodily mechanisms that serve it. Thus, with the years passing by, productivity (psychological, social, cultural) of physical time and organic time may increase, the adult making, virtually, a temporal densification of creativity, analogous to temporal densification of morphogenesis in early embryonic development.

Another approach to the character more or less capacious of "psychological time" starts by assessing the ability of consciousness to process a certain amount of information per unit of time. Various estimations (performed in our country by *Gh. Cartianu*, 1973) led to the conclusion that it can be processed, starting from the sensations, dozens of bits per second (although the brain receives, waking amounts to 9 orders of magnitude higher). The psychological experience of some people in the imminence of death, claiming that in a few seconds it was held in their memory a good part of their film vital, as some data on dreams, suggests that in certain conditions, the consciousness can work in unity of time, huge amounts of stored information. Such observations indicate the elasticity of "psychological time", it's exceptional virtualities.

Advantages and servitudes of the adulthood

We have shown in another chapter of this work that one of the main causes of the grown-ups' pseudo-knowledge was the confusion (rooted in the scientific thinking, and thus, in the current thinking) between "adult" and "man in general", respectively the characteristic "type" of the *Homo* species. That is why, the adult period was considered sort of atemporal, as a human "model" – and concretely "static", as a "stationary state" unlike the childhood or the old age[1] who are always seen in temporal, cinematic and even dynamically conduct (by causality, finality, motivations and conflicts). A proper understanding of adulthood involves overcoming the non-dynamic vision in its research.

In the previous chapter, it was suggested that, while pre-adult stages of life have an appointment and a biological limit (the body), subdivisions of the adulthood are to be assigned (or are constituted) by other criteria. Therefore, the adulthood study cannot be reduced to an ilikibiology (*Parhon*), a bio-morphosis or a bioreutics (*M. Burger*), but requires investigation, careful (perhaps prevailing) of a psychological, social, cultural factors.

Another methodology difficulty in the adulthood research comes from the fact that the human (and not even the human body) is not a system with a waveform "trajectory" in the sense of *V. Conta*, with an evolutionary period immediately followed by an involute period. On the other hand, adulthood cannot be considered as either a perfect age of organic homoeostasis because physiological, clinical and psychological research indicates a progressive decline (continuous regression) of some forms and functions. It is noted, however, that the phenomena of involution and decline are detected even before the end of the growing and maturing period; in fact, involution accompanies everywhere evolution since the early stages of development.

(Development has an "antinomy status" is a realisation of the dialectic of beings). Absolute chemical involution begins at puberty, but the maximum value of relative weight is reached at birth. Because of reasons whose firmness should be analysed in detail, we believe that the development of the reproductive system can find a biological criterion of the development of the body in general - but the human being presents, from this point of view, remarkable particularities, for example, menopause preceding decades' of (virtual) "physiological" age limit of human life. The great psycho-nervous development in humans would require a good biological thinking at shifting the focus to another source of searchable criteria. However, the "status," particularly of adulthood among the stages of human life, requires us to use a combination of methods unique to the study of growth, and development of unique methods of the study of the phenomena of involution, aging, and decline, as well as suitable methods of studying homeostatic processes.

The meaning of human life is not found in the biological sphere of the human species but the scope of its psychological, social and cultural activities. The psychological, social and cultural evolution and involution can be traced from subjective or objective platforms. In the first platform it could be distinguished (by *Erikson*): a young adult (20-34 years), characterized by the desire for privacy (and its realization); an adult age (up to 44 years), characterized by productivity, creativity, acceptance of responsibility for genitors then, the age of maturity, characterized by deeper integration of the ego, which begin to manifest some "psychological symptoms of old age". The times of "crisis" are now moments of the final stages, the confrontation of reality with the ideal of life. Such a time of "crisis" was immortalized by *H. de Balzac* in his novel "The Woman In Thirty Years".

It is worth mentioning that *I. Haţieganu* between 1930-1940 (hence a century after *Balzac*) described in his patients who were around that age, neuro-vegetative (and hormonal) disorders without gravity, proposing - for this clinical picture - the name of *Balzac`s syndrome*.

---

[1] *By J. Zeman (1958) information condenses, thanks to memory, so that will appeal to a logarithmic time, gnosiological time. If we have increasing amounts of information in successive identical units of physical time, we can talk about time dilation. Zeman also uses the model "dynamically time" (Milne) and refers to the density of the events as a speed equivalent.*

From the objective platform of achievements, activity, initiative, *Charlotte Buhler*, has admitted the succession of phases: growth (up to 25 years), mature (up to 45 years) and decline. Maturity could be regarded as stable growth (not progressive), the changes are offset deficits are covered. The decline is the period of "regressive" growth where the regenerative power of tissues is exhausted. However, the Genesis aspect (and regeneration capacity) admits a periodization with other time limits (from this point of view the decline is set to 50-55 years). On the psychosocial level, the accumulation of external events are divided into the following successive stages: the rapid growth of growing less rapidly, landing, decline; but the decline still stands here late (from 63-68 years) and this phase extension is probably due to an intellectual compensation of faculties in biological decline. Incidentally, in sports, the culmination is even more delayed as the sports variant relies less on purely physical capabilities. As with aging, wishes are decreasing, and the sense of duty is increasing.

It is a phenomenon of "transfer of dominance"; who was privileged to work at a certain time hides behind another less selfish. The highlight of life measured in the complex, through its fecundity on a family, work, cultural level, etc. it is generally up to 48 years. From 45-50 years we can speak of "negative acquisitions"; Economic and body losses occur (such as surgical ablation) irrecoverable loss of parents and friends; in many cases, we meet professional and home changes as difficult attempts of "re-cutting" of life. The individual becomes more introspective, sometimes lonely, sometimes philanthropist. Decreasing social dimensions begins only at 63 ~ 68 years, with a preference for entertainment (and not for business), possibly for rural life and cult of the dead.

The second part of human existence was recently analyzed and *Linden* and *Courtney*. Following these authors, maturity is a "most efficient organization of experience." The young are looking for particularly rewarding selfish impulses; the mature or older adult seeks to dominate, thanks, to culture (social environment characteristic respectively). The authors call evolescence the lifetime where development takes place using natural growth (it would end in 30 years). Subsequently, development continued by other means. At the same time, there are changes in the way of resolving conflicts. The evolescence – as the senescence[2] – do not go without critical "interruptions." One marks the reorientation from development to compensation, or that the effective compensation to the poor. Senescence reaches senility, and this word means a return possibly eruptive author, domination instincts.

Involution and damage are not evolution "inside" of what was purchased before; not lost in reverse order; Some purchases are final; persistent alterations occur (and not only regressions), compensation, etc. The decline in mental life is the expression of wear and damage brain mechanisms that make up the infrastructure of psychic life. However, it is not rare that confusion is created, as in respect of interests between decline and refocusing it. Regarding behavior, as also in the interests, concerns, attitudes, costumes there are "age rules" imposed by society. The individual can have, therefore, the impression that during his life he walks through final turns and as such, there would be "the last opportunity" to do this or that. *J. Stoetzel* notes that at 35 years, many women feel too old to get married; at 55 years a man gets too old to believe for social promotion, and at 20 years a student can be considered no longer young enough to deeper mathematics. However, these "norms" vary from one social environment to another; they are changing through the course of history, and strong personalities dare and manage to face. At 80 years, *Michel Angelo* he began studying Greek. I recalled the book of *W. Pitkin* (book well thought) *Life begins at 40 years.* In fact, for many - a life of achievement and satisfaction may start even

---

[2] *Regarding this, it was argued that the central nervous system itself involutes since adolescence because there are massive constant losses of neurons. To this, they have answered with a hypothesis in which the numeric and mass neurological losses can be seen as a progressive structuralization of the neuraxis, just like marble losses are mandatory when creating a statue. Regarding the observation in which memory loss starts with the first youth, it was answered with the variation of memory types, from which some develop for many decades.*

later. In fact, in linguistic expressions relating to age and aging, the resultant conventions and ideas submitted, we find the source of many prejudices. After *Techniczeck* the psychological age is given by the measure of psychological adaptability; Sociological age is expressed by how the individual meets its social obligations. I remembered that after *Galtung, Fr.Mahler*, and others, age is presented in a sociological point of view, as a decrease of options for a specific "role." The 'essential' options are made in youth, or before. Add that traditional societies granted a certain social status during each elderly stage. Sociological age would have many components, including grip and externalization (through behavior) of a social status.

We believe that the psycho-sociology of age is a complex area, infinitely more complex and our contribution of today is trying to suggest some coordinated from an interdisciplinary perspective. We feel that the mental age is not the reflex of biological age, but the social age. Social age does not take so much of the choices that were made, but how the attitudinal factors matter. Attitudes towards social ideals and models proposed to requirements, obligations, responsibilities, and constraints; towards their option, their role, and status; to his own personality; to immediate and mediated social environments - structures (evolutionary, rigidifying or involutely) person. It again appears the usefulness of the axiological age concept proposed to refer situations in terms of spiritual dominance. If biological involution, the 'closure' of mental configuration or "monopolistic" tendencies of social status do not receive a compensating riposte, springs from a combative attitude towards them, the person is likely to undergo senescence early and accelerated whose etiology should be placed rather, in the spiritual sector than the physical one. At the same time are firmly demanded: the tendency of becoming against homeostasis tendency: the trend of overcompensation, of "good use of disease" (*Pascal*) and of complexes (*C.G. Jung*) against the line of a minimum resistance, of demobilization, and impoverishment of personal life.

In the same style, we draw attention to an aspect capable of generating an optimistic correlation. The first part of life "wave" knows - physically – an endogenous programming determinism, fatal to the extent that depends on natural laws, biological, laws beyond our control (which can, however, be used, for example, medical, to influence the course of ontogeny).

Moreover, on a psycho-social level, like education and schooling, it is socioculturally scheduled beyond the control of child growth and development. We cannot choose as individuals in regards to the date on which the premolars appear nor regarding the date on which we get vaccinated or go to school. Adulthood is not essentially biological or social-cultural programmed. Circumstantial factors, or random, or personal decision - play a decisive role. This affirmation is particularly the case as we stand in the context of a more developed society, as an organization, in politics or as a culture We are increasing largely free to choose the tempo and mode of aging, not only cultural, social and psychological, but also biological; the way to travel in adulthood.

Another new characteristic for the psycho-sociological model of "adulthood" that we propose is the coexistence of different ages (and even both the sexual polarization) within the same individual. The idea that maturity must exclude childhood from us seems wrong even from a biological and ethological point of view because the species *Homo* appears as a neoteny species (pedogenetic), resulting in a phylogenetic process of "fetalization" *(Bolk)* and the long childhood compels parents (even for their own good!) to maintain of infantile traits *(G. Echeim).* The "infantile type" curiosity and the ability to wonder were seen as levers of scientific investigation. But not only reactivity (*Homo Ludens*) or childish or adolescent fantasy type persist into adult life, but also the aspirations and ideals (as such or transfigured) the adult life being the time of effectively achieving some of them.

The biosocial status of man, on the other hand, is not incompatible with some feminine "softness." According to some axioms of "*transactional* psychology" *(E. Berne),* in every person coexists the psychic of a child, adult and parent, the interactions between people is "the result of" interactions between these components.

It is necessary to recognize the relative autonomy of the different sides of evolution and involution of the human being. The curve of evolution must distinguish: the growth, differentiation, development; maturing, simple memorial acquisition (learning), *mimesis*. You must know how to make a distinction between what is happening standardized, such as teething, what leads to customization (idiosyncratic), such as an unusual biographical event. In this way, we can understand, for example, why some adult may have a well-developed body with a remarkable abstract intelligence, but immature emotionally and with some complex (inferiority, etc.) that it decreases the allowance yield. A young "soul" may dwell in a worn body. However, if the different sides of the individual have an involution and evolutive relative autonomy, they interact functionally. A fundamental question is of mutual repercussion of ages; calendar, biological, psychological, social (age).

A specific dependency of calendar age, meaning the measure of time physic astronomical would be expected only in the phasic processes dependent on the sequence of seasons, like the rings of a tree trunk, and with a programming determinism strictly physical-chemical. It has been talked about "biological clocks" - but less about the biological calendars. Comparative research of the evolescence phase and the subsequent ones makes us think that in the past, there are gerontology and pathological phenomena of nature whose occurrence is a function of physical time; *Burch* 's mathematized data advocate random nature of some autoimmune diseases and signs of aging (tooth loss, the appearance of white hair). In other words, if the first part of the curve of life occurs during physical in a determinist way - the second part comes not only probabilistic but also at random.

The social importance of the calendar generates another addiction (of "normative" order) to conduct a person's life, of physical and astronomical time. The social status of age, in civilized societies, is established after the calendar year, not the biological age, virtually impossible to determine. The "procrustean" coefficient, in this case, is mitigated through medical exams. Non-literal societies, marked the beginning stages of age were not only social occasion of celebrations, but also the result of the successful passing some ad hoc trials or some initiation rites. A known "prestige" of figures 5,7 and 10 suggested dividing the stages of human life linked to specific calendar age. Lately, it has sought to justify such astrophysical phenomena periodization by more or less regular, such as solar activity. Comparative study of biographies, genuine or apocryphal, seems to bring out the "fateful" ages, such as 33 or 29 years for men, suggesting the "critical" period of the adult life.

Attitude towards the calendar ages with numerological significance has consequences on the organization of psychosocial life as the biological life (by psychosomatic effect and self-suggestion). The body's biological age is a result of biological age that characterizes subunits integrated into the body; the physiological ages of organs and tissues; biochemical ages etc. From a certain point of view, it expresses the rate of wear of the body, which increases its vulnerability. The body deficiencies are highlighted by the chart performance of low functional organs (with decreases linear or exponential function after power). The accumulation of waste products correspond to linear or exponential growth; increased vulnerability manifests itself through exponential growth, age, mortality rate (the law of *Gompertz*) and increasing (by parabolic function or power functions) causes some mortality (e.g., by certain diseases). In addition to functional impairment phenomena peak performance of youth, biological age is marked by phenomena of decreased homeostatic capabilities, which manifests itself in stressful situations. The deficit functional organs, seen in isolation, making them more vulnerable and finite: hence limiting progressive resistance exercise and the "excess." The decrease of homeostatic capacities is a lack of integration and body control, hence limiting the progressive assumption of unbalancing, adaptability to new conditions of life; eventually, syndromes can be shaped in "Biocybernetics" essence which *Merloo* called with a suggestive term, "cybernosis."

Naturally, the body's homeostatic capabilities are based on functional compensation of organic deficiencies. The body is built on the principle of morphofunctional surplus (reserve), the "redundancy" of biological material, such as a decrease in functional capacity of organs, brought to light by special laboratory samples, there can be no echo in the daily life of the individual, held in average or reduced request parameters. Is not what decreases performance vital, but vitality is (*Peatniţchi*). Compensation is an Intra organismic adjustment to poor and declining deviations. As a result, the compensation function that can provide the appropriate level or from a lower level to a higher level: in the latter case we are talking about over-compensation. For the first time, the phenomenon has been described in detail by *Alfred Adler*, the early twentieth century, the works - classical remaining - the organ inferiority (meiopragie). However, in the analyzed cases by *A. Adler*, overcompensation riposte was produced by the intervention of personality through a conscious attitude and persevering through an exercise (and ambitious) - and not by inner visceral automatism. Thus, small refractive defects can cause a sharpening of visual perception, speech defects small, defeated, are found in the biography of speakers; a degree of deafness can contribute to the encouragement of music, etc. *A. Adler* was referring primarily to teenagers and younger children but - *mutatis mutandis* - the principle is applicable to meiopragie of age.

Compensation may, therefore, be made after the plan strictly various anatomic and physiological principles on the psycho-organic plan, the plan personality, etc. Decreased physical force may be offset by a "tactic" superior movements; what is lost in the area may lead to a gain in depth etc. If you cannot always talk about the advantages of decline (or involution, the "degeneration" - *Gino Lombroso*) can almost always talk about good or bad about the use of things, including good use of disease.

Embrittlement organic disease even requires a restructuring of how to live with and time-saving forces with a physical restriction of energy waste; lead to a more accurate assessment of ourselves body and an enhanced based care for it; Switching to concerns, for the cultural sphere, in fact, specific human sphere. Accidents morbid (mild or moderate) of adult life have scored more than once among the causes of fertile turns from culturally and spiritually.

It is stressed on this occasion that vitality can be trained - so what *Peatniţchi* called (1969) "regulator vitality type" and what by the same author, it denotes vitality "tolerant type." The concept of *Peatniţchi* falls from this point of view, at the opposite conception of *H. Selye*, after which everyone is born with a fixed amount of "adaptation energy" each of which consumes one hand stress. As for us, we consider that stress "moderate" followed by conditions that favor the restoration, is the very condition of maintaining vitality.

It noted that some organs reduced their functional activity to the needs of the entire lower body in living conditions "artificialized" monotonous routine, the operation (i.e., request) and maintained the vitality of organs. So dropping those capabilities, is not only the result of cellular deterioration and loss (damage "structural"). There is an interdependence between organs that and say. Also, intervene and deficits regulating organs and functions. The passage of time brings damage to organs, but also a certain workout which means better control and greater biological effectiveness (part of the damage is compensated thanks to some good adjustments and a proper training). If a large part of the young human performance is a performance to adapt to the outside world, in human adults and elderly, they are increasingly directed towards offsetting losses, injuries, metabolic and functional disorders. Therefore, one cannot equate the anatomic changes of an organ or disease - which is a situation of inadequacy to the requirements of everyday life. Therefore, the study of capacity ("resilience") adaptive effectiveness and timeliness adjustments must be taken into account when deciding on "biological age." For the same reason it is important physiological functions training (of course, avoiding excesses systematic training, ex. Gymnastics). It is advisable, therefore, quenching; is dangerous life taken too rigid habits and stereotypes that narrow the range adaptive. It is to avoid "veil" not to be confused with the necessary protection of a fragile body. It is understood - in the light of the written above - and it is precisely why functions often employed age later: are functions involved. It is also understood why the professional capacity of older adults can be maintained despite a general deterioration. Moreover, detailed physiological and psychological research has shown that the progress that can be achieved through exercise and workout sometimes masking age changes. Decreasing adaptability caused by lack of exercise may be more serious than predicted age. Once again we emphasize that living organism is born with a fixed amount, limited to "adaptation energy" that spends a living. The role of lifestyle is overwhelming. It was also revealed (*D. Postelnicu*) that some adjustment processes may improve after 40 years, exemplified by neuropsychological aspects (e.g., Some neurasthenia heal with age; social adaptability improves to the brink of old age). Not all bodies are "aging" in the same tempo and pace. This idea is today a scientific conclusion; but as intuition or speculative conclusion, we find authors and older. Asynchronous aging ("heterochromia") is studied by *C.A. Philites* early nineteenth century and is postulated by *C.F. Constant* in his treatise in 1839. Recently, it insisted that the development of different organs is not proportional (or isometric, but allometric) - resulting acyl imbalances characteristic. Studies by *V.V. Frolkis* led him to the view that with increasing age, lower influences on nerve tissue; instead increase their sensitivity to humoral factors (and hormonal). In other words, the minimum dose required to produce response decreases; which does not mean that it would increase "reactivity" (answers are usually smaller). The nerve centers would weaken the connections between neurons but would increase sensitivity to humoral factors. Command and weakening influences nerve stimulation on the endocrine glands; their secretory activity decreases as well; increasing the sensitivity of tissues to hormones compensation would be an example of the situation presented. *Șt. Milcu* stressed that regresses asynchronous endocrine glands. Moreover, for many hormones secreting glands, there is a change in the balance between them. Thus, secretion of adrenal hormones by changing the ratio between anabolic and catabolic.

A faithful interpretation of "differentiated" biological phenomena after three aspects of matter (substance, energy, and information), there were identified (1962, 1969) different ways of organismic aging for an individual: through injuries (e.g. Atheromatous, sclerosis); functional energy deficiency; adjustment disorders (the "cybernosis").

Restructuring bio-organisms occurs during adulthood, sometimes very obvious by changing the constitutional type. How often is this phenomenon? Systematic studies are few. *P. Ramneantu* (1973) who researched somatotypes in a relatively isolated area of the Apuseni Mountains revisiting the population within 33 years, concludes that the somatotypes do not change with age. Individuals with micro splanchnic or brevilineal type asthenic, a slight deposition of fat around the age of 40 years, but after 5-10 years return to the previous conformation. Towards the age of 50, all somatotypes become more flexible, except micro splanchnic bracing (called "chondroblast"), which remained rather slim. Brevitype asthenic type individuals accumulate fat but not exceeding 10% (compared to standard weight). In these cases, we can identify a genetic component (or family). At 60 years of age (or older), both sexes show a tendency to lose weight probably dehydration. *P. Ramneantu* notes, however, that the population studied was formerly chronically undernourished.

In 1973 *Maria-Elena Rosca Gramatopol-* researched aspects of change with age of sexual dimorphism in a rural population in Maramures County; collected data (from a cross-cutting research) would be suitable for a constitutionalist type processing, which is to be made.

Dan-Cristian Popescu in 1973 presented but longitudinal observations (urban environment) showing net type transformation chirotope (weight evenly distributed, including limbs) in a "somatotrope" type (storage truncal), even weight control. It is plausible percent increase fat.

* * *

In connection with the biological aspects of growing older, adulthood can be described in a proper medical point of view. From this point of view, the passing years could be characterized by increasing ailments and disease by increasing severity, the association of several diseases, by hindering of recovery, with increased risk of complications and chronic through an attendance thickest of medical offices by an increased consumption of the product. Attitude to health and disease is gradually changing. For their own health care reaches an increasingly important concern. Rest, relaxation - are increasingly preferred blood, effort, activity. Some diseases are especially common in elderly adults: atherosclerosis, coronary arterial hypertension, glaucoma, autoimmune diseases, chronic bronchitis (especially tobacco), spondylosis, prostate adenoma. Cancer is not a disease of old age such as the period that precedes old age. The causes of cancer are still at less than those of atherosclerosis: some cancers are related to endocrine imbalances, chronic local irritation, etc. Hormone-dependent cancers in adulthood and old age, are, for example, the breast, the uterus, the prostate. According to some theories, cancer - to a point - is a process of clearing regenerative failed by anarchy and atypical proliferating cells.

The above considerations allow us to understand why the passing years, age is not a process that all individuals act exactly the same species and we refer not only to the identity of tempo, but also the mechanisms and manifestations. In general, it can be said that adults and older adults are more different from one another than younger people. Diversify his "life experience" and vicissitudes of life, customs, and professions, as well as diseases. Diversify its clearing capabilities that are equal.

There are differences by gender in the phenomena under discussion (and longevity). Gender is biological in nature; but in humans, gender is also an element of social differentiation - in the occupations, clothing, etc. It seems that, biologically, women are more vigorous than the male; gender "weak" is actually a stronger gender in most species studied, the male has a shorter life than the woman. In humans, morbidity and longevity vary by gender - not only in terms of biological endowment but also in terms of historical, socio-economic, and cultural. Aging faster and shorter life of the woman shows primitive social relationships, a low level of civilization and economic misery. In general, women are more often sick than man, but man suffers more frequently from serious diseases. The average lifespan is now higher in women in most countries, but the process of senescence often installs faster in women than in men; especially during and after climacteric, aging can mutate rapidly. It is also the time when women begin to suffer their illnesses hitherto characteristic of men (as atherosclerosis, myocardial infarction, and hypertension).

Climacteric is a period otherwise arising in the two genders. The woman stops menstruating (menopause) and the ability to have more children (fertility); often during the transition to other endocrine balance, women complain of neurodegenerative and mental disorders. Male genital function decline is gradual, procreation ability is maintained longer; subjective and objective accompanying disorders are rare. The wrong opinion after menopause causes aging; soon it might say that the closure is a measure procreative function sparing the body is no longer so young and who would bear heavier load applications. Women freed from servitude procreation are not necessarily someone who has lost femininity. In any case, it has released energy for family and social benefits. In many cases, menopause achieves a favorable turning point in the life of a woman, a true psychosocial maturation. Prejudice then vitality and value of a human person are expressed by what is happening in the strictly biological sphere - and especially sexuality creates countless complex, mature individuals approaching climacteric or passes through this stage. In reality - beyond the climacteric (and even in the absence of sexual vigor) there is a long string of years in which man is capable of staying active and socially valuable and capable of providing satisfying and varied thanks. For the people of intellectual labor, old age begins today across (or beyond) sixty years. With these considerations, we approached but psychological and social aspects of adulthood. Changes in adulthood of the human psyche were seen from several points of view: the performance of some "mental functions," isolated the overall performance efficiency (e.g. creativity); as manifestations of character; that mentality changes; less problematic mind that changes as changes of attitude and that restructuring. Characteristic of the first view is researching intelligence. Authors who have dealt especially this (as *J.L. Horn*, 1967) appeal to the distinction between intelligence fluid intelligence crystallized and these types are affected uneven ripening of acculturation and altering database physiological (brain) alteration once the age, stress injuries. The physiological basis is declining exponentially (auto-attenuated) since childhood, a trend which is almost symmetric gain the cultural (acculturation). Maturation (ripening), reached late teens, entered a slow decline curve; a similar curve, but with a more pronounced downward slope, describes fluid intelligence. Instead, crystallized intelligence is continuously growing and is not capped (the author claims) than in older age.

Regarding creativity, some references were made in another chapter. In one of his works, *Al. Rosca* (1972) cites data by *H.C. Lehman, W. Denis, Hilgard* and *Atkinson* et al. There are (statistically speaking) ages that are a favorable performance in certain areas. Naturally, sporting activities, the highest frequency performance is superior early (25-29); after 44 years, the frequency is very rare for some sports, although - for shooting and pool, many champions have won major titles after 44 years: are sports that call for greater precision than the strength (or resistance physics). Superior performance in chess has a maximum frequency around 33 years; the decline was very limited until the age of 50 years. In science, literature, and art, productivity begins before age 30 years and continues after 40 years. The maximum frequency is important contributions to various sectors, the following:

1. 25-30 years old – chemistry, lyrical poetry, instrumental music;
2. 30-35 years old – mathematics, physics, practical inventions, technical surgery, botanicals, satirical poetry, comedy, symphonies, oil painting;
3. 35-40 years old – geology, astronomy, bacteriology, physiology, medical discoveries, logics, ethics, aesthetics, pedagogy, general philosophy, camera music, opera, sculpture;
4. 30-40 years old – genetics, entomology, psychology, economic and political sciences;
5. 40-45 years old – operetta, cantata, musical, novels, best sellers, modern architecture, contemporary oil painting;
6. 35-45 years old – social philosophy;
7. 50-70 years old – political and military leaders.

After *Ch. Bühler*, performance early creative are the sectors where needed vitality rather than experience (poets, mathematicians, athletes); the maturity (inventors, explorers, business) need maximum social opportunities; those with successful experience delayed require - (scientists, philosophers, politicians). A graph (*Lehman*) of the age distribution of 359 higher contributions in the sciences, mathematics, and invention shows a maximum frequency around the age of 33, after 80 years and continuing productivity. It presents the same maximum and distribution by age, of the 1086 patents for inventions made by *Th. Edison* (*A. Anastasi*, 1938). After *Lehman*, aged productivity decline is explained by factors such as reduced flexibility, the decline in physical vigor in sensory acuity and health. Also, changes in motivation, because of external circumstances (family responsibilities, financial difficulties, etc.).

In some cases, with increasing prestige, grow and tasks of an administrative nature, which reduces the time devoted to their creation. However, promotions in a leadership position usually multiply the number of virtual and actual collaborators. Personal research showed that, for the scientific work of *N. Iorga*, maximizing productivity falls at the age of 44 years. For *C.I.*

Parhon, a first maximum score earlier, but the number of certificates signed up again when becoming head of the department and director of the Institute.

Al. Rosca cites cases of late manifestation of creative skills, which however is not independent studies and deepened concerns persevering in manifest creativity. Also, there have also been no provisions for those skills. *J.J. Rousseau* wrote his first important work at 38 years of age, Russian writer *Aksakov* began writing at 56, *Cervantes wrote Don Quijote* at 58-68 years old. *Milton* wrote *Paradise Lost* at 57 years, and *Paradise Found* at 62 years. *Mark Twain* was 71 years old when he wrote the *Eve`s Diary* and *The $30,000 Bequest*. *Graham Bell* perfected the phone at 58 years. Created masterpieces in old age *Goethe* and *Verdi* (which, however, were said "in" or "out of" youth. *Verdi`s* most productive years are between 25 and 45 years).

The relationship between age and creativity meet contradictory aspects. Some authors wonder how it is possible, so late manifestation of creativity: *Lawton* brings as argument the thesis after which constructive imagination does not follow memory decline and other mental functions that decrease with age. Others, however, question why creativity decreases with age. *F.A. Osborn* criminalizes emphasizing the role of skills, which tend to make a more rigid approach to problems. *D.C. Peltz* and *F.M. Andrews* notes that specialization sided hampers creativity (what happens and if a greater diversification). The authors of the most productive are those with a moderate diversity in content scientific activity; *Al. Rosca* deemed advisable regular change of field research. By *W. Dennis*, a high scientific productivity to higher ages are found in those who started early to be more productive, as the eminent scientists, even if this was achieved eminence itself later. Of course, it should not be ignored dependence creativity of organizing life, "the methodology of the daily lives," as shown, for example, the analysis of painter`s diary, *E. Delacroix*. Creativity is largely a role of "permanent self-education"; the last issue (especially regarding sociology) was dealt in our country by *Leon Țopa*.

It should not be ignored any typological difference between individuals. The early twentieth century, *W. Ustwald*, parallel research dealing with biographies of great physicists and chemists, distinguished scholar romantic guy, with outstanding performance in his youth - and a classic, performing-maturity. The first is exhausted, often quite rapidly; last, retain creativity through the years. The differences between these types concern, however, especially in their style and creative scientific work.

H. Thomas proposed (1970) cognitive theory of personality and its development. This theory is based on three postulates:

1. Perception of change rather than the change may be related to behavior change;
2. Any change in the situation the individual is perceived and evaluated in terms of the individual's dominant concerns and expectations;
3. Adjustment, the passing years is a function of the balance between the cognitive and motivational structure of the individual. Passing years (aging), as a system of processes is either a system for maintaining this balance, or a system to reconstruct (restore) this balance. The balance can be achieved either by restructuring goals cognitive schemas that define "desirable" or "fulfilled" either by continuing the work. Cognitive restructuring is possible, sometimes through self-essential extension is "self-concept" (which in current terms, can be expressed as "opinion of himself"). Maintaining this self-concept is a homeostatic process or compensation, which requires a sustained effort. Balance to which we refer is essentially unstable. But in this case we believe we can distinguish different than those of her once-satisfied themselves of the eternal dissatisfied with himself by demanding Autoconstruct, of the discontent that did not correspond to improper aspirations etc. *H. Thomas* argues that some of the negative attitudes of the elderly towards younger generation come from continuous confrontation with the "stereotype" it (*Lehr* and *Merker*, 1969). In a society focused on youth, such confrontations can be stimulating, but also painful.

Havighurst K.J. (1968), concerning the passing of the years all of a socio-cultural perspective, put the same emphasis on restructuring (continued) adaptive. Suitability (fitness) you are asking performed for "aging" success is between personality, social environment, physical body. Matching is maximized when the personality is strong but flexible when the social environment is supportive, and when the body is vigorous. Adapting process parameters are, therefore: personality, social interaction, norms and expectations "sub-culture" in which the person lives; economic security, health and vigor, social provisions to support adaptation. It should not be forgotten the meaning of "life`s history," the biography. It can be said that everyone adapts to present them regarding their history. Passing years do not follow, therefore, standardized, but we can talk about ways (patterns) of "aging" (*B. Neugar,* 1964). Some authors go even further, saying that the deployment mature and postmature life is not standardized, it is idiosyncratic.

Mandelbaura D.G. (1973) draws attention to the interest of the anthropological study of biographies (Life Histories). Anthropologists have studied almost exclusively the life cycle stages (of life passage), with emphasis on events and "rites of passage" (*Van Gennep*), meaning ways of socialization and enculturation of young people, to make them useful members of the community. The comparative study of these events and habits left apart dynamic and adaptive aspects of life experience, relationships between one step and the next life, personal experience relevant to social institutions, the impact of personal choice, etc. Taking the example illustrating the life of *Gandhi, Mandelbaum* differs:

a) dimensions (biological, cultural, psychosocial);

b) twists and major transitions, the person will assume new roles, enter into other social relationships, acquires a new conception of itself;

c) adjustments (continuous adjustments and adaptations periodic changes in order to ensure continuity).

Havighurst R.J. (1971) stresses the importance of interactions change the meaning of social mobility: the passage of a class (or strata), the family he was born in another. We will emphasize again that the coordinated design of individual lifetime is not only age but at some concrete historical time. Ten years in the period 1960-1970 are not equivalent to ten years of a century ago.

Topa L. concerned about the issue of permanent education finds that "Teaching adults is (barely) in *status nascendi* "and "deplore the fact that too few psychologists are aimed at training human experimental studies from early childhood to old age" if we exclude species of novels called by Germans *Bildungsroman*. Method "life history" (socio-biography) was used far too little.

By *H. Hubert* (1961) is useful to distinguish between young adult (18-25), access to adult life, they obtain a professional qualification, or proper (if the young man became a student) is "set" jump on methods learning. From the point of view psychosocial, he enjoys an almost unlimited personal freedom. Widen social contacts; emotional fixations occur, it outlines socio-political activity, begins to act in full "school of life." Intellectual interests tend to stabilize. Generosity is a frequent note. Dreams and aspirations are alive and strong.

Moers M. (1964) wrote, for pedagogical lexicon, an adult "periodontology." For this author, until the age of 30 skills and performance stated "boisterous and colorful." Only between 31-40 years can speak of a consolidation, with a maximum capacity of organized labor, with a tendency towards activities targeted sewage, certainly shares with the balance between plan and execution. Between 41-58 years, actions are directed to maintain the conquered positions. "Crises" that appear in this period (in some respects, similar to those in puberty) are focused on the struggle between the ideals of youth and experience in social and intimate life. After 60 years there is a soothing, sometimes a heightened sense of life, sometimes a restructuring, often slowing of physiological processes and soul.

K. Gardini, which he considered the old adaptation to educational processes, recommended up to 30 years, the joint work and demonstration. Adult between 31 and 50 years of special interest (only) what experience does not contradict its work. Therefore, the successes are the "free unions" on professions, jobs, concrete problems. Concrete details are more popular than "things in themselves." The advantage is the action of universal interest. After 50 years only, it appears (or it reappears) desire (and even a "euphoria") theoretical knowledge, the thirst for understanding the "meaning of life."

J.A. Simpson (1964), predicting an "androgen" as a complement pedagogy recognizes Impressionist and too general character of such periodizations. Schooling previous profession, variations in environmental conditions determined motivation and aspiration. (We cannot forget, we believe, the differences in temperament, character, type "theory" is hungry for solutions philosophical or abstract, throughout life.) *Simpson* notes that the success of a program of adult education depends largely on the way in which we can link the prospect of going beyond personal performance.

Henz H. (1964) argues that beyond puberty, teaching methods are recommended: Method "ascetic" (by *L. Topa* method conscious discipline, self-control, and self-education) method, integrative method "existential" and restructuring method.

E.L. Thorndike, who researched (1927) learning problem in adults indicated, as the height, age 25-26 years and claimed that "*no one who had exceeded the age of 45, would have to refrain from learning something, fear or belief that is too old to do it.*" Psychologists today believe only in 60 years becomes sharp fall intellectual level, the effect is considerably instruction. Among those optimistic about the development opportunities of adults cite *Urbanezyk, Zewzuk, Anamiev B.G.* (1969*), Pacaud,* etc. *Leon Topa* stresses that in order to ensure a proper efficiency in teaching adult education system must have youth some formative and informative structure.

The adult must cope options, tasks, encumbrances, frustrations, losses, accidents, incidents, changes, Exam (literally and figuratively), competitions, etc. The way they are reflected in different levels of the person, on its different "sizes," is highly variable. A study of "anthropology full" of this problem must include, in our view, sufficient self-examination, retrospective and topical ("live"), of relevance not only phenomenological but abysmal (psychotherapy). Method completed questionnaires, and surveys required biographical method (biography is much more than a history) and the autobiographical biographical method ("idiographic" method should be detailed, so by including "egologic" methods).

Among the decisive events of adult life, capable of having meanings biological, medical, psychological, social, economic, cultural and axiological - mention that marriage (option conjugal), childbirth (Option parents create tasks spanning two decades), divorce loss of close relatives and friends, change (home, profession, lifestyle, social regime), economic ruin; disease with serious sequelae; war. The transition to a sedentary life, like a birth (female) can lead to obesity. Promotion to a management position, endowed with privileges, can result in Axiological turning toward conservatism, the rigidity of manners, closing intellectual solidarity with elderly people (so a true "aging" inside). A religious or philosophical conversion may change family regime and food (vegetarian, etc.), as in the famous case of *L. Tolstoy*. It would be of great interest to change research complex hierarchy of values related to life events, so those able to influence and those arising as consequences of such changes. All these events generate emotional problems. *By L. Yockelson* (1969) the main challenges related to age beyond 40 years are focused on prospect or reality of loss. Losses ("negative acquisitions") occur more frequently from 48 years before, economic, plant and equipment (surgical ablations), people (parents, friends).

1. adult logic exploration difficulties were expressed, for example, in our research, in that investigation of 130 sheets, which ordered a brief retrospective of 25 years of the professional life of a peer group of graduates (physicians) with enforcement of anonymity, were returned only fifteen!
2. I just recently talked about axosomatic diseases; *V. Frankl* described neologisms

neurosis etc.

Out of all these losses, the loss of an ideal, and especially ideal image of himself plays an important role. The author draws attention to the cases which, in this picture, among many ingredients juvenile appearance. An equally important role lies with the infantile ideal of happiness. Happiness is not a "chronic state of contentment and joy, a condition that once reached, automatically eliminates all the problems and frustrations. Happiness is (but) a co-product of effort, rather than its target." *Yockelson* notes and recommended a hygienic shift from trying to reach our desires, the desire to do what we can. A genetics and biochemistry satisfactory condition, like philosophy (wisdom) and luck, are the ingredients of a productive life and continuous self-development - "targets" a reasonably mature age. Homeostasis "image" of himself (on which insisted *Murphy, Rogers*, etc.) seems to be rather an attempt to maintain a positive balance (according to the theory of *Thomas*) by homologous compensation, analog or nonspecific than adherence to a fixed frame, a retrospective narcissism. The process includes valuation "gains" and positive redefinition of "losses."

For *G. Murphy*, "life is largely an effort to preserve a self-portrait. A major aspect of the conflict can be difficult to maintain an (auto)-image desirable from pressures of all sorts, or the difficulty of deciding between two pictures." Portrait mutilation is worse than injury or damage to the person felt. Redefining autistic ego means (i.e., interpreting distorted reality, according to our desires) is a means of defending the current "self-portrait." *G.R. Rogers* aims aligns person with self-image. Replacing a "component" old picture of him with another is not always done gradually, imperceptibly. Sometimes the process is not a simple substitution with restructuring but includes position papers, attitudes more or less critical.

A frequent attitude is an exaltation of individuality pride, overrated, personality details, including dates of decline deficiencies. It is an attitude of social danger when it falls on the collective leaders etc. A dangerous attitude directly hue is a masochistic person, complacency and declining in regressive metamorphosis. Specifically, it may result in denial of their own health care by adopting dress and way of life of "old person" by withdrawing into a shell with few social contacts through disengagement. There rarely are interwoven shades sadistic behavior this way it is a system of moral pressure (or imposing encumbrances) by a close person, possibly envy. Total refusal of life (not just declarative) is part of a depressive syndrome.

"Philosophy" is pessimistic, however, more benign. Obsession fearful about the aging phenomena not only lead to issues phobic, all unnecessary, self-centred, selfish - but also issues of Contra-phobia with behavior that the individual wants to prove (or demonstrate) that is young: for example, with excessive exercise and strenuous activity with an erotic and sexual.

Routines evade life by changing the dwelling, city, occupation, family background, etc. It is relatively frequent. Relatively frequently, it leads to imbalances - and only rarely to "rejuvenate." The significance of such windings is not uniform. Sometimes the outbreak of protest?! Sometimes - highlighting some aspects of personality, excessive hitherto neglected (for example, with "valve" a hobby). An attitude that is worth mentioning is the transfer procreative: the person becomes "father" or "mother" in the hope that their children will achieve the goals that they themselves have not been able to achieve. Consolation is one of the "healthy" attitudes if combined with an active resignation. Restructuring conscious personality, regrouping forces and reconsider realistic goals - not an "act" easy to execute, but a process that requires not only willingness and goodwill but also scientific knowledge, as a profound self-knowledge (possibly through exploration abysmal). *C.G. Jung* was one of those who looked at from this point of view, dialectical development of personality. For *Jung*, the contradictions of life vanish if we get a broader horizon by adopting new ways of life. Personality development is a fulfillment rather than an improvement while being a metamorphosis and rebirth. In the first half of life, the main task is the fulfillment of certain regulatory requirements, employment in the community (such as pregnancy genitive); in the second half of life, acquiring authentic aspiration to be our personalities. Crises mobilize our deepest layers, creative unconscious and prepare reincorporation in our being conscious of layers or sides kept in the shade: femininity in a male anti-figural typological recognition of the "right to life" has other values. Neurosis would be largely the expression of an inability dialectical development, the difficulties of renewal and reconstruction of our inner life, a "sin" by uni-lateralization and rigidification.

* * *

As noted, the adult "has it" manifest or latent, all ages earlier (and previewed, ages virtually wait). *Goethe* said that some of the great creators manage to repeat the "puberty spiritual." *E. Kretschmer*, commenting this aphorism wondered if what you mean by "normal maturation" is not a model of adherence to multiple life limited and limiting.

The relation between "inner ages" that coexist at a point in society is complex and requires analyzed to understand the significance and purpose of such co-existence." Age pyramid" that traces the statisticians have not only a demographic interest (on the future of the population) or economic (the percentage ratio between the active, productive, and the population is maintained). The set of relationships between creativity and age make us suspect a repercussion in the cultural dynamics. Blossoming (renewing) of *Florence* during the Renaissance was traced to the demographic situation since, as *D.M. Plopşor* found that in history more distant epochs of life (average) higher, with several elders. They are more stable erased with material culture. Indeed, until our time, cultures were prevailing post-figurative (*M. Mead*) - where children learn from their parents and grandparents. (Today, Western-style culture is co-figurative or even pre-figurative.) Interactions between age groups were studied especially regarding conflict between generations, insisting (improvers as *P.P. Negulescu*) on complementation of age (with their specific mentality and psychology), social and cultural dynamics. However, the "conflict" is not only the immediate interests, or mentality - but has perhaps the deepest roots in the human psyche. Abyssal roots - argued *S. Freud* ("complex *Oedipus* ") and *S. Eisler* (the "draw" the concept of s dormant from parent to child, expressed Bible - the mythological intention slaughter of *Isaac* by *Abraham*, the sacrifice of *Christ* by *God* – The *Father* and - specifically - in many wars triggered by elderly in dying young).

Ethological Roots - claim today *K. Lorenz* (intergroup aggression is "canalized" on vertical generations) and *I. Eibl-Eibesfeld* (non-acceptance rank correlation - old, ancient - present in primates; refusal to accept authority, though, ancestral, there is in us the need to obey a hierarchy, as an antidote against insecurity). Such a study of the problem is incomplete because it excludes the child interaction. The child itself, as a "child in all of us" play a liberator, buffered, a balanced and anti-aggressive role whose roots are psychological and perhaps ethologic.

Dublineau J. (1948) believes that adulthood is a "crisis pubertal development of" mobilization of the "kosmotropic" energies, with the emergence of a tropism and a "socio-spiritualization" toward equilibrium. Old age is a deployment of "climacteric crisis" with the withdrawal of energy from external investments Heterosexual tropism, painful and risky, may be prevented precisely because of the emergence children (the old grandfather). In the child is were the old man finds his complement: expansion forms compared to its retraction, kosmotropic instead of interiority, affirming the biological courts instead of "discarnation" ("spiritualize"). The couple "old-nephew" is thus a balancing socio-physiologic factor. However, the child is not "useful" only old but also for young and adult (retraining obligations and their valences of *Homo Ludens* and affection directed toward another, balancing it by centering it affective). Especially for women – the child brings a "fulfillment" to justify physiological and ethological female body with countless architectural details and functional procreative finality. Ethologically, child function is multiple notes morphological and expressive child having a positive, anti-aggressive affective signal - among others *K. Lorenz* and *I. Eibl-Eibsfeld* has long insisted on the role of "behavioral regression" mimicking infantile attitudes, acts to block the attack and generating acts of solicitude. In light of these data, it is no wonder that poor relationships between parents and children were in a lot of early aging, six times more frequent than in a control group (*Al. Ciuca, Sanda* and *I. Belea,* 1967).

Systemic approach and "systematic" approach

The systemic approach in *Anthropology* must be distinguished from the taxonomic-systematic approach and organismic-systemic approach.

A) We will understand the taxonomic-systematic approach, as the traditional approach of classifying human phenomenon using classical biology schemes. The variety of living creatures extreme human spirit undertakes the development of guiding criteria, allowing the identification of specimens and rational understanding of this diversity; involved in this operation, it is a nomenclature anger and justified. Facing the similarities and differences, owing to the existence of individual development cycles and empirical and experimental genetic criteria (lineage), we come to characterize species, genera and higher taxonomic units. These classifications beyond teaching present philosophy investigation. It is enough to remember that these classifications are divided into artificial and natural.

An artificial classification is arbitrary and has a high degree of conventional thinking. A classification artificial proposed either as a *faute of mieux* either to an end "virtually" (classifications "pharmaceutical" in ancient botany, botanical classification of *Linnaeus*, allowing fast diagnosis - "determination" - species. In the first case the aim was practical use and in the latter classification was "practical," i.e. anger).

A natural classification is justified rationally, taking into account trends rationalization (i.e. "naturalized") of classifications that were manifestly, for example, shifting the focus from external morphology anatomy (morphology indoor); from a small number of features (beams striking) the number (as) the wide range of characteristics; or summative assessment illustrative of characteristics in assessing their hierarchical etc. A significant turning point meant an acceptance of evolutionary vision of *Ch.Darwin*, which almost led to the identification of the 'rational-natural "with the phylogenetic (or suspected-phylogenetic). At the moment, systematics tend to confuse the living world with the systematic presentation of historical or phylogenetic. Because in the history of life on earth, organisms have progressed natural classification is identified, however, with a presentation ontogenetic. It is easy to show that systematic presentation of the living world today is primarily a (panoramic) presentation diversity, criteria logic - and this presentation is only partially parallel and congruent with a historical overview (paleontological), ontogenetic or phylogenetic. Development of life on earth was done according to a linear model, life climbed from stage to stage shapes and adding new functions to the old, nor did disappear stages "outdated." Life has developed a model branched complex, making countless forms of temporary success (ephemeral) preserving - for the sake of saving the biosphere - forms and functions of (almost) all levels, achieving partial successes on its various ramifications ontogenetic, etc. The numbers of major ontogenetic and adaptive windings do not coincide with major taxonomic units (e.g., Switching to terrestrial life forms evolved in almost all taxonomic units). Logic our exposure is important to remember that the biosphere contains many lines exploratory ontogenetic, which will allow us to look for analogies significant between representatives of "taxes" and "clade" more spaced from the point of view of kinship morphological (e.g. organizational type) or phylogenetic. For example, the pre-eminence of life evolved factor information can be researched on examples of insects as the examples of mammals.

B) We understand the systemic research-organismic approach "systematic" an organismic system after organ and tissue groups connected functionally, such as "appliances" and "systems" traditional anatomy and physiology, nervous system, cardiovascular system. These "systems" are viewed as subsystems within the body system. The grouping criterion is, as I said, physiological and morphological - and kept the old anatomists to distinguish between "apparatus" and "system," the degree of homogeneity histological bodies forming a subsystem. A body-systemic approach is largely a concrete approach. In the traditional spirit of biology as "natural history" it was understood mainly as a scientific description of specific details and specific.

Addressing organismic-systemic, examined the comparative point of view, and especially from the point of view of biology General (generalized), leads to a question, central to clarify the role of an approach abstract life sciences: it is the function of a "manifestation" substrate morphology or morphological substrate of benefits functional is the condition *sine qua non*, appeared in an environment ecological time for the manifestation of life: when we talk about "dialectical unity of form and function", we do not, sufficiently, point to "i ". For life to manifest itself, it needs some substantial metabolism and energy in one and the same type of environment (ex. The insect tracheal breath, pulmonary respiration in mammals). Life is characterized, therefore, by means of a number of functions carried out in various plants and animals of various organs, each with its particular physiology. A scientific study of biosphere diversity of mechanisms in the body can be - we believe - and a presentation beginning at functions ("abstract element") by morphology and physiology. In this way does not cause any "breaking" the function of form, but rather highlights we talked about the dialectical unit (a unit is contradictory dialectical unity). It is shown, that is to say, the same function can be fulfilled by formation distinguishable from one another; reverse (as a complement *aces* lime theses) can show that usually, the morphological formation is the support of several functions, physiology is "multivalent." This last sentence (a sentence which is "mutual") makes obsolete the traditional groups give some organs "systems" and "appliances" (metabolic organ and hematopoietic bone are therefore not classifiable rigid musculoskeletal). Such an approach does not mean abstract primacy over Anatomical physiologic because it is postulated primacy of functionality that is not coincident with physiologic, in terms of semantics. Naturally, it is absurd to argue that, in this way, biological thinking is "broken" by its substrate material (substructure material is not reducible to anatomy - but, coming down today, molecular biology and sub-molecular. The substrate material is not nor reducible to describe stable, the "elements" concrete, tangible, viewable or dosage, it involves, obviously, and relationships between elements; and functional relationships cannot be "seen" only "mind's eye").

We prefer to call them functions to distinguish them from Math "functions," which we frequently meet in the pages of this paper. Respiratory function characteristics are the characteristics of the environment. Of course, the dialectic of traditional biology (back when "Biology" was "Natural History") follows, with sufficient fidelity, the historical road of development of this science, which was first descriptive-intuitive, requiring especially the spirit of observation. However, today is theoretical biology, asking increasingly as abstract thinking, deductive spirit (and not only the inductive), quantitative thinking, etc. We can afford to do remark that biology is no exception to the "type" development of other "natural sciences" - and chemistry began as descriptive, giving details on the terms that the organoleptic characteristics (color, taste, smell); It became increasingly quantitative and abstract thinking they "practice." Thinking chemist today is a systemic thinking; he talks about atoms and molecules facets more than the qualities of macroscopic substances - and this allowed him to be a "materialist militant and creative," abstract, the scope functionality. Terms contraction, secretion is physiologic sphere, a sphere more concrete note, creating new combinations of materials.

C) The systemic approach we understand the special case of Anthropology, Human analysis with theoretical tools (concept) of a general systems theory. In other words, we consider man as a system, not to use a new terminology for facts known a long time ago, but mostly to see if such an approach brings real contributions to the interpretation and understanding of the facts known as the methodology acquisition of new facts. Man, as a system, is, in our acceptation, an attempt Anthropology abstract for proximity human phenomenon will be starting from the abstract to the concrete, rising from abstract to concrete (as a general methodological indications given by *K. Marx*). Essentially, the process that we expect (and we are trying to achieve, to a first approximation) is as follows: Man will be defined, note by note, by fitting it into the "system classes" into classes defined in turn by the abstract characteristic (not just the overall). Such a path could lead us, first, the characterization by notes "characteristic" but nonspecific (or with varying degrees of specificity), but in the end, and its characterization by notes "specific" generic man. Based on the characteristics Generic Man, we could reach the individual characterizations. We will notify the concrete human being by "aggregating" notes abstract (in which case, the concrete is found at the intersection of abstractions) or by assigning quantitative values specific to certain parameters characteristics (a process that might be called "determination"). Notes characteristic, but non-specific, for example, those relating to the quality of the open system; Specific grades are, for example, those relating to self-improvement.

Taxonomic-systematic approach defines man "series" of concepts: animal, multicellular, vertebrate, mammal, placental, etc. concepts from abstraction (line apprehension common characteristics important paleontological parentage) of specific biological evidence. The systemic approach defines a "series" of concepts of biological and non-biological life, general-natural (physical we say, thinking of the etymological meaning of the word *physis* = nature).

Taxonomic approach - systematic allows us to stand the anatomic and physiologic man in the living nature. The systemic approach allows us to relate to cosmic-coordinated natural (ontological) more comprehensive; In this way, it can get any further characterization of "essence" that goes beyond the horizon of anatomical and physiological presenting it in its meaning's biosphere, social, cultural, even trans-terrestrial.

Some heuristic advantages of systemic approach

"System Theory" is a heuristic tool whose usefulness is not as understood by researchers. We can distinguish three main trends. Some of them (including *Sadovskii*) envisage the establishment of a "general system theory" understood as a metatheory, precious in various fields of development of theories about objects, events, etc. Others are concerned about the development of a rigorous mathematical formalism, especially valuable in different sectors of art (among them we mention *Zadeh* and in our country, *O. Penescu*). We rally those who see the systemic approach, an improved approach to research about concrete, practical applications ubiquitous. It is an abstract approach to the concrete, a transcript abstract concrete for a better understanding of its mediation between the two approaches abstract concrete. It is a way of enriching the special theories, inter alia through the mechanism of a "transfer" concepts and modelling; the same approach abstract systemic appropriate in two or more sectors of reality, establishes similarities (i.e., links) unsuspected who remain concrete plan intuitive, making it possible to study one sector by means other (or, at least, make it possible to formulate new issues suggested by the sector study "analogue").

System theory is valuable because thanks to them, is done sometimes transforming some heuristic model metaphors. Thus, the resemblance is old (poetic and philosophical) life with a flame. The metaphor of "caught consistency" with the discovery of substantial importance oxidization metabolism and energy (flame is "gas that burns," i.e., a gas that is oxidized; breathing is a slow burning). However, the value of this comparison model was revealed only once subsuming both flame and living organism, the concept of the open system. In the second half of the nineteenth century, they had some movement in sociology "organicist conception" (*H.*

Spencer et al.) that “identified” (actually comparing the interest heuristic) company with a body. Moreover, the followers of these concepts, especially critics, this comparison were understood, more or less, as a variant of biologism; criticism of such views was a variant of critics all doctrines reductionist. In reality, those thinkers representing a still insufficiently advanced stage of scientific thought and methodology, ascertaining the value heuristic analogy between the social and organismic system but did not understand the significance of methodological (modeling) of this analogy. They failed to rise to that level of abstraction that would have enabled the development of a general theory of systems, fueled among other things biology as sociology, the terminology “neutral” (or conventional) not give rise to misunderstandings and interpretations of “reductionist.” Such systems theory has revealed functional and evolutionary traits in common.

In our opinion, the essence is to use a systemic approach (operative and operational) to what we call law system. By law, we mean law system which expresses the functional and evolutionary characters of a structured set. Any structured set has a scheme of composition, connection and structuring of constituents scheme which, for example, that a radio is a radio and not an agglomeration inoperative circuits, capacitors, resistors, triodes, etc. What is very important for such a system: the presence of specific components or their way of structuring? Achieve in this way, the famous problem of “emergence” and “qualitative leap.” It might reply that is important, equally so and elements that make up the structure. However, functionally analogous structures (and evolving) may be obtained with another set of items; and items can be replaced not only by the like (to wear a radio valve, for instance) but also by other iso-functional. For an item to be “functional” in a particular system, it must have some conditions necessary and sufficient particular, according to “nature” (specifics qualitative) system. Any conductor, regardless of the quality of the metal (a “Member”), some of its quantitative characteristics, can meet the requirement of a link between two terminals of an electrical system. Any body insoluble in water, a particular geometric shape, and a certain size can “work” as a stopper, preventing leakage of water from a pothole. We understand that there is a law system relative independence from nature constituent elements of different natures can be constituents, it has the ability to enter into those relationships specified. In a systemic approach, which is interested in the functional and evolutionary role of the elements and not, primarily, the details of which he specifies the composition and morphology. The systemic approach that is more interested than counterparts’ analogies. In biology, analogous bodies are those with similar functions and homologous organs are similar embryological origins and phylogenetic, or tissue cell structure are also similar. Butterfly wing and sparrows are analogous organs, wing sparrows and man are homologous organs.

May that system laws are the defining quality of a system specifics. Nature and society meet two extremes, many intermediate situations. In some cases, the resulting system is “spontaneous” free of interaction components. Interactions are sufficient elements to explain the genesis, persistent to, depending on the operation and developments to take system. Where (apparently) is the birth of atoms or crystals. A certain complicated systemic signed possible complicated if complicated and only if the complicated interaction of purchasing complicated certain components. In other cases, the resulting system “forced,” “constrained” by the external energy. Interactions elements are powered energy and this power, like other external constraints, largely explains the genesis, persistence, operation, and evolution of the system. A certain “configuration” is possible through the systemic interaction of components whose nature is not bound by any particular way. There is a “free” choice of components, but it is “paid” with an uneven energy investment (and a “risk” unequal).

The systemic approach is not only near all structured, the “forest” ignoring “since trees are trees” of the forest. Epistemological and praxeological basic usefulness is our opinion that given the attributive classification (e.g., characterization system as an open system, or as a self-organizing system, etc.). Such an assignment to "abstract class" is made by finding some qualities (notes), necessary and sufficient. This step is a qualitative characterization-systemic. Such a characterization is "deducted" as belonging to that scheme, and other notes specific to that class of systems. Special theory of that class reveals "deeper reason" the link between all these characteristic notes.

The systemic approach will investigate in a proper relationship between parts and whole. Namely, will examine the "power" of each individual component, insofar as it satisfies the requirements of incorporation. It can analyze how the quality characteristics are reflected in the systemic nature of the components (substrating), and insofar as there are easements of "law system," or the existence of deploying systems to these components." It may study other aspects of the dialectic between "element" and "organization."

An important chapter of the systemic approach is the analysis of driving forces concrete, two-way, functional and evolutionary. Every constituent will be appreciated, as such, its role in the functional processes (synchronous) and evolutionary (diachronic); positive role, negative or neutral. Distinguish, further features that we call qualitative or quantitative-extensive: volume, which can be viewed in terms of metric or sub statistically:

- metrically (volume in narrow meaning) means quantity, mass, space extension, "size" (meaning large or small);
- statistically, it means number, crowd (meaning more or less); a system may be considered as a population (the system "man" is also a cell population).

The "volume" is important at least for the following drivers:

- Expression of a certain specificity requires enough volume;
- Passing over the effect of the fluctuation like for neutralizing the accidental and incidental perturbation requires enough multitude;

Any progressive evolution claims for a minimal volume, required for self-consistency, polarization, attraction, and assimilation of what is "foreign."

* * *

The systemic approach can have different degrees of concreteness. Alongside qualitative characterization abstract-systemic, the systemic approach will lead to a qualitative characterization-specific in terms that reflect the specific quality of phenomena manifested (e.g., In biological terms). Systemic thinking, as is thinking operators will tend toward a synthetic coverage, the report assumes a functional whole teleonomic thinking - and not only a causal thinking; thinking deterministic networks (including the "causal circuits") and not thinking in the "spirit linear causality '; determinist dialectical thinking, the need is intertwined with the story - and not strictly causal thinking. Systemic thinking cannot be thinking the element-centrist element that uses the dichotomy/environment but inter-relationality thinking. The systemic approach can reach an idiographic analysis. This term means, as we know, a scientific description relative to an "object" 'singular. From *Aristotle*, it stayed thesis that science deals only with the general (and "universal") - but this sentence was not always properly interpreted. Knowing concrete signifies usually know the particular individual, even singular, but it is using general concepts (with varying degree of generality). Can there be a science of a particular object? Since there was a geography, geophysics, a selenology, etc., the answer is yes. The argument seems perfect idea that science can be about a particular person (e.g., An "Eminescology"). Moreover, it would appear that such science is obligatorily or sketched by any psychologist who wants to individualize treatment or work of *counseling*. The custom is being us, so it is legitimate to talk about anatomy, physiology, and psychology 'own," by, for example, reactive "idiosyncrasy." Addressing the concrete is usually a multi- or interdisciplinary approach. Concreteness natural (and not only he) is not usually differentiated by the criteria that led to the differentiation of traditional scientific disciplines! In reality field there are phenomena rarely "pure" natural or "pure" chemicals. When a man is no specific anatomy, physiology when, when psychology when culture. There is a systemic understanding that, as far as we are concerned, not sympathy: the overall system is considered a "synthesis" or "interaction" of issues recorded by the views of traditional scientific disciplines. If we are talking about, for example, about the influence of psycho-somatic do as a teacher compromise, because we cannot ignore the value of the notion of movement a perceptive routine, the usual. As we will show, they require a systemic approach needs examination and characterization of viewpoints us, "heretical." One of the most precious reviews is one that uses "methodological triad" substance - energy - information. The systemic approach (i.e., cross-) is, moreover, one that manages to clarify some issues related ontology for beams and evolution - and to emphasize the heuristic value of the concept of "information."

A comprehensive definition for "system."

Proposing its own definition for the system, which we will discuss contradicts other accepted definition, but (in our opinion) unsatisfactory from the point of view that we stand. We understand the system a lot of "elements," including suppose, find, establish relationships or enthrone apt to be defined. Explicit:

1. a) between the components, relationships can be "presumed"; for example, *Ptolemy's* geocentric astronomy sistem is not true, but it was upheld centuries

b) between the components, there is the task of science to find relationships;

c) between the components of a machine able to project, engineers and builders will establish topological, functional relationships, etc.

"Relationships fit to be defined" means postulating our cognitive capacity, modeling, etc.

The definition that we propose continues in a first classification.

A) We call those systems gnosis systems which we establish relationships between elements of the plan gnosiological: relations of similarity, analogy, ordering, symbolization; logical relations, quantitative, etc.

Taxonomic systems, the Periodic System (*Mendeleev*) systems are exemple gnosis.

B) We call ontic systems, those systems which actually exist interaction between elements of the plan goal ("material" ontological). The solar system or biocoenosis are ontic systems.

C) In addition to the ontological and gnoseological plan, we have to consider and plan the median between elements of a system in which interactions are virtual or optional. Alleged relations, or in place can be found, for example, genetic relatedness, or they may occur due to certain rules (e.g., A good part of the relationships in "linguistic systems").

We could call nominal system, the system that helps Gnosis classification, systematization orientation. In these systems, we can include both taxonomic and typological systems and also "family trees." Approach intercession nominal systems is a systematic approach (in the narrow sense.) We might call real system an ontical system that requires com¬ple-xitatea studied its internal and external relationships. Addressing real systems in accordance with the principles of systems theory it is a systemic approach.

The items within a system can be ideal elements (e.g., mathematical objects, literary characters) or real elements (existing concrete, e.g., A certain cell of a living organism). The "mid-plane" lies, for example, abstract and abstracted elements which retain the "juiciness" by reference to appropriate concrete (which are therefore valid abstractions).

Relations in real systems (ancient) are causal relations conditional relationships, relationships teleonomic (finals), genetic relationship: the causal relationship corresponds practically formula "to produce, causing phenology B". Conditional relationship corresponds practically formula "If α, β then. Any causal relationship involves a number less than or equal to 1 conditional relationship; The relationship teleonomic corresponds basically reporting the benefits the utility effect against random efficacy, evolving, etc.

We will call utility against undesirable effects of suppressing random hap-plării. Cybernetic self-regulation is largely a settlement against random; producing an effect we call effectiveness with some efficacy, producing a particular effect (effect target) efficiently produce a specific effect with optimal energy expenditure, material, time, etc." Efficiency" is a concept akin to the "yield";
we call evolution, the timing of the existence of system parameters with irreversible changes its status; the genetic relationship refers to the production of a system (or a system) over another (A, a) pre-existing. Not every interaction is "systemic" (narrowly), but any non-accidental interraction may suggest a new approach systemically.

An accidental collision of two objects is a purely external interaction - not a defined relationship; Instead clashes billiard balls on a pool table, are particularly suitable for treatment "systemic." Lack of relations can be regarded as a borderline case of existing relationships. Also as a borderline case can also be considered an element relationship with himself. A chaotic mass of "perfect gas" completely devoid of structure, and the interactions between molecules occur only when clashes and are instant - is, however, a system (in the same way that right can be regarded as a circle a ray of infinite length, or the certainty is a borderline case of probability). In literature, the system sometimes means a mathematical model, an abstract object reduced to a set of values *u* & *U* representing the "inputs" to another set of values *y* & *Y* representing "outputs," the crowd *x* values status and applications called transfer function which connects *y* to *u*. Status is the parameter which sets a certain relationship $u \rightarrow y$. A system can only have one (some) state at a time. Scheme system would, therefore, be a black-box scheme (black box) system structure is expressed by the parameter status and transfer function $y = f(u)$. Description concrete systems in this way is a parametric description.

In biology, methodology "black box" was used systematically by a behaviorist who was limited - the study of animal behavior - recording the relations established among response (response) and excitation. Methodology "black box" has been restored (after a period of fierce criticism) by cybernetics. Under that Restore is at least triple. On the one hand, it is necessary to understand that some results of scientifically valid can be obtained without knowledge of the structure and system. Correlative scientific results can be those set out in the phenomenological perspective, without resorting necessarily to study the mechanism. Sometimes the results are also very important - and they risk being overlooked, or not sought by researchers concerned with analyzing the causal relationships between structures and components.

On the other hand, the method of 'black box' allows a synoptic view of the entire system in which the components are grouped into functional sub-systems, and effective connections are "flagged": this is the block diagram. The analytical approach, purely causal (without being filled with the teleonomic) hardly makes himself effectiveness of the complex relationships of affection. Thus, the researcher analytical will present an array of conditions and causal results on organ physiology; but it will not be easy to determine which is the result of concrete processes in the body and what role "played" organ in the body. Block diagram shows a connection between functional and teleonomic "black boxes." Finally, the black-box method, fruit of functional thinking, explains a sentence of analog thinking, insisting that the results were identical, or very similar, they can be given different structural elements. It is an expression of thought that considers the laws of the system; law system should not be confused with the transfer function. Law system is expressed rather the block diagram, the topological graph connecting between them various "black boxes." Law system gives us relationships effectiveness - defining the class of systems that - between the functional elements of the system. They are operating laws, and as such, possibly a character dressed postulate (or even legal)." Postulates" are requirements *sine qua non*: if certain relationships between components are satisfied, then the system is effective. Among the "boxes "black relationships can be established equivalence. Two systems are equivalent if they have the same functional role, expressed among others by the same transfer function.

System and Structure

Parametric description, functional description and the description of "behavior" are just some of the possible presentations of the systems. The following descriptions will discuss the usefulness and possibility morphologic substrate and structure. In biology, the meanings of the terms "morphology" and "structure" are closely related. It should insist that contemporary semantics of the concept of "structure" in philosophy and general methodology of science has little to do with the composition of concrete, e.g., anatomy and histology their living systems. Vision and methodology "structuralist" refers, especially to systematic invariant relationships. Under the influence of mathematics, the focus was on invariation of certain "groups" of transformations (structure does not refer to the material being stored but relations persisting material and product exchanges). External shape and structure of anatomic pathology can be endowed with attributes "structural" as far as referring to all the constituents of the dynamic state of the biosystem. We remember the "vital vortex" of that French anatomist preeminent formations characterize this kind of matter. A whirlpool (vortex) in a river just has such features, like a flame, morphological appearance "figure" Space is maintained, although all other particulate matter consists of. This is, in both cases, open systems.

The abstract definition of the structure is a problem more complex than the parametric characterization of a "black box." Not only understanding (explanatory) the relationship between u and y is necessary to know the structure, but also for effective intervention to change at will the transfer function or repair of defective mechanisms that disturb the functional and evolutionary deployment of the system. We can ignore the structure when the system is "me-ontic," and its performance satisfies us; we are interested in the structure and "biotechnology" when the system is in "discussion" (disturbed, damaged, diseased). Neurologist and psychiatrist cannot be limited to a 'behaviorist' of the patient; neuroanatomy knowledge of normal and pathological brain centers as physiology, his knowledge of the laws depth psychology is usually essential to help to make a correct diagnosis and implement an effective treatment.

Throughout our exposure (exposure for our needs) we will consider the following aspects of a structural approach:

I. Composition we characterize abstract criterion homogeneity - heterogeneity. Heterogeneity, in turn, can be judged by the criteria of variety, complexity, entropy taxiologică, specification. Or a set of elements; variety is the number complicated ber of elements that can be distinguished between them. Such multitude (g, b, c, g, g, c) has a variety of three points (b, c, g). We can apply the distinctive criteria differentiate: for example, the multitude (b, c, a, a, C, A, B, a) has a variety of forms equally complicated five and a variety of letters equally with three. For many motives that cannot be discussed.

The effectiveness of stereotactic surgery is a striking illustration of interventions based on knowledge, not only topological and terrain but also surveying brain details.

W. Ross Ashby proposes that the variety is measured by logarithms of these numbers. (If the base two logarithms are taken, the variety may be expressed in bits - unit "information").

The complexity is after *A. Moles*, "the universal dimension of" structures." For this author, the measure complexity measure merges information 0 H - provided the message constituted by the assembly of N elements. So the pieces 3T "chained in a comprehensible" we have a complexity equal

$$C = \log_2 Nbiti,$$

when bodies are identical or "equally probable"; when bodies are different, the value is obtained using weighting coefficients that can mean frequency or probability:

$$C = N \sum p_1 \log P_1 .$$

A') – B'). We can use the characterization and the notion of diversity, the way it was introduced by *H. Margalef* in Ecology. In a set of N [elements] of the Class 1 N1, N2 in Class 2 NS in Class S, the entropy of the system is given by:

$$'B = \frac{\log N!}{N_1!N_2!...N_S!}$$

And the average entropy for an element would have the value

$$\frac{B_N = \frac{1}{N} \log N!}{N_1!N_2!...N_S}$$

Both BN and mutual value (I / BN "information medium") are indices of diversity. Suppose we determined the diversity index for the two points L and M. Mean Change in diversity can be expressed by a vector (which gives us orientation in organismic space)

$$\rightarrow H = \frac{B_N(M) - B_n(L)}{I}$$

The structure is manifested not only in the provision of its elements into space but also in its relations persistence and regularity over time. When complexity is expressed by the number of parameters required to define the full system, the order is dependent restrictions transition probabilities joining a state with one sequence. *Quastler* called integrating biological relationship between the number of possible states of the system and the number of states that appear effective. The toxicological entropy proposed by *G. Zapan,* index "energy information" proposed by *O. Onicescu* can express quantitatively (comparative) the extent to which, by the process of organization, could assert a preferential class of elements. Toxicological entropy is calculated by a formula derived from the information entropy (*Shannon*). Information energy index is calculated as a "concentration":

$$E = \sum f_i^2$$

Specifying imply a "referential" variants or virtual given consideration as a result of "fictitious election" of an assortment of variations on the same theme. The easiest is one combinatorial specifying the calculation: for example, many m elements can be present in m! Variants obtained by permutations; m! It grows very quickly, with m, reaching astronomical figures and hiper-astronomize soon." Information" contained in a system is a logarithmic function of the number of virtual versions of the class that owns the system. It is equivalent to the number of instructions required for the opacifying ambiguous binary system. For higher organisms, "structural information" reach> 10^{22} bits (if reported at the atomic level).

The appealing architectural structure is defined by a model system of "urban construction." In the architectural structure we have researched:

- Systemic inclusion relations: a system includes subsystems, an organismic biosystem includes organs, and apparatus, etc.
- Levels of organization ("floors"): organismic, subsystems, visceral (organ), histo-systemic, cellular, ultrastructural ("leptons"), etc.
- Topological relationships expressed in the classical law of organ connection.
- Topological relations are contiguous and continuous and can be summarized possibly in a "matrix of continuity" or a graph.
- Topographic relationships can be represented in two-dimensional sections in drawing work (according to the rules of descriptive geometry and proactive) in a matrix of contiguity.

The actual morphological structure can be captured in the following ways:

- The plasticity of the surfaces, exterior, and interior, is characterized by geometrical means (synthetic, analytical and differential), explained in part by biophysics interfaces (in the spirit of the works of W. Thompson d'Arcy)
- The topography of anatomical details
- Typo-stylistic organization plan (radial or axial symmetry, dissymmetry, etc.)
- Allometric relationship matrix available during growth.

The functional structure may be defined:

- by a topological graph, a block-schema, etc.;
- a matrix of correlations (concretising the classical law of organs correlation), current or virtual.

For those correlations' functional specification, use models and flowcharts as analog models, called mathematics "analytical" (analytical expressions, "equations" that are actually functional expressions in the mathematical sense of the concept of "function"). To specify what is meant by excitation, permissive action, synergism, etc. - We need symbolism (formalism) logic. To determine which variation of a reply "function" of variation of excitations, we need a mathematical function (Algebraic or, especially, 'transcendent' '- such as exponential, logarithmic cosine). Some systemic characterization of the human being:

1. Integrated System

In systems theory, literature has circulation term or fully integrated. It is understood by a number of factors that have, by assembling new properties defining; they cannot be attributed elements. In a mass of gas macroscopic characteristics meet the "Pressure," "Temperature" and "volume" which do not belong to individual molecules. Such qualities are resultant expressions "integral" incremental contributions; they belong to the whole and not the elements (or constituent parts). With all the reservations that may cause nomenclature, taxonomic need to remember to use it (or use an equivalent nomenclature).

Additive combination may result in attributes (scalar or vector) or non-additive, the characteristics of the elements. They are expressed, often at a different scale of observation. If a mass of gas state parameters (p, V, T) are sensed on a macroscopic scale. The scale defines manifestation sometimes the phenomenon (the positivists claimed erroneously that scale creates the phenomenon). The mass of the gas passage is a statistical ensemble, and microscopic macroscopic corresponds to the accumulation of a sufficient number of molecules in order to ensure the validity of the laws of statistical mechanics (which are probabilistic laws). In other cases, the size is the occasion for expressions of the predominance of certain natural laws. Dominates the microscopic laws of physics molecular such as those expressed in the phenomena of absorption and surface tension. The dimensions of the order cm, dm, m dominates the gravitational laws. A drop of water is nothing but a macroscopic mass of water. The first surface is convex surface last is horizontal. For biology, a dimensional scale that determines the predominance of a particular type of law is essential. Intracellular biology, cytology, histology and anatomy macroscopic "live" in different physical worlds. Completeness can be understood but in otherwise by the parties in compiling the necessary solidarity system. A lot of sand is nothing but a living organism; a living organism has other "organic structure" than a car mechanic assembled the parts can exist independently. I have separated *(1966) macrosystems (with conglomerate parts) and holosystems. The living organism is a holosystem.*

2. Heterogeneous system

Physics homogeneous and heterogeneous systems are different systems. From this point of view, the defining element is a continuous or discontinuous variation of traits, in its system. Living matter is a heterogeneous system (dispersed), primarily because it is a substantially colloidal system and secondly because it is structured at many levels superimposed.

Heterogeneity is thus conditioned and over-physicochemical physicochemical. Heterogeneity is over-physicochemical cytological, histological, anatomical.

Over-heterogeneity is the result of physicochemical processes:

1. Differentiation scheduled;
2. Interaction partially random environmentally part of having aggressive interactions (harmful);
3. Interaction function between levels of organization;
4. Alteration random somatic mutations etc.

Differentiation is done orderly and teleonomic heterogeneity. In relatively rare cases, it leads to aberrant differentiation and failing disteleonomic (malformation, etc.). From a heredo-biological perspective, differentiated cells retain the "seal" of genetic information from the egg cell from which updates only one hand. Meet situations where the body is *ab initio* "heterogenised" in this regard. Are examples of chromosomal mosaicism in which the constitution is not the same everywhere. Artificial genetic heterogeneity - Information can be obtained by grafting (at the organ) and by introducing foreign cells (chimeras). The heterogeneity of this type can generate contradictions type immunoassay. It can manifest phenotypic appearances mosaic responsiveness uneven influences endocrine, nervous, pathogenic, etc. Somatic mutations carried islands 'foreign' in the organismic system. These can be termianted by means of auto-immune enclaves that may persist as benign, which may be the starting point of a benign or malignant proliferation.

3. Anisotropic system

Isotropic properties mean qualitatively and quantitatively identical in the different dimensions of space. Anisotropy is a substantial property of living matter, the organic components essential. Anisotropy living matter is other than that of crystalline organizations (which are homogeneous systems). It is found, become more complex on every level of organization of living matter, depending more than anatomy, as we rise to a higher level. In fact, a complex of biological structures is anisotropic components. Striated muscle microstructure is a classic illustration of this principle. On the other hand, the degree of anisotropy depends on the functional state. In the connection between the phenomena expressed "mecanostructures" meet macroscopic and molecular conformation. A cause biomechanical underlying molecular conformational changes. By mechanical actions on anatomical elements influence reversible molecular conformation. Living systems use both crystalline components and non-crystalline components, to achieve adequate functional structures. Noncrystalline-crystalline transition is reversible functional means precious, whose prototype meets variation microstructures even water.

4. Geometric system

As a geometric system, the human body has volume, three-dimensional, shape (= surface defined by separation from the environment), symmetry, etc. When the absolute value of the metric sizes, the adult human body are within the meters (10^{2} cm), it (the value) and is thus "macroscopic" in all the higher animals (vertebrates). Situated in this area has been possible thanks to the development of pulmonary respiratory and circulatory (insects with tracheal breathing, can only be "small"). In this area, the corresponding volume is a selective advantage. Life is but the resultant macroscopic organisms billions of microscopic cellular life, physical and chemical phenomena dominated by the sub-molecular (macroscopically and signaling dominates mechanical phenomena).

CHAPTER V.
GENOTYPICAL AND PARATYPICAL INTERRELATIONS WITH IMPORTANCE IN INTERPRETING THE CONSTITUTIONAL TYPE. APPLICATIONS IN MEDICINE AND SPORTS

The substrate material of heredity is located on chromosomes, which are located in the nucleus; They are molecular structures of nuclear material in the specific activity of the division; outside breeding cannot be emphasized because they lose their morphological appearance without losing their molecular structure.

Chromosomes after form and their number, are constant features of each species, causing her karyotype. Human body cells have a double number (diploid) chromosome, which comes from the egg dividing diploid gamete resulting from fertilization of a male and one female, each with gasket haploid chromosome. Gender differences materialize mainly by the female presence in the cell of a pair of homologous chromosomes (XX) and male of a pair of chromosomes unapproved (XY). These are the gender chromosomes or allosome, unlike the rest of which are autosomes. Girls are homogametic (symmetrical), producing gametes in the reproduction of the same gender (X + X) and male gender is heterogametic, producing gametes of different gender (X + Y).

Note that not only gender but also determines heterochromosomes genes responsible for sexual characteristics. The body goes through a bisexual phase, and finally through a complicated process reaching the final at XX karyotype or XY, the taking of gender. That each somatic cell has 23 pairs of chromosomes, including 22 autosomes and one pair of gender chromosomes. Each chromosome has many genes arranged linearly, each gene occupying a given position, called "locus." Human Chromosomes are 46 in number, arranged in pairs. Cells containing two from each chromosome are called diploid, sexual ones you have one set are called haploid. Homologous chromosomes are a pair, and each locus is represented on both chromosomes of a pair. In the last decades, it has been shown that heredity is materialized not only in the nucleus, but it exists and extranuclear (cytoplasmic), located on epitomes all chains consisting of nucleic acids. Epitomes between chromosomes and complex relationships of mutual influence. The chemical structure is the genetic information of nucleic acids: deoxyribonucleic acid (DNA) and ribonucleic acid (RNA).

DNA is composed of two polynucleotide chains parallel helically coiled around a common axis; phosphodiester bonds between nucleotides is determined. RNA consisting of single-stranded polynucleotides. There are three kinds of RNA:

- MRNA (messenger) protein synthesis takes information from the nucleus into the cytoplasm;
- RRNA (ribosomal) is in ribosomes, where protein synthesis;
- TRNA (transfer) carrying amino acids at the site of protein synthesis.

Chromosomal material submitted by the two gametes is halved before fertilization through the process of maturation divisions (meiosis or haplosis), ensuring consistency seal chromosome generally more numerous species are always organized; the human species has 46 chromosomes, including 22 pairs of autosomes and two heterochromosomes (chromosomes), namely, XX for females and XY for males (*Painter, Tjio* and *Levan*, 1956), also called gonosomes (fig. 29).

Biochemical mechanism of realization forms involves, first, the mode of action of genes that have the ability to synthesize proteins specific to each organism, proteins, as observed *Engels*, the very essence of the living matter, defined by him as "mode Albuminoidal substances existence." This key issue normal and pathological Genesis could be clarified thanks to three major findings:

- The demonstration of *Sanger* that a protein, insulin, has a specific, well-defined chemical structure expressed by its amino acid sequence;
- Elucidation in 1953, the structure of DNA by *Watson* and *Crick;*
- Work of *Benzer*, în1955 on gene structure fine.

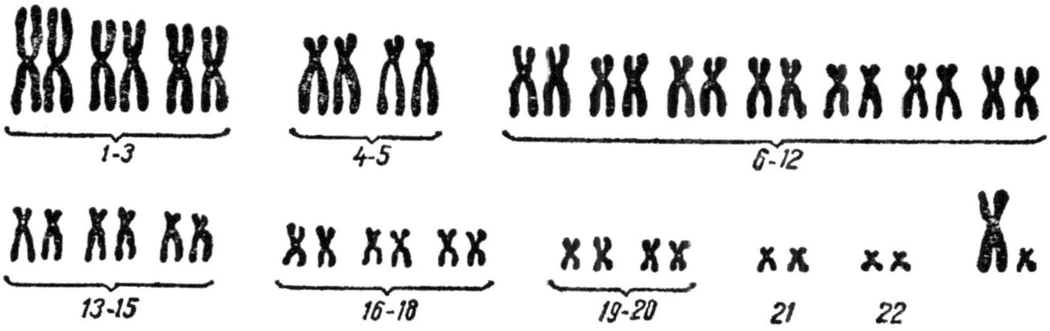

Fig. 29 Normal karyogram.

We do not insist on RNA structure, but mention only this gene is, morphologically, a fragment of the chromosome and biochemical a portion of the DNA that constitute chemical substrate chromosome. The entire specific and individual morphogenesis are determined by the structure and chemical composition of the zygote leptons, which is an essential part of the dowry chromosomal double nucleus and cytoplasm of the various components. The entire biochemical specificity of the development and function of the human being is, in interrelation with the environment, fixed genetic sample cast - the nucleus - and the responsiveness of the zygote cytoplasm. The whole body individually in shape and function of complex, interlocking is made of many "chains of gene action" in a real "action network gene" (*Kuhn*, 1955).

The question is how gene manages to transmit genetic information leading to protein synthesis. The answer to this we give it our code systems which explain how the sequence of DNA bases constituent induces a certain order in the settlement chain amino acids into polypeptide sequence responsible for a specific protein. The fact that an unidimensional setting of bases of the nucleotide can control the pleating of the complex of polypeptide chains is explained by the theory of the sequence of *Crick* (1968), which shows that there is a need for further information as to cause pleating in addition to specifying the sequence of amino acids in the polypeptide chain.

Effective realization of protein synthesis by genes is a complex process. DNA is the gene at a time; he separates the two filaments. One of them leads to replication of a molecule of messenger RNA (mRNA), which then falls off the encoded DNA filament and passing through the pores of the nuclear membrane, cytoplasm where it snaps reach the ribosome. DNA filament then meets with his counterpart, reconstructing the DNA molecule. The fact that the two chains have base sequences complementary DNA raises the question where the code is RNA chain, and hence the protein cannot be both because they have outstanding chemical polarity. There are numerous explanations among which we quote: the existence of exclusivity on one of the triplets' chains nonsense (Brenner), quadruplet's existence, not only DNA that codes for the amino acid and nucleotide sequences but has structural controls. In the cytoplasm, mRNA is fixed to the ribosome containing ribosomal RNA inside, believed to be intended to fix amino acids, which are part of the ribosome that determines the fixing of a specific messenger RNA ribosome. The cytoplasm is found RNA soluble (RNAs), which has a spiral shape, one end having a loop that is a triplet variable, the other end being fixed for all RNAs, triplet ACC (adenine, cytosine, cytosine). By means of the loop is fixed complementary RNAs of mRNA triplets, while the ACC group was combined with various amino acids (RNAs there are 20, one for each amino acid). The difficult problem is how to combine ACC group differently with the 20 amino acids, being the same? It seems that this is a specific enzyme for each amino acid that catalyzes this union or that there is a specificity amid the spiral RNAs. Once achieved this fixing using RNAs, amino acids of mRNA occur an enzyme that catalyzes NH-CO bonds of the amino acid, another protein and then opens the polypeptide chain thus formed. The mechanism is more complete, with the possibility of control of protein synthesis and its speed. Genetic systems are made up of R (regulatory gene), O (operator gene), S (structural gene), and there is a direct interrelation between O and S and one reverse interrelation between R and A, by a repressor substance. Genetic system is illustrated by the degradation of lactose. The emergence of a bloc genetically different causes reasons a dysmetabolic of galactose. R is influencing the quantity, while quality.

Things are more complex by the intervention of trigger mechanisms. This mechanism requires the existence of a genetic system ($R_2O_2S_2$), more specifically, its operator, the gene regulatory system other genetic ($R_2O_2S_2$). In these circumstances, blocking the functioning of the system two genetic operon activity will attract 1 and vice versa.

This led to an assertion by *Delbrück* the "law balances the flow," which shows that in developing organisms, producing a dynamic balance between various genetic systems under interrelated, so regarding malfunction of one, occurring disorders other disorders in the chemical mechanisms that ultimately translate into the emergence of dysmorphia. Likewise, pleads "axial development theory" *of Waddington*, showing that the development of the embryo craniocaudal (axial gradient) or dorsoventral (gradient cortical) is the result of balance and interrelationships between different systems and different gradients with enzyme inducer.

Speed control protein synthesis is performed by inductor and repressors, which carries functional circles, similar to those described by *Hoif* and responsible for maintaining homeostasis. In each stage of the synthesis, protein molecules pleated to form a particular shape that blocks the next edition amino acid. Speed synthesis depends on the probability that the system can get rid of this configuration. A repressor molecule, by combining with a chain partially synthesized, may force her to such a configuration; an inducer molecule can take place either competitive repressor or act directly on the protein. The importance configuration makes us conclude that protein synthesis rate is a function of its amino acid sequence and genetic mutation is under control. Mention that the functional unit, leading to the synthesis of protein, called cistron.

We must point out that, besides the ability of protein synthesis, which underlies the entire body structures, materials essential gene has the ability to reproduce identical, the same specific model is carried from generation to generation through cell division of the zygote. Building tissues and organs of an individual by multiplying zygote and blastomere differentiation is stabilized based on hereditary human species through its long existence, which extends through biogenesis until Precambrian. However, there is great variability, which is explained by the ability to alter the genetic material under the influence of the environment and the very act of fertilization, bringing dowry chromosomal manifold two lines, maternal and paternal. Particularly this type normal biological variability may occur, and some of the genetic basis of hereditary changes called mutations, which may affect the genome fully chromosome number and structure, and genes. After *Brenner*, regarding biochemical changes nucleotides sequence is the change in position of a particular nucleic acid, leading to the production of abnormal proteins, and the subsequent process, the appearance of dysmetabolic and dysmorphia. They recognize essentially disturbing the mechanism mentioned by the break, usually blocks of partial genetic, that disturb the normal sequence of intermediate stages in the chain reactions protein synthesis. The entire activity is phylogenetic morphology and thus directed the suite bio-physicochemical processes, protein synthesis, marked by the individual characteristics of polypeptide chains. In fact, this is biochemical individuality embodied in Intra- and interspecific variability great. This infinite variability was notified bodies since *Hippocrates* almost 2500 years, to assert that diseases are not possible outside of this variability bodies. Also, *Galen*, about 600 years after *Hippocrates*, considered that for the onset of diseases, we need a receptive individual in times close to us, *Osler William* asserts that "it is important for the doctor what kind of patient has a certain disease than to know what kind of disease a patient is." *Draper Georges* wrote in 1944 monograph Constitution human medical clinic, from which we derive the following assessments on individualization of the human biotypes in their relationship with certain predispositions to disease and capabilities sports:

- Dividing people into two main groups: the majority, 95%, with properties within normal range, and a small minority, 5% which can be considered as a deviation from the norm;
- Practically every human being, however, present some deviations, some more obvious and more important than others, or masked detectable at birth, which later may underlie susceptibility to disease;
- There is variability about the nutritional needs of people, bradytroph or tachographs, which may be the manifestation of an individual receptivity emissions.

Roger J. Williams in a monograph (1974), studying biochemical individuality, genetically determined, and its implications for the production of congenital and acquired diseases. We will return to this work, of which we use several examples to demonstrate the theory of biochemical individuality of the human body. This individuality, specific first and then typological, is the product of a long evolution, which crosses the first world invertebrates and vertebrates than the world, culminating in the human species. It consists in the individualization of many enzymatic processes, morphogenetic and functional, which make, despite progress in this area, the boundary between normal and pathological remain undefined. It is a task of human genetics and medicine in the future predispositions to detected endogenous individual variability relative reactivity against various toxins or drugs, ultimately genetically conditioned and thus biochemically. From this point of view, we distinguish genotype resulted in chromosomes gametes, summarizing the entire evolution biochemical ancestors, and the para-type which concentrates all external environmental influences. The paratypes together constitute the entire genotype and biochemical phenotype material. Synonyms used for these determinants: genotype: genome and homeostasis; for para-type: plastidom (Plasmon and plastom) and peristalsis; and for phenotype: biotype.

If the type is specific and even individual genetic condition, influence the environment should not be neglected, it can alter the course of ontogenetic development. It follows from the above that heredity is a process of transmitting genetic information, which is conducted according to objective laws leading to the building of genetically determined characteristics, which are in a close relation with the external environment.

In the absence of the appropriate genetic information, those properties will not perform even in the most optimal outdoor conditions." Objective laws of genetics" - writes renowned geneticist *B.L. Astauro* - "tell us that exercises and the developing body are subject to the hereditary constitution (genotype) of each person."

Ultimately, every feature of the body depends on heritable traits and those falling under the strong influence of the environment. A hostile environment exterior hides unsuspected possibilities hereditary forms and leads to a sensitive and undeveloped instead favorable environment open doors of opportunity hereditary potential of a constitution, developing to the highest level. There is, however, an upper limit and lower the possibilities of the individual hereditary and what is very important is that no exercise, no conditions favorable or unfavorable to the development of hereditary human body does not change the basis on which acts.
More information about the influence of hereditary factors and the influence of environmental factors on body development were obtained during research conducted on twins.

It was established so that hereditary reflects the stronger influence on body size compared to their weight. Monovular twins showed that even if their early separation, record correlation between height, head circumference, the length of hands, face.

Sergienko and *Aleksiejeva*, based on research results of a large number of scientists have classified attributes that characterize body and motility, according to the closely related genetic factors and environmental determining the order of occurrence dependence cited by these factors. Characteristics under the strong influence of hereditary factors are:

1. morphological - body height, the length of the lower extremities, trunk length, the circumference of the upper extremities, lower and upper extremities chest and length;
2. The mobility of joints;
3. Reaction time;
4. Special resistance (anaerobic) and general resistance (aerobic);
5. qualities of traction and force;
6. Force the muscles;
7. incremental movement speed - skills.

All the features listed were set during run-denominated selection for the practice of sports.

The group characteristics that depend to a large extent by environmental factors, suitable for training, there are:

1. Body weight;
2. The frequency of movements;
3. Force the regime speed.

Underlying sporting driving characteristics is an appropriate use of somatic and physiological characteristics of the locomotor system and other systems and appropriate psychological predispositions. With this genetic predisposition, it is necessary “to create a chance” and highlighting their training. *Galton*, noting kayaking in higher institutes, confirmed the result of genetic predisposition sports.

Grebe and *Gedda*, between 1954-1963, argued that the differences between MZ twins (monovular monozygotic) and BZ (dizygotic biovular) are lower for sport entirely, except for a certain discipline and results. The degree of genetic predispositions conditioning for a particular sport is varied from person to person. A high coefficient of genetic conditioning, line the various generations of practicing the same discipline (genealogical research) prove: fencing, boxing, shooting; lowest coefficient presents: football, gymnastics and light athletics (*Szwarz*, 1976). It follows that one can speak of a talent driving genetically determined, due to the chances of obtaining high sports results. There is a reluctance to sentence based on the “homo olimpicus” phrase refers specifically to the predisposition for sport, concrete. This can be compared with the ability to study the phenomenon. Success in each area depends on the talent, skills, and abilities under the influence of the environment. Because talent to occur, there must be not only genetic predisposition (for sport: morpho-physiological), and adequate social conditions. It can be said that sports results are conditioned genetically from other points of view, thus noting progress in getting sports results from different samples. When comparing the percentage increase sports results, results of 80 years ago, obtained the Olympics, we get the following data (Table. 1).

It is noted that the latest evidence of the table is those which involve moving speed, they are subject to a high degree of genetic standpoint, but progress is lowest.

Tabel 1

Discipline	Growth after 80 years in %	Average growth in 10 years in %
Discus throw	56.81	7.10
Pole jump	40.00	5.00
800 m run	26.57	3.32
1.500 m run	24.65	3.03
Long jump	23.95	2.99
Triple jump	20.71	2.59
High jump	19.56	2.45
100 m run	19.28	2.41
400 m run	5.51	0.69

At the other end of the table is throwing the disc. The explosive force of upper extremities is an example of the driving characteristics inherited a small proportion. Of course, the question may arise that ownership should be preferred in the selection for the main sports? It should be regarded qualities that are inherited in a high and constitute basic attributes for every discipline. We must remember, talking about sports result that heavily conditional attributes are genetic traits driving incremental rather complex. Mathematical analysis of the effects of environmental factors and hereditary factors in the development shows that if the height of the contribution of heredity amounts to 81%, and in the case of body weight, to 78%.

From research conducted on athletes-twins and the observations on family (genealogical comments) leading athletes, sports skills that are hereditary. There is evidence that children of famous athletes on average 50% of cases it is possible athletic talent. From his data, *Gedda* concluded that over 70% of twins resembling monovular acquire sports scores, while biovular twins phenomenon occurs in 25% of cases.

Zaciorskj and *Sergienko*, defining the influence of heredity and environmental factors on the development of traits drivers of human reveal essential conditioning hereditary during latent reaction driving in tests of strength and speed (long jump from a standstill, running the distance of 30 m), depending on muscle strength and maximum heart rate.

Conditioning prevailing environmental factors absolute force occurs when the muscles in the frequency of movements, agility indices. Based on these findings, the authors concluded that the simplest actions regarding coordination are based on the premise hereditary a greater extent than complex movements.

From the researches that the integral index of respiratory capacity is conditioned primarily by genetic factors. Comparative analysis of the index twins mono and biovular the hereditary conditioning was established at a rate of 79% and environmental factors conditioning only in the proportion of 21%. Similar data were obtained by other scientists (Table 2).

Table 2

Genetic conditioning of the respiratory capacity to twins

Authors	Heredity index %
Szwarz, 1970	79
Klissouras, 1971	93
Gedda, 1972	66
Zaciorskj, Sergienko, 1975	73

Szwarz revealed the existence of essential differences between monozygotic twins skiers on the distance of 2-3 km and concluded that respiratory capacity index is genetically determined. Other studies have established that the influence of genetic factors, to some extent, there is more to the functions of the cardiovascular system than in the case of the respiratory system (intensity, breathing capacity, the maximum ventilation of the lungs depends on the external environmental factors). It was also established that the indices anaerobic transformations, as well as the adenosine triphosphoric acid and lactic acid, depends on genetic factors. Genetic factors define not only developed the traits of the organism, but also hereditary reaction time in response to environmental conditions or "upper and lower limits of the possibilities of a person's hereditary" and training opportunities, training, and sports.

In his research *Klissouras* was shown that the influence of special training at one of the monozygotic twins was an increase in maximum oxygen consumption, not found his brother, who has trained. From the point of view of premises hereditary exercise does not lead to a significant increase breathing capacity index. During observations of 32 pairs of twins of the same gender (five pairs of students at institutes of physical culture, aged 18-21 years, and 27 students in Smolensk, aged 9-16 years), there were established major indices hereditary conditionings driving characteristics, respiratory capacity and autonomic functions (*Wotkow*).

Closest indices were obtained when maximum oxygen consumption, 89.4%. Genetic conditioning has been reported for simple reaction (84.2%) and complex motricity reaction (80.8%) and in performance tests of strength and speed (long jump, high jump and 30m running) 76, 1.79, 4, 77.1%. The genetic links are also indications of the length of the breath stop (82%) and the degree of oxygen saturation of arterial blood (76.9%). Torque measurements of clues hereditary force of the left and right hand amounted to 61.4, and 59.2% and back strength indices were 64.3%. From research carried out on twins have issued conflicting opinions on the genetic strength and speed conditioning. Some authors have concluded that speed and power are as genetically caused (*Eysenck* and *Prell*, 1951), and others say the speed is more genetically determined than the force (*Sklad*, 1973; *Szwarz*, 1976). There is also the view that force is more genetically determined than speed - this settling all based on the study of twins.

Osato and *Avano* state that the biggest differences between pairs of MZ twins and SZ appear in throwing the ball, then force back and shoulders and lower running speed. *Cratty* supports a correlation powerful dynamic force and then speed. As it is known, the main characteristics behave the highest correlation coefficients between parents and children. In speed tests, it was reported that the highest degree of heredity is manifested in jog 10 m (*Nikitjuk*, 1973) then jog 20 m, 30 m (*Zaciorskj* and *Sergienko*, 1976).

Regarding labor, the degree of heredity is manifested most pronounced in her hands and force back muscles, and the lowest for explosive force if the disc throwing and ball. Arguably, the strongest genetic determination is manifested in her hands, where reaction speed, speed in a jog on very small distances. The explosive force measured when the pole is highly conditional jump genetic instead of upper extremities explosive force measured by the distance throwing the ball or disc indicates a low degree of heredity. These results obtained from research on twins still require confirmation by other methods.

An interesting result of the research method twins was obtained by analyzing the fast moving so-called "tapping" of the lower extremities and upper. Most authors state that these movements are very strong genetic influence. Heritability coefficients of lift further relate to flexibility and shoulder joint movements; they are smaller and very small backbone system of the hip joint. These three genetic factors decrease during the period from 12 to 17 years. According to his research results *Wolanski*, visual-motor coordination is highly conditional genetic correlation coefficients tall observed between nine and 12, as well as people mature. This analysis provides the biographies of key data athletes twins. From these results, the following: masters of sports in judo, I and O. Pierminow (the birth year 1959), currently have the same height, 1.82 cm, and weight is 84 and 82 kg. The first to the training was *Igor* (Class VI - discus throw), after a year, he began training in athletics in the semi fond runs, *Oleg*. In Class VIII *Igor* went to the polling judo, a year later and *Oleg* took the same section. Despite the great influence of environmental factors, two brothers have almost the same index of maximum oxygen consumption: Igor - 4867 ml, *Oleg* - 4612 ml, with a share of 94,8% *(Wotkow)*. Much like the reaction parameters are driving, simple and complex (172 and 179 ms - 96%, 286 and 302 ms - 91.8%).

In 1979 both brothers won the master category in judo. It can be said that heredity defines physical development to a considerable extent, defines movement skills training, the aerobic and anaerobic capacity of the body. From this point of view are interesting data obtained from analyzing the characteristics of families of athletes. Many examples can be given that children of former athletes have achieved the same remarkable results in sports, for example: father and son, and so on Known also high results of brothers and sisters: *Majorow, Ragulin, Golikov, Holik, Stiasny, Lebiediewow.* Undoubtedly, besides genetic information, an important role in the formation of these famous athletes have had other factors - family views, traditions education at a young age, practicing sport very early, etc. Recognizing the importance of genetic factors, no diminishing the role of the environment.

It was shown that genetic information could be realized when it will be associated with environmental conditions that can have a big influence at this stage of ontogenesis. In various stages of development of the organism influence of external environment, in collaboration with the genetic information and the changes that have occurred in previous stages have different effects. But not all environmental factors correspond to the development of body and allow exploitation of accumulated reserves. About the great role of the external environment on the formation Athlete speak multiple facts gathered during the investigation. Investigations undertaken by some significant groups of high-class athletes show that subjects who achieved high results in sporting strength come from families with many children (Wotkow). In these circumstances, resistance is formed, the desire to an end, employment, and skill to organize leisure time. Environmental factors and, primarily, children's education conditions play an important role in those sports that are an essential strength, effort, skill to overcome difficulties; Generally, it can be said that only closely linked to the external environment and hereditary influences ensure achieving an appropriate upper limit of genetic adaptability. The means and methods of training should foster ongoing maintenance skills, conditional hereditary of young athletes. Also, there is some correlation between the age hereditary qualities of parents and offspring. It is a common opinion that parents of famous thinkers, scientists and artists were elderly. *Wolanski,* based on his research *Steckel*, drew attention to the existence of a relationship between parents' age, the age difference between her and the level of intelligence of children.

He showed that children born to mothers aged 25 to 31 years and fathers aged ~ 31 years, and parents whose age difference exceeds one year (the father of age) are more intelligent than children whose parents other ages, both young and old. From his research Wolanski that parental age at birth of the child exerts an influence on his development. The researcher, however, fails to elucidate the genetic mechanism satisfactorily. The author draws attention to the report evident between body length new-born and father's age and the correlation between the age of the parents and the state of development of the new-born. Wolanski stresses that there is an essential relationship (established based on statistical data) between aged parents and child development (between four and 14 years), and signals the existence of environmental differences.

Thus, in urban areas grows best babies of mothers aged 25-32 years and fathers aged 30-35 years, when the father is older than his mother three years or more.In the villages the optimal age of parents when children are born amounts to 20 to 25 years for the mother and 40 years - for the father (*Wolanski*).

In the literature, there is no information yet on relations between parents' age and level of development of natural endowment and sporting successes of their children. Research carried out by a group of 100 sprinters show that (*Wotkow*) fathers of the best representatives of the group (15) had the time of birth of their children, 32 years and mother 27 years. The parents from the athletes` weakest group of 15 were younger - fathers by 3.38 years and 2.04 years for mothers. It should be stressed also that the elderly parents had sons-athletes in the top ten (35.9 fathers, mother of 29.9, the age difference six years), the second group of ten sprinters had fathers 32.6 and mothers 28.7 years (age difference six years) and in the third group of ten – fathers were 31.5 years and mothers 27.8 (difference in age, 3.7 years).

The youngest parents had sons-athletes in the last group of ten (28.7 years have fathers, mothers 25.3 years, 3.4 years difference in age).

The biggest age difference between mothers and fathers (six years) occurs in parents' groups best 10 sprinters. Data presented above are to some extent similar to those we obtained *N. Wolanski*. The coefficient of correlation between fathers' age and performed during the race at the distance of 100 m amounted to 0.26, and the correlation between maternal age with the same time is 0.24; In both cases, the figures are the same statistical sources.

Age fathers and mothers do not correlate with times on the distance traveled by their sons 200m, and in both cases, this dependence makes the same correlation. One should underline that the age of the parents influences the children's sports, but in general, we cannot say with certainty the existence of this report.

Collaboration for understanding genetic factors and environmental factors has great importance to so-called "critical periods of development." Speaking of this, we consider a precisely defined stage in the development of the individual (child's age, the young, etc.) and the period characterized by the greatest appetite for action from environmental factors, factors favorable or unfavorable action. This is the period when consensus between genetic factors and the environment is plenary.

Knowing the critical periods and the optimum period of influence, can lead, deliberately, the main features of the body can determine an individual program development. That there is a very "profitable" in developing driving characteristics confirms the dynamics of uneven development of these properties and the effects of education and training in various periods. It was found, for example, that for the formation of skill, age is the most appropriate from nine to 14 years. It was noted that progress in skill development should record to 8-9 and from 10 to 12 years. According to *D.P. Bukriejewej* (1955), the largest yearly growth in the maximum movement tempo occurs about 7-9 and 10- 11 years, and 11-13 years later. *Korobkow A.W.* (1958, 1962) provided the information that a significant increase in the latent time of reaction motion is observed from the age of 6-7 years up to 9 -11 years.

Analysis by age in muscle force development dynamics confirm the substance of what was said. According to *A.W. Korobkow*, 16-17 years develops under optimal conditions, maximum muscle strength, closely related to muscle mass. To elucidate the role of critical periods, particular importance is accorded to the research of *G.I. Obrazcowej*, which stresses based on the experiences of animals, the existence of periods of high reactivity. They are characterized by intensive maturation processes in nerve tissue morpho-physiological and biochemical. It is known that the instruction and training success depends to a large extent on the ability of the central nervous system. Accelerate the development of the generation phenomenon is in full ascent involves some corrections on limited critical periods. Therefore, to ensure as far as possible a more efficient exploitation of these periods, it is necessary to consider the environmental changes that can lead to significant changes in developing morpho body. It should be remembered that this character, uneven, maturation of morphological structures in the main system functions of the body, binds changes that have occurred in the collaboration between the body and the complex social and natural factors.

Scale environmental influence of each factor is defined not only the parameters characteristic of quantity and quality but also the specific development of that period, in which this phenomenon takes place. The critical characterization age limits should not lean on calendar age but the biological age. In assessing the biological age of children and youth, starting from the development stage, teeth from skeletal ossification period, the sexually mature, etc. In practice sports, incomplete analysis of the relationship between biological age and coach sports results often wrong in assessing the true stage of development of the athlete.

In conclusion, we can say that a knowledge of constitutional type (phenotype), its components and genotypic para-type, has special significance for sport, whereas the cultivation of certain innate qualities or acquired depends on the success of practicing sports. Furthermore, the selection sport should be performed on the basis of science in which genetic investigation must occupy a considerable share. The very whole methodology and conduct training should be based on a deep knowledge of constitutional type, the genetic potential of the body, so that by the convergent action and directed the environmental factors (exercise, food, climate, etc.) to obtain maximum return on the sport.

Constitutional typology

By constitutional typology we refer to all morphological, functional and psychological types that define a particular human being. This division into three categories is made, by teaching reasons, the human being is but a whole, which explains the limits to this view, contrary to the truth yet formulated by Aristotle, then, in biology, the whole is not the sum of parts. Considering the Aristotelian truth, we analyze the constitutional typology through these three main groups of characters defining but bearing in mind the possibility that the typological resultant is to be achieved through a compensation function of various parts of the body without generalizing by the arithmetic value of any constituent parts. Being of a particular interest to us the constitutional typology problematic and its correlation with the performance value - both for the purposes of judicious sports picks, and an individualized training – we will follow, in defining the constitutional type, the main morphological and physiological aspects (somatic type) and aspects regarding the quality and bio-motricity skills, some of them being conditioned mainly by orthostatic (motricity type), some aspects of the psychical activities area (psychic type). The existent conditionalities between the level of these characters and individual biorhythms, so in the end and during each section analyzed, there are correlations between constitutional type and athletic performance. The entire presentation will highlight the essential element, namely, the constitutional type (phenotype) consists, in all its components, the genotype, i.e., hereditary inheritance, and para-type or what is acquired under the influence of the external environment.

History, evolving concepts

The concept of constitutional type dated back to antiquity and evolved until today. For some researchers, this notion relates exclusively to genotype, for others the term refers to phenotype, as indeed is more useful since our investigation concerns both genotype and paratype. Also, the content of the concept of the constitutional type performed initially it encompasses only the morphology of the human body, then covering and scope of functionality, physiology, because, in the modern vision of *Tanner*, it contains both morpho-physiologic and psychic (personality and intellect). In his performance *Tanner* is modern and precise, for which we will adopt in presenting the content of the concept of constitutional type, being consistent with the requirements of a typology useful performance sports.

We present below, in chronological evolution and history of the concept of constitutional type, and in the end to make a few general considerations. Constitutionalist views of the early ideas were done under the influence promo wool philosophers Hindus and Greeks. According to ideas of *Ayurveda*, the universe is composed of three elements: air, fire, and water. The same elements compose the human body. From their joints is born health or illness individuality and especially human. The notion of the constitution understands a set of mental and physical properties, specific to each individual having a permanent lifelong, modifying only due to external factors. The man is born with a constitution definitively determined, but only with pre-made for its development complex in different directions, which is achieved during ontogeny. The constitution refers to human attributes, considered as a whole, a psychosomatic cohesion while having features characteristic morphological, physiological and psychological.

In the opinion of modern science, the human body functions as a unit and connection with this statement, distinguishing the essential aspects of individuality, it is not fair; however, the classification of the type used further as a diagram convenient for conducting research and experiments. Constitution or biotype, how to say some authors (*Pende*, 1955; *Tanner*, 1964) depends on the biological laws of heredity, first; It also depends on the environment acting on the genetic basis. The concept of constitution is interpreted divers. For some researchers, this notion relates exclusively to genotype (many of the doctors and anthropologists' German school), for others the term constitution refers to phenotype as the only phenotype can be observed and described. Another problem is to establish the concept of constitution. Some authors understand this notion only body construction, so morphology (*Bunak, Poire, Pende*). For others, like *Vida, Martiny*, the concept of constitution includes morphological and physiological traits, separating them on the personality or intellect; *Tanner* and other researchers believe that this includes the entire human individuality. His performance is one of the most modern and precise, regarding physical education and sport." The appearance of the construction, function, and behavior, which changes from day to day or from year to year, to a great extent in most individuals, we call constitutional characteristics" *(Tanner*, 1964). From a medical standpoint, "constitution represents all the physical and mental innate tendency on which provision of the individual to certain diseases or resistance to certain pathological factors" (*Konopka,* 1948). The notion of building typology of the body means systematizing genres and types of body building in terms of individual similarities and differences. Type of construction as the entire body constitution is genetically caused. Constitutional peculiarities are not inherited in directly, but predispositions in order to develop them. Compliance genetic influences on the construction of the external environment, climate, social, lifestyle, nutrition and - very important regarding physical education - moving factor. Certain features of the building are more or less subjected to the action of external stimuli, and it depends on their plasticity. Strong construction of genetically caused features is those which relate to the overall size of the body height, the development of long bones and the skeleton as a whole. Moving factor can have a negative role in the evolution of body constitution.

Thus, overtraining force exercises can have negative influences on the development of excessive bone or stagnate their development. For this reason, it requires special attention in the use of force exercises, especially the young followers of the sport. Rational use of proper exercises can stimulate development and can hasten puberty leap of some features, however without affecting body size terminal (*Milicerowa*, 1964). Individual height is finalized after the period of maturation and theoretically does not change in the next stages of life.

Very sensitive influence of the environment is the development of soft tissue. Under the influence of intensive diet and exercise develops muscle fibers and fat tissue behaves different variations depending on these factors throughout life. The amount is defined genetic muscle fibers and is supposed to remain unchanged during ontogeny.

Adipose tissue mass is increased either by increasing the size of existing fat cell, and the process is reversible, either by increasing the number of fat cells, and this process is irreversible and strong genetic condition. Intensified appears (as shown in some research) in the last months of embryonic life in the early stages of childhood and the pubertal period preceding the jump.

Typological differences and genetic predispositions deepen after maturation. Thus, if we look at the three types of construction - the ind vidual "fat with a high-fat anabolism, its opposite, the individual" slender "type" athletic "- that each reacts differently to an intensive diet. This is where the psychological factor that influences the reaction deepens. Active, athletic type, the action intensifies and enhances muscle development. This individual may acquire a silhouette of "bodybuilder." Bold type - weak-muscled the large quantity of fat cells - can increase fat mass, becoming increasingly difficult, refusing effort, and in extreme cases can reach monstrous dimensions. A slender individual who possesses fewer muscle fibers and fewer fat cells under the influence of intensive diet and exercise will gain less weight. Civilization and change the environment acting on the phenotype, and genetic predisposition plays a key role in his training. Construction of a human body can define varied depending on the look you consider. Thus, we can use:

a) overall criterion size (weight), height and weight;

b) criterion exterior proportions, for the purposes of measuring the proportions of body segments in biomechanical evaluation report;

c) the criterion of body tissue composition, which is important in terms of adipose tissue weight, the active tissue.

These various aspects, the construction of the body, find expression in different typological systems created by different researchers' constitutional issues. In this vision of complex constitutional typologies, where we highlighted the existence of typological features physiological somatosensory, motricity and mental enroll personality and model morpho-physio-psycho-cyber proposed by Dr. *Mircea Rázusa* that can present high-value applicability in sport, regarding its computerization. It starts in establishing this model, from the research of Acad. *Manea Manescu*, showing that, overall, through a modeling process appears the next triplet, A, S, M, where A represents the system studied by the subject S, with the help of model M. The same author using the model shows that the modeling process begins with analyzing the original system and identification in this way the properties P 1 (a), P 2 (a)... P n (a) that characterizes it. In the proposed model distinguish morphological, functional, psychological and psychiatric cyber, from which, implicitly at least four categories of properties:

$$P^1{}_1(A),\ P^1{}_2(A),\ P^1{}_3(A),\dots\ P^1(A).$$
$$P^2{}_1(A),\ P^2{}_2(A),\ P^2{}_3(A),\dots\ P^2(A).$$
$$P^3{}_1(A),\ P^3{}_2(A),\ P^3{}_3(A),\dots\ P^3(A).$$
$$P^4{}_1(A),\ P^4{}_2(A),\ P^4{}_3(A),\dots\ P^4(A).$$

Given the complexity of the system approached, it must tabulation of these properties on a basic matrix whose columns are formed of criteria for structure (neuron junction bi-neural junction multi-neuronal ganglion center ... overall) and the lines topographic-forming organic criteria (periphery marrow, bulb... cortex), symbolized above properties being arranged on the basic plan in the form of columns that reshapes, horizontal levels of the classes of properties.

Molecular biology of embryonic development - the foundation of constitutional type

All multicellular plants and animals reproduce sexually start their development from egg or zygote cell-cell have its nucleus initial entire genetic information of the species. The multicellular body is composed of a wide variety of cell types. For example, in a mammal differentiate nerve cells, muscle cells, thyroid cells, cells of the blood elements, etc. These cell types must appear on an extremely orderly in a same original cell. In some organisms, specialization starts from the first cell division of the zygote. Other bodies, a large number of divisions appear before these cells are to fix their destiny tissue and organ. Regardless of the exact differentiation occurs, it leads to the transformation of the initial cell in a large number of cell types progeny. The zygote is itself a specialized cell, performing specific functions that cannot perform any mature cell. Gametes cannot survive if there is no merger of the opposite sex, her not being able to divide normally and die:

- Egg, due to excessive enzymatic equipment with hydrolytic action;
- Sperm, because of its poverty in the cytoplasm. Partogeneză cases (ginogeneză or androgeneză) are rare in nature and meet, usually in the plant kingdom, androgenesis being found exclusively in plants;
- When joining in the fertilization, egg and sperm reinforce each other, resulting zygote, starting point for the development of a new organism.

Successive divisions of the zygote, called cleavage divisions, result-great for many cells. They suffer first accurate determination even in the early stages of embryonic development, giving rise to cell clones which will then undergo differentiation to become liver cells, renal, neural, etc. Immediately after fertilization, the egg frog undergoes 12 divisions cleavage, very fast, characterized by very short periods of interphase, when DNA synthesis occurs with a very accelerated. It is most often irreversible differentiation in the cell as a whole. The culture medium is increased; the differentiated cell cannot synthesize proteins other than those found in it. Differentiation is not due, as a rule, loss or gain of chromosomes, but tuning gene activity. At the nuclear level, the difference is usually reversible, as shown by nuclear transplantation experiments. Cytodifferentiation is in the process reveal a memory that makes a primary cell determined in a certain direction to undergo further differentiation, for the direction that has been determined. The memory cell, as opposed to engrammatic memory, the nervous system is not affected by cell division. Status determination or differentiation is maintained even when cell division occurs. Conversely, the neuron, according to the cellular engrams would disintegrate. Consequently, to preserve its engrams, the neuron is no longer divide.

Semiconservative replication ensures that each daughter cell to receive identical copies of each gene, but the gene sequences cannot, by themselves, specify whether a gene must work or be decommissioned. This is achieved through a variety of mechanisms:

- Diffusible regulatory factors;
- Served covalent modifications of DNA (CpG methylation dinucleotide);
- Changes in local chromosomal proteins, active and inactive regions of the chromosome.

Any of these mechanisms can contribute each cell daughter to inherit a characteristic pattern of genes active or inactive. We do not know what happens at the bifurcation of replication, i.e., whether parental duplex binding proteins remain associated with the gene when it is replicated. It could be that some, but not all proteins remain weakly bound to the sugar-phosphate DNA strand (template), while its bases are used as a template by DNA polymerase synthesis reply. They then would unite closely to duplexes daughters. This would explain the possibility of genes active or inactive status during differentiated cell division. DNA methylation usually accompanies (there also are exceptions) the differentiation state, most active or potentially active genes are methylated, at CpG sequences level.

Cytoplasmic irreversible differentiation, accompanied by loss of ability to divide, is found in reticulocytes - blood cells in birds. In mammals, cells are disintegrated nuclei of such cells and thus only specialized in the synthesis of hemoglobin. The same happens in adult plasma cells that produce antibodies specific: they do not divide, produce specific antibodies, several days after dying. It can be inferred that cell division is a condition sine qua non of life. Exceptions are neurons which, although no longer divide, live many years, their nucleus is functional only in genetic transcription, synthesizing RNA involved in all cellular processes, including, in this case, and memory processes. A certain protein synthesis takes place at very low (basal) for the continued functioning of all cells. This synthesis can replace aging proteins which are targeted destructions by the proteolytic system, and ATP-dependent ubiquitin. The state of cellular senescence is installed when altered protein disposal system is not effective.

The complex stable transcript synthesized on the template DNA, the genes by all three RNA polymerases, eukaryotic, representing the transcripts associated with transcription factors, is the stable association DNA, as soon as the transcription factor binds stable gene, then that particular locus is activated and can be transcribed by RNA polymerase III repeated. The same is true for RNA polymerases I and II.

Thus, transcription complexes provide a possible mechanism for maintaining the state of differentiation interphase, that is, between the successive cell divisions. Transcription and replication, however, cannot take place simultaneously. Not all cells give rise to identical cells by division. Stems cells - stem cells-line - often divide asymmetrically, as the line hematopoietic stems, resulting in a daughter cell line that continues evolving towards different strains and erythrocyte. It will live 120 days after dying, being replaced by other erythrocytes. The spleen is considered “old cemetery erythrocytes.”

RNA polymerase III is a transcription factor that binds TF III preferentially to the coding strand of the 5S rRNA gene and can remain connected even during replication. Chromosome-son who will inherit the parental DNA strand will inherit factor and, along with it, and gene transcriptionally active state. The Catena which is noncoding, and that will go in the other chromosome-son will inherit the gene idle. This can be packaged in Nucleosomes and thus can be repressed. A nucleosome segregation conservative parent at the bifurcation of replication, provide another mechanism for generating two cells, of which only one gene is active. Chromosomal reshuffling linked to cell differentiation in eukaryotes are found both unicellular and multicellular those. During the life cycle, the cilia extensive DNA rearrangements occur, especially in the evolution macronuclei with extensive gene destructions. The most difficult problem is that modern embryologist to explain how terms may be converted to molecular genetic information represented by a one-dimensional sequence of nucleotides in the DNA, in a complex organization, three-dimensional, of an adult body. Classical embryologists, they realized that egg and sperm are not entirely devoid of form and symmetry. In some way, these germ cells, the union which arises cell (zygote), the starting point for the formation of a new body must contain either a version miniaturized plan body adult or a biochemical mechanism for the production plan this body refreshed with every generation.

In 1700, this concept led to a preformism theory which held that the ovum (in oocysts' opinion) and sperm (in spermists' opinion) are really tiny adults, a *Homunculus*, in the case of *Homo sapiens*. In this case, the main function of the development is to make it bigger this little creature hidden in the egg or sperm. Although people today look with superiority to these speculations, they must recognize that there is some truth in the basic idea of this concept. We know today that certain models (patterns) are performing in egg development and that other mechanisms are determined by body shape, in fact, enabled by fertilization.

Insects, like amphibians, early embryogenesis occur so quickly that there is not enough time to be held cell growth. Instead, the point of early embryogenesis is to split the large egg into small cells so that morphogenesis can commence. In Drosophila, as well as other insects immediately after fertilization, zygotic nucleus undergoes rapidly about nine divisions, resulting in 512 nuclei to take place without the divization process, meaning the separation of the egg in the cell cytoplasm. Syncytium egg becomes a gigantic literary syncytial means a single cell with many nuclei filled. After the ninth division, nuclei migrate to the surface of the egg and dividing synchronously a further four times. Invaginate the plasma membrane of the egg, so that each core cell is separated from that present in a cell membrane. It follows blastoderm.

Complex folding of the balloon ellipsoidal cells arranged as a hollow gives rise to a segmented larva, called instar, which has a head, three thoracic segments (T1-T3) and eight abdominal segments (T1-T8). The *instar* is the first of three larval stages, separated by molts, leading to the formation of a creature similar to a worm that is voracious, eating and accumulating enough biomass to build a midge adult. After the third instar, the larvae pupate, to provide a protective environment for the pursuit of metamorphosis. During metamorphosis, the larvae digest many of their tissues (histolysis) which it replaced by structures of adult (histogenesis). However, signs segmentation adult body keeps larval stages. Surprisingly it appears that adult organs (legs, wings, antennae, etc.) are built not from larval cells differentiated in small groups but relatively undifferentiated cells which retain the ability to proliferate and were called imaginal discs, a name derived from the word "imago" that means adult. The 19 imaginal discs (a new form of a genital disc and a pair merged) are distinct very early during embryogenesis. Each disc is also intended to provide organ-specific adult (left leg, right leg, left eye or right eye, etc.).

Imaginal discs remain in a relatively undifferentiated larvae body to the surface, until, by changing hormone levels during pupation is triggered the differentiation with carrying out morphogenesis. Thus, most of its basic body plan is established during embryogenesis the fly, long before imaginal discs distinguish adult cuticle structures to create enveloping internal organs of the animal. To understand morphogenesis, modern biologists almost always start with identifying genes and gene products affecting the visible aspects of the body. It was also the strategy used in the analysis of lambda bacteriophage capsid morphogenesis and T4.

Dorsalization genes from *Drosophila* are well studied, enabling understanding of the mechanisms governing morphogenesis in higher eukaryotes. Unfertilized egg from *Drosophila*, as in other insects, is surrounded by a shell of the egg, highly structured, called the chorion. Front and rear, like the front and rear (ventral and dorsal), are easily distinguishable. This suggests that external differentiation egg itself possess polarity and anterior-posterior dorsal-ventral, as evidenced by biochemical and genetic analysis.

For the construction of a dorsoventral polarity of the egg with the corresponding gene products are required for at least ten different genes. If the mother does not have a wild-type copy of any of these ten genes, a dorsal embryo cannot be duplicated by a single copy of the gene wild-type (normal), made by sperm during fertilization. Obviously, it is too late to be reconstituted egg, using wild-type gene product, brought by the sperm; in this case, a gene also carries what was called maternal effect. Thus, father's genotype is completely irrelevant to the original embryo morphogenesis. For recessive mutations in the genes of the ten dorsalization, maternal effects are observable only in homozygous her eggs, which both copies are a defective gene. Eggs female wild-type, heterozygous, on which a copy of the wild type normal gene product can produce are completely normal. This is because essentially all mRNA and factors present in the egg mature are produced in the cytoplasm of the egg by 15 diploid nutritious, or cells-nurse (nurse cells) mRNA dorsal, for example, it may be identified in cells nutritious before he appears in oocytes. Transcription of the haploid nucleus of the egg contributes little if anything helps in storing enormous amounts of the cytoplasm of the egg. Almost the entire capacity of the egg is inherited from the oocyte, from the mother.

The appearance of a fully dorsal embryo is amazing. This appears to be entirely accounted for by the back (dorsal) and does not have the front (ventral). The embryo cannot survive, because it lacks structures such as the dorsal-lateral *Filzkoper* (breathing tubes) and ventral structures, as denticulate bands, rows of bumps that help the larva to swim. Instead, dorsal structures extending around the body of the embryo.

Geneticists were able to identify mutations in such genes that have led to the loss of some, but not all ventral structures. The existence of such intermediary embryos (partial dorsal) suggests that the polarity dorsal-ventral in the unfertilised egg is defined by a gradient of some sort, most likely molecular. *The task of collecting various genes dorsal is to generate this gradient, giving cells able to interpret their position in the gradient, and thus to vary the molecular corresponding to the determination that a previously suffered.* Surprisingly, mutations occurring in some of the ten genes may be partially or completely dorsal "saved" by microinjection of cytoplasm taken from an early embryo, wild type before cellularisation of the blastoderm. The rescue, at least five of the mutant seems to be due to mRNA molecules. Moreover, embryo RNA from a mutant with a defect in the gene dorsalis other and vice versa. Thus, each of the ten genes contributing dorsalis seems a distinct gene product at the molecular machinery responsible for generating dorsal-ventral polarity.

Particularly relevant is the finding that saving ventral structures in embryos homozygous mutation in one of the genes dorsalis occurs only when injected wild-type cytoplasm in the ventral part of the embryo mutant. This means that the embryo dorsalis has already established a gradient of positional information along the dorsoventrally its axis but in the absence of dorsal gene product, the cells are unable to perform their position within the gradient and differentiate properly. Equally interesting is the finding that injecting cytoplasm wild-type posterior region underside of an embryo dorsalis where forms breathing tubes in the wild type, save Filzkorper site, while injecting region middle ventral (where head to the wild-type structures form) restores sensory organs of the head. Thus, the mature egg Drosophila has also established a gradient of positional information, the anteroposterior axis. These two gradients seem to be independent of each other.

Toll gene product determines the morphogenetic polarity gradient.

The dorsal-ventral polarity of the fact that the egg is determined by a gradient of some type is supported by the behavior of dorsalis gene mutation, a gene known as *Toll*. Recessive mutations in this gene, like the other nine genes dorsalis produce embryos free of ventral and lateral structures. The gene product Toll but that should behave differently from other new products, gene because it was possible to isolate dominant mutations in the *Toll*. Funny is that these dominant mutations that cause ventral structures to expand throughout the dorsal side of the embryo. This suggests that the gene product Toll can be really morphogenic (or generate morphogenic) which is to form ventral structure. Mutations *Toll* dominant (ventralizing) will result in overproduction of the gene product Toll, at the site of the ventral normal or expression occurs failure of the gene product, Toll, throughout the egg, so that the cells are put in a position to produce structures ventral places wrong.

Cytoplasm microinjection experiments are wild-type embryos to restore Toll, support the interpretation that the gene product Toll is (or produce) a morphogenic. As seen in Drosophila embryo has the same polarity as the normal eggshell (chorion). When mutations in any of the other nine genes dorsalizării are restored by microinjection of normal cytoplasm embryo achieved or partially achieved retains the same polarity as the chorion, but for mutations Toll, rescued embryo polarity is determined by normal cytoplasm injection site. Injections dorsal polarity reverses normal egg relative to the coating. Thus, in contrast to other products of dorsalizării new genes, which only helps to interpret their position blastoderm cells in a dorsoventral gradient of the pre-existing gene product of Toll appears to determine the polarity of the gradient itself. We do not know if this information the positional may be encoded by a gradient of a morphogenic such as AMP in Dictyostelium (which makes the adherence of the cells to the cell foundation of the colony to form the body of the fungus), or the like of an electrical potential, such as the force proton motive or impulse propagation from bacteria to higher eukaryotes nervous, polar interactions of cell surface glycoproteins on adjacent cells by large cytoskeletal structures that cross the entire embryo, or mechanisms that we cannot imagine now.

By recombinant DNA technology, different genes have been cloned and mutagenized in vitro dorsalis. The capacity of such gene products dorsal mutagenized to restore embryos may then be tested in vitro or reproducing mutagenized genes into the germ line of *Drosophila* using P element-mediated transformation studies can reveal the physical nature of the positional information and the way the cells interprets their position in a gradient of development.

Regulatory architecture of the genome

Cis-regulatory elements can be considered as units of information processing, caught in the regulatory network so that they receive multiple inputs, in the form of numerous transcription factors that bind within.

Input APIs (entries) vary depending on which gene is functional in a given cell and the process of development in which it is activated. Output CPC (out of the system) is "instruction" given the basal transcription apparatus that determines whether a gene must be silent or be active with certain intensity. If the gene encodes a transcription factor, output CPC leads to cis-regulatory elements all others, where there are functional target sites for the above quote factor.

It is said of it as connected 'downstream,' while input APIs are terminally toward a regulatory gene and cis-regulatory system of their own is what makes him able to "process" different stimuli (inputCEs) he receives, converting them into a single response (output). Only by checking the functional significance of the sites target specific transcription factor in an item cis-regulatory understand what it means genomic DNA sequence of an item and the functional significance of a sequence of genomic DNA could be considered the most important issue in bio -science. Information processing function of a cis-regulatory element is a link between the various circumstances that occur in the cell and response capabilities are incorporated in regulatory sequence of organisms with bilateral symmetry. A general feature of cis-regulatory architecture organisms with bilateral symmetry is that different phases of expression of certain genes are frequently mediated by cis-regulatory elements different, called "modules." The use of such a term instead of "enhancer "has advantages because the functions of these items can be complex and integrative than those suggested by the verb "to amplify" and, in fact, in some cells, some modules work soon to the Represa than to stimulate transcription.

Morphological structures of organisms with bilateral symmetry is never the product of a single gene or single regulatory systems. Direct measurements on the complexity of RNA and data on EST (acronym derived from *Expressed Sequence Tagged*) obtained by analyzing cDNA banks for certain tissues, confirming the assertion that hundreds and often thousands of genes must be expressed to direct matters create a particular tissue, a specific body part or a multicellular structure. These genes are controlled in space and time for development of large networks of genes regulating development. In the conception of *Davidson* (2001) is organizing network architecture connecting links regulators cis-regulatory elements by cis-trans interactions and, until today, begin to decipher the true nature of these networks. Genomic changes that alter this network creates new directions in the development process, as they may affect the activities of large sets of genes. For example, the emergence of new molecules entering or cis-regulatory in the vicinity of a gene that controls other genes battery makes these genes are expressed in different spatial areas of an embryo. Likewise, changes in cis-regulatory sites target genes lead to adding to existing batteries of genes, as changes in the target site without sub-items under the control of various functions of the network signals. The network architecture is most often specified by the identity of the target sites of cis-regulatory elements all participating. Analysis of genomic cis-regulatory systems and the interrelations between them allows understanding how genomes are encoding properties of organisms.

Developing genetic program execution is to build a body of a particular species. Until it reaches the final shape of each element morphological body of an organism during its ontogenetic development, genetic sub expressed in progenitor cells are transient, representing stations in the path leading to the final stage of spatial organization. Transient control involves a temporal precision. There cis-regulatory systems that only work for a few hours, the entire life of the organism, and only for these few hours are necessary functions mediated by genes that are activated during this time; they are not necessary at other times of the individual life. For example, setting the asymmetry of dorsal/ventral (D / V) in the frog embryo can occur during a crucial period that lasts about an hour, during which genomes are activated at the end stage of the blastula. Genes encoding transcriptional regulators of a particular homeodomain as well viz, twin and goosecoid are then transiently activated precisely, specifically on the dorsal side of the embryo. Moreover, cell signaling events regulated by these factors are still needed before the start gastrulation. Similarly, certain gene products function in certain types of differentiated cells in different stages are only required only in those specific cells. For example, the proteins 'sticky' are produced in the salivary glands of larvae of *Drosophila*, just before the pupa stage (*Backendorf* and *Kaftos,* 1976). These adhesive proteins, encoded by a small family of genes coordinately expressed are needed to secure the larva of a dry, to begin metamorphosis insect, and consequently, they are synthesized only in the last few hours of the larval period of four days, and there will never be synthesized during one's life, either before or after this time. The nature of the signals (inputs) of a particular type used for such control to be exercised transient gene expression, for the determined target sites is linked in cis-regulatory systems of these genes. The formation pattern acquis is a term commonly used as spatial patterns occur at every level of biological organization from the subcellular to the body. In functional genomics, it is applied specifically to the development process in which the areas of spatial cell unspecified designated as "state of adjustment," creating finally fields of cells that will give rise to different parts of a structure, an organ or organism. Early events of the training pattern acquis establish the basics of body plan such as metameric segmentation that occurs early in embryogenesis the fly, or axle front/back (A / P) and left-right asymmetry of a mouse. Subsequent events forming pattern fixes may define detailed and smaller items such as arrangement sensory hairs on midge or fingering limbs in mice. Formation processes pattern acquis are progressive, meaning that as development occurs, specific spatial elements are refined to high resolution. In all cases, the formation pattern acquis in areas deserves its existing cells, new subdomains, having a place of their successive partition.

The core mechanisms of the *pattern* acquis are the regional specification. The new subdivision of an existing cell area is created by the expression of one or more transcription factors, within a bounded region. It sets out a new regulatory state in the region, differentiating it from other cells and preparing programs for the development of the following events. In the process, intervening cis-regulatory systems that perform the crucial function of integrating signaling, lineation and other *input* defining specific regional areas to suffer. In turn, the transcription factors that control it provides its *input* specific transcriptional activities of other downstream genes, regulatory network to the next level. Genes encoding transcription factors involved expressed space and elements of intercellular signaling systems. From this cascade of gene activation events resulting progressive nature of the process of forming the pattern acquis. All metazoan produce differing types of cells, but only those with bisymmetry side give rise to strings morphological dimensional cell types differentiated terminal which we call "organs" and only body shapes adult bilateral layers or tubes of cell types mesoderm differentiated constitute components all major body parts. The bilateral cell differentiation is performed accurately, so that, under normal conditions, such cells can carry out other functions, and, when they retain the replicative capacity, they give rise only to cells of their similar. There are very few cases of highly-differentiated cell transdifferentiation: differentiated cells undergo differentiation because then suffer a re-differentiated in another direction. Cells that are characterized by what embryologists have called employment since they underwent terminal differentiation present stabilizing functional mechanisms that block certain *pattern* transcriptional instead deploying other summaries specific to them. The paths of such a stabilization circuit feedback network gene that regulates cytodifferentiation are diverse changes in the conformation of the domain structure chromatic including systems-regulating of relevant genes, methylation local or demethylation local DNA, reducing the turnover of RNA, loss or inactivation of the total of the entire apparatus transcriptional nuclear, from the moment the cell was loaded with enough types of specific mRNA, as is the case inactivation of the transcriptional nuclei red blood cells from birds or solution choice extreme - elimination of the cell nucleus - such as is the case erythrocyte in mammals. Terminal differentiation may be defined in terms of a specific set of genes encoding the differentially expressed proteins, such as those for hemoglobin and red blood cells of vertebrates or enzymes in the cell surface receptors signals the effector cells and molecules of the immune system. The realization of such an organization regulating genome provides expression coordinated t of such sets of genes, each with a specific function very accurate intervenes so-called "battery of genes" - a set of genes are in a linkage of functionally powerful expresses concert. The term "battery of genes" is due to cis-regulatory elements relevant to the four functional genes in muscle cells to amniotes. It can be seen how several types of transcription factors that bind to DNA regulatory systems are also used: viz, a bHLH factor MyoD family of specific muscle (MDF); SRF ("serum response factor") and MEF2 factor specific muscle. Thus, the basic principle of gene battery is Linc Linc organization of genes in a gene battery by the presence of cis-regulatory target sites for common sets of transcriptional regulators. This principle is based on the peculiarities of structural organization of the genome that cause certain genes to become part of certain batteries gene, both during development and the evolution of species body. Transcription factors activate gene regulatory elements of the battery. Sometimes the trigger is singular factors which genes are activated terminal differentiation. Sometimes several different positive factors may act synergistically. When the boundaries of space in which to be cast functions, terminals were organized upstream repressors outline of these boundaries no longer are needed, so elements cis-regulatory functioning in this situation are devoid of any target site for repressors spatial. Cis-regulatory elements are often compact terminals, and if a gene is scheduled to operate in several different cell types, they may, in the same way, sites for various activities which are present in these cell types. Further still, terminal differentiation processes often mediate expression to very high levels, gene products that control them sometimes being present in huge quantities. The classic example is that of globin genes in mammalian erythrocytes. In some stages, such genes provide more than 90% of protein synthesis in these cells (*Hunt*, 1974). Very high levels of transcription imply that the particular features of cis-regulatory mediate maximum rates of basal transcription initiation device that can be adjusted both quantitatively and qualitatively. The whole band that provides the "logic" of such an organization regulatory component is entered into the genome of a nucleotide sequence of DNA.

If the morphological features of an animal are the result of process development and process of development of each being controlled by regulating genomic program, the progression of the evolution of these animals is the consequence of genomic adjustment programs. Regulatory genomics and comparative genomics will provide such data and rhythm essential in understanding how biological evolution. When we are in functional terms that are specific tuning components genomic elements that ensure morphological differences between two organisms have a common ancestor, then we will see exactly what the differences are essential causes of the DNA of these organisms. Thus, understanding how these development programs ontogenetic and evolution, will be giving a precise interpretation of fundamental evolutionary mechanisms, little or no understood at present. Differences in regulatory network architecture are due phylogenetic diversification.

Anthropological schools and constitutional typologies

Hippocrates was the first constitutionalist, in the broad sense of that term (the fourth century, BC). He believes individuality a set of morphological, physiological and psychological. His views were transmitted to us through his Galen and it is not known exactly which of them is thinking utterances of Hippocrates and which ones were introduced by Galen. The foundation's constitutional criteria Hippocrates is represented by humours and temperaments - these concepts have survived until modern times. Hippocrates spoke of the existence of four temperaments:

a) blood - active, serene, living reactions;
b) choleric - explosive, excitable;
c) melancholy - apathetic with reduced mobility;
d) phlegmatic - balanced, less excitable.

In building the body, it distinguished two extreme types:

- Habitus phtisicus - with a slender build;
- Habitus apoplecticus - with massive construction.

In the views of Hippocrates find findings that can be considered the beginning of scientific observations on individual reactions of the body to every man according to his temperament, influence action on the environment and the individual response to this environment.

In II century AD, *Filostrates* was busy studying the interdependence of body building and exercise. He analyzed the peculiarities of athletes in terms of proportion body of his vision tempers after *Hippocrates*, indicating the specific methods of training depending on the competition. In the Middle Ages interest in the constitution of the human body disappears. In the early days of modern history Current appear interested in physiognomy, which were no scientific basis for scientific research of constitutional issues. False tests are known typology's *Lombroso* and his school, which led to racism, in the worst sense of the word. The nineteenth century brought a new breath in the development of natural sciences and interest in the man, in terms of the place it occupies in the world of living beings, of its evolution. Develops anthropology in the broadest sense of that term, which is concerned, inter alia, construction, and typology body.

Goethe creates word morphology; while appearing the disciples of the typological school: French school of descriptive morphology, based on the observation body construction; Italian school is developing, which is concerned with anthropometry; and German constitutional school, studying the influence and action of endocrine glands.

French School. Precursors are French school *J.N. Hall, F.N. Troisvévre, and L. Rostan.*

The first two still rests on the notion temperaments; Halle defines in general temperaments: active, muscular and nervous. In his views of *Troisvévre* are felt influences of *Lamarck* (if the organ or body part is used, develops, if not used, disappears).

The real founder of the French school is *C. Sigaud* (end sec. XIX). He distinguishes four anatomical systems of the body, which is formed under the influence of the environment: respiratory, digestive, muscular and nervous. Each of these systems remains in regular contact with such external factors:

1) Atmospheric conditions act on the breath;
2) Nutrition affects the digestive system;
3) The world of physical objects produces muscle reactions;
4) Social environment generates psychological necessities of life.

In terms of building body muscle type is characterized by a strong development of extremity muscles, the chest is well developed in the form of trapeze; developing chest and abdomen is proportional ends relatively long hair growth is enhanced. The face is rectangular.

The predominance upper torso on the bottom characterizes the respiratory type. Chest in the shape of a trapezoid but longer has a diamond shaped face.

Digestive type is characterized by a large abdomen, waistline slightly contoured, narrow shoulders, extremities short and poorly muscled, a front triangle with the highly developed jaw, neck short and thick.

Brain-nervous type is characterized by a large head and lower part of the face, underdeveloped gives triangle position opposite type of digestive. The overall construction is slender, delicate stems and narrow basin, relatively long extremities. These types do not remain final set; they may change during life. Children are respiratory type encountered in young matured - muscle type. A man in his prime matured returns to the newborn digestive type. *Sigaud* highlights the strong influence of the environment in the formation of these types, and his successor, *Mac Auliffe* (1925) develops this concept, illustrating it with examples. Thus, the type of breathing is common among nomads, living in the open, under the open sky. Type digestive meets amid privileged social class and agricultural areas. Muscle type and environmental influences workers' physical and type of cerebral nervous is specific intellectuals.

Sigaud`s successors were *L. Mac Auliffe* and *A. Thooris*. Both authors convey notions of tonic and atonic in body construction. Some concepts we encounter and other researchers (sthenia and asthenia construction).

Thooris conducted a synthesis model of the clinical morphology of *Sigaud*, technical morphology of *Saron* and physiology of *Pavlov*. It shows in his work, *La vie par le stade* their dependence on the construction of the physical body and skill, exemplifying with data collected from French sporting competitions. *Thooris* stresses the importance of the length of the lower extremities for some athletic sports easier and uses the nomenclature of *Manouvrier*. Body building in "fours," in *Thooris`s* vision, consists of three types;

a) brachyskelic;

b) mesoskelic;

c) makroskelic.

In addition, *Mac Auliffe* (1926) and *Thooris* (1923) divide individuals after their phenotypic appearance in uniform or corrugated types, flat and round. They believe that these types are determined by gel protoplasmic water to soak differential. Flat type is tall and slim, with flattened gel, less avid liquid. The round, brevilineal, short and bulky limbs type are oppositely determined by the quality of the gel.

Italian school. While typological French school relies primarily on morphology and chemical research, the Italian school is based on anthropometric measurements, which is the foundation of typological systematics. Italian school was the precursor Frenchman *Manouvrier*. He classified according to body type, building relationship between body length and height of the lower extremities. The skelic index, widely known height - the height of a seated position - classifies people into brachyskelical (with short legs) - the index is up to - 85; mesoskelical- the index is between 85-90, and makroskelical (legged), the index value of 90 passes.

Giovanni (after *Verdun*, 1955; *Comas*, 1960) is the first and true representative of the Italian school. Using the technique anthropometric method, established some ideal proportions.

Building the ideal proportions of the body, after *Giovanni* is:

• Size = shoulder length;

• The circumference of the chest cavity height = 1/2;

• The height of the abdomen = 1/5 of the circumference of the chest cavity;

• The length of the pool - 4/5 of the height of the abdomen.

The best-known representative of the Italian school is *G. Viola* - who has made a great contribution in the use of anthropological measurements accurately. He introduces the concept of volume, determining the three-dimensional components of the body (length, width, height).

Viola typology is based on 10 measurements anthropological very intricate (heavy) and impossible to use in practice. However, the contribution of *Viola* in anthropometry development is very high. He introduced:

a) the term average time;

b) three-dimension measurements, the notion of volume;

c) very accurate measurements;

d) a new typology;

e) a new concept of morphological differences between form and volume.

Anthropologists and doctors' views on the typology of Viola are divided and even paradoxical. Some authors consider it accurate and scientifically valuable; On the other hand, the same researchers admit that the typology is exclusively theoretical and impossible to use in practice. Therefore, the typology of *Viola* remains only in the sphere of conquest theory and not practice.

German school.

Bauer - the most prominent representative of German school - defines components as a constitutional predisposition to developing organ systems. He places great emphasis on the role that it plays in the formation and constitution glands components.

Kretschmer`s typology. It first approached the problem from the standpoint of psychiatry constitution. He tried to demonstrate a correlation between the psychic and somatic structure between the constitution and mental pathology. Based on empirical observations, Kretschmer established three main types that correspond broadly classical classifications. The predominance lengths distinguish the leptosome. Thin and pale skin covers a fragile skeletal mass and a weak muscular system. The thorax is flat and has protruding ribs. The abdomen is small and secluded, small head and oval face.

A harmonious and powerful whole body distinguishes the athletic type. The head is high, oval face, elongated, with well-defined relief. The picnic is characterized by a great development of circular diameter of the head, thorax, and abdomen. Excessive fat deposition. *Kretschmer* described a rare variant, dysplastic, which has placed several pathological forms: eunuchoid giants, infantile, and cretins. Psychosis exists between morphological types and biological affinities net. On the clinical level, *Kretschmer* concludes that there is a strong affinity between the picnic and manic-depressive syndrome, and schizophrenia between leptosomes and athletic. Contrary, between and among leptosomes, picnic and schizophrenia and manic-depressive syndrome affinity missing. Other research has shown that there is a correlation between athletic dysplastic and epilepsy.

Russian school. In Russia, *V.V. Bunek* created a typology personal, interesting.

Bunek lists seven characteristics of the morphological type of constitution and defines four types of construction:

- Stenoplastic;
- Metaplastic;
- Europlastic;
- Sub-plastic.

Pavlov studied the types of nervous system in dogs. Using different experimental conditions, he distinguished four types of central nervous system: weak; strong, unbalanced and excitable; strong, balanced, mobile; strong, balanced, inert.

Certain characteristics distinguish each type. Thus, the type animals weak, conditioned reflexes snap hard and are inconsistent. The second characteristic of this type is the lack of balance between excitation and inhibition. However, the predominance of excitation has a relative character. Animals' excitable processes can be distinguished with a high degree of stability. The strong balanced type there is an equivalence between excitation and inhibition. However, these animals placed in various environmental conditions have different adaptation speeds. Depending on the mobility, strong types were divided into mobile and inert. At first, it snaps conditioned reflexes quickly and just as quickly, it changes according to the environment. Type inert conditioned reflexes change a difficult and adapting to new experimental conditions is difficult. After *Pavlov*, the same types are found in humans and are known under the generic name of temperaments. Pavlovian temperaments are broadly overlapping the Hippocratic. Thus, melancholy temperament type corresponds weak, unbalanced and strong excitable type is synonymous with the choleric type balanced and strong temperament corresponds mobile blood and strong, balanced type corresponds inert phlegmatic. These types were very rare in humans in their classical form: usually people belonging to intermediate tempers.

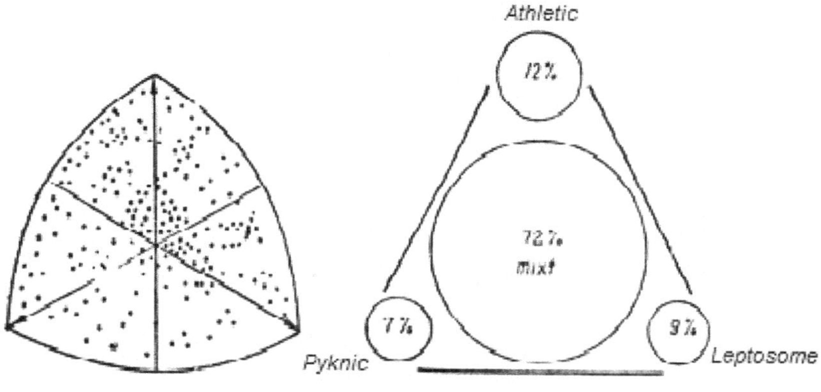

Fig. 30. Constitutional type (by Sheldon).

Anglo-Saxon and American School.

The US emerged some typological conceptions based in particular on the notions of building sthenic and asthenic. After the Second World War, the US and Anglo-Saxon countries have spread a new typology founded on principles different from the other - *Sheldon* somatotypology. *W.H. Sheldon* - psychologist and psychiatrist, making an analysis of the typology of *Kretschmer*, said that only a part of the human population, 20%, with features extreme could be defined by this method, the rest remaining typological undefined. *Sheldon* requires a new conception of individuality somatic and claims that every individual, there are three elements of construction.

He thus creates a variety of somatic types encountered in the human population; there are only three different but a continuous type of construction of the body. The names of the three elements (components) of the building, which Sheldon links them to develop flakes embryonic - endomorph, mesomorph, ectomorph - have generated many reservations among morphology, in terms of their character imprecise since not all tissues entering composition components come from the same embryonic leaf. (Fig. 30)

Endomorph is softness and roundness of forms, the domination of fatty tissue, fat and viscera, the storage capacity of fat, trunk size preponderance of the extremities. Depths trunk dimensions are large in relation to the cross, wide hips, calm front lines, small hands, and feet.

Endomorph type can be identified with the type of digestive of the French school. Construction of athletic mesomorph is a strong skeleton, musculature strong. The hinges are well connected, especially in the extremities, face shape is square, thick skin. Extremely athletic mesomorph corresponds to the type of other authors' typology, even if *Sheldon* states that not every mesomorph can be an athlete.

Ectomorph is the preponderance of suppleness and delicacy construction. The body surface is large relative to the table, big brain, central nervous system well developed, domination ectodermal tissue of origin. Appear, therefore, cerebral type classifications similarities with other authors. *Sheldon* considers the notion of gynandromorphy, which defines sexual characters conflicting presence in each individual. A high degree of gynandromorphy is met mainly in men, and endomorph and mesomorph mainly in women. *Sheldon,* in its principles, emphasizes the great interdependence between the construction of the body and the psyche of the individual. This part of his conception is severely criticized, especially by psychologists, and it has not spread equally known as body building typology. His method is to assess each individual building components based on photographic images estimated. Initially, Sheldon intended to make the photographs measurements required for a summary of the value of a given component scale of one to seven. The measurement system was not yet used to assess the three components is "eye" at the scale of one first, then scale 1/2. Of proxies emerged height-weight index:

$$\frac{\text{Body height}}{\text{Body weight}}$$

The value of this index to individuals' ectomorph's minimal changes during life, in contrast to individuals' endomorph, decreases with age, with increasing layers of fat, especially in women. Somatotype, each individual, is indicated by a code "of biological individuality" consisting of three digits, the first of which defines the endomorphic value, the second - the mesomorph amount, the third - on the ectomorphic. Thus, the extreme types will be presented in order: 711, 171, 117. The most common type and is built harmoniously expressed through the somatotype 444, with a balance of all components. Sheldon shows the process evaluation of the three components based on photos taken from behind, side, front, in detail. At first, appreciate silhouette entirely (first impression), then set the value components for each part of the body: head and neck, trunk and extremities, based on the proportions and size of the parts of the body, drawing muscularity degree of deposition of layers of fat, etc. This determination is based on models (see *Atlas* of *Sheldon*, 1954) and scale index suppleness, defining the ectomorph and whose values are to somatotypes individual's past in the *Sheldon*`s Atlas, taking account of age.

He alleged that the somatotype is genetically conditioned and is unchanged throughout life; it signifies not only what we see and measure a point, but also the expression of a certain trend towards a transformation that occurs with age. This determination is done based on models (*Atlas, Sheldon*, 1954) and suppleness index scale, defining the ectomorphic and whose values are to somatotypes individual's past in *Sheldon*`s, taking account of age. He alleged that the somatotype is genetically conditioned and is unchanged throughout life; it signifies not only what we see and measure a point, but also the expression of a certain trend towards a transformation that occurs with age. In *Sheldon`s* typology, he considers the age of the individual. Thus, he states that if a young individual, the layer of fat will express a higher degree than an individual endomorph older. Endomorph hungry, losing fatty tissue will always be an endomorph, changing the only appearance in an ectomorph.

The number of fat cells remains the same, only that they will be lower. The graph of the somatotypes can be represented by a somatogram the form of an equilateral triangle. Each peak of this stage somatogram expresses extreme (maximum) of one of the three components that stage gradually decreases as the distance from the top, and the values of the two remaining components are increasing (from 1-7). Amid the somatogram, figure 44 expresses the most harmonious elements. This method is alleged the following:

1. component names are inadequate;
2. somatoscopy method is biased;
3. somatotype genotype is not equal because we can only appreciate what we see, so phenotype, there and genotypic characters, which we cannot ignore exclusively;
4. somatotype as interpreted by *Sheldon* informs us about the absolute size of the individual, are only its proportions;
5. *Sheldon* proposes the same rating scale for both women and men, which causes feminine somatotypes immeasurable progress on somatogram.

Followers of the method of *Sheldon, R.W. Parnell, Barbara Heath, L. Carter* amended and even corrected it. *Parnell's* desire is to objectify the method of *Sheldon* with features subject to measurement. Based on averages and standard deviations of anthropometric measurements performed on a group of students, he builds "charter Mh" evaluation scale representing the three factors of construction. Factor expressing the phenomenon of fat deposition is the sum of the three layers of epithelial fat- fat weight factor (musculature and bone building) and suppleness factor expressed by index:

$$\frac{\text{Body height}}{\sqrt[3]{\text{Body weight}}}$$

.

Analyzing materials obtained from research conducted on women, *Parnell* proposes using somatogram the focus of value 433 as being closest to the average female construction. *Parnell* gives up the entire psychological weight and states that we can only momentarily define the body`s building situation and not it`s genetic fundamental and note that the somatotype is not unchanged. He used the concept of phenotype instead of the notion of somatotype. *Sheldon`s* assistant, *B. Heath* does not share the same concept, noting that this term already has a larger value in biology and should not be used to define the body construction. *B. Heath* (1963) to undertake changes in her classic somatotypology transformation, changing "Mh's charter" by *Parnell*. Charter's Heath used to determine the construction of mature persons, regardless of age or sex. Thus, the image evaluation of a somatotype, in most cases, will turn age.

Another main change made by *Heath* and *Carter* (1968) consists of seven-scale expansion in both directions, from 1.2 to 20. Scala processed by *Sheldon* on American students does not include all somatotypes and opportunities and those groups that can probably reach values (related to individual factors) off the scale. (Such groups are *Nilotic* - who evaluated the new flexibility in ectomorph groups (tribes) of the Admiralty Islands, mesomorph whose value exceeds seven, and fat women reach a 12-13 in endomorph). From here comes the need to extend the scale. Although some changes were necessary *for Sheldon`s* somatotypology, he makes a valuable contribution introducing the notion of "building components" instead of "type" and is thus in line with the fundamentals of modern genetics. All types that followed *Sheldon* define continuity considering the construction of hull forms to different groups of individuals.

Modern biotypology. The development of science in the first decades of the twentieth century was echoed on constitutional anthropology. The strongest influence they have exerted, of course, endocrinology and genetics. Due to these influences are waived schemes so simple and much used by anthropology, in the nineteenth century. New achievements of medicine are based classification systems of human variability. Thus was born the modern biotypology.

The broad description of modern biotypes belongs to *Martiny* (1948). For him, the explanation of differences in form between individuals lies in the uneven development of the three skins embryonic, ectoblast, cordomezoblast, and endoblast. It is thus formed which is characterized by the predominance of the type of tissue or organs derived from primary tissue, with the participation of two other normal or defective tissues. Thus, the type endoblastic is hyper endoblastic with normal or deficient nephroma and ectoblast low forever. Mesoblastic has ectoblast deficient and ectoblastic is characterized by a significant lack the two other tissues. The only type that is cordoblastic tissues is balanced. These four types correspond to older classifications of French morphologues.

The endoblastic or digestive type of *Sigaud*, or asthenic brevilineal of *Pende*, has a variable size, sometimes high, sometimes deficient, is cumbersome, prone to obesity. The legs are short, small and large hands. The face is a pale-looking infant with less developed bone relief, because of a lack nephroma. Mandibles are large, so the lower floor of the face is prominent. This set of characters coming the lymphatic, the endoblastic of the old constitutionalists. Endocrinologic finding an adrenal insufficiency, translated by a decrease in blood pressure and a reduction in body hairiness. Endoblastics also have a pituitary and thyroid hyposecretion. Thyroid failure is due to the decrease in basal metabolism and tends to hydrophilic tissue.

Martiny says that the endoblastic is hypo-evolved, pseudo-infantile with strong hydrophilic tissue. From a biochemical criterion, he distinguishes the anabolism nitrate through a low-carbohydrate and lipid anabolism stronger. Endoblast hypercholesteremia is so frequently. They, however, many private mental notes. I am calm, sedentary, with patience and a lot of fantasy. Endoblast supposedly would have a power of concentration lower than other types.

Meroblastic equivalent type of Sigaud respiratory and invigorating brevity of *Pende*, is distinguished by a middle class often under relatively heavy. The trunk is wide, strong, with long limbs, and muscular. The skull is large, hexagonal face. Middle respiratory prevails floor. The thorax is strong and covered with profuse hair growth. Regarding endocrine meroblastic hyper-adrenocortical is an element that generates a strong musculature, and a hyper-pituitary element that favors the development of strong chin and muscles. Only sometimes, shows signs of thyroid insufficiency. Due endocrine hyperfunction, this type is strong, permanent asset. Cordo-mesoblastic corresponds to the older muscle type (*Sigaud*) or bracing longline (*Pende*). His whole development is harmonious. It has a high waist and slender, long hands, muscular fingers thin and fine. The skull is strong, top right. The face is rectangular, with good bone shaped reliefs. Prominent nose is straight or concave, round type. From an endocrine glandular cordoblastic reflects a balance. He has a strong and balanced metabolism and mentally. As meroblastic, cordoblastic is violent, but a violent cold.

The ectoblastic, cerebral type of *Sigaud* or sthenic long-shaped of *Pende,* is a man of medium height, gracile with tight trunk and flattened. Frequently meet deformities of the spine: scoliosis, kyphosis, and lordosis. Hands are long and thin, hypotrophy. The face is underdeveloped, triangular, due to the predominance top floor and floors subjacent failure, and respiratory tract. From an endocrine view, the ectoblastic is hyperthyroid, hyper-medulo-suprarrenal, hypo pituitary, hypo-adrenocortical, hypogonadal and hypo-parathyroid.

Somatotropin hormone deficiency explains the weakness characteristic of this biotype, and deficiency of parathyroid explains spasmophilia, common among ectoblastic. The ectoblastic is catabolic with lowered blood sugar, hypocholesterolemia, and hypocalcemia. He is always emotive with an imagination vivid and abstract. Biotype includes the whole being, with all its somatic and psychic; He is shown graphically as a square pyramid supported by a genetic basis. Each of the four sides comprises one of the fundamental aspects of individuality. The face is identical morphological morphotype, biotype the most obvious aspect. It includes relations and body segments. The physiological face is the modern expression of what the old constitutionalists called temperament. *Pende* believes that the last two-sided, intellectual and characterological are distinct. The first relates to instinct and affectivity, the second - in intelligence. Biotype thus conceived is a result of interaction between heredity and environment. A process takes place in uneven rhythms. As such, it can differentiate biotypes of children, adolescents, and adults. During the process of growth and sexual differentiation biotype may undergo significant changes. Therefore the clinical anthropology most numerous and most used schemes are those in adults. The best known is *Pende* biotypology, dealing with “study architecture and engineering individual human body.” Its purpose is practical. To establish biotypes, *Pende* uses two criteria. The first is the proportions of the body's mass and Stena characters or asthenic body. He distinguishes an environment type, characterized by a harmonious constitution, around which morphotypes have heterotypic: long-shaped, normolin, brevilineal, hypersoma, normosoma, hypo-soma, sthenic and hypo-sthenic.

The second criterion is the functional aspects of the body: tone vagosympathetic nervous, the endocrine degree of reactivity. With these elements, *Pende* divides people into four basic types; a certain morphofunctional structure characterizes each type:

1. long-shaped sthenic, tonic or hyperthyroid hypo pituitary are individuals with good adrenal and gonadal activity;
2. long-shaped asthenic, hypotonic are hyperthyroid a constitutional deficit adrenal or parathyroid gonads;
3. brevilineal sthenic, tonics, are hypogonadal or hyper-adrenocortical. All their organs are well developed.
4. brevilineal asthenic, hypotonic, they are hypo pituitary, hypothyroid, hypogenitalism and hyperinsulinemic. They are characterized by a predominance of fat deposition.

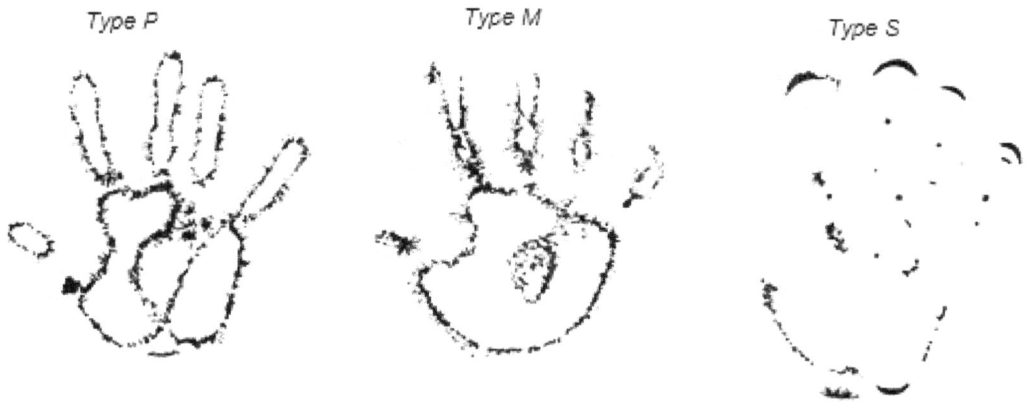

Fig. 31. Electromyography of the hand.

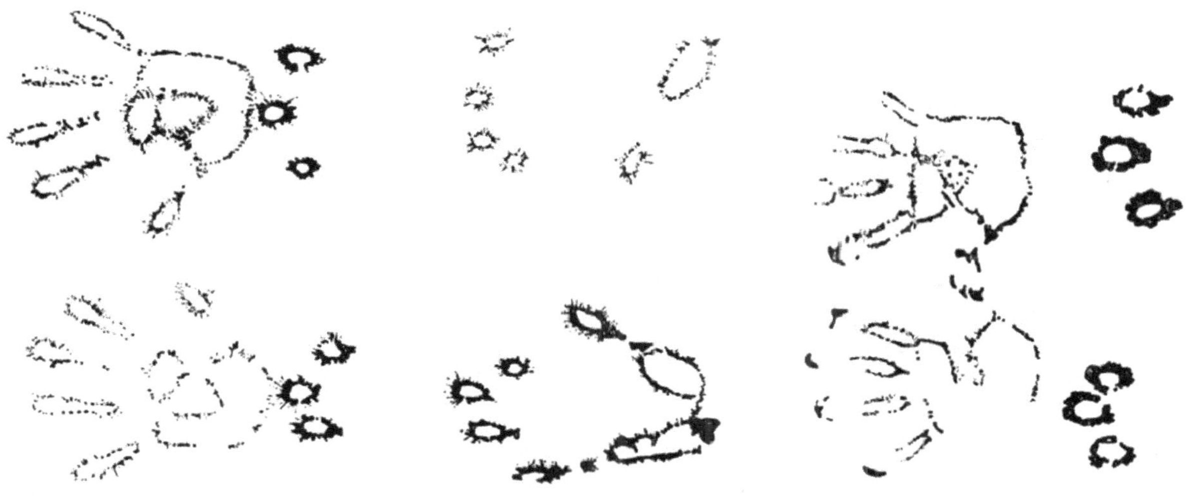

Fig. 32. Various electrograms of the palmar region of the hand.

Bioelectric typology. A typology is the bioelectric constitutional perspective, developed in our country by *Cornelia Guja*. (Fig.31, 32). Electromyography rearrangement performed in images of electrical characteristics of a body. Electroretinographic first recordings were made in 1777 *Lichtenberg*, through the mobilization of very fine powders between two electrodes with different tasks. Subsequently, the graphic image was produced by photographic record. At the end of the nineteenth century, *Tesla* shows that around the human body exposed to electromagnetic fields, radiation appeared bright. Luminescence obtained Electroretinographic first images in 1892, the Polish doctor *Markiewich*. In 1939, The Soviet *Kirlian* noted that the human body exposed to electromagnetic fields where ultra may cause the appearance of bright pictures on photographic films; in the same year mentioned research by the Polish *Schlemer* and *Prat* (1939), who used similar methods to those of *Kirlian*.

In 1961, he filed the first patent of *Kirlian*. Electroluminescence phenomena were concerned, in the coming decades, various research teams Soviets, like the Americans, Polish, French, etc. Based on electrophysiological research on human skin and shell structures to effect *Kirlian* technique, Romanian doctor *Dumitrescu* put in place in 1975, a new method: Electromyography. The essential feature of this method lies in emission control, propagation, and conversion of energy to release electrons of a single pulse in a living organism exposure device. In our country, *Cornelia Guja* investigated palmar surfaces. Recording technique is performed by the original method patented in several countries and recorded at the National Institute of Industrial Property of France under no. 7628301 (*Dumitrescu,* 1975 No. Publ.2325352).

It consists of obtaining an image emitting a single pulse in the conversion of the measured and electro-nooptic, over long converters placed inside dielectric layers. The electroluminescent effect has been recorded on a radiological cliché. Of the three distinct aspects characterizing such a picture, and examined particularly skin effect (downloading marginal) as well as environmental aspects proximal dielectric. Electronomorf appearance is less obvious in our investigations.

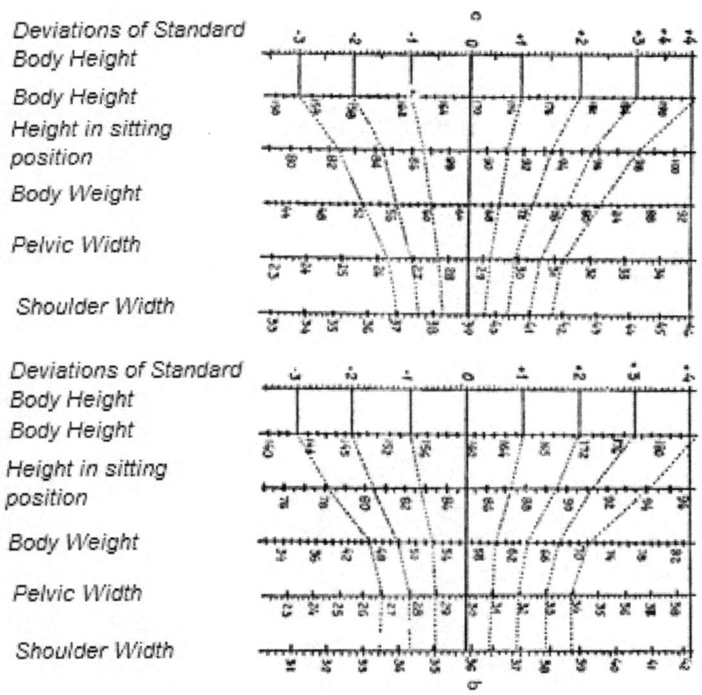

Fig. 33. Olivier and Pimeau Morpogram (a – gender masculin, b – gender feminin)

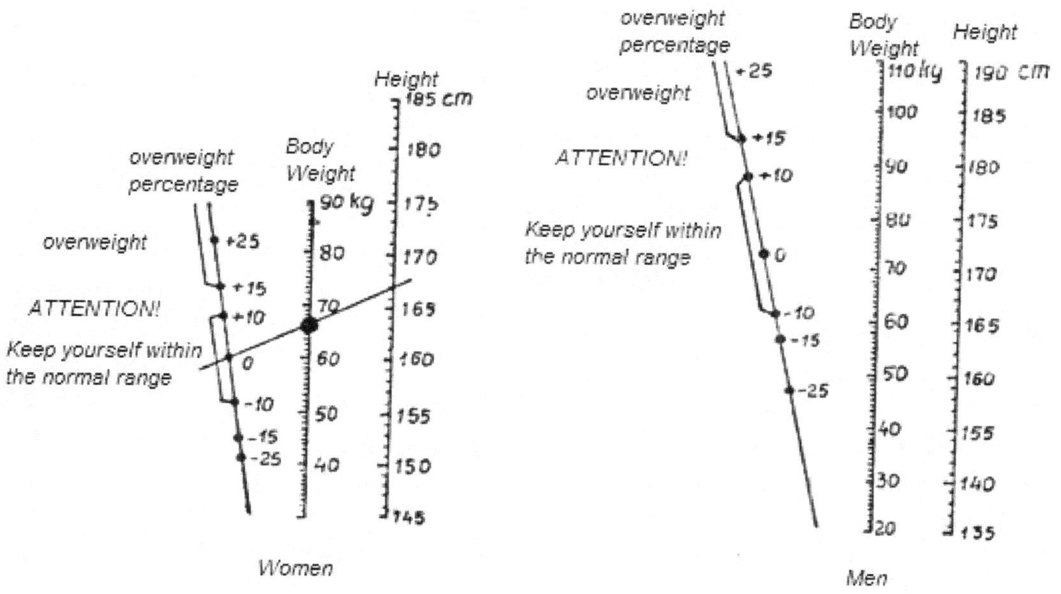

Fig. 34. Nomogram of the proportion height- weight at grown-ups (the weight and height unites, and it can be observed in the area on the basis of overweight, are within the subject investigated.

The following indicators, useful in the classification of the material, have been established.

A) Average drop density along the palm contour. Depending on this criterion, we have noticed three major categories that we call fundamental bioelectrics (fig.33, 34)

1. Type Dmax, with the maximum average density of the discharges. It is easy to appreciate given the continuity of downloads along the entire par-course; The contour of the image is well delimited by “streams”; He was named by us and type P (strong);

2. Type Dmin, with minimum mean density; The image is characterized by a series of dots or spots, without “streams” (beams, luminescent wave); The picture does not suggest any clear contours; It is also called type S (plate);

3. D medium type, with intermediate mean density, given by the intermittent discharge of lengths of the palm contour, or type M (mean);

The analysis of the series of electrons produced for the same individual over a long period of time (days, months, years) has allowed, despite all the qualitative variations noted, to keep the individual within the same fundamental type, in proportion of fish 80%, which leads to the conclusion that the appreciation made is a permanent basis for the individual.

B) Structural elements of the phenomenon of electroluminescence;

C) Combinator of the two polarities;

D) Degree of “polarization” of two electronic images;

E) Right / left symmetry between images with similar polarity of the two hands;

F) Homogeneity or Heterogeneity of elemental discharges.

The analysis of the results reveals an important variation in the distribution of the fundamental types, starting at the young age (6-7 years), where the percentage corresponding to the Dmin type exceeds 50%, and until the adult age, where it decreases sensitively, reaching an average of 19. It is possible for this aspect to accompany the child's development and maturation process. The decrease is mainly in favor of the Dmed type, which reaches an average of 39.4%.

From the research done by *Cornelia Guja,* it follows that:

- There are standard exploratory conditions to capture the dominant characteristic types of individuals;
- Bioelectric types that are highlighted may be the expression of a typology of the neuroendocrine function of different human groups;
- It is possible to establish a characteristic coded pattern corresponding to certain categories of diseases determined by specific metabolic changes.

The method can be used successfully in sports selection, given the correlations between its electrical and endocrine type. This interesting bioelectric typology is correlated with the androgynous one, established by the *Bailey Bayer* method, proving the existence of palmar bioelectric correspondences to each androgynous type (*Cornelia Guja*). Also, a comparison of the type of growth, the androgen type (*Bailey Bayer*) and the bioelectric type, electronically evidenced by longitudinal research on a sample of subjects studied from 8-10 years to 18-20 years, reveals the existence A stability, a constant of a typological structure, which justifies considering the anthropological variant from the early ante pubertal age.

These conclusions are of particular importance for sports activity and especially for selection, making it possible to estimate the degree of androgyny (masculinity) or ginoidity (femininity) in the initial selection stage, in the prepubertal stage, by the *Bailey Bayer* method correlated with the electrographic method Perspective, essential for performance in a number of sporting disciplines. It is also necessary to complete the criteria for the optimal anthropological status of the sporting sector, with elements from *Bailey Bayer's* gender typology and electron scanning. We also mention that, according to research conducted by *Cornelia Guja*, a number of athletes show that there are electronic images specific to performers in different sports disciplines, which opens great prospects for selection.

Lindegard's typology. *B. Lindegard* capitalized on the notion of factor (components) introduced by *Sheldon* in the somatic typology. He emphasized, first, the tissue proportions of the body, which condition the type of construction. *Lindegard* seeks an objective method, based on concrete anthropometric measurements, noting that *Sheldon*'s somatotypology allows the researcher too much freedom of interpretation. The development of three basic components defines body construction: bone, muscle, adipose tissue. The quantitative development of these components is dependent on the action of four factors:

1. The length factor (bones) leads to the formation of long and thin bones;
2. The weight factor (bones) influence the development of the massive skeleton with short and thick bones by straining the bone tissues;
3. Muscular factor defines muscular development;
4. The fat factor decides on the amount of fatty tissue.

Lindegard assesses the action of these four factors on the basis of several anthropometric measurements by which the muscles are defined by the force of muscle measured by a hand dynamometer and the amount of fat resulting from the regression equation as a residual after the decrease in the general body mass, the weight of bone and muscle tissue.

On the basis of the values with deviations from the arithmetic mean, *Lindegard* builds the body construction profile defined by the four factors.

Skerlj typology. *Skerlj* introduces the notion of vectors of body construction. Their meaning approximates to some extent to the notion of *Sheldon*'s components (figure 35). At the opposite ends of each vector, there is the type of construction, "ideal, abstract."

The intermediate values of the extreme types are deployed along the vectors.

Skerlj proposes four aspects of construction:

1. The aspect of gender dimorphism, the vector of which is between the extreme masculine construction M and the extreme feminine F;

2. Aspect of body proportion - based on the notion of types (after *Weidenreich*): eurysome (E) and leptosome (L);

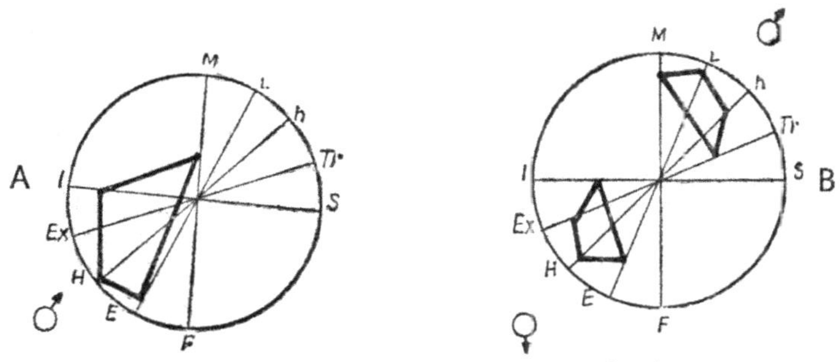

Fig. 35. The vectors features after Skerlj
A. Man with many feminine qualities; B. Male and female type.

3. Plastic appearance - aimed at the formation of soft tissues; its vector switches from the hyperplastic type (H) to the hypoplastic type (h). The author proposes several methods of defining the degree of plasticity of the body;

4. Distributive aspect defines the development of adipose tissue. It is expressed by two vectors defining the deposition of the upper body (S) adiposities in comparison to the lower part (I), as well as the trunk fattening (Tr) in contrast to the extremities (Ex). Extreme types, as in other types of typologies, meet as seldom. In the graphical representation, the vectors of all aspects are the diameter of a circle, in which, in the form of a polygon, one can represent the construction of each individual; uniting, on separated vectors, the points defining the differences, each vector is divided into ten segments.

Conrad's typology. Among the modern methods, published in 1941 in Germany, it is worth mentioning *Conrad*'s typological method, which used the characteristics of body building of athletic groups. This method uses two notions, related to the definition of body construction: the proportion, the length of the body width and the notion of the plasticity of the construction. The first defines the so-called matrix index, an index that represents the ratio of body height to width and depth of the chest box. The values of this index range from +2 to -2 and are divided into nine classes, after the alphabet, from A to I. In this classification, the extreme types are: in an extreme pyknomorph (class A with index values of +1.7 and more), in the other extreme leptomorphic type (class I, with values from -1.7 and below). They correspond to *Kretschmer*'s leptosome and picnic types. The plasticity of the building, its solidity (index plastic) is expressed as the amount of three anthropometric measurements: the width of the shoulders (a-a) circumference of the palm and forearm instead of the solid. The values of the plasticity index are on a scale of one to nine; the smallest is for the hypoplastic type (class 1), and the largest ones are for the hyperplastic type (class 9). Both indices have different values for men and women.

The development of the types of body construction is graphically represented as a square; The hyperplastic - hypoplastic type is read vertically, and on the horizontal: leptomorphic - pyknomorph. This graphical representation of *Conrad's* types can be compared to *Sheldon*'s somatogram, with the only difference that at *Conrad* there are four combinations of extremes of construction, and in *Sheldon* only three. Besides, due to the different reference points for men and women, *Conrad*'s graphical system allows an easier reading of similarities and differences in female gender, since the average distribution of the female population is equal, and the concentration of individuals only appears In the case of groups selected in terms of construction, while in *Sheldon's* somatogram, women are usually more concentrated on the endomorphic surface.

Wanke's typology. Until the Second World War, no original typological conception emerged in Poland. The *Kretschmer* typology, which was the most popular in Europe during the interwar period, has a strong scientific foundation. It was only after the Second World War that in the 1950`s appeared in Poland the first typological method and method proposed by *A. Wanke* (1954), who wanted to create a taxonomic method, eliminating all subjective assessments.

The author extracted from a series of features only those that he intuitively recognized as the most important to define body construction and based on them established five taxonomic indexes of construction, working on a group of 3000 men. *Wanke* thus defines its types:

- the first type has a short trunk, wide shoulders, narrow basin, flat thorax box, a body weight quite high in relation to height;
- the second type has narrow shoulders, wide basin, slightly curved chest box and middleweight;
- the third type is characterized by a short trunk, wide shoulders, wide basin, curved thorax box and middleweight;
- the fourth type is of a weak construction: long trunk, tight shoulders, flat thorax box and low weight.

The silhouettes of these types are similar to the letters V, A, H, I. Every subject whose construction is expressed by the five indices occupies a definite place in their typological space. The distance from each of the four somatic elements allows the somatic structure to be defined. The smaller the distance to one of the four elements, the greater its likeness to this element - and vice versa. The resemblance of the subject with the somatic element is therefore inversely proportional to the square of the distance of its settlement. The sum of the inverse squares of the distance - to all somatic elements - defines the somatic structure of the subject, the contribution of each element in the body construction. This amount is expressed by a unit, and the contribution of the main somatic elements is expressed as a percentage.

Wanke's method can define typologically each individual, groups and entire populations, considering the arithmetic means of a given group, normalizing them in the same way as the indices of the settlement of the elements. *E. Kolasa* (1969), using the same method, defined the somatic elements for the Polish female population, based on the research on 3162 women - conducted by the anthropometry commission from 1955 to 1956. Many groups of young athletes were tested using this method. *Wanke*'s typology relies, first of all, on measurements made on the bone system. The only index referring to the formation of soft tissue is the *Rohrer* index, which does not say anything about the internal tissue proportions or the silhouette of the construction. It seems that this typological method, despite the high degree of mathematics, is less precise and does not reveal the essentials of typological differences to a satisfactory extent.

Typology based on natural indices. It was proposed by *Perkal* (1953) and used for the first time to define the construction of the *Milicerowa* (1956); Is not only a new typological classification system but also a new statistical method, allowing a characterization of the internal proportions of body building of each individual or groups of individuals.

The natural indices resulting from the calculation of the values of the normal characteristics in statistics are called standardized indices (*Guilford,* 1960). This statistical method is considered to be one of the best for defining the type of body construction under its various aspects and that is why it was widely debated.

1. *Standard features.* Body building features have various denominations (kg, cm, etc.) and numerical values; thus, the 2 cm difference in body height is not a large deviation, whereas the 2 cm gap in the elbow width gives a large error of interpretation because the measurements of these features are expressed in strict and non-comparing values. To eliminate these difficulties and to express all the characteristics in comparative values, we use a statistical calculation, the so-called normalization in arithmetic mean 0 and deviation of standard 1:

$$Z_{ij} = \frac{X_{ij}^{-x^2}}{S_j}$$

Zij - the value of the normal characteristic of the individual j;

Xij - the value of the characteristic and the individual j;

Xi - the arithmetic mean of i;

Sj - deviation of the standard i.

We thus obtain the value of the characteristic and individual j, expressed in the number of standard deviation units. The values of the expressed characteristics can be compared to each other and can be used in the mathematical calculations.

The arithmetic mean of the characteristics we are normalizing represents for us a point of reference; The + or - sign, before the normalized feature, informs whether its value is higher or lower than the reference point, and the numerical value defines the magnitude of this difference. When we want to check the proportions of a child's height in relation to other children of the same age (12, 25), we normalize his characteristics in the average reference group. For example: the body height of a boy Xw = 158.7 cm and body weight Xc = 37.8 kg. The mean value of the height of the body in the reference group is xw = 147.3 m and the arithmetic mean body weight xc = 37.9 kg, the standard deviation for body height is Sw = 6.6 cm, and for body weight Sc = 6.3 kg.

After using the model (model), we get both standard features:

$$Z_w = \frac{X_w - x_w}{S_w} = \frac{158{,}7cm - 147{,}3cm}{6{,}6cm} = 1{,}73$$

$$Z_C = \frac{S_C}{X_C - x_C} = \frac{37{,}8cm - 37{,}9cm}{6{,}6cm} = 0{,}02$$

We notice that this boy is higher than the average of his age, but at the same time it is easier than the others with 0.02 standard deviation units. These values, compared to each other, expressed in units of the same kind, allow us to affirm that the boy, studied by us, is characterized by a very slim construction. As a point of reference, on the basis of which we normalize, we can take either the arithmetic average of the specific group as in the given example, or the arithmetic mean of another group.

Thus, for the athletes of the Olympic groups will be standard groups, and the ones of the university youth who do not practice intensive training will be reference groups, on the background of which will draw the silhouette of the athlete's construction. In this way, we receive the answer to the question: by what traits and to what degree does an individual differ from the average of his group and the average of the reference group? Analogously, we can treat the normalized characteristics of a group of individuals and make calculations based on the arithmetic mean of the group - as we did with the individuals taken separately. The normative characteristics are presented graphically in the form of the so-called structural profiles, where, on one axis, we note the specific characteristics of the construction, and on the other axis, we note the scale of the normed characteristics.

We point out the normalized values on the lines of those attributes, join these points together, and thus show the body construction profile. The method of natural indices often links the notion of body building factors - which was first used by *Milicerowa* in 1959 to define body construction in children and youth. Unfortunately, this notion is not always precisely defined and established. Using the notion of factors in the description of body construction by the natural factors method, we will serve the normalized characteristics and include them in factors - which calculate the index **m** in comparison to **M** - for the entire body construction, for each factor, for example: for the factor Flexibility, massive construction - we calculated the **M** index for all characteristics together. The arithmetic mean of the value of the factors of construction gives us the value of the index of the general construction **M** of the individual j:

$$M_j = m_{j1} + m_{j2} + m_{j3} + \ldots m_{\pi j}$$

where π = the number of factors. In cases where, with the help of construction factors, we want to express the typological models, for simplicity, we can use the *Sheldon* typological scale (with the seven elements) and transfer the values (with the deviations of the standard) in which ***m*** factors are expressed as *Milicerowa* did in his 1959 paper, using classification according to the statistical tables, so that each grade corresponds to the same fraction. In practice, this example looks like (Table 3). The normalization method and the natural indices method are welcome when analyzing the bodybuilding of the growing groups (development) because they allow the acceleration of influence on the chronological age by normalizing the individual characteristics.

Tabel 3

Points	Values with standard deviations
1	X to 1.07
2	1.06 to - 0.57 - lower values than medium values
3	0.56 to - 0.18
4	0.17 to + 0.18 - average value
5	0.19 to 0.57
6	0.57 to 1.06 - values higher than medium values
7	1.07 to x

Morphogram method. In contemporary France, the method of defining the type of construction using morpho-grams is prevalent (*Olivier* and *Pineau*, 1961; *Decourt* and *Doumic*, 1950); Based on them, some anthropometric features, expressed in standard units, are reported at the height of the body.

Lines that link significant points to the value of these features form a profile, allowing the body type to be read. These morpho-grams are built separately for men and women. *Olivier* uses this morpho-gram technique. The units of measure of the characteristics are found on the parallel, vertical lines. The first line indicates the height of the body and the other sitting height, body weight, basin width, width of the shoulders, expressed in standard values, multiplied by the correlation coefficient of these characteristics and the height of the body. The scale points are merged transversely forming some channels, which represent the construction rules corresponding to a given height. *Olivier* presents a very simple and very clear typology; He distinguishes three extreme types of construction:

1) longilineal, slender type and two massive brevilineal types;

2) muscle type - with a strong construction in the upper part of the trunk;

3) digestive type - having developed the inferior region of the trunk. (This type corresponds to the endomorphic type.)

Olivier pointed out that among the representatives of these extreme types is the whole scale of the types expressing only a tendency towards a certain extreme, and in the center is the intermediate type - the normotype.

Ross's typology. In 1974, *Ross's* new concept of body building assessment was published, which notes that there must be a common reference point that allows a univocal comparison of the varied features of body construction for the entire population. Thus, *Ross* proposes a general human model with a symmetrical construction common to both genders.

As a starting point for the measurements of these silhouettes, *Ross* arbitrarily takes the body height of 170.18 cm. This value corresponds to the mean body height in the conception of the Heath and Carter's somatotypes. The standard deviations corresponding to these values are calculated on the basis of the very large variability coefficients of *Gault* and *Kennedy*'s 1975 anthropometric material.

Average mean deviation values of other peculiarities are adapted to these data by correcting body height corrections. For example, body weight is calculated from *Behnke*'s data as follows: Body weight = body weight. (After *Behnke*), that is:

$$X = \frac{Body\ Height}{170{,}18}$$

The author believes that all anthropometric measurements of populations can be used according to the following model:

$$Z = \frac{1}{S}\left[1\frac{(170{,}18)^d}{h} - p\right]$$

Z - the proportional value of the normalized characteristic, variables;

1 - the value of the freely chosen variability;

S - deviation of the standard for the given variability, using the body height of 170.18;

H - the height of the body for the individual under investigation;

D - the exponent of the height, which amounts to:

1) for measurements of height, width, circumference and fat layers;

2) for surface measurements;

3) for weights and volumes measurements;

P - the value of the variability given.

Ross presents for his model the values of typical measurements, considering the height, length, width, circumference, cephalometry, construction indices and essential tissue components in the sense of anthropometry. Its model serves to evaluate body construction in children and adults. We present the following values - obtained from the measurements made:

- body height (cm)	170.18	6.29
- body weight (kg)	64.58	8.60
- weight of the slim body (kg)	52.45	6.14
- weight, fat layer (kg)	12.13	3.25
- percentage of layer, fat (%)	18.78	5,20
- Body Density [g / cc]	1.056	0.0111

- Air that penetrates into the lungs (e)	1.053		0.265
Body height (cm)		42,42	
Body weight (kg)			
Body height (total)		23,58	
Body weight (fungi)			
Body weight (kg)		12.83	
Height (cm)			

Pluricaracteristic method of analysis. It was initially used in solving psychological problems; Towards the end of the 1930s is used in research on body building and has spread very much after the Second World War. This method belongs to the sphere of statistical methods, allowing objective quantitative measurements. Analytical techniques are varied, but in each case their basis is represented by a matrix of correlations of some assemblages of characteristics, and the results obtained depend to a large extent on the selection of the characteristics. One of these methods can be considered factorial analysis - used by *Tanner* (1964) - referring to 15 anthropometric features. The analysis distinguishes four factors of the construction: the layout of the fat layer (adiposity), the muscularization, the thickness of the bone extremities and the length of the lower extremities. Another method is that of the essential components of *Hotelling* - distinguishing the factors that characterize the somatic construction.

Schreider (1963), using this analysis, obtained a high similarity of results in groups of 11 different populations, which confirms the permanence of some correlations and linkages in the morphology of the human genus - as a unit. The factors and components of pluricaracteristic methods are abstract notions - that is why they can hardly be translated into a biological language.

* * *

Taking a balance sheet of the typological conceptions set out here, we must affirm that each typological system is conditioned by the concerns of its creator. The endocrinologist builds his system from a certain point of view, looking for the correlation between the body construction and the action of the internal secretory glands; another is the point of view of the coach, who is looking for champions among the youngsters with a height and the proportions of the body corresponding to the sport competition. Other are the criteria of the artist's classification, which is looking for the appropriate model for sculpture or painting.

From the time of *Hippocrates*, in all morphologically typological systems, we find similar concepts about the body construction model, whether they are called types or the outcome of the action of the factors. In classical typologies at the end of the 19th century and the beginning of the 20th century, the groups became individual types with a well-defined construction. In these classifications, the types and intertype appear (e.g. in *Kretschmer*), and if we treat them as individual groups, a large part of the population (e.g. *Viola*'s typology - 40%) does not fit into any typology, remaining in Undefined. The new vision of the factors or components of the construction refer only to the intercorrelations of certain characteristics and not to their close interdependence. The notion of components in *Sheldon*'s conception allows us to define and assign numerical values to each individual.

Sheldon's constructional constructs, as well as *Lindegard*'s factors, though intuitively constituted, represent a qualitative leap in relation to the notion of "types" of authors from earlier periods, because they allow a precise characterization of each individual.

Reviewing some typological systems, where reference points are imposed from the beginning, and normotyping set by the system itself, such as *Sheldon*'s somatotypology - processed on the basis of bodybuilding of 4,000 university students in the U.S. Higher Education Institutes. - We can conclude that this reference point has proved to be unsatisfactory for some human populations. *Sheldon*'s somatogram has been expanded to include extreme types of fattening, muscular, suppleness. If in an initial somatogram, a particular population surveyed is found to be very fat, slim or muscular; we must remember that it is so in relation to the American student population, which has been taken as a reference point in this typology.

Decourt and *Doumic*, who have dealt with gender genders, and have built a type of morphograms and defined male and female types of construction based on the construction of the body of 100 firefighters in Paris and a number of 100 models for a picture. These are fewer representative tests for the whole population.

Wanke has based his typology by researching on 3000 recruits - as a point of reference, similar to that of *Sheldon*'s students. The use of such a method implies a critical attitude towards the results obtained. Statistical methods, as well as the norm or method often used in Poland that of natural indices, allow the free choice of the reference point, depending on the researcher's problems. When we want to characterize individuals individually on the basis of their own group, we normalize their particularities according to the arithmetic mean of the features of this group, and such a reference point will not generate any doubts or reservations. Thus, we must take into account:

1) gender-specific selection;
2) selecting the appropriate age;
3) specific population selection from the genetic point of view (within the same breed) and the environmental point of view (rural, urban).

Turning to the constitutional concept, we must finally highlight some important issues.

1. Considering the immense number of constituent variants of the human body, it logically follows that they can never be "closed" in some constitutional types, but there are many intermediate forms. It follows that pure constitutional types are deviations from the average, which, according to the rule of biological variability, are all the rarer as they are expressed (*Leng*).
2. Constitutional determinations have been made more of men, so that female typology is less well defined.
3. A good correlation of morphological and physiological parameters is also required in defining the constitutional type (*Conrad*).
4. Each of the presented typologies shows limits related to the human model that has been achieved, under these ratio net benefits of the typology that uses natural indices, which allows a choice as required by reference control groups.

* * *

Endocrine typology (*C.I. Parhon - Şt.M. Milcu*). Bio-typology tried to understand the factors generating human diversity by appealing to all the explanations offered him contemporary science. One of the fundamental explanations was the endocrine projection models.

C.I. Parhon stressed for the first time in literature, the existence of relationships between endocrine and somatosensory mental constitution. He admitted that every gland directly contributes to the development of the body; according to the development of either gland, the body can develop in different ways. According to *Parhon,* the differences between individuals are carried out by operating glands, more or less. The Constitution itself becomes, as interpreted his broad limits, comprising individual entirely different plans: somatic, physiological and psychological. Balance the endocrine glands ensure a harmonious development of the organism. The emergence of a hypo or endocrine hypersecretion body gives a characteristic shape. It forms hypo and hyperthyroid such types, and hyper-pituitary, hyper or hypogonadal and hypocoristic- adrenal.

Hyperthyroid type is characterized by the predominance of the values of length width. Hyperthyroid sufferers are tall and lean, with a narrow waist, with long thin muscles. The skin is warm, easy hyperpigmentation, abundant hairiness. Basal metabolism is increased, and hyperthyroid sufferers often have a tendency to tachycardia. They are hyperexcitable and have a great lability of the nervous system.

To differentiate the pathological condition of the constitutional function of glands it has been proposed (*Şt. M. Milcu*) the term hypertonic or hypotonic. In this regard, one may be ill or suffer from hypothyroidisms hyper, hyper or hypo-hypophyseal syndrome and a healthy individual can only have a hyper or hypotonic pituitary, thyroid, etc. *The hypothyroid type* is brevilineal with shorter stature, often below the average population. Reports offer tangible values translate dominance on the length and width of the trunk of the limb. The head is large, with a round face and features less prominent. The eyes are small and less expressive. The skin is rough and poorly pigmented. Dental disorders are common; teeth are small and irregularly. Often there is a marked tendency to fatness, especially on the face, neck, and abdomen. Physiological processes are slow, which explains the apathy so characteristic of this type.

The hyper hypophyseal type is the consequence of excessive secretions of the pituitary gland. Hyperhypophyseals are tall, with limbs relatively larger than the trunk. Distal parts, hands, feet, and face are massive. The mandible is long and thick, pushed forward with strong teeth, often with small spaces between them (diastemas). The skin is thick, abundant hair growth on the trunk and limbs. The muscles are strongly developed. Adiposity is poor. Hyperhipophyseals have frequently hypertonic and intestinal hyperperistalsis. This corresponds to an incipient but acromegaly. Most times, hyper hypophyseal types are distinguishable only by emphasizing facial features and the development extremities, nose and lips.

The hypo hypophyseal somatic development type is characterized by insufficient and often exaggerated by adiposity. Adolescent and adult to child ratios are maintained and puberty, the legs are relatively long. Men have flattened or slightly rounded face. Facial features are gracile. The lower jaw is underdeveloped. Sometimes presents some female characters; insertion pubic hair, fat disposal areas, gynecomastia. In women, there is a weak development of breasts.

Hypergonadism type is characterized by the appearance of early puberty. Therefore, teen has a relatively large frame height and strongly muscled, hypertonic. The particular nature of this type is formed by the discrepancy between the abundance of hair on the face, trunk and limbs and his head rarity. Hypergonadism adults are relatively short, well developed somatic, muscled and strong abundant. Women have a relatively wide basin, but the breasts are small.

The Hypogonadal type is characterized by an above-average waist and moderate development of sexual characteristics. Skull and face have small diameters. The mandible is relatively prominent but gracile. Head hair is abundant, but pubic hair growth is rare in men and women available. Women are sometimes observed the weak development of facial hair. However, the pelvis keeps infantile female characters.

The Hypercorticoadrenal type has a massive body, muscled, developed and abundant hypertrichosis. Women often stand abundant male pattern hair growth. *The Hypocorticoadrenal type* is tall and thin, with weak musculature, skin and hyperpigmentation hypotrophy, especially the parts discovered. Due to poor development of muscles, hypocorticoadrenal often have visceral ptosis. They have described hypoparathyroidism or thymic types, but their characters are not well-defined somatic.

The more common Endocrine type are hyper and *hypothyroidism*, associated with secondary influences of other glands. Thus, a heavy frame, developed especially in the extremities, distinguishes the hypothyroid-hyper-pituitary type. When, in addition *hypothyroidism* note and adrenal hyperactivity, muscle is strong and abundant hair growth. *Hypogonadal-hypothyroidism type* of thyroid insufficiency adds to character development and a marked sexual apparatus. *Hyperhipophyseal- hyperthyroid* type is characterized by an increase in somatic characters, which may sometimes go to the development of an acromegalic image.

Concept of constitutional type and physical sports in the anthropological vision

Above, we presented the concept of constitutional type, the evolution of concepts and methodological and practical aspects of determining the parameters that define it. When defining the content of the concept of constitutional type through the requirements of anthropology motive, whose primary objective is to determine the type anthropological optimal specific to each branch of sport, follows three important sections of biotype sports: somatosensory physiological type motricity and psychic which we present below. Incontestable that the delimitation of the three components of the notion of anthropological sportsman is arbitrary and do it educational reasons, the human body is a whole and the sum of its parts, as stated since antiquity *Aristotle*, not equal sum of the parts. Hence, the limits of both the presentations and the applicability of the concepts we possess today on the human body. The fact remains that every organism is an individuality and typology constitutional, although help us achieve a better understanding of the body, the potencies, and its valences in order to maximize the guidelines socio-professional, in this case, the choice of sports they can obtain performance, it still presents great limits, and data interpretation should be performed strictly individualized.

• *Physiological somatosensory type*

The concept is rooted in somatic type reading specialist, referring to the totality of morphological parameters that define the human body. We believe, however, that there is, as substantiated Professor *Francis I. Rainer*, rector of the National Academy of Physical Education at the Department of Anatomy and Anthropology A.N.E.F. (1930-38), a close interdependence between form and function, “the science of anatomy form alive.”

Through this morpho-functional concept, founded in our country by Professor *Rainer* and adopted worldwide, we cannot make a separation between form and function.

As a result, we cannot define the somatic type, strictly morphological, apart from its functionality. In this context, it is necessary to introduce the notion of type somatosensory physiologically sport the vision is of major importance. Thus, the somatosensory physiological type is defined by all the morphological and physiological constitution entering the human body. Of these, we will stop only on the main parameters of importance for the sport, as follows, without detailing the morphological and physiological content; this work is the subject of strict morphology and physiology.

a) *Morphological parameters.* These parameters are represented by body height, scale size of various segments in body proportions and their shape, weight, the chemical composition of tissue - which, in particular, interested in body weight active muscle mass, the amount of free water and intracellular structure histological and histochemical fiber visceral elements that define the somatic constitutional type. These items are detailed in the anthropological methodology as major anthropometric indices on which structural - detailed by different methods also in the same chapter - defined constitutional type. There is a close correlation between the types of somatic so defined constitutional and sports performance.

b) *Physiological parameters.* These parameters aimed at the functional level of the various structures assessed by morphological parameters. In essence, they define the entire functionality of the body. Educational and sports activity, especially for the selection and conduct sports training, the most important physiological parameters the following quote, without detailing the contents of this section without the list in order of importance. (Special attention is given to the main hormones that react to effort respectively thyroid - cortisol, and catecholamines to which we add androgens and estrogens) (N.A.). Type endocrine thus determined by establishing dominance and subdominant certain endocrine glands (*Şt. M. Milcu*) is correlated with the morphological type rules settling individual effort dosage and correlation with the requirements of the different branches of sport, for optimal performance.

Both the physiological and morphological parameters recognize a good degree of genetic conditioning, so at their establishment is required to determine the level of genetic conditioning. This is particularly so since the selection in sport, making it to age very early, about the necessity properties while skills driving and complexity of the various branches of sport, requires to establish a typology constitutional age groups, depending stage of selection, initial, secondary and final typology deciphering the genetic conditioning - to specify the extent to which the subject will become anthropological or not optimal for the sports branch prepares - is essential. Also, apart from physiological somatosensory global typology which, in its complexity, is increasingly being deciphered, currently pays particular attention segmentation and typologies of importance in various branches of sport.

Thus, for example, the morphotype of tha plantar has a huge significance in the performance of different branches of sports (athletics, sports games, etc.) or brachycranial type is essential in football for achieving effective head blows. Regarded as compared morphological and typological somatosensory physiological type, defined by complex characters morphofunctional, it is of paramount importance in holding sports performance.

The osteoarticular and muscle system	– various functional groups muscle and individualized muscle strength – joint mobility – muscle tone
sensory organs	– visual acuity – chromatic sense – visual field – auditory acuity – kinesthetic sense (Weil method) – the sense of balance – the type of nervous system
CNS	– determining the dominant hemisphere through the Pardue-Pegboard test – excitability determination through EEG, EMG, cronaximetry – determining the reactivity of the reaction time, the execution speed of the load motricity at a simple or complex (Csinady method), the rate of repetition through the Tapping test – neuromotor coordination determination through thermometry, the tracing test, etc. – determining functionality by measuring the time lag synapses peripheral (neuromotor plaque) and Hoffman reflex

endocrine system	– determining the functionality of the endocrine system through the hormonal dosage related to endocrine typology presented (by Șt. M. Milcu). Of these the most important focuses on the radioimmunoassay growth hormone dosing, ACTH, thyroid hormones, correlated with basal metabolism, the Achilles reflectogram and the creatine-creatinine variation ratio serum hormones adrenal cortex and especially 17 cetone-steroids hormones, adrenal or catecholamine, by fluorometric method, androgens, including, in particular testosterone and estrogen hormones, respectively, estriol, estradiol and progesterone
respiratory system	– thoracic mobility – respiratory rate – vital capacity
cardiovascular system	– heart rate – blood pressure – cardiac output
metabolic parameters	– aerobic capacity – anaerobic capacity

• *Motricity type*

For optimum branch statutory anthropological type of sport, great importance is determining the level of motricity qualities. Physical attributes are characteristics that define the movement. Essentially, their content, they express possibilities and act metric conducting substrate. Long driving qualities were regarded as enshrined musculoskeletal, and especially its muscular component. With the evolution of biomechanical concepts that have passed through the stages of physical-mechanical and muscle function, it has seen that the movement is a fundamental result of the whole body as a whole. In fact, the movement can not be separated from matter, as interrelated, so, on the one hand, the act motricity engages and expresses the activity of all systems and organs components of the human being, and on the other hand, act motricity evolved during phylogenesis being achieved in humans understanding, which entailed a series of structural changes specific to an upright posture existing only in humans and that allows a certain structure biomechanics of great complexity of the document motricity.

From this point of view we should emphasize the importance of building human movement during phylogenesis movement is, in fact, the intimate nature of the living body, hence its value capital for vital processes. If therefore, the movement and offer within phylogenesis of orthostatic led, ultimately, to structure the human body, we must emphasize that, while movement is the result of the functioning of the whole body. Thus, if the motricity act is performed by musculoskeletal system, this effector functions-based command trains the nervous system and the functionality of all systems and devices (cardiocirculatory device respectively, excretory, digestive) that ensures general metabolic substrate. In making, the motricity act can consider biomechanical body system as a whole. Hence, the name of qualities that driving is insufficient, only expressing strict musculoskeletal belonging to motoricity So the physical qualities which excludes, by definition, nervous system or psychic activity, for which we propose nomenclature biomotricity (suggested by coaching Prof. *Tacota George, Petrisor Costica,* and

Caraiosifoglu Leonida and work on potential biomotricity of school population developed by conf. Dr. *Nicu Alexe*), such as to express the complexity of these characters, in the view of the body seen as an integrated whole.

Considered classics of physical attributes are speed, stamina, strength, and skill. In the following, we present some issues of importance for anthropology motive, namely selection, and training on these qualities biometrics.

1) Speed. We understand the ability to run fast speed movement under the circumstances. This quality is manifested in four major forms: responsiveness, execution, repetition, and displacement. *The reaction rate* is the time to achieve the physiological and biochemical processes that occur in the application of a turn and lead to a simple response reaction. Phases of these processes involve the following steps, which, incidentally, we encounter, other types of speed:

- During reception of the stimulus that causes depolarization of the cell membrane receptor bound by the stimulus, and the transformation of the influx nervous stimulant, which lasts an average of 3 to 5 seconds;
- Efferent transmission to the central nervous system (duration is variable - for pulse visual, acoustic, olfactory 5-10 ms, and for those cutaneous or proprioceptive 20-25 ms);
- During which are central to analysis, synthesis and development command at C.N.S.; it takes on average between 70-82 ms. This time is improved through training, resulting in dynamic driving stereotypes are formed, which have much lower central time. Rapid formation of the stereotype depends on the determination of structural genetic nervous system and training;
- Efferent transmission, ranging between 8-10 ms, from inland cortex pyramidal periphery;
- The effective, lasting about 25-35 ms, consisting of neuromotor plate depolarization and contraction of muscle fibers. This time is much longer act as the motricity is more complex.

The execution speed expressed during the performing of any motive complex or a higher degree of difficulty when stimulus and execution contain unexpected elements (e.g., The stimulus is a moving object, and the onset of the reaction cell performance is based on choosing one of the several possible variants, etc.). The phases are the same as the speed of the reaction increases with the difference that they are related to the complexity of the movement, respectively, of the cases shown; for example, unexpected behavior change related to the partner. Training stereotype in reducing the value of time is central in this case, a crucial significance.

The maximum possible movement of repeated voluntary acts having special importance in driving cycle, simple or complex, gives speed repetition frequency. It is conditioned by the ability to deliver stimuli to the nervous system, repeat the sequence of these operations and the ability of effector muscular energetic-metabolic, motricity act to achieve.

Travel speed is a complex form of manifestation of speed, expressing the time of making full driving acts such as running, swimming, etc. and is in an interdependent relationship dialectic of the elementary forms of expression of speed.Thus, a run comprising the reaction speed when it begins, execution in moving from the block start, repetition in conducting cyclical movement.

This kind of speed is conditioned as previously described elementary forms of speed, power and muscle force under speed, neuromotor coordination, speed strength under some structural biomechanical characteristics of the segments moving. Biomechanical speed has two phases: increase the speed based on acceleration after start and phase relative stabilization speed the process, the first phase being conditional upon the level of force as a matter of speed, and the second, resistance under speed, coordination of movements is essential in both phases. In these circumstances, a functional view, speed is conditioned mainly by two fundamental elements:

1) nervous system and mainly of the cerebral cortex, which takes place during office

which performed throughout the command, coordination and movement control;

2) metabolism in the muscle which provides energy for muscle contraction under anaerobic conditions.

Provided the energy needed if anaerobic effort, resulting from the breakdown of ATP to ADP and phosphoric acid in muscle, while maintaining the requirements to achieve coupling excitation - contraction. Restoring the macroergic phosphate bond is initially on account of a link similar to phosphocreatine (CP) and still occurs anaerobic glycolysis, leading to the release of energy by converting pyruvic acid into lactic acid, which accumulates in muscles, as Following the large oxygen debt (movement and breath may not provide sufficient O_2 in a short time as the effort is conducted), and negative burden on the capacity of muscle contraction.

It follows therefore clear that, in an effort to speed the second essential element, after the C.N.S. functionality is anaerobic capacity. We also note that, as compared morphological, has proven that muscle fibers are fibers that provide speed white, rich in mitochondria and enzymatic redox equipment. The proportions of these fibers are genetically determined and can be set based on muscle biopsy. Starting from this remark that morpho-physiologic substrate, forecasting sports perspective for tracking speed and rate of progress achieved by training, are of particular value following determinations:

- Reaction time (*Demeter*'s research certifies classification following sports: up to 180 ms - well, up to 190 ms - good; 210-230 ms - environment, more than 230 ms, weak). There are numerous types of apparatus for these determinations including one of the best is the chronograph Electronic Eng. *Gagea A.*
- Chronaxis;
- Typewriter test repetition speed (speed of pressing the keys of the typewriter 85);
- Anaerobic capacity;
- Muscle biopsy;
- Typological tests that determine the functionality of S.N.C. and analyzers (presented when describing somatic-physiological type);
- Stopwatch contained in the national selection (*NICU Alexe* et al.).

Given conditioning, the nervous system, or by the anaerobic capacity, speed, point out that speed it is one of the biomotricity qualities with the highest level of genetic determination.

1. The speed of leg movements more clearly highlights the role of a hereditary factor than the speed of hand movements. So to assess the qualities of speed development is preferable *Tapping* test for lower limbs.

2. Period aged 9 to 14 years Rest and 9 to 12 years for legs is characterized by a reduction of genetic control on development speed movements. It can be assumed that at this age, pedagogical actions, properly organized, prove more effective for improving the qualities of speed (Table 4).

2) Force. Strength is the property of musculoskeletal that by moving its segments after muscle contraction triggered as a result of nervous system activity, to overcome different external resistors or even the weight and inertia of parts of the body. This biological definition is complemented by the notion mechanical, physical force, which represents the product of mass and acceleration (F-MXA – Second law of mechanics after *Newton*), which essentially expresses the change of state of motion of the body and even its shape above. These aspects of computing and defining force are detailed in our mechanistic monograph, so we will not develop. Classification various aspects of labor mention:

- Power can be *general*, expressing the main muscle groups or *special* ability concerning certain muscle groups;

- *Explosive* force (expansion), expressed by the maximum force achieved in a minimum of time by a sudden contraction of the muscle groups (jumps, throws, etc.);

- The *dynamic* force, achieved by isotonic contraction can be in overcoming regime or regimen failure;

- *Static* force, which is assessed under isometric contractions, essential in wrestling, weightlifting or global regarded with speed and strength in a variety of sports such as rugby, rowing, swimming, etc. In this mode the maximum force is assessed;

- The force *under stress* or speed.

Regarding morpho-physiologic substrate for achieving the force, we recognize two main segments of the body, which, of course, add work of all other systems and devices:

a. - Nervous system;

b. - Muscular system.

Table 4

The correlation coefficient between each pair indicator Holzinger frequency hand shake (I) and legs (II) 7 twins 16 years

Age (years)	I			II		
	MZ	DZ	1-1	MZ	DZ	1-1
7-8	0.64	0.373	0.245	0.683	0.455	0.512
9-12	0.593	0.635	-	0.662	0.456	0.463
11-12	0.38	0.584	-	0.705	0.500	0.410
13-14	0.691	0.528	0.345	0.837	0.383	0.735
15-16	0.734	0.272	0.634	0.436	0.274	0.223

a. The nervous system acts through two main mechanisms:

1) *Putting into action a greater number of motricity units.* Party motricity unit is composed of peripheral motricity neuron together with its extensions dendritic axonal plates together with all related neuromuscular muscle fibers that innervate the (*Sherington*). It is known that, at rest, are Contract 2 5% of units in efforts least 10 30% 40 60% strenuous efforts, and activity sports performance, 70 75%. There is a 30 per motricity units constituting 35% genetically determined reserve, which can be even lower or higher in exceptional cases. Genetic selection based sport seeking to find subjects, from this point of view, have a reservation, genetically determined, the motricity units as small.

Operating a greater number of motricity units depends on the ability motricity cortex, the area that pyramid, sending nerve impulses as more and more precise, to determine depolarization of motricity units. This is due both training and the nervous system and genetic determination of genetic reserve value determined by motricity fibers. Of course, mention that putting into action more motricity units with increased excitability crust front leads to a higher frequency of nerve impulses efferent essential in achieving contractions of muscle fibers, which in a large number of pulses may fall even tetanus contraction. It is known today that a muscle contraction occurs at 5:10 pulses per second, and maximum values reaching 40 50 pulses/sec.

2) *Assemble unit active motricity units.* Central nervous system, namely motricity cortex, is the functionality that synchronizes motricity units because, initially, they come into action under various conditions on their degree of contraction and later by increasing nerve impulses that reach 45-50 / sec, is reached achieving maximal contraction force. Training increases the capacity of the nervous system synchronization. The reticular formation of the cerebral trunk, the *Renshaw* neurons in the spinal cord, which are involved in the motricity backbone mechanisms - the paraphrase cortical areas, the rhinencephalic zones involved in motivation, etc., are involved in the realization of these nerve mechanisms that condition the force. (Details are found in the *Human Anatomy Atlas* - Volume III).

Starting from these nerve mechanisms of driving the motricity units, it is clear that medium and small loads have low biological value, sub-maximal loads determine 15- 25 pulses/sec, the activity of motricity units is asynchronous (motricity units depending on fatigue, Act asynchronously and will especially increase strength under force), and maximum loads will have a maximum biological value, effectively increasing the force. Supramaximal charges can induce inhibition of protection, restoration, sometimes followed by overcompensation phases.

b. Muscle is the second main element which makes the force.

We emphasize, from the outset, that the force developed by a muscle is directly proportional to his physiological section. So increasing the physiological section and, respectively, muscle hypertrophy is one of the main ways of increasing the force. Muscle hypertrophy occurs by increasing the synthesis of muscle power for hexose phosphate esters, which in turn is subject to the colloidal state of muscle protein.

It is known that in biological systems and thus also in the muscles after the excitation is a step of inhibition, the recovery processes which take place by anabolism, raised above the level of the excitation function, performing the so-called over-compensation. The more intense, the higher excitation is overcompensation. Hence the need for the strength training to use loads close to the maximum amount (maximum load, although very high value, may rise just once, but usually without repeating itself, at close intervals, their value is somewhat less under low loads less than the maximum but may be repeated). The principle of gradual increase in effort is essential. Based on these considerations morpho-physiological, ways of achieving muscle hypertrophy and thus force growth are two categories:

1) methods using isometric contractions (static)

2) methods using isotonic contractions (dynamic);

Force, given her determination by the central nervous system and the quality of the muscular fibers, is considered as the weight of heredity is substantial heritability coefficient is above 0.80. Although we do not share this view, we note that there are authors who feel like having a force greater than the speed genetic determinism.

3). Resistance. Is the quality of the human body to perform a certain activity, motricity, mental, intellectual, etc., a certain level of intensity, a longer period of time, without loss of efficiency without causing fatigue or tiredness conditions matched that we can overcome. After the kind of stress that is placed on the body or taking into account the biochemical processes that constitute the substrate activity, we recognize the following types of resistance:

- *General* resistance motricity, by which we mean the possibility of doing a certain amount of mechanical work, with the participation of almost the entire muscular system;

- *Local* resistance motricity when work is done only by certain groups or muscle chains;

- *Intellectual* resistance when work is predominantly neuropsychiatric;

- *Sensory* resistance, the requirement has at various receptors for longer;

- *Vegetative* resistance, by which we understand that the maximum load is at the various visceral and autonomic function entering the constitution of the human body;

- *Aerobic* resistance when energy needs are provided during the activity of aerobic, with an intake of sufficient oxygen molecule ATP resistance;

- *Anaerobic* resistance, the activity level is so high that it can not provide the oxygen needed energy processes and ATP resynthesis is initially done at the expense of phosphocreatine (10 -20 sec), and then make way anaerobic glycolysis (30-40 sec), the accumulation of lactic acid and catabolic loss. In fact, considering these forms of resistance is only a vision dictated by grounds staff. Since the activity is not exclusively motricity, or intellectual, but preponderant and engaging the body as a whole, is true of every form of activity, resistance expresses a complex equation in which all systems and appliances constituents in the body, so biomotricity that this, like the others, is a result of systematically looked morpho functionality body in his unit. In physical education activity, we refer in particular to the general motricity resistance manifested aerobically. At the beginning of the effort, the energy will be provided about anaerobic (one-two minutes), then mixed aerobic- anaerobic (two -five minutes), and then, six minutes is almost entirely derived from aerobic. So regarding resistance, the decisive factor will be the performance of maximal oxygen consumption (VO2 max) and aerobic capacity. Maximum O_2 consumption (VO_2 max) is expressed in liters/minute or reported in kg (in ml/kg/min) - maximal aerobic power (*Margaria*) - will be conditioned by two sets of factors:

1) factors relating to anatomy and functionality especially cardio-respiratory, ensuring intake of O2 in the vault;

2) biochemical factors which relate muscular system especially where changes occur metabolic energy release.

Anatomic and functional factors are:

- Lung volume and alveolar-capillary surface (information corollaries of these elements provide us anthropometric exploring the chest, with diameters and perimeters determine its expiration and inspiration, and the measurement of vital lung capacity, and total waste);

- Radiotelemetrically determined cardiac volume (700-750 ml has values in normal adults athletes reaching up to 1 300 -1 400 ml);

- The concentration of hemoglobin in the blood (normal adults, between 14 and 16g%) - from athletes values rise by 19- 20g% especially given training at altitude. After effort, values reduced by hemolysis;

- The volume of total sanguine;

- Respiratory capacity maximum (the maximum amount as may be inspirited per unit of time - usually per minute - determination is made on 15-20 / sec to not produce phenomena alkalosis, normal values are 120- 150 liters/minute). Determinations are using spirometer and of nomograms. Chest muscle strength conditions the value of this determination;

- Expiratory volume per second (UPMS);

- Maximum cardiac output, which reaches 45 to 40 l / minute and is conditioned by the amplitude of contraction of the heart of the fiber, which causes primarily systolic flow rate, and heart rate. Of course, these parameters, especially those functional, are conditioned not only by cardio-respiratory, whose capabilities they express but also a nervous system that coordinates the functionality of these devices. Equally intervene and digestive system, which involves the intake of nutrients necessary metabolic energogene processes and appliance export of material (especially the renal apparatus), which ensures that catabolite, whose concentration in the body in various sectors somatic and visceral, trigger mechanism of feedback, very important for the whole organic functionality and resistance in particular.

Biochemical factors. Lately, histochemical research proved that main element in the existence of a high threshold of motor resistance overall is the ability of muscle fibers to use a larger amount of O2 and provide energy to perform mechanical work on the path aerobic processes phosphorylation oxidative. This capability belongs to, in particular, red fibers containing an increased amount of myoglobin and mitochondrial oxidative large capacity high. The amount of these fibers in the muscles is genetically determined, hence the usefulness of muscle biopsies while selecting and guiding the appropriate sporting future - according to the proportion of fibers red, which is the substrate resistance and strength on the one hand and fibers White, who speed conditions - corresponding to the branches of sport sportsman biomotricitye qualities.

It was proved lately that resistance effort leads to the biosynthesis of proteins large mitochondrial ribosomes and cytoplasmic neoformation respectively mitochondrial RNA. These processes occur in the fibers called intermediate-DESCO perished soon and had a structure between the fibers and the fibers red white resistance effort in turning them red fibers. Note that resistance effort must have a high intensity and so not only high volume (*Miron Georgescu - A. Demeter*). The intensity should not be too high and should pass in the anaerobic energy because then triggers other mechanisms of intracellular but must be at the top of aerobically at the border with anaerobic reaching that threshold aerobic-anaerobic called area endurance effort (steady state condition). The intensity of effort that will reach body in the endurance depends on the genetic structure of muscle each subject, and it must be individualized. This zone of aging is characterized by the lactic acid concentration in blood of 4 m mol/liter. When the endurance level is at 90% of maximal oxygen consumption, aerobic capacity is very good; values of 80 85% is already unfavorable situation.

For practical purposes, since dosing the lactic acid in the blood and even determining the maximum oxygen consumption are not always possible, we routinely resort to established correlations between these parameters and pulse. Thus, to 140- 150 beats / minute touches 70 - 75% of maximum power consumption of O2 and we are in the area strictly aerobic (*Demeter*) at 155 -165 pulses/min we are at the upper limit of aerobically when the effort is getting an exciting functional strength, and between 165- 175 beats/minute endurance we are in the area. Stamina training will be conducted in this area until the pulse will start to shrink, which will indicate a better adaptation to stress the possibility, while growth effort. This is to apply a more exciting functional strength, which is an exciting biological able to determine the biochemical changes in the muscle fiber, such as to raise the quality of resistance value motricity body. Incontestable that alongside these biochemical mechanisms by obtaining neuromuscular synapses occur durability or neuromuscular plates that are put into action the way nerve centers and pyramidal motricity units. Hence the great importance of central nervous system activity and, in particular, areas of rhinencephalon behavior where, according to recent research, there are centers of volitional that - by commissioning of receptor systems endocrine intracerebral - have an important role in maintaining activities neuromotor plate, despite the fatigue caused by the accumulation of lactic acid in muscles. The consequence of that resistance, although biomotricity perfectible by transforming the way training fiber intermediate red fibers, is genetically determined both by the existence of the plan peripheral a percentage of fiber intermediates in muscle and size anatomical apparatus cardiopulmonary (*Williams)* and marked by determination genetic brain and nervous system functioning especially its rhinencephalon areas.

Heritability coefficient for resistance is also determined by the degree of heritability quite high (over 0.75) aerobic capacity, which is the functional substrate of this biomotricity.

Apart from sports events which indicate objective and improving its resistance level, more appropriate to measure corollary of this quality, the following determinations:

- Somatofunctional mentioned determinations;
- Aerobic capacity;
- Reserve rate index (*Ozalin*):

$$RV = \frac{t_d}{n} - t_{em}$$

RV= speed reserve

td = time spent covering a distance

–resistance coefficient (*Lazarov*):

$$CR = \frac{t_d}{t_{em}}$$

tem = best time

n= standard full length

–resistance index (*Cunton*).

4) Skill is considered in the classical and even currently adopted by most specialists in physical education and sport (coaches, doctors, psychologists, etc.) as a motricity quality attribute of the musculoskeletal system, the content of which is expressed by the precision movements, ie, muscle contractions and their adaptation to the conditions imposed by the requirements of sporting victory, especially for achieving a more efficient driving replicas opponent's actions. The existence of this quality is on the forefront in sports games, in fencing, boxing, and other sports, the answer to the opponent motricity is essential. Quality, according to our experience, is subject to the greatest extent of cortical activity, respectively, on the command received muscle inland motricity cortical and much more than muscle itself, which is important only insofar as possessing certain properties of speed, strength, and resistance even to respond promptly to order cortical received.

For this reason, we will not count as a biomotricity there is a relative balance determining the proportion of different systems and devices, including the nervous system, but we will tell psychoneurotic quality as its net determining dominance is the nervous system. In these circumstances we will present with constitutional mental typology is closely linked to the nervous system and general intelligence researched subject.

• *Type of neuropsychiatric constitutional typology*

Typology on issues of constitutional envisages the necessary references neuro-psychological I did when I presented the evolution of concepts and different ways of establishing anthropological types in their entirety. Reference is now particularly interested in issues that anthropology sport without addressing the complexities raised by psychological aspects not covered by this publication.

We emphasize from the start that motricity activities, like the whole morpho functionality of the human body, is controlled by the central nervous system is the extent of its complexity, in a direct proportionality with the level of efficiency of activity of nerve superior, whose coordinator is the supreme bark cerebral. It follows, therefore, that skill, as viewed from the angle of psycho-neuro-motor and driving around skills training is major conditional - along with mental activity - by the morpho functionality of the brain (brain). It stems so that the sport - especially in sports where, in the foreground, it is necessary to acquire additional skills or particularly complex motricity skills - and the nerve activity type upper high threshold for the cortical function is essential. There is the acting musculoskeletal sports victory in these cases, but the intellect and hence the need for the highest possible level of intelligence.

The cortex is the result of a highly complex development process in which genetic and environmental factors between very closely. It proved the existence of a genetic control of brain development structures on macro and microscopic constituents. Number, type, location and main network connections of nerve cells resulting in sequential expression of a genetic program which runs autonomously during embryonic life. It remains to be seen whether inequalities between native skills of normal individuals also explained by differences in the structure of the cerebral cortex, differences that would then be more subtle and would put on another scale.

It could be the degree of branching of cellular extensions, the number of contacts which they can establish with other neurons. We know, for example, that brain cells - whose total number is around 14 to 18 billion cortical neurons - begin to differentiate to end this fetal differentiation life and continues during the first years of postnatal life. They grow, branch out and connect with each other at synapses, to form a complex network of nerve unimaginable. There are a number of 1014 - 1015 synapses in the human cortex (*Changeux*) per mm^3, a neuron having from 1 000 to 10 000 synapses. Pyramidal cells of the cerebral cortex, for example, emit: inwards, an axon that penetrates white substance in it and myelinations later, and toward the surface, dendrites.

These branches increasingly more abundant and are covered with an increasing number of thorns, long 1 to 3 microns; eventually, they reach a few thousand per neuron. The level of these dendritic spines, especially pyramidal cells endings is in contact with axons of other neurons and synapses knotted (each pyramidal cell could be linked to thousands of other neurons). Structural refinements corresponding progress psychomotor development, and intellectual child. At birth, fewer nerve structures are concluded, both in terms of establishing connections between neurons and myelin fibers. It is about enabling those first movements, first reflexes (sucking, swallowing). Then, little by little, as the structures progress, the senses are sharpened, gestures diversifies and improves. It becomes possible to learn how to walk and awakening intelligence, language acquisition. Consequently, the plan histologically inequality genotypes could be expressed by an uneven density of nerve connections in different areas of the cortex, so through a different number of thorns (per unit length) of the dendrites. However, it is possible that the expression of a genotype more or less favorable to occur at the ultrastructural level: for example, the breadth of contacts synoptic between the button terminal axon of one hand and somatic or spin dendritic on another hand, would be larger or smaller.

There is a genetic control of brain metabolism. Based on the research of lately it has shown that the brain is a huge gland, endocrine, of which there are many receptors. It is assumed that a part of the gene that controls the driving intellectual skills and regulates the production of these receptors and enzymes existing in the brain. It has been shown, for example, the temporal lobe acetyltransferase enzyme activity that synthesizes acetylcholine is strictly genetically determined (*Mandel*), there is also a correlation between the behavior and the enzyme. Begins to decipher increasingly biochemical substrate of some psychiatric genetically determined. There are also proven a correlation between genetically determined threshold levels of certain hormones, sex hormones, and thyroxine or intellectual capacity. It proved that the presence in the blood that irrigates the fetus, an amount higher than the standard hormone androgen (testosterone) or hormone with androgenic effect secondary (progesterone) - and this within a certain period of intrauterine life - could increase intelligence in a meaningful way (*Money*, 1971).

Begin to prove the existence of genes that neurogenesis conditional branching dendrites and multiplying their interconnections or over the whole cortex or in one or another area of *Brodmann* other enzymes that regulate the production of nerve metabolism specific or general metabolic reactions; then others favoring (or hinder) the development of the meningeal that of their endocrine secretion etc. Moreover, because - in a first approximation - these genes, or at least some of them, differ from one subject to another, intellectual potentialities are not the same at all. Pleiotropic genes, i.e., their property to control not one, but several characters further complicate the picture. So, a plurality of factors - it is a complementary aspect - which condition each particular anatomical or physiological. Of course, when considering whether genetic morphology and functional brain there are still many unknowns, as otherwise there for the entire anatomy and physiology of the brain, but is certain that there is a heredity marked the central nervous system and hence the need to take account this reality in the selection and conduct individualized sports training. We will address further some aspects of intelligence and skill are essential for defining the type of athletic activity and mentally.

a. Intelligence. The term intelligence is increasingly used to describe operative side and the value of thinking. *Pieroni*'s dictionary gives them four meanings: 1 - the faculty, along with sensitivity and will constitute the whole mental life; 2 - mental level as a whole, as a result of development; 3 - the general factor skills, common to all mental operations and innate cognitive activities; 4 - problem solving capacity in comparative psychology and differential. As noted *Ursula Şchiopu* (1969), the term intelligence served to treat thinking from a different point of view other than the old associationism, which features reduced to simple combinations thinking of ideas and concepts. Considered complex mental aptitude, intelligence is equated with the operating effectiveness of thinking. She is regarded as a relational capacity or intellectual activity, or, short, straight or bi multifactorial capacity or faculty.

Factorial theories and skills of intelligence led to attempts to evaluate through an intelligence quotient (Q.I), a term introduced by *Stern* in 1912, which expresses the ratio of mental age and biological age determined by tests of the subject. Three-dimensional model of intellect given by *J. P. Guilford* (1966) developed the theory of three-dimensional character of the intellect, the factor structure of thought is given systemically in a single vision. The basic dimensions are accountants groove, operations and results of thinking, which results from combining theory intellect factors. In the model proposed by Guilford are five operations, four types of content and six kinds of products, leading in theory to 5X4X6 = 120 skills or intellect factors. Current research, however, failed to detect than 55 of these, the behavioral factor is sometimes unthinkable (fig. 36).

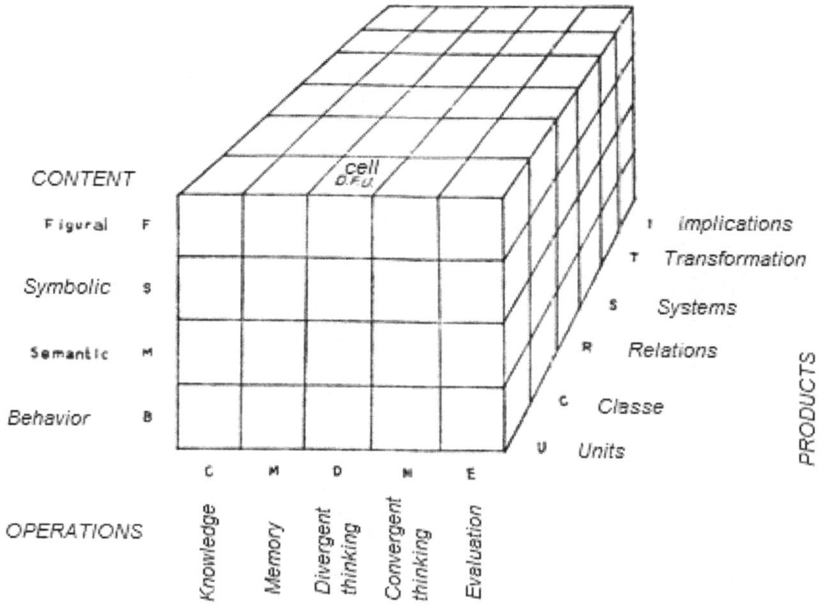

Fig. 36. Intelligence components (after Guilford)

D. divergent thinking, creative skills contained in operation, the main issue is the variety and quantity "outputs" system;

N. Convergent thinking, in which the processing operation information received regarding one and the most acceptable outcome;

E. Evaluation, assessment includes judgments or rulings regarding the satisfactory nature of the information received (correct, appropriate, adequate, etc.).

Broad categories of types of information that the individual can differentiate are:

F. Figuratively - the concrete form of information perceived as an image or updated. Organization comprises perceptual visual information spatial, kinesthetic, etc.;

S. Symbolically, the information is in the form of descriptive signs without significance of themselves, such as musical notes, codes, etc. conventional notation;

M. Semantic represents a certain meaning or significance of information and words are spoken or thought. Some images (photographs) may also contain semantic information;

B. Behavior, comprising mainly Non-verbal information included in interaction subjects, expressing attitudes, needs, desires, intentions, thoughts of others or oneself.

The form they take information as a result of individual activity are:

U. elements of information, relatively isolated units or circumscribed to an "individual" character;

C. Classes grouping as notions of information by virtue of common properties;

R. relations established links between information elements, based on variables or contact points that they have;

S. Systems, organizing or structuring the information elements in groups, interacting or complex parts are interrelated;

T. transformations, changes of various kinds (redefinitions, transfers or changes) of information;

I. Implications extrapolation of information in forms of expectations, predictions, history, concomitant or consequence - known or suspected (*Guilford*, 1979)

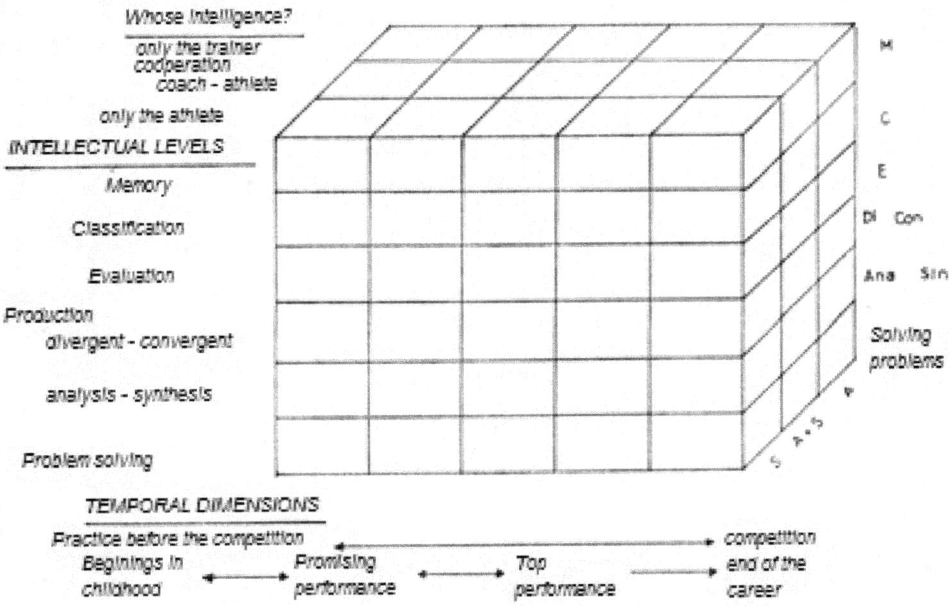

Fig. 37. Elements of intelligence (M. Epuran).

Operations, content and products correlations. The application gives mentioned operation products (results) mental, the content of which is also expressed in different forms. Social intelligence is associated with the behavioral content, understanding the behavior of others and one's own (*M. Epuran*) (fig. 37). As a global expression of nerve functionality, so important in sport and especially in certain sports, intelligence is required to be at a higher level to athletes. This goal is conditioned by two elements:

a) determining IQ parents as having a high degree of heritability enables us to select for sport, subjects with a high level of intelligence, which is essential, especially in certain sports branches such as games, fencing, boxing, where their opponent requires rapid adaptation of the actions of movements;

b) Whereas the environment and the in particular capital have an extra big on genotype intellectual, potentially leading to the development of intellect to the upper limit of adaptability genetic, it is very important that, in preparing the athlete, even in training, to be paid socio-cultural educational importance factor.

These elements are essential to achieving parameters as heights of intellect, are very important because of the work at the top level of the brain depends on the one hand, the threshold of what it can achieve psycho-neuro-motor quality skill, on the other hand, the ease and speed fixation of complex motricity skills. On practical aspects of testing intelligence and its heritability coefficient will return in the next chapter on the anthropological genetic determination of typological character, as we consider a basic element for performance in sport.

All the more so since we cannot make a distinction between general intelligence and mental and motricity. There is an interrelation between these two manifestations of intelligence, so intelligence motricity is ultimately an intellectual stereotype of general intelligence. The fact is attested by new ways of training, starting to be more and more scientifically; exercise starts with acquiring theoretical aspects biomechanical, which involves a deep knowledge of trigonometry, mathematics, physics, and after reasoning intellectual - on which foreshadows schemes tactical - were acquired, it goes into the ground where the training is forming motion skills and whose assimilation is even better as the athlete is more intelligent, with a higher cortical function. In fact, it is proven that the brain works as a whole, based on multiple connections between all its parts, as we will detail this issue with the presentation quality skill.

b. Skill is a psycho-neuro-motor quality whose definition and content they have presented in the description type motricity. We note at the outset that most researchers, including his quote *Malina* (USA) *Nikitjuc* and *Szwarz* (Russia), *Wolanski* and *Sjopa* (Poland), *Eiben* (Hungary) and others, consider that there is a directly proportional relationship between this quality and general intelligence. That we fully justify the thesis, based above regarding the need to test the degree of intelligence, both for the selection of sports - focusing on her character determining the genetic - and for tracking the progress in training because, as observed environment also has a major and decisive role in achieving the upper limit of genetic adaptability.

At the recent Congress of the International Federation of Anthropology and Genetics Applied Sport was also concluded, that the skill called by other researchers and skill, is subject primarily to the functionality of the nervous system and is under the control of the nervous system, representing 'ability to adapt to different changes to the external environment "(*Malita*). On the structures that determine skill, we notice the nervous system, endocrine system, and muscular system. We will follow in detail how the systems involved in the development of this quality. I. Observe absolute predominance of the nervous system, acting mainly through certain segments.

1) *The cortex* is undoubtedly the main element in achieving fine motricity controls, and motricity responses appropriate actions opponent. It works by several areas:

- *Prefrontal area*, where departs a pyramidal beam, leading the conscious voluntary motility.

- *The region* consists of a voluntary motricity function and extends endorsement, precentral and neighboring Giri, close to the lateral cerebral sulcus and the pars operculars of the frontal and parietal lobes. Also, extends over the upper edge and ends of the hemisphere and the rear part of the paracentral lobe. Throughout the region arises path pyramid (corticobulbar tracts and tracts corticospinal).

- *Extrapyramidal cortical areas.* Outside the system effector pyramid, with two beams, corticospinal and corticonuclear there extrapyramidal system, whose party controls are under the whole neuraxis in floors subcortical: nuclei striated subthalamic, cvadrigemeni colliculi, red nucleus, substantia nigra, nucleus vestibular Oliva cerebellum - regulating organ par excellence, vestibular and proprioceptive receiving inflows. However, these centers operate under the influence of bark and, in turn, by the circuit complicated influence cortical activity, extrapyramidal system is a servo motricity which regulates the influx from the common final pathway. In this active substance complex cross-linked part, the fiber goes up to the crust, while the other goes down in the brain stem and spinal cord.

- *Areas inhibitors*, so named because they can inhibit the functioning of the area motricity main are located on both sides of the area precentral (4s, two frontal lobes, eight in the occipital lobe around the area 19, 24 gyrus cingulate onto the inner hemisphere). The influx of these areas reaches the globus pallidum then caudate nucleus, where it is referred to in precentral cortex (areas 4-6); while the nervous influx from ventral pallidum is sent to the nucleus of the thalamus and then the side previously, fiber talamocorticale at cortex. It is corticostriocortical repressive system, acting as a filter thalamus.

- *Areas integration circuits* serve the neocerebelos engine. Neocerebelulm achieved second adjustment mechanism of cortical influx. He has two great beams related to the cerebellum bark, frontopontin (*Arnold*) and parietotemporopontin (*Tűrk Meynert*).

Lately, besides this representation, the pyramid and para-pyramid motility cortex in the neocortex, several areas of representation of the arhipaliumul, of particular importance to achieve precision, finesse and adapting maximum act motricity conditions environment were discovered:

- *Representing integrative own body assembly*. The man sometimes aware of his own body in different ways: touch, allowing us to feel the shape and consistency; by inflows proprioception, which informs us on the attitude and situation in space; by visual inflows; by inflows aids, which allow us voice recognition etc. It has been shown that the sensitivity areas (parietal), listening (temporal), visual (occipital) connects to the body lying in the projection area surrounding the rear end of the convolutions of *Sylvius* and the first furrow fissure time. Also in the region is projected pulvinar, which takes turn receives inflows from the lateral geniculate bodies and medial and posterior ventral lateral nucleus of the so diencephalic tract relays auditory, visual and tact.

- *Cortical fields related to the ability of foresight*. Action requires foresight. *Penfield*'s research is proving links with the core medial prefrontal cortex, thalamus, cortex engine at the touch of the occipital and temporal. These anatomical elements associated with clinical facts suggest some areas of forecasting at the anterior portion of the prefrontal cortex, the prefrontal region is proven that intervention is done in relation to mental processes which will lead to actions that are expected.

- *Fields of cortical sensibility*. Electrophysiological and clinical research done in recent years, begin to allow deciphering of cortical areas of sensibility. Emotional feelings and emotions are most often inflicted by sight, hearing, smell, etc. Emotions trigger motricity and autonomic manifestations. Two regions of the cortex are directly linked with centers regulators of motility and nuclei hypothalamic respectively prefrontal cortex and the area cingulate (limbic), which, based on research electrophysiological and clinical facts, concluded that these areas are the representation sensibility. It found a number of receptors in the brain and endocrine substances that are responsible for the behavior and the overall functionality of the brain (cybernine, etc.). It defines, therefore, four areas (a d).

a) *The prefrontal cortex* is linked with the two-way precentral cortex and posterior nuclei of the hypothalamus (ergotropic which produce hypertension, tachycardia, and reactions of anabolism).

b) *cingulate cortex area* (*Broca*'s limbic lobe) by its anterior part, is an inhibitor of motricity activities through its action on the caudate nucleus and the brainstem reticular substance. Cingular area receives all areas related to suppressive cortex (frontal, parietal, occipital) and the hippocampus, the way nucleus of the anterior thalamus. This last conduct shows that the rhinencephalon can trigger autonomic effects through the fibers onto the anterior hypothalamic nuclei (trophotropic - *Hess*) and through direct action, through the cingulate cortex, the subcortical motricity centers afferent the cingulate cortex, the subcortical motricity centers. Cingulate area, such neo activated and sends archicortex in turn, inflows from centers inhibitors, the place where assembly takes place mechanisms that translate condition called emotion (*Papez*).

c) *The first middle temporal convolutions* (projection area of the fibers before cochlear) for verbal deafness.

d) *The angular area* around the finishing of the first temporal convolutions, occipital lobe before, for verbal blindness. Among the four areas are associative fibers whose injury causes aphasia involvement processes. Some authors believe that there is an ideational area, which assembles the work of these four areas (*Delmar*). Also, the fact that the four areas exist in both hemispheres, but that only the left hemisphere in right-handed and right to left-handed intervention in language associated with that muscle phonation entirely - with representations motricity on both sides - part synchronously raises number of issues to be elucidated. We also notice that these areas work in close correlation with each other and with behavioral areas and other cortical areas, brain forming a functional unit as a whole.

2) *Extrapyramidal system*. Consisting of all formations nerve, ultimately, by way downward, they send impulses to the motricity unit (via peripheral motricity neuron), providing fine adjustment movements and muscle tone. This system, which is controlled cortical constitute an effector to achieve the highest level of skill. It consists of bundles subrospinal, tectospinal, nigrospinal, olivospinal, reticulospinal, vestibulospinal (*Atlas of Anatomy*, Volume III).

3) *The substance mesh*, which is a formation nervous comprises a plurality of neurons, particularly in the brain stem - on one hand - the area was called the system activator upward, keep the tone of cortical, including the areas of motricity, and through another area, descending inhibitory system adjusts called motricity impulses coming from higher levels adapting them outside environment requirements and giving them the necessary precision.

4) *The cerebellum*, which is involved particularly in motricity circuits as follows:

- Neocerebellum adjusts smoothness and accuracy;
- Paleocerebellum regulates muscle tone;
- Archicerebellum regulating the balance.

Between these segments of the central nervous system integrated circuits and cybernetic (feedback) reafferentation are made which is substrate anatomo-functional of precision, finesse and adaptability of the motricity act; they essentially express neuromotor coordination and skill so (for details see *Atlas of Human Anatomy*, Volume III – coord. *Mircea Ifrim*).

5) *The vestibular analyzer* involved also in achieving skill because, by its segments reception, management and projection cortical it ensures the maintenance of body balance: skill behaves to man keeping in position orthostatic inappropriately making it impossible precision movements. For these reasons, the major skill involved, along with cortical structures, and whole vestibular analyzer.

It is undeniable that other *analyzers*, especially the visual, auditory, kinesthetic, through the information they provide cortex is involved in making skill, so their integrity structural and functional - with a higher degree of acuity - are very important for achieving maximum parameters of skill.

Regarding functional cortical mechanisms involved in skill, we will not repeat those known on brain physiology. We particularly insist on the role of the balance between excitation and inhibition processes, concentration and irradiation. Inhibition of differentiation is one of the basic mechanisms of the nervous system that determines the skill, the selective contraction of muscles, controlled cortical is essential. Also forming dynamic stereotypes that express, in fact, intelligence motricity, motricity skills is essential for printing. However, the process of thinking and reasoning, which are beginning to be deciphered their morpho-physiological aspects, but are far from being understood, are essential to the driving skills that require reasoning and answers in action driving fast opponent. Knowledge tests based on the type of nervous system over which we have previously insisted is essential to have information on these processes and the potential skill of an athlete. Thus, balanced type of cell is optimal in fencing, boxing, sports games and other sports, skill is on the forefront. However, fatigue strength of nerve cell is essential for skill with the ability to fast recovery. Only in terms of freshness nerve cell skill is full. It has also been demonstrated that nerve cell, because the blood-brain barrier, they operate in anaerobic metabolism. Are interesting from this point of view the research of *Malina* (USA), showing that athletes who have a high anaerobic capacity and a high skill and high intelligence. The fact is all the more interesting as anaerobic capacity has a very high coefficient of heritability, as proof, once again, by the fact that the nerve cell metabolism is anaerobic conditioning strong genetic brain activity.

II. Secondly we must view very close *neuroendocrine correlations* involved in nervous system function: thyroid and gonadal hormones in particular, are involved in higher nervous activity (see *Atlas of Human Anatomy*, Vol. III); hypothalamus, pituitary and its correlations are also very important. Hence the need to establish the type described and endocrine branch corroboration with the sport practiced. Hypothalamus region of the neuraxis is also important phenomena which occur with secretory functionality important role in maintaining homeostasis of the nervous system and body. Secretory products are neurotrophic, neuroregulators and psihoreglations. Secretory phenomena from the diencephalon are neurosecretion, Neurocrine and ependimocrinia.

Neurosecretory. It turned out that groups of magnocellular paraventricular nuclei supraoptici and have endocrine activity. These neurons produce an neurosecretory which descends along axons to the posterior pituitary (*Scharrer*). Neuro-Crete is accumulated in the pituitary and then released into the blood; it seems that oxytocin, vasopressin, adiuretina have their place in the pituitary gland is not developed, but in the hypothalamus. It also secretes hormones hypothalamic nuclei passing tube-Rian in the region, stimulating and regulating the activity of the anterior pituitary function and especially corticotrope.
Equally, it is considered that there is a hypothalamic neurosecretion walking on nerve fibers dispersed in the pineal region, the midbrain and amygdala.

Neurocrine. Neurocrine is meant by the phenomenon of excretion, within the nervous system, a product produced by glandular or secretory organs that hypo-metaphyseal, or ependymal epiphysis (opposite the hemocriny term, by which we mean glandular secretion discharge blood). It is a reverse phenomenon to neurosecretion

III. Addressing the issues of skill, we emphasize that the bio-psychomotor quality is subject to two essential elements of body functionality.

1. Formation driving habit, subject to the central nervous system functionality.

2. The extent to which the device has other biomotor muscle, speed, strength, stamina, which allow a proper reception of orders cortical and therefore a correct execution, if the muscle more correctly the whole body, not possess these qualities in the corresponding parameters (accuracy, timeliness and the adaptability of the movement). In essence, the realization is encumbered for guiding fulfill-negative.

A. *On first appearance in this vision of skill* emphasize some aspects which determine and define motricity learning and corollary have a high degree of determination on skill development. Driving skills are complex conditioned reflexes based on improving links between internal organs (apparatus cardio respiratory, digestive, excretory, endocrine system etc.) and locomotor system, being conditioned mainly by the central nervous system functionality. Training process improves the reflexes ensuring the adaptability of the entire body to the requirements of the effort being put in. A clear definition of driving skills is made by Prof. *M. Epuran* after that "skills are components of voluntary activity which, through practice, achieve a high yield index based on improving execution (coordination, precision, speed, automation, etc). The physiological mechanism of habit is the activity of the cerebral cortex assembly, according to the laws of interaction of two signaling systems, training complex conditioned reflexes and coordination mechanisms of the central nervous system. The concepts underlying the notion of motricity skill, we note that phase has passed it is considered that learning is achieved exclusively through the connection of external stimulus and triggering the adaptive response (*Behavior*). Today it is considered, on the nervist theory, Pavlovian, in which building habits of a series of intermediate variables in the upper floors of plasticity and functionality S.N.C. plays a key role. We emphasize also that using current notions of skill and motricity skill, sometimes creating confusion. We agree with *M. Epuran* showing that "voluntary human activity is complex and consists of abilities and skills that overlap and complement each other, meaning that some abilities and skills are made, and no skills can exist without understanding."

Vanek add that it "defines skill as a step equivalent to the finishing stage, with end stage of differentiation of motricity skills training, is actually better use of dynamic stereotype obtained during the primary automation." Summarizing the views in the literature, we consider that learning motive elementary or complex represents the first stage of formation of dynamic stereotype, because the skill to be an upper stage, the subject, fully realized, is able, thanks to function cognitively logical SNC, combine and use creative and appropriate driving habits formed. Hence the need for the training to pay adequate attention to respect differences in anthropological age, so as not to block the nervous system during stereotype, training only healthy habits, but to develop the ability of creative and training motricity (for example: tactical action games, *M. Epuran*), enabling rapid assembly of complex and cortical neurons, absolutely indispensable in achieving quality parameters senior bio-psycho-motor skill that determines the performance of a series of sports activities.

In this context there is a danger of creating stereotypes in learning skills driving, especially in children and youth, which fit very consolidated habit driving can be an obstacle or a "barrier" net, limiting the ability to adapt, conditional on the formation of acts new elementary existing driving skills. Such cite "speed barrier" that can occur under a bad workout conducted in children and youth. We emphasize that driving skills training an important role, along with environmental factors, educational, training, returns heritable genetic determination of the nervous system, in terms of its structure and functionality. But completed by research lately that certifies that in addition to biological heredity - which consists of the transmission of genetic information under the mendeleen laws (heredity closed) - there is a heritable behavioral model called heredity open. It had such a close correlation between motricity learning and metabolism ribonucleic acid (RNA) and other brain proteins. It is proved that inhibition of RNA synthesis stops any motricity learning. The first driving molecules responsible for the transmission of information have been isolated experimentally on animals, by *G. Ungar* and were named scotophobine.

These studies open new perspectives in elucidating the complex mechanisms that determine genotype, so important to know for selection. Making it studies the quality genes, it is recognized that the majority of subjects, 68% are carriers of medium quality, 16% above average and 16% below average (*A. Gagea*). The possibility of combining genes from two parents above average increases to the extent that they are the possessors of great quality and great talent is born when the gene is the combination of genes characters above average. It's a rare situation quite large, bound and that *Terman* (USA) shows, on an experimental basis, that there is a genetic tendency to return to the mean.

It thus appears that genetic determinism of vocational skills and motricity corollary, the skill, play a particular role as heredity closed, genetic, and the open, represented by neuropeptides produced in the brain, able to facilitate the establishment of neural connections and engrams driving. These facts explain the superior driveability of the subjects remembered the families of athletes of great value, with a family tree as deep as possible. Of course, these mechanisms add information intellectual exclusively own the human being, the only owner of the second signaling system. Programming and driving habit formation, conditioned as compared potential genetic mechanisms exposed, as compared morphological and neurophysiological depend, ultimately, the full functionality and integrative nervous system, ability and cortical plasticity of the cerebral cortex. In this context, we emphasize the following components of C.N.S. building habits that contribute to driving.

a) *related component* which receives, by way of various analysis, external environment, or those stored in certain stages of S.N.C. (Especially in subcortical areas) and transmits cortical floor. Also on this level acts and cyber reafferentation mechanisms (feedback) that continuously adjusts central responses based on changes in the periphery. We note that this component related, in terms of subsystems contained in them is requested depending on the specific differential branch sport (eg visual analyzer in the shooting, proprioceptive analyzer in gymnastics, etc.).

b) *The central component cortical* performing synthesis, anticipation and image global motricity, cognitive response logically likely to develop adaptive control for the locomotive periphery.

c) *Effector component*, represented by the efferent cortex transmission and muscle contraction coupling excitation, biomotricity conditional qualities and the metabolic muscle (fatigue etc.).

To these are added:

d) The vegetative component, expressing the full functionality of other systems and devices that provide metabolic levels, anabolic and catabolic neuromuscular necessary functionality, in terms of the human body viewed together as a complex biomechanical system. Of course, request that the share of these components in building habits driving varies by sport practiced. Thus, a player will be required all components and is hard to say which comes first (in our opinion appreciate priority central component followed by the effector and related to the conditioning by the autonomic), while a player chess is clearly dominant central component. Depending on the selection of components will be both selection and training methods by sport.

We also appreciate that approach Prof. *M. Epuran* on the types of skills and corollary skill - then distinguish: smart driving habits, where, in the forefront, driving the skill development and thus quality skill bio-psycho-motor cortical functionality ranges (eg in sports games, fencing, boxing, etc.); proprioceptive driving skills, the neuromuscular coordination and balance are on the forefront (gymnastics, rowing, etc.); sensory motricity skills in some analyzers are required in particular as visual analyzer in the shooting - it is helpful in addressing scientific sports training and differentiated selection of sports branch. To these we add skills with a high degree of stereotyping and request vegetative major component, which makes the very possibility of achieving the stereotypes imposed by the pace and speed with performance, as in some field events (sprints, throws, cycling etc.). This category of skills, qualities biomotor speed, strength, stamina - depending on the specific sample - have a decisive role in obtaining performance, especially since the complexity of the skill driving cortical and the requirement of creativity in achieving it is not maximum degree of cortical request. Of course, that is added in this case, as well as in other types of skills, personality components, the psychic type, which are critical to performance.

B. Regarding the *formative stages of motricity skills*, we mention the following stages:

1) *Step unnecessary movements or preliminary properties - cognitive* (generalization of excitation), the cortical ideomotricity image includes a greater number of neurons and is imperfect coordination both at cortical interneurons and motricity coupling and wide. There is risk of formation of stereotypes as, for example, speed barrier, and too long breaks are not indicated. The movements are undifferentiated coarse. This stage dominates the ante-pubertal and puberty periods, is explained by the peculiarities of the nervous system at this age.

2) *The strained movements execution step of specified properties - organization (concentration partial arousal)* when, although we are dealing with a cortical higher concentration, however there is more cortical areas acting in achieving movement. From a metabolic, biochemical, energy costs are high, sometimes exceeding even the first step. Fatigue occurs rapidly and neuropsychological stress is high. Movement is made rigid, uptight. At this stage it is necessary to work analytically, individually and correct executions to be immediately reinforced through repetition. If this step is not outdated quickly, we deal with a subject lacking the necessary genetic qualities performance.

3) *Phase correct execution of movements - the strengthening and improving the skill (differentiating fine movement).* It is the merging processes strictly nerve cortical areas concerned, and energy savings with maximum functional effect characterized habit. Movement is done selectively, exclusively for optimal muscle groups necessary technical execution. At this stage it is necessary to increase the number of repetitions and should focus on removing small imperfections. This phase coincides with the phase post-pubertary and anthropological peculiarities are explained by this age.

4) *Phase detailed properties of the movement (automation habit*). Is the phase that forms and reinforces the stereotype motricity is based on a chain of conditional and unconditional reflex that automatically triggers a repetition time, respectively workout. This phase is compulsory for all driving documents.

Training stereotype right may be encumbered negative the existence of reactions vestigial quartered in floors subcortical, especially in the *putamen and pallidum nucleus* of extrapyramidal system reactions that are either innate or acquired by an incorrect execution in the early stages, which must be observed and corrected patience through initial awareness chain driving acts forming the stereotype.

Once stereotype motricity format, bear in mind that if he begins to fire in its entirety, outside awareness, although precise and saving energy, it constitutes a brake on creativity so necessary in sport. Hence the need to maintain the skill and execution personal plasticity, which is achieved in practice through various executions, different opponents and further difficulties to seek new populations of cortical and consequently stimulate creativity athlete. The fact is imposed even in stage performer of the highest class to avoid capping and routinist. More so avoid stereotype motricity consolidated itself on the way to the high performance as it can hamper an insurmountable limit to the sporting process. We note also that skills training entails following the workout, a series of morphological changes of which we quote: increasing capillary network strokes by 20% enrichment innervation of muscle fibers, increase the area button Synoptics, increasing the volume of motricity neurons to about 34%. As regards the stability of driving skills, we note that the innate, such as walking, running, climbing, persists throughout life, although impractical long time (illness), decrease in efficiency. The same is true for some acquired skills, such as cycling, skiing, swimming, which, if they are no longer practiced for a long time, remain only in terms of basic structure, coordination of fine movements is lost.

Similarly, the driving skills of high-tech performance sport after a break in their execution, they lose accuracy, smoothness, high degree of neuromotor coordination. While it is possible that an interruption to allow the restructuring of the skill to a higher level in terms of loss of a series of acts facilitating acts motive and driving us higher quality, which is built on the basic structures remaining from the old habit. Hence the effectiveness of longer breaks in training, strictly individual branch of sport and trained subject. We note also that in determining the development, strengthening and, ultimately driving habit execution, an important role all factors stress positive or negative type, which acts on the nervous system. It results from the above that skill, seen as quality bio-psycho-motor, depends, on the one hand, the training of the driving conditional functionality of complex nervous system over which we insisted, and the quality of bio-motor of body which, ultimately, are also indicators of locomotor function of which depends on the extent to which cortical command can be received and executed correctly.

From those presented on skills which ultimately determines motricity learning, it is clear that learning in corporal activities include an "intelligent learning built in acquiring notions, concepts and creative learning" *(M. Epuran)*. Intelligent use of higher learning mechanisms of the human intellect, thinking mechanisms that direct the process of reflection of reality, as a reflection of logical relationships and essences phenomena is a cognitive learning. This fully justifies the selection, athlete intelligence testing, and training, nurturing and development.

Thinking conditioned by intelligence, as an expression of overall functionality of cortical provides orientation to the environment through its operations of comparison, analysis, synthesis, abstraction, generalization, being able to have a number of qualities, including critical thinking, flexibility, speed and the breadth, which gives the possibility of a human subject responses to environmental changes or if physical education and sport, action driving more efficient and adapted to various situations on the ground. In these circumstances, it is clear that thinking skill condition essentially seen as bio-psycho-motor quality. Between intelligence and learning ability motive there is a positive correlation with both greater as are more complex exercises. Some authors have even proposed a motoricity coefficient (M. Q) to designate time learning motricity skills of children. It follows therefore a very close correlation between the formation of the intellectual and motricity skills, both conditional intelligence. Tactical skills in sports have, in their content, both mental and motricity components, as they are a unit that reflects the body's physiological structural unit. Tactical skills are acts smart tactic being answered fully and effectively, individually or collectively, in a problematic situation (*M. Epuran*). Tactical behavior is the smart guy, the athlete cannot be considered a servo scheduled, but must have a high level of intelligence or creativity, to allow the reelection of an adequate response to the multitude of situations arising during the competition.

C. Third, skill is determined by the extent to which muscle fiber is able to respond to commands needed and, therefore, achieve neuro-motor coordination. In this sense, depending on environmental conditions, requires skill to achieve speed motricity act (eg. hitting the ball in a game, quickly and accurately, before your opponent gets to her), power (a blow and precise box that i slammed his opponent to the floor) or resistance (possibility muscular system to resist until the last minute of the game, preserving precision and smoothness of movement, given that, in terms of muscle fatigue, response to commands cortical muscle is imprecise, several units muscle inhibition is able to compensate for metabolic reserves; neuromotor plate itself does not have an adequate permeability, making it harder to depolarization. In this view, in our opinion, in muscle, skill is conditional on other biomotricity, so necessary for maximal parameters of this quality to develop, to pursue other qualities driving, depending on the requirements of industry sports practiced.

As regards the possibility of assessing and forecasting skill, besides stopwatch made, well established in the national selection (Nicu Alexe), we expect the following tests concerning the neuroendocrine system, muscular system and vestibular analyzer:

Neuromotor coordination skills tested by:

- Pegboard Pardue test,
- "tracing" test
- Thermometers,
- coordination and dissociation hand shake test;
- The ability to inhibit the differentiation can be tested by determining the threshold of fusion, based on the difference threshold;
- Mobility nerve processes are tested by determining the capacity of rotation per unit time;

-Reactivity S.N.C. is tested by:

- Reaction time,
- Speed of execution on a simple motricity task,
- Repetition speed test (Tapping)
- Achilles reflexogram, providing information and on thyroid function;
- Excitability S.N.C. can be tested by:
- Electroencephalography,
- Electromyography
- Cronaximetry;

The type of nervous system is determined by:

- Psycho pedagogical medical observation,
- Psychological personality tests;

Determining the dominant hemisphere is done by:

- E.E.G., EMG and Pardue Pegboard test;

Sense of balance is tested by:

- Statokinezimetry (Gagea A.)
- Romberg test,
- General determination of the center of gravity (see Anatomy and Biomechanics physical education and sport - M. Ifrim et al.);
- The permeability of the synapse is determined by:
- Latency,
- Hoffmann reflex;
- Anaerobic capacity;
- Clinical and laboratory exploring endocrine glands, especially the thyroid, pituitary and gonads;
- For other biomotricity skill that conditions in the branch of sport using tests presented to each of these qualities;
- Exploring visual, acoustic and kinesthetic analyzers through current methods

We also emphasize psychomotricity skills diagnosis which made, in most cases, along with the motricity skills, the authors operated here distinction between the two categories of skills (M. Epuran). Fleishman (1964), the famous researcher of driving ability and psychomotricity uses a large battery of tests consists of practical examinations and laboratory sample.

Of the laboratory samples used by Fleishman may be mentioned:

- Sample of pulling and pushing, to determine the effectiveness general driving;
- Evidence of coordination complex, precision targeting self-control;
- Sample dissociation of movements, to study ambidextrous abilities;
- Speed of response;
- Tapping for measuring the speed of repetition;
- Push the lever type samples, in order to know the speed of the arm;
- O'Connor test, measurement of finger dexterity;
- Test type thermometer for measuring precision hand arm. Herbert (1911) and Denisiuc (1967) using field samples in order to know the driving ability of children.

The research intended to assess “skills fundamental driving,” Ludwig Denisiuc recommends a battery of tests that actually measures the overall motricity skills, psychomotricity skills and the level of learning of motricity skills and may not however appreciate the weight that each of these have on the yield obtained from the sample topic. Therefore:

- Speed - defined by the author as faculty to perform fast movements - measured by test running 30.40 and 60 m. It is obvious that in this case, as to the evidence on a very short distance, the student who can take start right will achieve a much better than another with a higher “faculty to perform rapid movements,” but with a lower level of training;
- Power (in English power), considered the subject faculty to execute actions with maximum force in minimum time, jump height was measured by extension arms (Sargent's test);
- Force by throwing the medicinal ball (one or two kg) overhead;
- Flexibility or faculty to execute movements with large amplitude is highlighted by bending forward of the trunk;
- The strength, the power to execute a long-term work with full load, measured by the number of executions (squatting position, throwing legs back, return to standing position) made in the time allowed (30“ for girls, 1 min. for boys);
- Agility, regarded by the author as faculty integration of the various movements into a whole and the ability to move quickly from one act engine to another is measured by a composite sample of several elements: race over a distance of 5 m, race around obstacles, roll forward and walk on all fours.

The research department of Prof. Michael Epuran on psychomotricity capacity to six students 18 have revealed a battery limited diagnostic value of evidence: tapping for measuring the speed of hand and foot rehearsal; senzomatory distance appreciation for coordination; kinezimetry sensitivity for diagnosis (hand and foot) Matorin test for overall coordination knowledge and skills test for the diagnosis of rhythmic percussion.

With this battery could appreciate the peculiarities and psychomotricity development capacity between six and 18 years in children who do not practice organized in any branch of sport and the differences between them and those who practice a branch of organized sport. Our results were confirmed by research carried out under the leadership of our collaborators Fl. Dumitru, El. Badea, I. Iminovici. Results of research on psychomotricity skills can be a serious support for selection work in sport, physical education programs for compiling and individualize training. Given the high degree of heritability of these tests the skill and skill in exploring analytical report and determining its constituent elements, necessary and recommended by the literature (*Malina* et al) that these determinations to be made and parents, thus constituting a valuable perspective sports forecasting a selected topic.

- Personality (by Prof. Dr. *Michael Epuran*: physical education and sport psychology.). Addressing the issue of mental type, we need to make a few references on the personality, which has a decisive role in getting sports performance and medical act correctly; they constitute a common denominator for achieving great results across all sports.

There are many definitions of personality, as that concept is essentially a synthesis of the whole biopsychosocial traits that characterize a human individual (*Meili*). We appreciate that the definition issued by Allport, after which personality is "dynamic organization within the individual of those psychophysical systems that determine his characteristic thinking and behavior" is quite conclusive. The structural components of personality are also viewed differently according to the author, The majority view, however defining personality: temperament, skills and attitudes plus character (*M. Epuran*).

- Temperament is expressed by energy and a dynamic personality that is characterized by being impressionable index of impulsiveness, inner feelings, rhythm, tempo, changes in mental and psychological expressiveness (*Ana Tucicov*). These characteristics have inherited a great deal of determination, being very stable.

Correlations between somatic type and temperament meet in Kretschmer's typology and especially that of Sheldon. Also, the study of ambidextrous ability attests that training in the administration entails extra motricity skill is sometimes decisive victory in sports. Sheldon sees the temperamental type as a set of physical and mental traits. It defines the key dimensions by which individuals can be ordered. Somatic type depends on the value of the three physical components of the individual: endomorphism (grade digestive organ development) Mesomorphism (grade development somatic structures) and ectomorphism (nervous system development). If every feature is denoted by between 7 and 1 are theoretically 343 types (73). In fact, through case studies, Sheldon finds only 76 different somatotypes.

The temperamental type is determined from all of the three dimensions: viscerotony (general relaxation, sociability, sociopfilia, hunger for affection and approval, equality emotional flow, easy communication of feelings, the need for another in case of conflict, etc.); somatotony (desire for physical adventure, energy, desire to dominate, the trend towards risk, physical courage in battle, competitive aggression, unrestrained voice, the ability to act alone etc.) and cerebrotony (retained movements, excessive mental tension, anxiety, control the emotions, voice retained, chronic fatigue, introversion, loneliness desire to failure or conflict etc.). Sheldon found significant correlations (over 90) the following types of somatic and temperamental:

- Viscerotony and endomorphism;
- Mesomorphism and somatotony;
- Ectomorphism and cerebrotony.

All other correlations being negative, reaching affirmation of the link between somatic and temperamental types for which correlations are positive and significant. Like any typology, those discussed above have much questionable, arbitrary. Even direct binding of the somatic temperamental type has no justification. Heymans and Wiersma try to create a division on the basis of mental temperaments. Starting from combining three fundamental characteristics: activism, emotionality and the repercursivitaty (first, second), established eight temperamental types (Table 5). The main lack of all classifications cited results from ignoring the role of nervous system activity and, in particular, higher nervous activity in determining the type temperamental.

-*Type of nervous and temperamental activity.* Scientific understanding of temperaments is precisely linked to the criterion of physiological nervous. Keeping division and terminology of Hippocrates, Pavlov link types temperamental peculiarities higher nervous activity, type of activity nervous top. These kinds result from the combination of three specific features of manifestation of the fundamental nervous processes (excitation and inhibition), namely: strength, mobility and balance them.

Table 5

temperament	criteria		
	excitability	activism	primary / secondary
amorphous	nonemotional	nonactive	primary
apathetic	nonemotional	nonactive	secondary
nervous	emotional	nonactive	primary
sentimental	emotional	nonactive	secondary
phlegmatic	nonemotional	active	secondary
blood	nonemotional	active	primary
choleric	emotional	active	primary
passionate	emotional	active	secondary

P. Popescu Neveanu (types of nervous activity superior to man, Ed. Acad. R.P.R., 1961) gives indications which may be estimated after three typological characteristics experimentally.

1. intensity nerve processes:
   - Subjects' performances in heavy burdens in a short time (working capacity);
   - Level of stress that develops inhibitors of protection;
   - Resistance to disruptive excitation;
   - Report concentration of nerve processes irradiation intensity excitations they induce.
2. Mobility nerve processes:
   - Speed of onset, discontinuation or conduct nerve processes;
   - Replacing a process other characteristics;
   - Peculiarities of formation and restructuring of dynamic stereotype.
3. To balance nerve processes:
   - Comparing the performance of subjects in developing positive and negative reflexes;
   - Assessing the phenomena of induction (positive and negative). This phenomenon occurs with greater intensity in the excitable type;
   - Analysis of the phenomena of overloading, which lead to an intense unbalanced type overexcited.

Type of nervous activity superior physiological basis of temperament, but not identical with, because temperament is both pro-social influences shower educational who acted in the course of life, on the individual. Pavlov even shows that innate characteristics of the type of higher nervous activity (genotype) are added traits acquired during the life of the individual (phenotype). They also show that in humans, these qualities are dependent and particulars of relations between the two signaling systems, resulting in the specific human types: thinker, artistic and environmental.

- Features temperaments according to Pavlovian typology. The division into types of temperament is approximate because of the temperament of each person lists numerous individual variations in turn influenced by other traits of personality, such as the skills and especially character. The main features of psychological temperaments were shown by various authors, including *Paul Smith Neveanu* (1978), whose wording reproduce. Choleric is distinguished by the relative weakness of active inhibition, where the trend irrepressible self, impulsivity, restlessness, impatience, emotional explosion, the impetuous oscillation between activism and depression, propensity for exaggeration and alarm condition, etc.

The sanguine type is characterized by speed, quickness, calm, intense emotions and shallowness of feelings, longing for change, instability interests and inclinations, distribution and concentration slight attention, maximum adaptability, strength through restructuring easy to difficulties, relatively still maintaining strength and psychic balance.

The phlegmatic type calm has the relevant features, slowness, poor emotional reactivity and durability of feelings, natural patience. The melancholic type is characterized by reduced working capacity, neuro-psychological resistance weak and by an acute sensitivity. *Eysenck* observed a high correlation between this temperament and introversion. Towards the end of the activity, *Pavlov* completed after how special temperaments typology higher nervous activity, the relationship between the two signaling systems:

-The artistic type, the prevailing first signaling system - intuitive reflection of reality through concrete images with emotional, volitional, synthetic attitude towards the world;

- The environmental type - equality of the two signaling systems;

- The thinker type, the prevailing second signaling system; a reflection of reality by logical emotional connection type; analytical attitude towards reality.

Diagnosing the temperament is essential for sport, for which we present some elements to facilitate its setting (*Epuran*) (table 6)

Skills, as defined by *Rubinstein*, are human traits or qualities that make it apt for the successful completion of certain activities, recognize a genotyping and paratypes. They can be classified, in our opinion, by the application of systems and devices constituting the body and interest in the sport, the mental intellectual (attention, memory, intelligence, etc), psiho-bio-motricity (endurance), biomotricity (strength, power, speed). Typological features of these anthropological issues, which are embedded in the content of the concept of personality, aptitude take the name has been detailed in previous pages.

Character, defined synthetic orientation, and behavior are significant human individual, is mainly expressed through what man does with the value for the community in which he lives. Properties of character fundamental emotions (dependence subject object) activism (the influence of the subject on the object), the repercursivity (resonance of an event on the mental sphere of the subject), attitudes (ideals, beliefs, attitudes assessment evaluation, attitude towards society, labor, people, to himself), will (orientation purpose, consistency, determination, self-control, courage). Of the mentioned briefly that personality, defined by temperament, skills and character is essential to sport performance. Appears important in selecting knowledge of particular temperament and skills, and training full development, the upper limit of adaptability genetics, these parameters defining of human and especially education, on the way to the high-performance character sportsman, representing side the most perfect, especially personality. (Table 7, 8)

Table 6

Temperament identification guide

CHOLERIC (loud, excitable, mobile)	SANGUINE (strong, balanced, mobile)
1. Restless, agitated.	1. Cheerful and optimistic.
2. Impulsive, irascible.	2. Energetic and enterprising.
3. Anxious.	3. They do not finish what they start
4. Harsh and honest in relationships with people.	4. Inclined to overestimate their abilities.
5. Determined and full of initiative..	5. Able to seize the new.
6. Stubborn.	6. Fickle in interests and inclinations.
7. Ingenious in discussions.	7. Easily withstand troubles and failures.
8. Work in leaps	8. Adaptable to various circumstances.
9. Prone to risk.	9. Responsiveness to new things.
10. Do not hold grudges and do not stay upset for long	10 Calms down quickly when activity lowers their interest.
11. Fast talking, passionately and with intonation.	11. They learn quickly.
12. Inclined toward risky actions.	12. Negatively affected by monotony and painstaking daily work
13. Rowdy and aggressive.	13. Communicative and serious.
14. Impatient to shortages.	14. Patient and hardworking.
15. An expressive pantomime.	15. Speak aloud, quickly waving hands.
16. Able to think and find solutions.	16. They keep their composure in dangerous situations.
17. Yearn for new things.	17. They are always full of life.
18. Movements are violent and sudden.	18. They fall asleep and wake up easily.
19. Persevering to achieve the goal.	19. They are hasty when they need to make a decision.
20. Their mood changes suddenly.	20. They treat things lightly.
PHLEGMATIC (strong, balanced, inert)	MELANCHOLIC (weak)
1. Calm, cool.	1. Shy.
2. Consistent and serious about everything they do.	2. They become flustered in a relationship wit strangers.
3. Cautious, prudent.	3. They have a difficult time establishin relationships.
4. They know how to wait.	4. Little self-confidence.
5. Silent.	5. Easily put up with loneliness.
6. They talk calmly with stops without mimic.	6. Depressed and disoriented after a failure.
7. Can take irony.	7. They have the tendency to become closed off.
8. They don't waste they energy.	8. They tire quickly.
9. Abide by a certain way of life.	9. They talk softly.
10. There are less sensitive to praise and reprimands.	10. They have a hard time adapting to th character of the person they're speaking to.
11. They easily repress impulses.	11. Very impressionable.
12. Constancy in relationships and interests.	12. Overly receptive to praise and scold.
13. It takes time for them to fall into a new activity	13. Very demanding of themselves and others.
14. Equality in relationships with others	14. Predisposed to suspicion and mistrust.
15. Punctual and disciplined.	15. Very sensitive.
16. It's hard for them to adapt to new situations.	16. Very vulnerable.
17. They are inert, heavy, and indifferent.	17. Closed off, they do not share their thoughts.
18. They know how to keep themselves calm.	18. They are not very active and they are fearful.
19. Can control their impulses.	19. Very docile.
20. Thy finish what they start.	20. They tend to stir up compassion around them.

Tabel 7

Correspondence between skills and athletic capabilities and intellectual capabilities (according to Cratty)

Intellectual abilities	Specific sports skills
1. Memory – long term; – short term.	Updating habit components to incorporate them into a total action. Updating rules.
2. *Rating:* appreciation of own self and the environment, discrimination differences, placing people, events, and objects on different scales of assessment.	Assessing own assessment skills teammates and opponents, the coach's assessment, tactics, training regime components, mechanical principles analysis, the technique of individual sports (e.g., in sports competitions).
3. *Convergent thinking*: ability to extract the best solution to a problem, several possible alternatives.	The decision on the best alternative during the game, the decision about tactics, etc.
4. *Divergent thinking*: perception of all possibilities to a certain situation.	Establishing viable strategies in the field of all possibilities of the game.
5. *Synthesis*: to unite, combine the parts into a whole.	The decision on the best course of action under the circumstances.
6. *Analyze* ability to dissect, to differentiate.	The skill analysis, interactions of team skills and weaknesses of their opponents.
7. *Flexibility:* solving problems: rapid adaptation to new alternatives and act on their perception etc.	The ability to change tactics when the situation demands, to use a variety of skills and habits change according to the situation.
8. *Social intelligence*: analyze the interrelationships of group, to fit into the group, and their participation in society and others	Ability to analyze interactions in the team, personal relationships with the team and the coach, the perception of hierarchy.

Correlation between constitutional type and, on the one hand, the medical act correctly, on the other hand, the anthropology of sports

A. Typology Applied Medical

Also sciences, biological disciplines have felt they need for their systematization and classification of the huge living material, in view of practical guidelines in its bosom. It is, moreover, one of the characteristics of scientific thinking, to seek, in pursuit seemingly chaotic nature plan for the type of single or few basic types, around which crystallized the multiplicity of reality. It is what Goethe, a particular biological specimen balanced thinking, my designation rightly “Urtyp” meaning prototype. Any biological discipline must be able to fit reality, they want to study in a series of prototypes, lines corresponding guidance adopted by the very natural evolution. “Infinity causes working in nature,” said Allendy, “are grouped at random without order and without plan. Prodigious complexity of plants that grow on the earth's surface is dissolved in a number of fundamental types, which are families. Botanical family is still an object of direct experience: its specific characters are intimately mixed with others accidental, to be removed, to be able to remove individuals from the comparison synthetic idea.”

Neither zoology nor botany could definitively resolve the disturbing problem of the origin of life, and even the chip conclusively, that of the evolution of species. This has not prevented him achieve an overview of the biological reality, in a synthetic vision, the principle of typological classification:

- The animal kingdom - divided into five clades, which are the five prototypes of animals: vertebrates, articulated, mollusks, radiated and protozoa (last four grouped under the generic name of invertebrates).

- The plant kingdom - divided into four clades, which are four prototypes of plants: phanerogams, vascular muscinee and thalophyte (last three grouped under the generic name of cryptogame) cryptogams.

Table 8

Stages of motricity skills development (adapted and completed by *M. Epuran* after *Harre*)

Stages	Physiological (*Krestovnikov*)	Morphofunctional (*Meine*)	Regulators (*Cihaidze*) Biomechanics (*Bernstein*)	Psychological (*Rudik, Zapan, Lopez*)	Methodical
I	Irradiating excitation processes, leading to generalized answers.	Movement in its fundamental form. Coordinating is in its fundamental form.	Neutralize reactive forces that distort the conduct of the movement.	Training representation and execution of preliminary motion. Execution based on verbal briefing (basic understanding). Implementation of the strains unnecessary mistakes.	Arming motion picture
II	Differentiation. Development of inhibition of differentiation	Corrections finishing and differentiating the movement. Coordinating fine movements.	Unleashing a series of degrees of freedom which disturbs less reactive force deployment motion.	Acquiring stated motion; adequacy the task (skill advanced). Execution on Visual control movement. gradual elimination unnecessary movements, selection and judicious use of the useful.	Acquiring direct movement
III	Concentration of nerve processes.	Fixing and adapting to varying conditions. Stabilizing the movement.	Unleashing total degrees of freedom needed; use movement to achieve reactive forces of neighboring segments.	Learned movement is conducted easily, economically appropriate and automatic (skill). Executions based on kinesthetic control. Attention movements successfully completed.	Perfecting the movement
IV	Dynamic stereotype formation. Stabilization and automatic reactions.			Well-learned movements with possibilities to adapt to changing conditions (upper motricity skill)	

Two great kingdoms biological could be so divided each into several clades which in turn could be subdivided, as we know, in groups increasingly narrower known as: order (class) families genera and species. Species, in turn, at least some of them, could also be divided into varieties, races. In the hierarchy of terrestrial life known to man is the more evolved species of animals. It questioned whether humanity, that the human species must be considered as a plurality of individuals can be assigned only to a certain number, but questionable human races, or if this typological division could be pushed further.

In this regard, especially medicine, discipline essentially biological felt this need to integrate diversity seemingly infinite individuals, healthy and sick, in a logical system of categories or patterns of biological determined based Physic Morbid dominant group. Morphology and research biologists have demonstrated, in a positive sense, the possibility of such systems typological classification of human individuals.

On the one hand it found that each human individual is a perfect biological unit, whose features and functions found in the closer and more harmonious interdependence. There is no local phenomenon with general visibility on the body, as there is a general phenomenon, without adequate local organic expressions. Hence the predominance of a particular function prints the individual peculiarities anatomical, pathological and psychological physio, whose knowledge allow to draw conclusions valid for the entire behavior of the individual. It is exactly what he did Cuvier, who knows that could restore the peculiarities of an animal from a single bone examination thereof. Each type is so individualized to the smallest details of his work. On the other hand, the number of normal human types morphological and physio-pathological, it is not unlimited, but, on the contrary, it is restricted to a game relatively small number of patterns, due to functionality, as is well known that they are not they limitless. Human typology of modern works on the following two fundamental postulates:

1. All human individual peculiarities are determined in relation to its general type.
2. Possible types in normal order are always limited in number, making them knowable and describable.

It follows, therefore, that the morphological, physiological and psychological human gather by the rules, we discover the constitutional types, tempera-mental, drug, etc. Therefore, it is given two or three details possible with a sufficient knowledge of the law classification, to draw conclusions on the temperament of the individual and thereby to provide much of the undesirable organic and mental effects (*Allendy*). Medicine knows not only one, but also numerous typological classification systems, each taking account of other criteria of differentiation biological individuals. Here also the main classifications:

1. *Types of homeopathic medicine.*
2. *Types of constitutional temperament.*
3. *Types of poisoning.*
4. *Other types: endocrine, autonomic, astrological etc.*

These classifications without exception and without restrictions, have all course in homeopathic medicine, some exclusively (giving the drug, infectious toxicity typology), together with other allopathic medicine (temperament-constitutional typology, typology endocrine etc.).

The fact that there are several such systems of classification and not one must not lead us to underestimate the value typological principle.

All systems of human typology together, and each of them separately, constitute both adjuvant equally legitimate, valid and valuable for medicine practice, because all addressed to the same realities biological human species, which ranks in order to useful guidance, not from one point of view, but from many diverse points of view, adopting different criteria.

Therefore, in medicine, any of these systems can show typological useful if it is adopted as the basis of theoretical and practical medical activity provided to be thoroughly known and consistently applied. But whereas allopathy medical typological classification has a function more speculative and theoretical decorative, almost devoid of any recovery practice, homeopathy, on the contrary, it is the very backbone of this doctrinal and therapeutic disciplines. This is why the possibility of typological classification of individuals based on characteristics of their fundamental physiological, although there and allopathy not acquire its true framework than within homeopathy is medicine par excellence of individualization, ie sick and not disease, or specifically expressed: a disease seen only through the prism but the sick.

In the following pages we explain the basics of the main human typological classifications mentioned before, focusing mainly on systems that have a common circulation in homeopathic medicine and therapeutics. It is normal, moreover, for any homeopath to know fullest typologies commonly used in the branch of activity.

- Types of homeopathic medicines

Current elementary typology in homeopathy, without which this therapy could not even be conceived, is the classification of individuals based drug. Typology of homeopathic medicine is a classification based on the criterion analogy between certain individuals, more or less ill, current experience in everyday life and similar types made by various drugs poisoning.

On this basis, homeopaths have come to individualize the great mass of human individuals, a number of types morbid fundamental, known types of medicinal wearing each name remedy (generally a polychrest), which presents the greatest analogy events morbid. Applying human typology that nomenclature drug, homeopathy underlined two categories of facts, namely:

1. In terms of semiotic, ie the pathological manifestations, each human morbid can find correspondence or similarity more or less perfect in an otherwise morbid, led by a certain drug intoxication.

2. From a therapeutic standpoint, it is this particular drug substance and this is the proper remedy able to rebalance the individual's physiology, functional abnormalities and changing it in normal health.

Such types are homeopathic drugs:

- Phosphorus Longiline
- Graphites obese,
- Aurum picnic,
- Abdominal Lycopodium,
- Emaciated Natrum muriaticum,
- Loquacious Lachesis.
- Pulsatilla shy,
- Sepia bleak,
- Sulfur bustling etc.., each with peculiarities of morphological, physiological and psychological, so thoroughly described in textbooks.

Homeopathic medicinal prototypes are mentioned in the part knowledge remedies.

These are the basic principles of homeopathic medicinal typology, to which they could, however, bring two main objections:

1. The first complaint and could refer to the legitimacy of reasons capable of justifying stability correlation between toxic types caused by drugs and morbid types encountered in clinical practice. This objection is could answer simple yet concrete, the analogy between the two categories of types morbid (medicinal and clinical), it is an objective finding recorded by any

observatory closely, and that she would remain a fact certain and incontestable no matter how shaky, precarious or insufficient would seem to be his current scientific explanation.

In reality, finding doubtful of such parallels or analogies between the two sets of facts, apparently diverse, it seems to constitute in itself a strong evidence that the number of mechanisms morbid human body is not unlimited, how wrong they might think, and that morbogen processes (whether infectious microbial and non-microbial toxicity or drug intoxication) are forced to externalize through the intercession of the same (few) great opportunities morbid fundamental expression. Morbogen various causes, the body seems to keep them available only a relatively limited number of types react. In this case, the correlation between clinical type and type of medicinal gets through this understanding, a very logical justification, both the harshness of the same mechanisms similar results physio-pathological living body, the causal factors of the most diverse. Morbid picture (syndrome), the morbogen body is the same morbid picture (pathogenesis) caused by the remedy in toxic doses. In both cases the body is the common factor expresses both patient symptoms and those of the remedy.

2. S homeopathic medicinal typology could bring another objection: if homeopathy is truly a clinical and therapeutic individualization medicine to the sick, is it compatible with that statement describing the various human medicinal own not a single individual but an entire category individual? This objection may be based, if the concept of individualization would homeopathic an absolute sense.

In reality there is no contraindication between the trend and the establishment of individualized homeopathy drug prototypes, precisely because the concept of individualization may not have completely understood than a biological relative.

In fact, while speaking about individualization and always in homeopathy though mainly there are as many individual syndromes, many individuals are actually sick syndromes represent individual classification categories but not individuals, groups or species clinical therapeutic. So, in reality, there is one individual that meets syndrome Nux vomica or Chamomilla times Sulfur etc., but also a multiplicity of individuals, very close between them, though not identical.

Each type or homeopathic syndrome is an individual expression so sick, but a multiplicity of individuals with syndromes similar to each individual so that they can all be embedded in the same category typological bearing similar names to remedy that. Itself this fact means another demonstration very conclusive statement above, the medium of the body seems to be in really limited, that is polarized around a relatively small number of mechanisms physio-pathological maneuvering appropriate number of small patterns expressive. Typology based homeopathic drug may be sufficient in very many cases to meet the needs of medical practice. But there are cases and circumstances in which the homeopath feels the need classification types and syndromes homeopathic typological units a broader comprehensive and therefore more general. It is not disputed that the types or syndromes homeopathic no stability than the limits very resilient: they are subject to always progress in a time longer or shorter, which makes them turn in terms of their expression morbid adopting characteristics of other types of medicinal or homeopathic syndromes.

An example of evolution homeopathic type: an individual Natrium muriaticum, moving, take the improvement or worsening Sulfur type characteristics, characteristics of the type silica or Arsenicum or Kalium carbonicum etc. Homeopath, however, has every right and even the duty to inquire, on the one hand, which takes place this process of change in the type medication, and on the other hand, for the sick Natrium muriaticum not adopt all going the same trend morbid but each a different direction morbid. Another example of evolving type of homeopathic syndrome: someone with measles can start by disease syndrome type Belladonna; during the state's syndrome may look kind Bryonia, and during terminal syndrome can become Pulsatilla or Sulfuriodatum.

Homeopath, however, it has every right to question, on the one hand, why this individual, unlike others, is particularly exposed to the disease called measles and, on the other hand, why, sickness is measles, must pass by this sequence of homeopathic syndromes and not through a different pathway. For what could say, homeopathy, homeopathic drug that types and syndromes, although absolutely indispensable medical practice, there would still be only a minor somewhat as typological units; because, in most cases, they appear to be static surprised than morbid phase in a certain time or a certain period of evolution morbid process. It therefore felt the need to integrate, in turn, these entities morbid practice of homeopathic drugs, other larger biological units that constitute true prototypes of framing the diversity of human individuals.

This role meets him, in homeopathy, based typologies based constitutional temperament and infectious toxicities.

- ***Patterns basic constitutional*** *temperament* (constitutional temperament diatheses)

Medicine former possesses an excellent principle of typological classification of individuals into categories constitutional temperament: quaternary classification of temperaments, transmitted to posterity by the great Hippocrates, who dominates 25 centuries medicine.

Along with-it s proposed constitutional temperament but other classifications, of which we quote: ternary classification of temperaments von Grauvogl, ternary classification of constitutions of Nebel Vannier etc. and classifications neuro-vegetative, endocrine, astrological etc. Before proceeding to the main display of the constitutional temperament classifications it is necessary to clarify in advance the precise meaning of the notions of constitution and temperament, and the related concept of diathesis.

- ***Constitution and temperament***

Broadly, the term is denoted by the constitution and temperament, all biological skills to a given individual, health condition as the disease state. In this regard, pathology books often talk of the constitution and temperament, as two synonymous expressions.

In a narrow sense, but it is customary to differentiate the concept of constitution so temperamental, using each of these terms in a certain sense his own. The Constitution represents the actual morphology of an individual, his appearance somatic: an individual can be fat or thin, tall or small, proportionate or misshapen brown or blond etc. The Constitution is, therefore, shape or somatic determinant of an individual, ie his element fixed, static and unchanging. Constitution covers the study of the skeleton of an individual of its shape and the relationship between its various anatomical parts. In fact, the constitutional immutability is a very relative concept, like any biological time any individual evolves, even in terms of somatic, but this process occurs quite narrow limits beyond which it can not pass.

Therefore, a constitution can be good, mediocre or bad, can become somewhat by worsening or improvement: a soft touch for instance, can plump or, conversely, an individual fat may weaken, but never a specific type fundamental constitutional can not be transformed into another constitutional fundamental: an individual instance, tall, slender, with long bones, asthenic and prone to tuberculosis, can never transform into a brevilin type, stocky, short, with bones short plethoric prone to apoplexy. It is true, however, that some types of constitutional instability can be found throughout the development of an individual over time (along with age).

Constitution may therefore vary, but within relatively narrow margins. In reality, the constitution is not an autonomous individual, which is a determinant of ways to react. The Constitution itself is not only an outcome or a result of temperament, namely: how somatic reactive nature of it. Proper is the physiological temperament of an individual, its functional aspect: an individual can be active or indolent, irritable or melancholic, healthy or sickly, prone to tuberculosis or cancer etc. Background or temperament is so functional determinant of an individual, ie its dynamic and invariable element par excellence.

Although each category corresponds to a specific constitutional framework of possibilities temperament, their free play is more flexible than their morphologic substrate: the individual living can not be fixed in a static formula, but is in constant evolution and transformation. What temperamental and wide dynamic aspect of an individual, that his body's physiological orientation is more important at a time than its morphological characters, but also evolving in much narrower limits. Broadly temperament of an individual includes all its modalities Reaction: physical (constitution), psychological (character), physiological (health) and physio pathological (disease condition). What it is customary to use the terms of temperament or constitution as synonyms, but the actual constitution always implied that one aspect of temperament, namely, one of the characters of relatively fixed.

In reality, any classification temperamental includes a somatic aspect, like any constitutional classification includes an aspect react. Moreover, any classification or temperamental or constitutional, always a third psychic aspect (character). This paper uses both the term constitution or temperament or synthetic expression fund temperament-constitutional, to designate the characteristics reacted personal to an individual, considered from three points of view: somatic (constitution), functional (temperament) and psychic (character) that are known issues are interrelated.

Fund temperamento an individual's constitutional assembly is thus its biological personal skills: physical and psychological, fixed and dynamic physiological and morbid inherited and acquired. Each individual is born with a certain morphological appearance and certain hereditary predisposition to work according to a certain pattern physio-psychological. This rhythm can be an equilibrium, if the individual is born with a healthy heredity: it can be in a state of imbalance, however, if the individual is born with pre-morbid provisions for tuberculosis, cancer, diabetes, neurosis and other diseases.

From the moment of birth, every individual is thus endowed with a certain morphology, physiology and psychology, corresponding to certain predispositions intrinsic, relative progeny heredity, race, gender etc. This combination of elements somatic react with an individual appears alive, that his luggage hereditary, it directs in certain directions, all its possibilities for further development constitutes what is called destiny, that his future probably unlikely.

But the very moment of birth, along with the influence of hereditary factors intrinsic begin to intervene actively and continuously extrinsic circumstances of life, and their various modifying influences: climatic factors, meteorological, cosmic, microbial, human, social, etc. All can alter physiological predispositions ancestral heritage and morbid or deepening them or creating new ones. Everyone is born with certain possibilities reacted personal experience that can continuously make changes. Fund is therefore a constitutional temperament resultant reacted skill, inherited or acquired, own a particular individual at a time. He is not a formula stable and steady, but once the biological eminently variable and can evolve to a same individual in relation to a multitude of intrinsic and extrinsic factors.

Knowledge of an individual's constitutional temperament fund is very important from a medical standpoint, because it allows only reason understanding the peculiarities that distinguish the living beings of the same biological group. Only this knowledge may explain why, for instance, in similar cases, individuals may react with different processes or, conversely, to different causes, with similar processes.

Knowledge of an individual's constitutional temperament fund is so useful because it reveals not only its morbid predispositions to contact a specific disease, but being sick, to evolve in a certain sense. Morbid predispositions, as well as physiological predispositions are therefore predetermined for each individual in a certain direction and according to a certain plan of possibilities." Not everyone can be a disease, but only one prone. Morbid side of a patient are not exaggerating his reactions than normal, ordinary "(Vannier).

In fact, between normal and morbid reactive manner to an individual qualitative difference and there is no precise limits, as there is no between health and disease state.

The body uses in both cases, the same mechanisms or reacted own individual ways, ie its possibilities constitutional temperament." Sickness and health are ways and different aspects of the same functions: human qualities of living" (Grasset).

Only constitutional temperament substrate knowledge may explain why two individuals of the same age living in the same house under the same environmental conditions, and exposed to the same possibilities of contamination, one contacts a pulmonary tuberculosis while the other remains healthy. The first has a constitutional ground tuberculin (phosphoric constitution) so favorable development of tuberculosis Koch, while the second can be healthy or in any case refractory tuberculosis (Constitution carbon or fluorine).

All data only constitutional temperament may explain why, of the two sick with the same illness in the same circumstances, a pulmonary tuberculosis instance, one evolves to caseoufication and worsening, while the other towards sclerosis and healing. The first can be a sanguine temperament, while the second can be a atrabiliar temperament (nervous). Knowledge of an individual's constitutional temperament fund is so useful because it reveals not only its morbid predispositions to contact a specific disease, but being sick, to evolve in a certain sense.

Morbid predispositions, as well as physiological predispositions are therefore predetermined for each individual in a certain direction and according to a certain plan of possibilities." Not everyone can be a disease, but only one prone. Morbid side of a patient are not exaggerating his reactions than normal, ordinary "(Vannier). In fact, between normal and morbid reactive manner to an individual qualitative difference and there is no precise limits, as there is no between health and disease state.

The body uses in both cases, the same mechanisms or reacted own individual ways, ie its possibilities constitutional temperament." Sickness and health are ways and different aspects of the same functions: human qualities of living" (Grasset).

- Constitutional temperament diatheses

Constitutional temperament reactions of individuals are important to study, from two points of view: health and morbid condition. In health, temperament prints each individual an amount of elective predisposition in some sphere or in a particular functional organic sector.

Hygiene is designed to prevent conversion to clinical reality of these virtual morbid predisposition. Basic hygiene is the duty of each individual to prescribe the most appropriate living his temperament. Living a balanced life with the rules of general hygiene and hygiene own type or temperament, any individual can maintain healthy happily ever after (or, more precisely, to the depletion of vital), naturally without being able to escape ever the physiological limits of his temperamental pattern.

The limphatic, for instance, which is a liquid-soaked, should avoid foods too rich in liquids or wet climates, unlike bilious type, which is a dry, by contrast, feels better than in such conditions. Unfortunately, however, in the many cases hygiene imperatives are ignored; due to these deviations from the rules of hygiene, morbid predisposition becomes latent ability to update pathologies, more or less coagulated. These morbidities but some are not, but their characters have certain, specific to each constitutional temperament type. There are so many kinds of voices in so many ways temperament or constitution can be differentiated in terms of typology. With the advent phase VOICE mission preventive hygiene, although remains important, however, it falls into the background in favor therapeutics.

Therapeutics is meant to actively intervene, to effectively curb this growth morbid, dangerous for the individual, reintegrate him in his normal state of health. Therapy, in this sense, is synonymous with homeopathy only or most effective method known until today to combat diatheses, by reintegrating the individual within its normal physiological.

- ***Temperament Hippocratic***

In ancient medicine works Hippocratic first large well known physician of antiquity, the doctrine of temperaments comes out once as an equally unified and consummate rennet that modern scholars have seen forced to accept, without any substantive changes, but only with additions of details. Temperamento -Hippocratic constitutional classification is based on two fundamentals:

1. The doctrine of the four prototypes basic quaternary (water, air, fire and earth), so familiar antiquity, and so little understood by modern subtle.
2. The doctrine of individuality humoral substrate

It differs in any body, four kinds of humors, each in relation to a specific biological function and some organic organ system:

- Lymph: chyliferis intestinal fluid that would liquefy nerves and mucous membranes, is humor nutrition, represented by the digestive tract.
- Blood: arterio venous fluid that would ensure nutrition is humor breathing and therefore hematosis represented by a heart.
- Bile: liquid liver which would remain open and would favor cocteau and emunctory food, humor liver function is represented by the liver.
- Atrabile: liquid hypothetical elimination products catabolism is catabolism humor and nerve functions represented by the brain and accessory via the kidneys.

These four humors would exist in any individual healthy or sick, but in certain proportions. Diversity of individuals would result in the predominance of a certain humors and therefore that particular function on the other. Their quantitative disproportion constitutional temperament creates four categories, namely four types of human traits, physiological and pathological various diverse humoral related to a formula: nodes, blood, bilious and atrabilious (also called melancholic or angry). The Hippocratic conception, physiology and pathology are problems with balance and metering between the four humors and functions to which they relate. But Hippocratic temperament varies not only by individuals but even the same individual, depending on age or even the season. So for example, childhood is dominated by lymph (nutrition), youth blood (breathing and hematosis), the maturity of bile (liver function) and aging of atrabilious (catabolism and nerve functions). Likewise, in winter prevails lymph, blood spring, summer and autumn atrabilious ball. Humoral medicine of Antiquity, like us today, temperaments represented the kinds frames elementary human characters based on their biological dominant fixed differentiated characters (somatic) and character varying (REACT), both subject to the law of evolution. This is briefly Hippocratic doctrine of temperaments in its original form. Note that all followers of Hippocrates, without exception, have accepted the doctrine of the four temperaments humoral as a basis for different topological variants proposed. Gradually, gradually, the doctrine began to dilute and to withdraw from circulation the scientific and the four temperaments, so familiar experience popular and recognized for centuries clinical observation, began to float at random in search of rationalize capable positivism to justify to the world.

Modern medicine began by rejecting the doctrine Hippocratic humoral considering data based on a hypothetical and entirely too insufficient scientifically. However, any of the assumptions could not cancel modern value and the most conceptions proposed instead they proved to be, inadequate, or return more or less disguised, the original Hippocratic tradition. Really, what else is, really, cholesterolemia, natremia, glycemia, uricaemia, acetonaemia, oxalemia etc., or admission syphilitic heredity of land, hectic, etc., than the modern version of the doctrine of humor.

"Despite the chaos theories, hypotheses, nomenclature and modern systems, the four types of classical Hippocratic clinical facts remain indisputable ideal models and bow mental frameworks classification of temperaments" (Allendy).

Before an exposition of the four temperaments Hippocratic viewed through the prism of contemporary medicine requires some clarification designed to facilitate understanding. The four constitutional temperament be considered as ideal models, which almost never meet in nature in its pure state. However, a closer observation will cause major tonality of an individual. Few readers will not be able to hold the overlap almost involuntarily and effortlessly, each of the four models temperamental image close some of their knowledge. In fact, not only is there no pure types, only the rule of mixed types. The four temperaments Hippocratic combine in reality, every human being, and their harmonious proportion is compatible with a normal state of health fundamentals. Theoretically there could conceive of an individual so completely as to achieve a harmonic balance and ideal anatomical parts of his body functions. Such an individual could not fit into any of the four major temperamental patterns, which, naturally, they would exceed their ideal synthesis personifying. In everyday life, however, each individual is dominated more or less by one (or more) of the four major mechanism fundamental functions of life: nutrition, respiration, excretion and catabolism. In fact, the individual ambient conditions require continual modifications and adaptations of its functional balance. Thanks to their predominant function, that function most frequently called during the life of the individual, and repeatedly requested and across generations that succeed, finds expression in somatic tissues or organs hypertrophy they serve and support." *Predominant function creates hypertrophy appropriate bodies" (Lamarck).*

In turn, development organizations exaggerated in some organic sector will naturally tends to use the resources that are richer, giving the hypertrophic sector, a higher average yield functional. Will present their physiology so a characteristic hyperactivity in some organic sector, both in health status and in the morbid state. The predominant biological function creates special skills in health, translate to certain physiological ways, and disease state by corresponding diatheses. So can distinguish four constitutional temperament types, valid for health: lymphatic, blood, bilious and atrabiliar. They correspond, in a morbid state, four major types of voices symmetrical temperament constitutional: lymphatic, blood, bilious and atrabilious. Wide exposure of the four temperaments Hippocratic synthetic translated into a modern version, largely reproduced after *Allendy* and *Sigaud.*

• **Lymphatic**, synonyms - ***phlegmatic, digestive*** (*Sigaud, Chaillou, Mac Auliffe*), ***abdominal*** (*Thomas Husson*).

A. General features

Inhibition excess lymph tissue, excessive moisture, soft meats. Quantitative digestive dominance life (Duprat). Type honest official, standing in a row eight o'clock in the office, but not for the sake of work, but the aversion to motion. Sober lack of appetite, cold cast by the senses, there is no opponent yet the food nor the pleasures. Generally prefer everything that does not require work or effort (*Duz*).

B. *Physiological morphological characteristics (temperament and constitution)*

Lymphatic constitution is characterized in particular by:

a. *Expanding the lower floor of the face*, meaning the jaw or digestive floor (gastrointestinal tract vestibule). The forehead appears small and low, nasal floor is also proportionally reduced.

b. *Abdominal hypertrophy*, hypertrophy digestive tract, the abdomen is wider than thorax. Distance bi increase is greater than the bihumeral distance, wide hips, narrow shoulders.

Short stature, rounded shapes and meat soft, puffy and prone to obesity, chest short and narrow shoulders sagging, wide hips, short limbs, white leather, fine, smooth, hairless, cold and wet to the touch, veins thin deep.

White face with expression puffy bliss, leading relatively small, fine hair, blond or gray, growing slowly and fall early, eyes light (gray or blue), less mobile, looking sweet and vague, and becoming mydriasis, very long eyelashes, thick nose and wings apart, swollen upper lip, lower lip and hanging soft, big teeth, wider than long, opaque color, irregular shape, regularly lined semicircular arch palate.

Pulse slow and weak circulation abundant and lazy. Digestion slow but complete, atonic stomach, mouth smell nasty tendency to flatulence. Watery urine and Abuna-relative. Late puberty in general.

C. *Dynamic Characteristics*

Gestures slow, clumsy, less expressive, walking slow, soft voice, veiled monotonous, speaks little conversation dragged on.

D. *Psychological Characteristics (Character)*

Character matter, soft, dreamy, indecisive and lacking energy. Regular life, persevering, patient without violent passions. Excellent memory, imagination poor, slow and deep intelligence.

E. *Morbid predisposition (diathesis lymphatic)*

Slow response of chronic diseases, torpid and weak with fever low resolution difficult convalescence late. Scrofula (tuberculosis torpid), lymphadenopathy ganglion and glandular climb chronic tonsillitis, bone tuberculosis, tumors White dermatitis (impetigo, eczema, acne, frostbite), gastritis, enteritis, diarrhea, helminthiasis, scurvy, ophthalmia, asthma etc..

Examples: *Montaigne* is the type of lymphatic psychology. Lymphatic temperament is common in the Nordic races, especially white, in cold and wet climates. Meets especially lymphatic temperament in childhood (under 15 years), the prevail functional digestive organs and lymph their system and endocrine thymus, thyroid and adeno lymphoid system.

Children have generally round shape, light hair, angelic appearance, undecided and dreamy. Lymphatic temperament differs earlier. Ageing get fat, the neck is short and thick, double chin, cheeks sagging abdomen ptosis.

F. *Remedies lymphatic diathesis*

The main substantive VOICE also homeopathic remedies are: Calcium carbonicum, Baryum carbonicum, Graphites, Silica, Pulsatilla, sulfuricum Natrium, Kalium carbonicum, Ammonium carbonicum, carbonicum Magnesium, etc. Carbo vegetabilis

• **Sanguine**, synonyms - ***respiratory*** (*Sigaud, Chaillou, Mac Auliffe*)**, *thoracic*** (*Husson, Halle, Thomas*).

A. General features

Hiperfunctie blood, depending on the dominance of breath (*Duprat*). Type lover of good food, pleasure and joy in all superficial (*Duz*).

B. *Physiological morphological characters (temperament and constitution)*.

Constitution blood is characterized in particular by:

a. *Hypertrophy of the middle of the face*, ie nasal or respiratory stage: long or wide nose.

b. *Hypertrophy chest*: chest is long and wide, with augmentation amplianţei and respiratory capacity. Distance shoulders bi bi is greater than the distance increases: broad shoulders, narrow hips.

Strong stature and thin or muscular, athletic type with States fusiform and thin, slender shape, white skin, moist and warm to the touch, with large veins, prominent and bluish.

Face rosy, Florida with golden reflections and warm features harmonious, expressing the welfare and health, brown hair or brown, rich, supple, with golden reflections, blue eyes with a tendency to prominence and sclera very white on the right, open nostrils, mouth smiling, round and red lips, teeth medium, well proportioned (the most beautiful teeth), yellow-cream regularly lined arch palate almost square, rounded to the angles. Pulse lively, regular, well beaten and full, active movement and hearty. Quick and easy digestion, big appetite, prone to excesses. Urine abundant, and often with reddish sediment. Sweating, especially on the forehead and chest.

C. *Dynamic Characters*

Brisk walking, vigorous, powerful but slow. Gestures violent and without grace, keeping your head goes up. Speaks sternly, broad and strong voice, emphasizing cheerful, open and loud conversation.

D. *Psychological Characters (Character)*

Character lively, cheerful, affable, voluptuous, versatile, courageous and magnanimous needed. Nature optimistic, accommodating, generous, expansive, but irritable, impulsive, violent outbursts of anger with fast transient and unrepentant. Very subjected instincts, gourmet, voluptuous, fiery and changing the affections. Normal memory, mild, keen intelligence, but shallow. Capable of energy but will short.

E. *Morbid predisposition (diathesis blood)*

Acute congestive states: hemorrhage, plethora, pulmonary congestion, aneurysms, heart disease, palpitations, headackes, insomnia, sunstroke. Violent inflammation: pulmonary tuberculosis, rheumatic fever, gout, erysipelas, eruptive fevers, angina, furunculosis, abscesses. Uricaemia diathesis. Rapid convalescence.

Examples: *Marc Antony* and *Alcibiades* seem to have been blood. Blood is often breeds temperament red temperate climates. Temperament blood often occurs in adolescence (15 to 25), when functional, respiratory and circulatory prevails, and endocrine glands and genital partial liver.

F. Remedies lymphatic diathesis

The main substantive VOICE also homeopathic remedies are: Sulfur, of iron, Arnica, Aurum, Kalium Bichromicum etc.

• **Billious**, synonyms - ***choleric, muscular*** (*Sigaud*)

A. *General features*

Excess movement, effort, activity. Food rich, required expense, driving (Duprat).

Type dominators endowed with great vitality, courage, love and misleading-lator with the same good faith, jealous and capricious, great lover of food, loving society, companionship and strong drink (*Duz*).

B. physiological morphological characters (temperament and constitution)

Constitution Bill is characterized in particular by:

a. overgrowth of the liver and liver region, ie upper abdomen, increased distance between the shoulders, the abdomen does not protrudes.

b. The face is rectangular or square, three-story proportionally equal to each other.

Height generally small, thin body shapes dry, emaciated and hard muscle energetic and well draw under the skin insertion fine leather yellow brown, with reflections green, hot and dry to the touch, rough to the touch, with large veins, very visible under the skin; hair system very well developed throughout the body. Square face, olive, expressive severe, with hard features and enhanced, leading relatively high, black hair, abundant, with reflections bluish eyes, dark color, black, bright, sunken, with sclerotic greenish stare, sharp and burning, sharp nose, with nostrils mobile, thin lips, teeth are more long than broad, the projection canines.

Rapid pulse, less full than the lymph and blood. Violent appetite, mouth often bitter, very contractile stomach. Dark-colored urine. Sweating rare.

C. Dynamic Characters

Active walk, restless, fists clenched. Sharp and precise gestures, sudden movements and vocal. Speech short, choppy, with expanses emphatic voice. Talk harsh and imperative, elocution fast and easy.

D. Psychological Characters (Character)

Always full of restless, energetic, generous, stubborn, irascible, passionate, restless, disdainful of money, tireless worker, crazy glory.

Character despotic, proud, ambitious, authoritarian, violent, insubordinate, vindictive. Strong-willed, unyielding, tenacious: carries out in any direction extreme activity. Very ardent passions, affections tyrannical, violent shades of jealousy. Memory has nothing remarkable. Very timely intelligence and brilliant imagination. Sleeps little, be deprived of sleep, but can not withstand the post.

E. morbid predisposition (diathesis cholemică)

Especially liver disease, acute, but long-term, easily degenerated into chronic conditions: infection and cholelithiasis, chloasma, xanthelasma, pruritus, urticaria, erythema, dry dermatoses, constipation etc.

Blood disorders hypertensive cardiac hypertrophy, spasmodic disorders etc.

Examples: Alexander, Caesar, Mohammed and Napoleon appear to be Bill. Bilious temperament is common in Nordic races and especially the yellow race.

Bilious temperament differs relatively late, only after puberty occurs mostly in adulthood (25 45) when dominates both functional and endocrine liver. For 50 years, this temperament Degen-bearing, usually in nervous temperament (melancholic atrabiliar).

F. Remedies lymphatic diathesis

The main substantive VOICE also homeopathic remedies are: Lycopodium, Iodum, Nux vomica, Nitric acidum, Cimicifuga, China, etc. Bryonia

- **Atrabilious**, synonyms: **melancholy, morose, cranial** (*Husson, Halle, Thomas*), **cerebral** (*Sigaud*).

A. General characteristics

All functions are, in general, slow and irregular. There is a hereditary tendency to self-poisoning with autogenous persistence of residues due to vitiations either a functional or a deficiency of emunctory (*Duprat*).

The type of devoted friend or ruthless enemy, despising pleasures and capable of any sacrifice to achieve their ideal.

Constantly tending towards a perfect world, concerned about the happiness of the human race, but unhappy himself, and ruin those around him; prey to misery, dreams about the honours of Capitol and finds it surprising that there is nothing. Eager for reputation and power-hungry is quickly disgusted by what he has (*Duz*).

B. *Morph physiological characteristics* (*temperament and constitution*)

The nervous constitution is characterised, in particular, by *the skull and brain hypertrophy*; the upper floor (front) of the head predominates in height and width, "*cap en toupie*."

Tall figure, thin shaped, poorly developed body and very emaciated, with little muscle reliefs, sagging shoulders, small and narrow trunk, short and thin limbs; smooth, shiny, hard, dry and cold to the touch skin, covered with black hair with large subcutaneous veins.

The face is matte, very dark coloured, with hints of earthy and leaden; excavated and dry cheeks, fine features, but crisp and restless, with a sad expression, in which all seem a darker colour; black, rough and thick hair, eyes a more or less darker colour, very sunken and dry, with a fixed and anxious stare; thin nose, thin lips, medium or small teeth, conical or flat, with sharp tubercles, grey or blue (very characteristic), irregularly lined or with anomalies, with the palatal arch being irregular, narrow, and sharp in a "V" shape.

The pulse is slow, small, tough and dry. The appetite is weak and capricious, with a slow digestion. The urine is abundant and turbid with sediment. Sweating is rare.

C. Dynamic Characteristics

Gestures are short, trembling and looking awkward. Walking seems difficult, studied and in general with a bent back and bowed head. It has a harsh, low, throaty, slightly stretched voice with an extinguished accent. The conversation is sad, slow, serious.

D. Psychological Characteristics (Character)

Poignant and wise character, prone to fear, sadness, anger and revenge.

A selfish, suspicious, vindictive, stubborn, character, seeking solitude; pensive, with a pessimistic, bizarre, concentrated, avaricious nature.

A complicated theoretician, a routineer, persevering in all his undertakings, tortured by abnormal desires. It has a difficult but tenacious memory. Although it has imagination and intuition, it is a systematic spirit, excessive, superstitious and sceptical. Difficult sleep, troubled by nightmares.

E. Morbid predisposition (nervous diathesis)

Auto-poisoning by insufficient emunctories: gout, lithiasis, diabetes, etc. The tendency to dehydration and sclerosis: emphysema, bronchiectasis, cerebral arteries, atherosclerosis, cataracts, dry gangrene, etc.

Mental and physical disorders: insomnia, neuroses (epilepsy, hysteria), nervous exhaustion, disgust of life, headache, painful tics, etc.

Examples:

Louis XIV was a characteristic atrabiliar. Atrabilious temperament is common in Oriental breeds and black breeds from tropical lands. He differs, generally after puberty, particularly in old age (after 45 years), when sclerosis and dehydration processes begin to predominate, and from a mental standpoint, there is a suspicious selfishness and complex susceptibility.

F. Lymphatic diathesis remedies

The main such homoeopathic remedies on diathesis base are: *Natrum muriaticum, Sepia, Alumina, Argentum nitricum, Conium, Causticum, Rhus Toxicodendron, etc.*

- **Ternary Constitutional Typologies**

A new typological doctrine appears in medicine in the late Middle Ages and early Renaissance, recognising only three types of morbid constitutions, each relating to a different chemical substrate: **hermetic dogma**.

The hermetic ternary system is a fascinating attempt, which did not remain without consequences because even today he continues to survive in some modern classifications.

Here are two such ternary constitutional types, chemically based, typologies who know quite a large spread in the medical world: the first is *Von Grauvogl`s* constitutional classification, the second is *Nebel and Vannier`s* constitutional classification.

- **Von Grauvogl`s constitutions**

Von Grauvogl (1868) distinguishes three types of morbid constitutions based on the dominance of chemical functionality: Oxygenoid Hydrogenoid, and Carbo-nitrogenoid.

- **Oxygenoid**

Relates more to warm constitutions: sanguine and bilicus. Oxygenoid is the arterial type, the basedowian. It is characterised by the exaggeration of the oxidants and metabolism through an over-activity of exchanges. This acceleration of nutrition consumes oxygen in excess, and it produces carbon dioxide in excess.

The Oxygenoid is an emaciated, and excitable individual, prone to fever and with ameliorated symptoms in bad weather conditions and cold air. Hyperoxygenation of the body leads to an active consumption of living tissues, which creates an elective predisposition for tuberculosis.

The main Oxygenoid diathesis remedies of homoeopathy are: *Phosphorus, Arsenicum Iodatum, China, Iodum,* etc.

- **Hydrogenoid**

It relates to the humid constitutions: sanguine, and especially the lymphatic. The hydrogenoid is the torpid lymphatic type. It is characterised by the augmentation of the body's water content by the dominance of the tissue water. Hydrogenoid is an individual pale, clumsy and slow, sensitive to cold that her condition worsens and causes any tissue and increase the proportion of water: moisture, residing near water, etc.

It is prone to oedema and pleural fluid (effusion). Bouts of diseases evolve.

The main hydrogenoid diathesis remedies in homoeopathy are: *Natrum sulphuricum, Calcium carbonicum, Dulcamara, Aranea Diadema,* etc.

- **Carbo-nitrogenoid**

It relates to the dry cold temperament: atrabilious (nervous). Carbo-nitrogen is characterised by insufficient oxidants and the retention of nitrogen and carbon in the form of autogenous toxins, meaning unassimilated results.

The slow trade of nutrients and the retention of unassimilated results creates the morbid framework, commonly referred to as arthritis. Carbo-nitrogen is the auto-intoxication type, prone to gravel, mania, gout, rheumatism, diabetes, asthma, suppuration, putrid processes, dermatosis, etc. The main carbo-nitrogen diathesis remedies of homoeopathy are *Graphites, Carbo vegetabilis, Lycopodium, Petroleum,* etc.

- **Constitutions of Nebel and Vannier**

The second ternary typological classification, chemically based, has been realised in our time by *Nebel* and *Vannier*. They distinguish three fundamental mineral constitutions, all on limestone, namely: carbon (*Calcium carbonicum*), **phosphorus** (*calcium phosphoricum*) and **fluorite** (*calcium fluoricum*).

• **The Carbonate**

A. General characteristics

Moderate mineralisation, slow reaction, torpid nutrition. Medium resistance to infections, especially tuberculosis. The carbonic is a rigid and upright individual, stiff gait, but always rhythmical, with sober and precise gestures. Inflexible in al acts of life, patient and tenacious, he is always clear, accurate and orderly, even meticulous. He makes his own mark by his own authority. He is the type of orderly and balanced constructor.

B. Morphostatic characteristics

Big guy, with soft and bulky meat, and with large and thick bones. Although he is of short and stocky stature, he is particularly remarkable through the perfect harmony of proportions of the body. His usual attitude is rigid, stiff, military, as in extension, never bending. The forearm and arm, both at rest and in hyperextension, even maximum, always make a slightly obtuse angle forward. Thigh and calf are in perfect rectilinear position. The teeth are small, white and irregular, in normal anatomical relationships: the upper incisors slightly exceed the inferior ones, which are in continuous contact.

C. *Dynamic Characteristics*

Regularity is the essential dominance of its movements, just like the resistance to fatigue and illness.

• **The Fosforic**

A. *General characteristics*

Emphasised demineralization. An energic reaction, even excessive. Accelerated nutrition. Very sensitive to infections, especially tuberculosis. The fosforic is a delicate and slender, nervous, brisk and cold individual, with a light and elegant walk, graceful gestures which are usually harmonious. He is an exalted person who suffers and vibrates intensely, with a sensitive and delicate nature, enthusiasm and despair just as timely, whose charm captivates and moves. He is the kind that creates art, dream and poetry.

B. *Morphostatic characteristics*

The type of guy that is slender, long-shaped, with long and thin limbs, long trunk and tight chest. His attitude is always variable, but always expressive and graceful, exuding charm and elegance, never rigidity, but always in a position that puts him in optimal aesthetic value with the least effort. Suppleness is its essential feature. Forearm and arm in hyperextension, are always straight, just like the leg and thigh. The dental arches are entirely overlapping, and the palate is always ogive.

C. *Dynamic Characteristics*

The dominant of his movements is elegance, distinction naturally harmonious attitude and gestures. All his gestures are natural, aesthetic and expressive; he is a very popular model for sculptors.

• **The Fluoric**

A. *General characteristics*

Hypomineralisation, tendency to sclerosis, very high resistance to tuberculosis. The fluoric is fundamentally unstable, with broad and messy gestures and attitude, with impulses that lack continuity. He is the kind that tends to be unbalanced in gestures, attitude and physical and mental activity. He is also the type of the intuitionist, often illuminated with a sprang of geniality.

B. *Morph physiological characteristics*

Individual with deformed, thick, dense bones that are poorly juxtaposed, with a highly developed venous system, and in particular with a great laxity of articulation and ligaments. For these reasons, his static is unstable and flexible; the right attitude is for him a constraint, he never stays straight, always bent, taking the shape of a Z or an S. The forearm and arm in hyperextension make an obtuse angle, opened backwards. The same goes for the thigh and calf which form an obtuse angle, opened forward. The upper jaw is protruding incisors and canine teeth on the lower jaw.

C. *Dynamic Characteristics*

The essential dominants for his movements are irregularity and disorder.

- Other constitutional typologies

The three major classifications revealed until now are the main constitutional typologies, commonly used by homoeopaths in current practice. They do not, however, cover this chapter, which may extend to other constitutional classifications, more or less similar, or different.

Some of them are just variations of precedents. This category includes, for example, the following types:

- *The Quaternary typology of Sigaud*: Muscular Respiratory Digestive Cerebral.
- *The Quaternary typology of Kretschmer*: Asthenic and Pyknic (short and stocky type) Athletic and Dysplastic.
- *Viola's ternary typology:*
- Brachial Mega Splanchnic Logotype
- Micro Splanchnic Normotype
- *Dualistic typology of Mac Auliffe*: Flat/ Round.
- *Corman's dualistic typology*: Dilated/ Retracted.
- *Dualistic typology of Pende*: Squat/Long-shaped.

Other constitutional types are based on other criteria of biological differentiation of individuals. Here are a few typologies, very briefly sketched in their guiding principles.

- Neuro-vegetative typology

Embracing it as criteria for differentiating individuals with the modalities of the autonomic nervous system, they have described three major types of neuro-vegetative temperaments that are well known in medical practice: sympathetic tonically, vagotonic and Amphoe-tonic, or neuro-vegetative mixed type.

- Endocrine typology

Another more interesting classification is provided by dividing individuals into constitutional categories, determined based on their humoral endocrine substrate. From this point of view, it can be described, in principle, as a series of pure endocrine types, each entailing two opposing net functional variants: the hyperfunction and hypofunction. Such types are known in endocrinology as **thyroidal, hypophysial, adrenal, reproductive** (male and female). However, in clinical reality we can only find mixed types, achieving real polyglandular combination with various variants through hyper or hypofunction endocrine. L. Lévy, especially, is the one that has striven to give life to these endocrine types, in a series of main clinical descriptions. Regarding homoeopathy is *Tetau's* merit to have proposed and implemented a constitutional distribution of remedies and individuals, based on the combination of autonomic and endocrine criteria.

- Basic poisoning typologies

A. Poisoning diathesis

Along with constitutional types, more or less classical displayed until now, there is also another category, somewhat peculiar, of morbid types, made by the great diathesis of human poisoning.

As it was seen in a previous chapter, in general, morbid causality in medicine can be studied from two points of view that are very different from each other:

1. **Analytical** (or **mechanistic** or *from outside in*) meaning in their apparently determining factors: microbes, ultraviruses, exogenous or endogenous toxins, known or unknown, cosmo-telluric influences, etc.

2. **Synthetic** (either **biological** or *inside out*), meaning in their real determining factors: pathophysiological state and reactive capacity of each individual living organism.

From the analytical point of view, it is undeniable that today we know a lot more causative agents than in the days of *Hahnemann*, thanks to advances made in the last 180 years, especially in bacteriology and biochemistry: microbes and ultraviruses, for example, the ones that replaced *Hahnemann`s* miasma. The mechanistic could not radically solve the problem of morbid causality for two reasons, which will continue to be available for a long time, if not forever:

1. From a quantitative perspective, because even today science and medicine continue to ignore a large part of morbid causative agents (and their mode of action).

2. From the quality point of view, because the living organism proved not to be a laboratory test tube, supporting passive and objective the pathogen reactions of the causative agencies, but a very dynamic factor, endowed with high capacity of individual responses, a factor that almost always actively interposes between the alleged morbid casual agent`s influence and their morbid effects.

Here is the reason why they always stress in biologic medicine that casual morbid factors, although fascinating, have less importance in itself, but mainly because of the active living organism, which remains the only judge indicated to decide in each case, whether it accepts or refuses to react in a certain sense to their influence. What prevails almost always in pathology is the reactional capacity with a personal character of a living organism, towards the diversity of morbid factors considered to be causal.

From this point of view, our current knowledge related to various morbid causes in the individual biological field, there are almost no more advanced today than in the days of *Hahnemann*. From a biological or synthetical point of view, *Hahnemann*'s conception of the poisoning diathesis substrate of maladies is, even today, as valid as in 1828, when he set them out for the first time.

The "Chronic diseases" of Hahnemann

At that point (1828), Hahnemann tried to provide an overview of maladies in the medical world, about the body state, meaning the poisonous land on which they grow and evolve. In this way, he concluded that the origin of several diseases is at least one of the following *three fundamental diatheses* **Syphilis, Sycosis** or **Psora**.

These three diatheses that *Hahnemann* calls "Chronic diseases", would represent three poisonous entities, with a very complex nature, which, if inherited or acquired, come to confer certain morbid traits peculiar to the land they impregnate. In this way, the body can become an elective land, receptive or conducive to developing a specific group of maladies, especially those who, just like a certain type of land where there can only be cultivated a particular type of plants, excluding more or less the others.

Hahnemann's concept, which assumes that at the origin of all diseases there are three categories of land diathesis, by a specific responsiveness, represents an accurate classification of morbid prototypes, poison based. Note that *Hahnemann*`s chronic diseases should in no way be confused with the chronic diseases of modern pathology: the Hahnemannian diatheses differs from them in that they have a much broader scope, constituting the substrate on which acute and chronic diseases of general pathology develop and evolve.

Acute or chronic, the various successive diseases of an individual`s life, don`t represent sporadic, anarchist and autonomous morbid outbursts. They are only phases or evolutionary, polymorphic and discontinuous episodes of the same diathesis substrate, due to which they are inserted in time, like beads on an axial string, or the islands of an archipelago on the same tectonic background.

"*Disease, states Glénard, succeed, in the individual, after a determined order in relation to the sequence of years and, therefore, relative to the phases of a morbid process.*"

"*There is a doctrine of general pathology,*" notes *Duprat*, "*based on vast observations, which considers logically that diseases* (except highly virulent infections) *are discontinuous manifestations of a persistent clinical morbidity, like being their actual substrate. This morbid constitution, underlying discontinuous manifestations is, in fact, one of the most common in humanity today. The morbid episode must be seen as a temporary manifestation of a chronic disease state, an effort to heal the body in a state of chronic suffering, a real crisis of disposal or purification "P. Carton's* statement. It should be recognised that the acceptance of this biological conception of *Hahnemann* is, at first glance, a very serious obstacle for an allopathic doctor who would like to enter the homoeopathy, because it fundamentally differs from current medical opinions. The Hahnemannian diatheses concept is an attempt more or less successful in the applicating of the morbid criterion, to study the individual biological field.

Even if it cannot be fully accepted in its original form, the knowledge of *Hahnemann*'s concept, in its revised version by the contemporary medicine, proves to be an invaluable support in the medical practice, as we will see later. Perhaps, the objections of the allopathic rises less against the principle of the dependence of diseases of an individual to a particular diathesis substrate, and more against the limitation of the diversity of the morbid land at the three Hahnemannian diatheses, apparently arbitrarily chosen and probably unprepossessing named.

It should be remembered, however, that *Hahnemann* was not a doctrinaire, but **a practitioner par excellence**: his conception is the fruit of lengthy observations transmitted through the ages, and confirmed by his own medical practice, and therefore by his many successors.

The principle of Hahnemannian diathesis classification remains valid even if the poisoning diatheses will be more numerous than the three morbid types, described the founder of modern homoeopathy. In our days we have already begun taking action in this direction, *breaking down, from the psoric diathesis, tuberculosis* - morbid entity net individualised only at the end of the last century when it was elevated to an autonomous diathesis. In this regard, *Vannier* distinguishes four categories of poisoning diatheses which, isolated or associated with each other, would represent all the possibilities of diathesis background, on which should develop all humanity diseases. These four poisoning diatheses are *tuberculosis, syphilis, Sycosis and psora.*

B. Applied motricity typology and medical typology

The idea of correlation between constitutional type and athletic performance has existed since a long time ago. It registered, for a time, a smaller accreditation in the eyes of the specialists, because athletes who did not fit the typology established parameters, achieved an outstanding performance. This was due both to the strictly morphological vision over the constitutional type, and the use in the typological determining of a shortage of investigated parameters. Today we know about the morphological, functional and motricity conditioning of the constitutional type and, at the same time, a correlation is realised – with both biological and technical sporting – of multiple parameters with obtained performance. Very complex, methodological and in its content, the link between constitutional type and athletic performance has particular value both in the selection and in sports training.

It is regarded, in particular, the possibility of compensation between the three analytical sides of the constitutional type – morphofunctional, motricity and mental – and their differentiated importance, depending on the specifics of each sport, where the performance has a differentiated conditioning compared with the morphofunctional, motricity and mental parameters.

We will present below some correlations between constitutional type and sports activity, based on own research and data from the specialised literature, without exhausting the problem, because in the national selection system developed by Conf. Dr *Nicu Alexe* and in *Medico-biological Selection in Sports*, developed by Conf. Dr *Ion Dragan,* the problems are very well explained. Without exaggerating anything we stand, thanks to these works, among the first countries in the world that were stipulated, on solid scientific basis, a selection system, based both biologically and through technical sporting evaluation tests.

We note that in our research we used: the *Briant* method, for establishing the constitutional type, the Biiliac angle (*Firea Elena - Ifrim Mircea*) for the estrogen or androgen level, conformation body complexes A, B, C, the index of active body substance, nomogram (*Milcu-Ciovârnache*), sole and palm dermatoglyphics, technical sporting control standards, establishing joint mobility, reaction time, aerobic and anaerobic capacity etc.

Gymnastics

Our data lead to constitutional typology elements described below, with the value in the selection of sports.

A. Sporting Events (women)

The optimal anthropological type for this branch in sports, age 13-16 years, is the harmonic micromorph, brevilineal, with a height of 140 - 155 cm, respectively with 15 - 17 cm below the average indicated by the general charts prepared for this age by our country. Elevated lengths (eg., Sst. -XYZ., etc.) to widths and depths, compared to the general graphs, are characteristic. The same findings also apply to ages between 9 to 13 years old, optimal stature standing between 119 cm - 140 cm. Regarding the proportion of limbs and trunk, we note that at the age of 13 - 16 years, the best type has legs longer than the trunk, the percentage difference is between 1.40 and 1.52% the same as the upper limbs, but with percentages between 1.11 - 1.15%.

Regarding the *biiliac angle* (*Firea E., M. Ifrim*), we consider that this is an indicator of the utmost importance since the conformation of the pelvis relies heavily on performance since it plays a major role in achieving balance. Many failures, along with the aging of the subject, are related to increasement of the rib cage and biiliac diameters due to establishing a hyperestrogenic endocrine type.

From the researches of the subjects covered in this paper we can see that the optimum angle is between 55 ° - 70 °, angles above 70 ° revealing the existence of a pelvis that burdens the performance. In ten cases it was possible to investigate the biiliac angle in young mothers, finding it a 95.4% concordance index, which reflects the value of the parameter of selection.

The complexes body conformations in subjects with high sport performances have the following semicircle values:

For

A= 534,35 – 564,45 B= 12,2 – 13,2, C= 4,5 – 5,8	comparing with the average	A= 633,70 – 714,85, B= 12,9 – 13,6 C= 6,2 – 7,5

Correlated with data obtained from parents, where it was possible to conduct the research, it appears that the data confirm the high degree of determination inherited by these coefficients, attested by *Tittel*'s research, which entitles us to consider that it could be included in the selection parameters.

Active body substance index shows that subjects who achieve high performances for a group of seniors (both male and female) have a quantity of fat between 7.5 to 8.5% of body weight. *Palm dermatoglyphics*, in top research subjects, indicates the existence of 4-6 whirlpools compared with 8-10 in ordinary subjects. The literature attests the existence of a correlation between these errors and waist and their high degree of hereditary determination.

The *sole dermatoglyphics* indicates the size of the sole from 20 to 23 cm, with 2 - 3 cm above average, and the angle between the anatomic axis and the functional one is between 10 - 15 degrees, compared with the average 15 - 20 °. The optimum sole type is *pes cavus*, with greater length and reduced width. *The heritability index*, especially those on the waistline, used in research, proves to be of great prognostic value, so researching ancestors or parents, states that, for selection in women's gymnastics the sum of the height of the two genitors must lie between 330 - 350 cm, the mother`s biiliac angle between 65 ° - 80 °, the optimum value beeing as low as possible and the complex body conformation - A = 710-740, B = 16, 5-18.5, C = 8, 2-9, 3.

Also, the angle between the functional axis and the anatomical axis of the sole, the parents must be between 12 ° - 17 °, the plantar configuration having a high degree of heritability.

B. Sports events (male)

The *optimum anthropological type* is the harmonious micromorph, brevilinear with a height between 1.58 cm - 1.72 cm, respectively situated with 20-30 cm below the average indicated by general graphs prepared for the age group of Olympics performers for our country. The raised values of the length towards width and depth, compared to the general graphs, are characteristic. For ages between 10 to 12 years (secondary selection) note that optimal stature ranges from 125 to 145 cm, so the values with 10 - 15 cm lower than the average observed in the overall charts. The proportion of limbs and torso indicates a greater length of the legs than the torso, lying between 1.42 - 1.57% and the upper limbs the same, ranging between 1.20 - 1.35%. Regarding the timing of puberty note, conversely than in girls, an early puberty appearance. In valuable performers, we found that puberty occurs at 11- 12 years of age or by 1-2 years faster than the national average. That correlates to where they could find with the advent of puberty earlier paternal, being able to discover an approachable criterion in the selection. The *value of complex body conformation* in subjects who have passed the final selection stage is:

A= 620 – 630,		A= 650 – 680,
B= 15,4 – 17,5,	compared with the average	B= 17,2 – 20,3,
C= 5,7 – 7,3,		C= 6,7 – 7,3.

The high degree of hereditary determination of these coefficients justifies, even on the basis of these preliminary research, their inclusion in the selection parameters.

The *active body substance index* indicates, for final selection stage, the amount of fat located between 9 - 11.5% of their body weight, compared with ordinary subjects, where this percentage is between 12% - 15%. We note the high degree of hereditary determination of this index, which justifies the effort to establish it even in parents. In cases where we could do research, the percentage was 15 - 20%, not exceeding these values. For secondary selection step (10 - 12%) the optimal percentage is between 8.5- 10% of body weight.

Plantar dermatoglyphics indicates the size of the plantar for the final selection stage, between 28 to 30 cm, with 3-4 cm above average and the angle between the functional axis and anatomic axis is 15-17 °, compared with the average lying between 18 - 20 °.

For the secondary selection (10- 12 years of age), the length of the plantar is between 26-

28 cm, with 2- 3 cm above the average, and the angle between the two axes of 13-15 ° as compared to an average of 15-16°. This indicator has a high degree of hereditary determination, and could use the heritability index to determine these parameters from parents, according to the formula:

$$\text{Boy`s plantar length} = \frac{\text{Mother`s plantar length} \times 1{,}003 + \text{Father`s plantar length}}{2}$$

$$\text{Girl`s plantar length} = \frac{\text{Father`s plantar length} \times 0{,}817 + \text{Mother`s plantar length}}{2}$$

The *Heritability index* proves useful clues with high prognostic value for selection in male gymnastics. The sum of the height of the two genitors must be between 350- 380 cm and complex body conformation -A = 720 -750, B = 18.5- 20.5, C=9.5-11.5. Also, the angle between the functional and anatomical axis of the plantar, the parents must be between 14 °- 18 °, plantar configurations having a high degree of heritability. We note that gymnastics is characterized by requiring all muscle groups, a mixed metabolic regime – aerobic- anaerobic -, volume and intensity of maximal and submaximal effort, request, in priority order of the nervous system, musculoskeletal, cardiorespiratory system. To this, we add the literature data on the dynamics of selection. The *initial selection* is made from 5-7 years to girls and 6-7 years to boys, height at this stage is between 106 -112 cm in girls, 112- 124 cm in boys; the wingspan equals height: a–a>tr–tr (biacromial diameter greater than bitrochanteric diameter); body weight in girls 15.5 -17.5 kg, 18-24 kg at boys. We also take the above tests of skill, speed, strength, endurance under force, intelligence, balance, neuromuscular coordination.

Secondary selection is made from 8-10 years for the girls and 10 - 12 years for the boys. The height is between 110-120 cm for the girls, 120 -135 cm for boys; wingspan is 115 -125 cm for girls, 125 -140 cm for boys; biacromial diameter is larger than the bitrochanteric diameter with at least 3 cm for girls and 5 cm for boys; fat is not more than 12-13% of body weight; Aerobic and anaerobic capacities have average values; good balance; skill, speed, strength, intelligence must be in the highest possible parameters; tests must be according to the mentioned methodology.

The *final selection*, in addition to those arising from our research, we emphasize the need for testing skill, intelligence, motricity coordination, balance, speed, strength, and resilience under speed, force (expansion). All these parameters must be at the highest possible levels: general skills test scoring 45-59 points; *Pardue Pegboard* test for motricity coordination, 20-43 points; the arithmetic traction motricity reactivity test, 58 points; by spatial perception test 'blend in space ", 14 points; general intelligence test for "verbal agreement", 16 points, etc.

Athletics

A. Runs (male)

In running disciplines (*Tittel*) average *body height* values varies between 170.5 cm (marathon runners) and 184.2 cm (110 m hurdles). It is found that the average height of the runner's speed increase from 800 m to 1500 m (174 cm to 179 cm), then with increasing distance decreases, so that marathon runners have the lowest height. First, we may find that among athletes, runners have medium height. Only middle distance runners deviate from this and certainly hurdler runners (those at 110 m hurdles, 184 cm; those from longer distances, 182 cm). If you average the six types of runs (except runners from 800 m), including Marathoners, it shows the following: unexpected the size of 200m runners is about 8 cm taller than the rest. So it can be concluded that the 200, 400, 800, 1500 m runners, the highest body height is around or above 180 cm (Fig. 38).

Corenti and *Zauli* (1964) showed how variable are the values in all subjects. Regarding the body height, for example, marathon runners at the Rome Olimpic Games (1960) took part runners with a variation in height up to 30 cm. At 400 m runners, the value varied by 16 cm. Except for hurdlers and race walkers, no other group does not delimit themselves from others by significant values. Similarly, on sprinters lots researched by *Tittel* (1963), body height and body weight were not distributed evenly. Thus, after excluding those with very few chances, the best of the rest were not differentiated by these two characteristics, so that they could not determine some optimal values for body building.

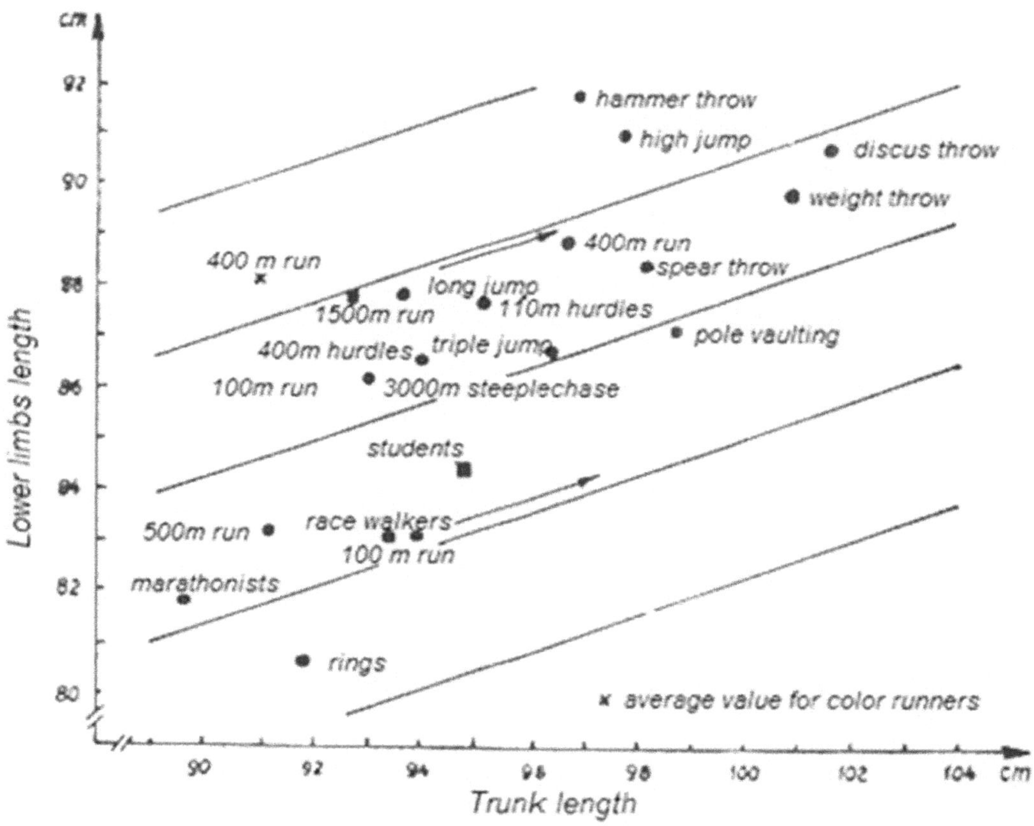

Fig. 38. *The correlation between the length of trunk and lower limb performers in different sports.*

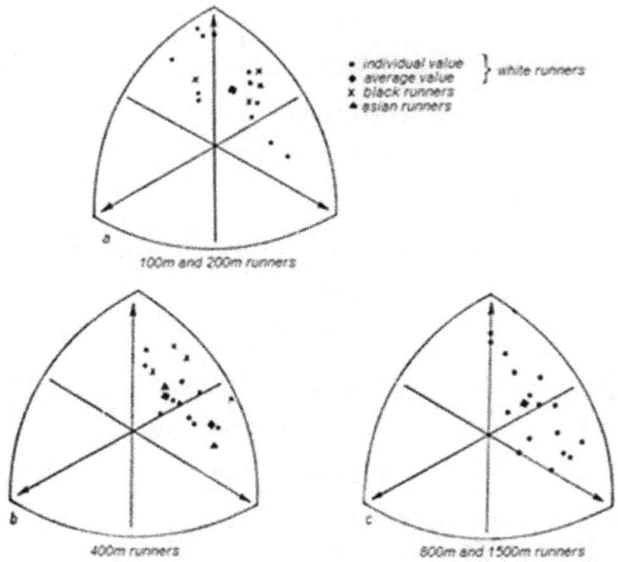

Fig. 39. Type of body building system Sheldon the best white, black and Asian runners (Tanner).

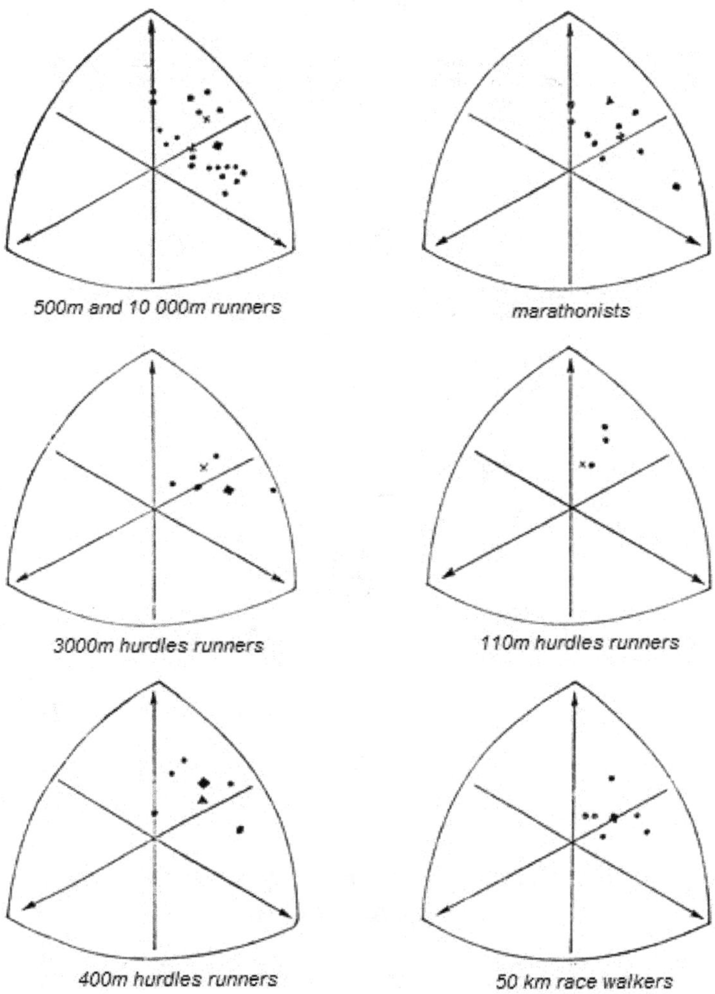

Fig. 40. The types of body building after Sheldon performers, in some disciplines of athletics (male samples).

The body *weight* 100, 200, 400 m runners varied very little (70 kg). Synchronously with increased length running, it drops. Exceptions are hurdlers, which weigh about 3 -4 kg more. Since body weight is closely correlated with body height (*Tittel*, 1963 r = 0.81), weight values can be better assessed after body height differential is compensated. Values used by *Quetelet* index explains the relationship of weight almost identical of 100, 200 and 400 m runners with those of hurdlers, 110 m, and 400 m., The height becomes the first feature of body differentiation on short distances, with a roughly equal weight. As expected, the *Quetelet* index decreases as distance increases (between 800 m and marathon) continuously so that relationships deducted from the weight of the runners of medium and long distances, compared to those for short distances, is a new diagnostic feature.

The *body building* type. Besides the weight - force relationships (the relationship between body height and weight), running performance is influenced by power - levers relations. In anthropometry; considering this, body proportions determines the representation of individual construction type.

The findings by *Tanner* (1964), *Correnti* and *Zauli* (1964), regarding the body construction typology have been made tangible thanks to the participants in the Rome Olimpic Games (1960) and by *Hirata* (1966) on the participants in the Tokyo Olimpic Games (1964). *Tanner* has assessed the construction of the runner`s body type discussed by *Sheldon* (1960) (Fig. 39, 40). The runner`s body type, regardless the distance, varies between the ectomorph and the mesomorphous, and out of them all, sprinters are the closest to the mesomorphous pole.

A marked hypoplasia characterizes long-distance runners. The hyperplastic trend of runners from the 3000 hurdles, which is a feature that relies on other body characteristics (active body substance with a high value). Research by *Conrad* and *Sheldon* showed that the pycnosome trend types are not suitable for running, and by the method of *Conrad* it was established that for running, only the extreme leptosome types have a chance, being either the hypo- or hyperplastic. A slight hyperplasia is advantageous for sprinters and hurdlers; in exchange for long-distance runners, a slight hypoplasia is advantageous. In other words: for runners it corresponds to a harmonic external shape, normal, medium to slender.

Factor analysis shows that most of the characteristics influence body height data so that it can be said that it could develop relative relationships between measures of body height dependent. The comparable graphical representation with two variables, show differences in the body build of athletes. There are proportions expressed in respect of trunk / lower limb length, foot length / long arm, shoulder width/ trunk length.

Tanner characterizes sprinters, compared to runners in medium racing as having short limbs, tall torso, and short legs. Extremity musculature is well developed. Runners in 110m hurdles are high, with long limbs, as muscular as sprinters from the 100m, but with shorter legs. The proportions of the limbs correspond to runners from 400 m to 1500 m. They, however, have calf muscles more developed than 100m sprinters. 400 m runners are characterized as large, with long extremities, broad and muscular shoulders.

Long-distance runners are characterized as small, with narrow shoulders, short extremities, and underdeveloped muscles. Between the two extreme groups (400 m runners / the marathon) there is no overlap in terms of body height, body weight or muscle development of the superior limbs, thighs or calves.

Differences in height show the dimensionality difference, and proportional variability (lower limb length), if the comparison is for the same height. The proportions of the extremities and the degree of muscle development are two criteria which the coach has available for prognostic evaluation and directional tactical measures which he has to take. Relatively long ends show an inclination for medium distance or hurdles, a degree of increased muscle development can be a predestination for short or long sprint tests, respectively 110 m and 3000 m hurdles. German athletes, *Wutscher* (1970) calculated active mass after *Parizkova*'s method, the so-called index AKS,

$$\frac{\text{Active body substance}}{\text{Body height}^3}.$$

Variable body height is compensated according to the *Rohrer* index. The sum of the thickness of the skin folds (and thus the percentage of body fat) is 51, 1 - 55, 2 mm = 8, 2 - 9.1% (except for the 3000 m = 45.6 mm - 6, 9%) for runners, which shows approximately equal values between different types of runners. The active body substance decreases - following the trend of losing body weight - with decreasing distance (70.3 to 55.3 kg). In the AKS index of average values appears another feature that shows tangible differences between sprinters for short (100-200 m) and those of longer distances (400 m) and medium and long distance runners. The first is characterized by a high index (1.21), which shows well-developed muscles in comparison with other runners (1.07- 1.11), of which 400 m runners (1.11).

From the multitude of individual body characteristics, the results of factor analysis guide us on groups of limited features and the focus on dependencies, relationships between body building and physical performance. Especially for children and young people, there are two factors as worthy to be remembered. The first group of factors conditioning the length and weight values (eg., Body height, extremities length, arm span, body weight, active body substance, circumference, etc.) shows that the development process is characterized by body size building which is always growing, and shows dependence performance of "biological age." The second group of variable factors, independent of body height (i.e., The relative length of extremities, the AKS index) is characterized by a conditional influence, largely limited to the proportions of age on body building. This way, any research can compensate by anthropometric methods, different degree of body development. In this regard, *Grimm* (1959) gives the example of a young swimmer with many successes and show how much performance depends on the accelerated development of body build in the same age class. As a result of this experience was found, however, that the differences in performance (11.7 sec and 13.3 sec) corresponding to body height and body weight about like (173.6 cm - 174.8 cm; 59.2 -60.7 kg). By direct comparison with other tangible measures (Table 10) emerged as the most representative variables of proportion factors and body build parameters set by *Tanner* (1964) by measuring the participants in the Olimpic Games (Rome, 1960).

B. Running (female)

The average values of body height to female runners from different distances vary only slightly (166- 168 cm); however it is found, in women as in men, that the hurdlers are among the highest (168 cm). Best height for runners is around the average value. At the 200m they ran with 3 cm longer than the others. Moreover, the average body weight varies slightly in runners (56 -58 kg), finding, however, that, contrary to men, lighter female runners have achieved better results. This trend is observed in the group of 200 m, on the basis of their big body height, being stronger for the athletes of 800 m, whose weight average decreased from 56.8 kg to 54.7 kg.

These data are grouped appropriately along with relative body weights, weighted in proportion to body height (*Quetelet* index). Female runners of 100, 200 and 400 m have, generally, the same high value. The best six runners from 200 m, however, remains below the average for their group. Meanwhile, female runners of 800 m have the lowest weight, while those on the 80 m hurdles, the biggest relative weight. A typology based on body established by *Conrad* (1963) there are several mesomorph types among medium distances female runners than through Sprint. *Klaus* (1961) determined based on measurements of students that, for short distance races and the long distance, are suitable for both sportsmen and women with slim bodies with an athletic body. The presented data related to the results offer us some conclusions on the motricity type.

The *speed runners*. The optimal performance age is 23 to 25; height is high, between 180-185 cm in men, 170 - 172 cm in women with certain body proportions between segments; lower weight (7 kg boys, 10 kg women); lower limb muscle strength and overall strength is very good; anaerobic capacity very high: over 52 for 75- 70 kg; over 56 for 85 -60 kg; low reaction time. *Middle distance runners*. Optimal performance age is 24- 26 years; height for men 180 cm + 2 cm and for women 168 cm ± 2 cm; weight 10 to 15 kg for the centimeters over number 100; Long legs and short trunk; The maximum fat 9 -10% of body weight; global force above par (200% lumbar, thigh extension and flexion of 100%, calf and thigh extension, 75% of body weight); maximum oxygen consumption - 78 ml - 84 ml (kg); anaerobic capaity 55 kgm / kg - 60 kgm / kg. *Long distance runners* get maximum performance for men 24-27 years of age and women 25-26 years of age. The majority are between 171-172 cm height, boys and women, 166-168 cm; fat, 8-9% of body weight; tested as indicated resistance at high parameters; resistance under speed, the same; maximal oxygen consumption between 78-82 ml O2 / kg. (Table 10-14)

Table 10

The results of the factor analysis on the relationship between sports performance and bodily characteristics in 800 m runners

Factor 1 (size factor, saturation = 0.67)

Variables	Factorial saturation	Coefficient	
		Performance	Body Height
1. The sum of extremities length	0.99	-0.67	0.95
2. Body Height	0.98	-0.69	1.00
3. Calf length	0.91	-0.57	0.88
4. Arm span	0.96	-0.73	0.95
5. Body caracteristics complex A	0.85	-0.75	0.85
6. Active body substances	0.84	-0.79	0.88

Factor 2 (proportional factor, saturation=0,46)

Variables	Factorial saturation	Coefficient	
		Performance	Body Height
1. AKS index	0.77	-0.31	0.09
2. Metric index	0.68	0.21	-0.15
3. Body caracteristics complex B	0.68	0.64	-0.62
4. Arm circumference	0.66	-0.7	0.65
5. Gradient length of circumferences	0.66	0.39	-0.17

Table 11

The results of the factor analysis on the relationship between sports performance and bodily characteristics in 100m runners

Factor 1 (size factor, saturation= 0.54)

Variables	Factorial saturation	Coefficient	
		Performance	Body Height
1. The sum of extremities length	0.97	- 0.47	0.91
2. Body Height	0.97	- 0.62	1.00
3. Arm span	0.92	- 0.56	0.89
4. Body caracteristics complex A	0.91	- 0.66	0.90
5. Calf length	0.88	- 0.34	0.82
6. Body weight	0.83	- 0.69	0.86
7. Body characteristics complex C	0.83	0.69	-0.83
8. Thigh length	0.82	- 0.34	0.73
9. Active body substances	0.81	- 0.72	0.85

Table 11 *continuing*

Factor 2 (proportional factor, saturation=0,47)

Variables	Factorial saturation	Coefficient	
		Performance	Body Height
1. Gradient length of circumferences	0.89	0.40	-0.12
2. Relative length of the inferior member	0.81	0.46	-0.25
3. AKS index	0.80	-0.36	0.01
4. The sum of extremities length	0.69	-0.64	0.69
5. Arm circumference	0.70	-0.68	0.71

Table 12

Skin thickness and fat tissue accumulation for runners (*Tittel*)

Body characteristics	Running	Running	Running	Running	Hurdles	Running
1.Body height	177.5	184.3	176.9	174.7	175.8	173.1
2.Body weight (kg)	74.6	76.7	65.7	62.6	64.3	60.3
3. Fat tissue %	9.1	8.1	9.1	8.2	6.9	8.2
(vol)	6.3...13.2	4.8...10.3	6.3...11.0	4.1...17.6	2.3...6.4	6.3...9.8
(kg)	6.8	6.2	6.0	5.1	4.5	5.0
4. Active body substances (kg)	61.8...78.8	7.05	59.7	57.5	59.8	55.3
Active (vol)	67.8	62.7...76.5	50.3...66.1	50.1...63.0	56.3...63.2	52.7...59.9
5. AKS index	1.21	1.11	1.08	1.09	1.10	1.07

(AKS value limits)	1.10...1.29	0.91...1.23	0.99...1.12	0.97...1.26	0.97...1.22	1.01...1.14
6. The value of skin folds (mm)	54.8	50.1	55.2	50.3	45.6	50.1
a. Tragus	6.0	5.5	5.3	5.4	5.3	5.6
b. Oral floor	3.0	2.7	26	2.6	3.0	2.7
c. Armpit	1.2	1.0	1.2	1.1	1.1	1.2
d. Rib 10	5.0	4.0	3.6	3.6	3.5	4.7
e. Abdomen	7.5	6.7	6.7	5.6	4.9	7.7
f. Fold	7.0	6.7	7.1	6.5	5.4	7.3
g. Back	8.2	7.0	5.7	5.6	5.3	7.0
h. Arm	5.4	4.7	5.6	7	5.4	5.3
i. Thigh	7.5	7.6	9.6	8.3	8.0	6.1
j. Calf	4.0	4.0	7.3	5.5	4.6	5.0

Table 13

The Athlete Biological Performance
Group I (speed and hurdles runners) (as *I. Drăgan* et al.)

Biological Index	Men				Women		
	100-20m	400 m	110 mg	400 mg	100-200m	400 m	100 mg
Age	23±4	23±3	24±2	24±3	22±4	23±3	24±2
Height	180±6	185±7	186±5	180±4	171±3	170±3	172±3
Weight	473±6	476±3	79±3,5	5 77±3	60±3	555±3	560±3
Torso	292±2	94±3.5	94±3	91±3	87±2	87±3	87±3
Arm span	5 186	188	189	185	175	174	175
Biacromial diameter	41±1	42±1	42±2	41±2	38±1	38±1	38±2
Bitrochanteric diameter	32±2	34±2	34±1 8	33±1,6	32±2	32±2	32±2
Toracical diameter	87±4	86±3	93±4	92±4	85±3	85±2	87±3
Abdominal perimeter	72±4	71±5	72±4	71±4	67±4	68±4	67±4
Buttocks perimeter	92±2	92±2	93±3	92±2	93±3	93±3	92.5±3
Arm perimeter	28±2,9	28±3	29±3	29±3	24±2	25±2	25±2
Forearm perimeter	27±2	28±2	28±2	29±2	23±2	23±2	23±1
Thigh perimeter	53±2	54±2	54±2	53±1,5	51±2	50±2	52±2
Calf perimeter	38±2	39±2	39±1	38±1,5	35±2	35±1	35±2
Strength of right-hand flexors	56±5	58±5	58±5	57±5	37±5	37±5	38±5

Strength of left-hand flexors	53±5	54±5	55±7	54±6	34±5	34±5	35±5
Scapular force	52±6	53±5	53±6	54±7	38±5	38±5	39±6
Lumbar force	157±25	160±	170±30	155±20	120±15	120±15	120±15
Size / Weight	405	30 410	420	430	350	325	350
Proportion of adipose tissue	10-7,3%	10-7,6%	11-7,9%	11-7,7%	10-6,5%	11-6%	11-8%
The active mass	62 kg	69 kg	72 kg	71 kg	54 kg	50 kg	54 kg
(Bust / waist)/2	2	3	2,5	1,5	2	2	3
Errisman	3	2	4	5	3	4	4

Table 14

The Athlete Biological Performance
Group II (medium and long distance runners and speed walkers)
(as *I. Drăgan* et al.)

index	Men					Women	
	800-- 1 500 m	5 000– 10 000 m	3 000 m obstacole	42 195 m marş		800 m	1 500 m
Age	24±2	25±2	24±2	26±3	27±2	25±2	26±3
Height	180±2	170±5	182±2	175±3	175±3	168±2	168±2
Weight	70±5	55±5	68±2	60±3	65±3	54±2	54±2
Torso	92±2	86±2	93±2	90±2	90±2	84±3	84±3
Arm span	183±2	174±2	185±2	178±2	178±2	171±2	171±2
Biacromial diameter	40±1	38±1	41±1	39±1	39±1	38±1	37±1
Bitrochanteric diameter	32±1	31±1	33±1	32±1	32±1	32±1	32±1
Toracical diameter	87±4	85±3	88±4	86±3	86±3	83±2	82±2
Abdominal perimeter	72±5	71±3	72±5	70±3	76±3	68±5	67±5
Buttocks perimeter	90±3	88±3	91±3	89±3	89±3	89±5	88±5
Arm perimeter	27±1	26±1	27±1	25±1	25±1	22±1	22±1
Forearm perimeter	27±1	23±1	26±1	23±1	23±1	22±1	22±1
Thigh perimeter	52±2	50±2	53±2	51±1	51±1	48±2	23±2
Calf perimeter	38±1	35±1	39±1	37±1	37±1	35±1	35±1
Strength of right-hand flexors	51±5	40±5	52±10	45±5	45±5	38±5	35±6
Strength of left-hand flexors	50±5	40±5	52±10	40±5	40±5	34±5	36±6

Scapular force	50±5	42±5	54±10	40±5	40±5	32±5	36±6
Lumbar force	175±10	140±10	180±15	140±10	140±10	120±10	120±10
Size / Weight	388	323	363	342	371	321	321
Proportion of adipose tissue	10%	9,5 %	11%	10%	10%	11%	11%
The active mass	90%	91,5%	89%	90%	90%	89%	89%
Bust / waist)2	2	1	2	2,5	2,5	1	1
Chest perimeter - stature /2	–3	0	+7	–1	–1,5	–1	–2

C. Jumping (male)

The best jumpers in the world are greater than short, medium or long distance runners, but are equal to hurdlers. The arithmetic average of *body height* varied in the disciplines of jumping between 195 and 181 cm. Jumpers who perform a long jump, triple jump and pole jump are about 5 cm shorter, with the same body height, than high jump jumpers. The top six athletes in each competition have shown that an increase in height above average result in performance growth, excluding the pole jumpers. Also, the body weight average increased most evidently at high jump jumpers (77.4 kg- 78.1 kg) and those from the triple jump (72.6 kg -75.0 kg). A more athletic expression of the best jumpers was also noted through their high performances, although height and weight were relatively higher. Jumpers differ greatly in height with high performance (*Quetelet* index - 411), then their less successful peers (*Quetelet* index - 41a). The relative weight of the jumper is equal and even exceed that of the short sprinters because, in jumpers, weight gain is not based on an increase in inactive tissue (fat), but his asset. No leverage ratios alone, but particularly power relations/levers determine the jumping performance.

This is the conclusion reached by methods of statistical mathematics, by processing additive factorial groups of characters, using primarily factors length - the length of the arm and leg - and secondly, circumference factors - the pelvis width, the circumference of the chest and arm circumference (*Tittel*). After *Tanner* (using *Sheldon*, 1940) jumpers, as all light athletes, are spread between mezzo and ectomorphs. The body build of performers who were investigated (by *Conrad*, 1963) corresponds to the leptosome type. Particularly compelling is the high concentration of pole jumpers in the fields E6 / F6, which shows that they, like high jumpers, have a slim – hyperplastic conformation. Through his research, *Tanner* proved the importance of length factor and its influence on the performance of the jumpers, which, relative to trunk height, have the longest light athletes extremities so that the center of gravity is located above. Otherwise, as an athletic allure, they approach middle distance runners. Relatively high body weight of the best jumpers shows that these athletes, in *Tanner*'s opinion, are the muscular type, this course only in the jumpers group. Jumpers from long jumps, triple jumps, and pole jump are identified in terms of body building, according to *Tanner*. For long jumps jumpers, *Tittel* noted with a certain probability (95%), that there are relations between the jump`s length, weight, and circumference, in particular between chest circumference and extremities. Regression coefficients, which indicate the importance of proportional changes to the above variables, underly the results.

Pole jumpers had, in *Tanner*`s opinion, the musculature more developed in the upper extremities, but otherwise the body measurements are - as long jump and triple jump jumpers – the same with 400 m runners, so that the body criteria to diagnose performance and propensity for a particular discipline is the body height (over 180 cm), length of lower limbs (relatively long) and a muscular, athletic expression. So that kind of base for jumpers corresponds to the length, as a medium-distance runner, and as athletic form -sprinter.

In the long jump jumpers, the size of skin folds is 54.1 mm = 8.9%, those of triple jump, 54.7 mm = 9.1%, therefore both are close to those of sprinters, and at the pole jump, 59.2 mm = 10.0%. The active body substance in the pole jump is based, however, on a higher body weight (74.5 kg). So long jump jumpers and triple jump jumpers differentiate from sprinters, i.e., the AKS index (active body substance relative to body height), 1.08 for jumpers and 1.21 for sprinters, although it was expected a closeness to these values because the length of the jump depends on the élan. However, the best jumpers have an index of about 1.17 AKS, but no linear relationship to determine the length of the jump in these collective. At pole jump jumpers there is a strong concentration of AKS index of 1.10 to 1.13.

Table 15

The biological performance athlete
Group III (jumpers) (as *I. Drăgan* et al.)

Index	Men				Women	
	High jump	Long jump	Triple jump	Pole jump	High jump	Long jump
Age	23±2	25±2	26±3	26±2	23±2	23±2
Height	195±3,5	187±2	188±2	181±2	178±2	170±2
Weight	83±2	74±2	77±2	73±2	65±4	59±1
Torso	97±1	93±1	95±1	93±1	90	86
Arm span	197±3	192±3	193±3	186±3	182±2	175±2
Biacromial diameter	42	40	42	40	38	37
Bitrochanteric diameter	34	32	33	31	32	31
Toracical diameter	91	88	90	92	88	82
Abdominal perimeter	76	71	74	72	70	66
Buttocks perimeter	96	94	97	90	95	89
Arm perimeter	32	29	29	33	29	27
Forearm perimeter	26	25	26	27	24	23
Thigh perimeter	55	53	54	54	56	51
Calf perimeter	39	36	38	40	37	35
Strength of right-hand flexors	60	50	58	59	43	40
Strength of left-hand flexors	53	48	55	55	41	38
Scapular force	44	46	48	55	38	36
Lumbar force	170	150	150	180	125	120

D. Jumping (female)

The female jumpers` size corresponds roughly to the ones of the great female runners, although the high jump jumpers (which is found the same trend as in men) are still somewhat higher than these. Body weight is lower in this group (-10, -12 for over 100 centimeters height). Regarding the value of the *Quetelet* index, female jumpers have a higher relative weight than the other competitors in the same event (the long jump, 348, respectively, 355, high jump, 351, respectively 365). From these numbers, we can see a stronger conformation for female jumpers (relative values, 355- 365) than female runners (relative values 314- 338).

The trunk is short; narrow thorax, longer legs, shorter thigh, located above the center of gravity and the plant cava (pes *cavus*), with an angle between the anatomical and functional axes 7-10° degrees; with a very low proportion of fat 9-10%. AKS index is 0.96, and its increasing leads to better results, a highly important fact for coaches and sports medicine doctor. Global Force has an index greater than one (Table 15).

E. Throws (male)

Our research data indicates the issues below.

The optimum anthropological type is the disharmonic long-shaped mega morph, with a stature between 185- 200 cm, for men and 175-182 cm for women respectively located above the national average with 20- 25 cm for men and 10-20 cm for women. Distinguish that, for hammer throw, stature lies, without prejudicing the event, in the lower limit (180 -185 cm for men and 170 -175 cm for women), while the discus throw, weight, and javelin stature are at the upper limit. (Fig. 41). Widths values are higher than average. Biacromial diameter for men is 44 -48 cm and for women, 40- 44 cm; and the bitrochanteric diameter, 34 -36 cm, in men and 35-36 cm in women. Body weight for men is between 104-114 kg, and for women from 75 to 90 kg.

The proportion of limbs and torso indicate a greater length of the legs to the trunk, the percentage difference being between 1.40-1.50% for the javelin throw, 1.25 and 1.35% for the other events; the same goes for the upper limbs, with percentages ranging between 1.25- 1.35% excluding the weight throwing, where the percentage climbs from 1.30 to 1.40%.

Regarding the *initial selection*, we consider that the orientation group of throws events to be made since the middle childhood (from 7-8 years of age), even if it is general training for other athletic events, the constitutional type is still the disharmonic long-shaped mega morph. The stature is 140 - 160 cm for boys, with 15- 20 cm above the national average and 130 -145 cm for girls, with 10- 15 cm above the national average; weight between 45 -55 kg for boys (5 -10 kg above average) and 35-45 kg for girls (5- 10 kg above average).

In terms of genetic determination we appreciate that, based on preliminary data, that the sum of the genitors` height must be, for boys, between 380 -400 cm and girls, between 350- 385 cm. *The timing of puberty* is at the upper end of the period, for boys around the age of 14 and girls around the age of 13.

Complexes body conformation show high values:

A= 765 – 820,
B= 21,5 – 22,5,
C= 12 – 14,5;

And for genitors:

A= 770 – 830,
B= 22,5 – 23,
C= 13 – 15.

Also, the research undertaken indicates some differences that seem significant in the four samples of throws, but will have to be confirmed in later research, which is why we do not present them yet. The active body has to be between 83.87% for men and 82.8% for women for the final selection stage. For secondary selection, made in the pubertal stage, our research values are 81 85% for men and 80% 84% for women.

Planetary dermatoglyphs indicate plant sizes for final selection, between 30-32 cm for men (4-5 cm above average) and 24-26 cm for women. The angle between the anatomical and functional shaft is 20-22 degrees for men, 1-2 degrees above the mean, and for women, between 18-20 degrees, the same is 1-2 degrees above average. It is enlightening to use for this parameter the heritability coefficient.

Palmar dermatoglifs indicate the existence of more than seven digital whirlwinds from the initial selection stage, constituting a precious genetic indicator for a stature over 190 cm in boys and over 180 cm in girls. The palm surface is large, with a longitudinal diameter of 24 cm 26 cm and a transverse length of 10 12 cm in males, 25 23 cm and 8-10 cm in women. The indicator recognizes a high degree of genetic determination and should also be tested in parents.

Rostandt's joint mobility test indicates abduction and adduction values in the scapular humeral joint by 20-30 degrees above average; Of flexion and extension, 25 35 ° higher, especially for hammers; Of the torso rotation, by 10 15 ° higher. Muscle force testing shows values in terms of weight for men 50-65% for flexors, 70-80% for scapular belt, 220-230% for lumbar muscles, and for women, 40% 50 for flexors, 60- 70% for scapular belt muscles and 200 180% for lumbar. We also mention that body weight has increased from 1960 to the present day in weightlifters from 106.3 to 117.3 kg; At discs, from 100.1 kg ~> 107.5 kg; In the hammers, from 93.8 kg to 101.4 kg, and in the spear throwers, from 84.8 kg to 86.2 kg (Tanner).

A basic anthropometric problem in throwing disciplines is the representation of the optimal ratio between athletic strength and body weight. The best six participants in these tests differ from other competitors not by higher corps height but by higher body weight. From this, the hammer throwers deviate, with the best six having a body weight below average (101.4 kg and 97.5 kg respectively) and the spear throwers (86.7 kg, Respectively, 86.2 kg). For this reason, the correlation coefficients between height and body weight, calculated by Iwabucki only for throwing weight and disc, show an independence of the two measures (p <95%, and in all other disciplines, p> 99%).

The Quetelet index has the following values: weight throwers 615, about 50% higher than sprinters and almost double than marathoners (these athletes have their maximum value); Disk drives, 580; The hammer, the 550 and the spear, 473. *Tanner* (1964) established (after *Sheldon*, 1940) that these athletes move away from the ectomorphic pole and approach the mesomorphic pole. He also points out that the throwers, moving away from the lepto or picnomorf pole, are grouped in the mesomorphic field.
Characteristic of the throwers is that, although multiple differences arise between them, the hyperplasic aspect is common, from which only the spear throwers, which have a development from the Extrem hypoplastic upward, deviate.

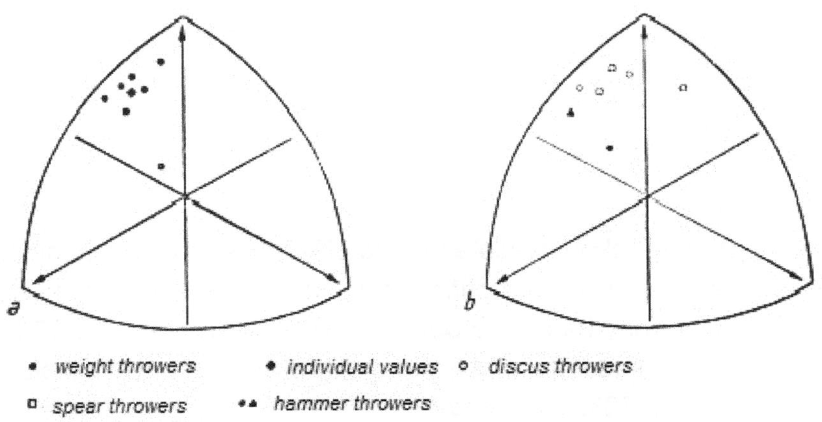

Fig. 41. The distribution of types of bodybuilding (Sheldon).

Tanner (1964) describes the throwers as long-lasting athletes, evident in hammer and disc holes, while weight and spear throwers fall into the mid-end group. In relation to the length of the lower limbs, the discs have the longest upper limbs and have the widest shoulders relative to the length of the trunk. They follow the weight, the spear and the hammer. Although on average, weight throwers also fall into these groups of body shape among them are short-track athletes who still have successful results (Tanner).

Tittel (1963, 1965), investigating the discs by measuring the biacromial, bicistric diagrams of "thorax circumference", "forearm length", thigh length, "calculated correlation and regression coefficients. Based on factorial analysis, factors have been established - in which body height, circumference, and body weight predominate - that reveals a prominent expression of body disc design. For weight lifters, the most important measure is the circumference of the arm. The large body weight of these athletes is advantageous only when it has enough strength to design its total mass. The value of the body of active substance is therefore a conditioning factor. The amount of skin folds to these athletes far exceeds that of all athletes so far. It varies between 70.5 mm (=12.3% - spear throwers) and 94.8 mm (= 16% - heavy toothbrushes) (*Tittel* and *Wutscherk*, 1970). With all the high proportion of body fat, the body's active substance is well above the average of the runners or jumpers (after Tanner). Body weight and body active substance are height dependent, as the AKS index indicates. Only hammer throwers reach the value of 1.26 of this index, while discs (1.18) equals that of non-loners (1.18) and sprinters (1.21). Spear throwers with a 70 m performance have a relatively high AKS index (1.17... 1.29), the best weight throwers have the same (1.24). The best hammer throwers are athletic hyperplasic type (1.19... 1.24). (Figure 41, 42).

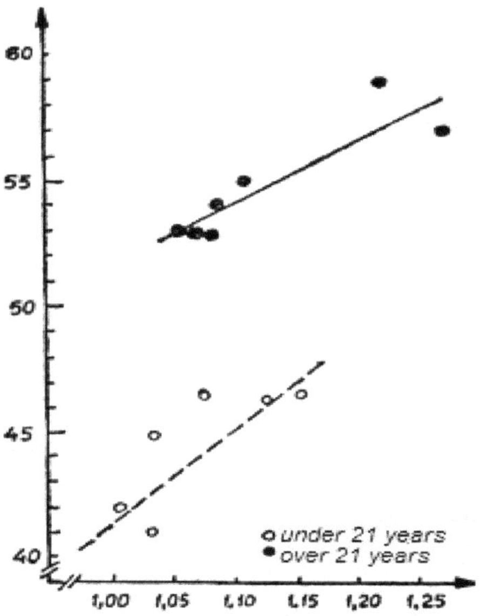

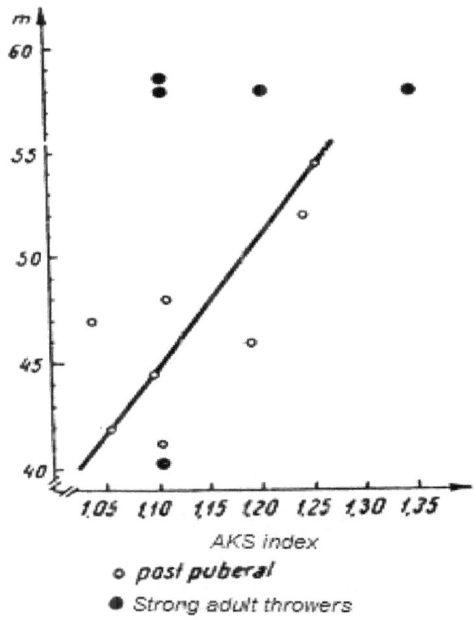

Fig. 42. The ratio of disk discarding distance to AKS index (Wutscherk).

In women, after *Conrad* (1963), weight and disc throwers have hyperplastic expression. There are many differences in the series of picnoleptomorph variations. The best throwers had a mezo picnomorphic to purely picnomorphic configuration, which, on the coordinate position, could be put alongside the men. They may also belong to the leptomorphic type by decreasing body density. The disc thalers are distributed between H9 (hyperplastic leptomorph) and D8 (hyperplasic mezo picnomorph) fields of this classification. In contrast, spear throwers are in a well-defined field, that is, athletes with mezzo-mesopic mesolifique leptosphere athletes. *Tittel* (1963, 1965) determined, at disk throws, the correlation coefficients between shoulder width, arm length and sport performance.

The data on body measures highlighted by participants in the Olimpic Games (1968) is limited to age, body height and body weight; The average body height is differentiated. We also mention in the throwers the very strong scapular belt with 46 cm diameter in men and 40 cm in women, the very large global force (indexes over 420), the large palmar surface, skill, neuro-muscular coordination and The balance at the above parameters, according to the indicated tests, good aerobic capacity and very high anaerobic capacity (47 kgm / min / kg) (see Figure 43.44).

Table 16

The biological performance model of the athlete.
Group IV a (throwers) (after I. Dragan, A. Popovici)

Index	Men				Women		
	Disc	Weight	Spear	Hammer	Disc	Weight	Spear
Age	28 ± 2	26±2	26 ± 2	26 ± 2	25±2	25±2	24±2
Height	193±3	194±3	187±3	185±2	179±2	178±2	176±2
Weight	114±2	117±3	98±3	115±2	88±2	89±2	74±4
Bust	99-100	101	97	97	93	93	91
Calibre	199	199	195	192	184	183	182
Biacromial diameter	45	46	45	45	40	40	39
Bitrochanteric diameter	36	36	35	34	35	34	33
Perimeter	101	102	99	98	92	91	90
Abdominal perimeter	92	95	90	92	78	82	74
Perimeter	99	99	97	99	98	98	97
Arm perimeter	37	37	36	35	31	31	28
Forearm perimeter	31	32	30	30	27	28	25
Thigh perimeter	64	65	60	65	67	66	65
Calf perimeter	42	43	38	40	41	41	37
Right-hand flexors` strenght	74	70	67	70	50	50	49
Left-hand flexors` strenght	69	65	63	65	48	48	46
Scapular force	67	65	63	65	48	43	46
Lombar force	220	200	200	220	180	180	145
Weight/waist	590	603	524	621	491	500	420
Proportion of adipose tissue %	15	17	14	15	15	17	14
Active proportion %	85	83	86	85	85	83	86
Bust – (T/2)	+3.5	+	+3.5	+	+	+	+
Perimeter	+	+	+	+	+	+	+
- (T/2)	5	5	3	2	2	2	2

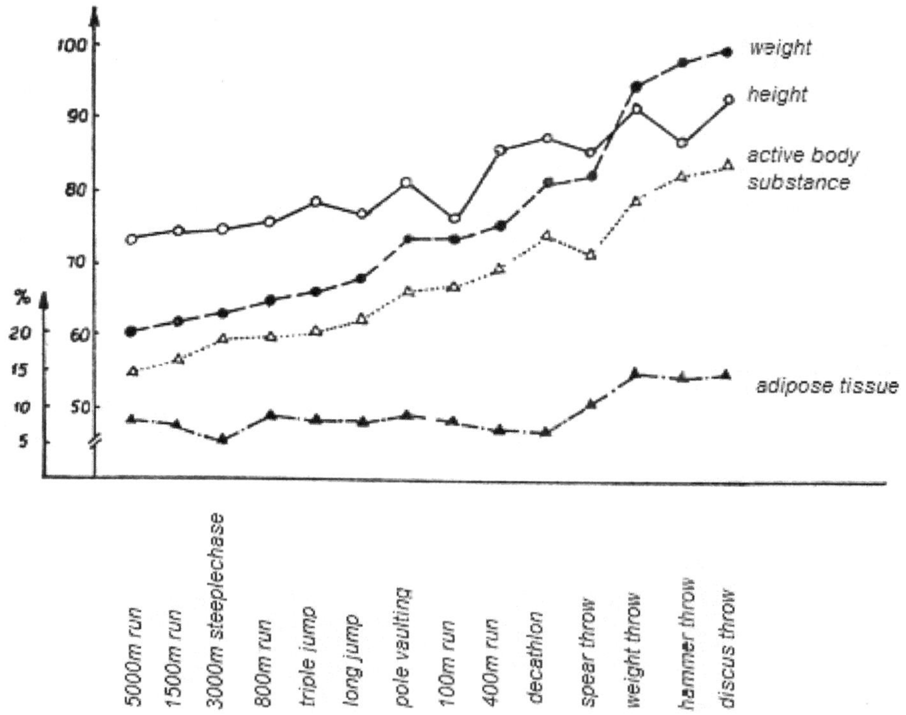

Fig. 43. Interactive diagram of height, weight, active body and adipose tissue in performers in some male athletic disciplines (Tittel).

Natation

Looking at the results of our research, we note the following:

The optimal anthropological type, resulting from the Briant method, for watering, is the disharmonic fractomegamorph, longilin, with the widths and depths prevailing.

For girls, the height is 14 to 15 years old, between 165 and 180 cm and 10 20 cm above the country average; 104/105% of the height, the bust being 45% 55% of the stature. For the age group of 16-21 years, the stature should be between 167 190 cm and 15 25 cm above the mean; Size, 102 104% of the height, the bust relative to the stature being between 42 and 49%.

For boys, the height of the investigated groups is for the age group 13 16 years between 158 185 cm, where we consider that this parameter is only valid in the limit of 170 185 cm, thus only exceeding the average for the country with Values between 15 and 25 cm. Also, on the group investigated in this age group, the size is between 158 188 cm and we conclude that, in order to be appropriate, it is necessary to be between 178 189 cm and 103 105% respectively Stature, especially for sprinters.

For the age group 16 22 years, the height is between 170 186 cm, so values between 2 16 cm above the country average, which still requires a selection to achieve higher values of the stature, which should lie Above the average of 10 20 cm, especially for sprinters, the funds being slightly lower. The range is between 101-104% of the waist, and it is still necessary to look for athletes with the highest possible range, giving good results in the water. In situations where the scale is equal to the stature, the results are mediocre. The bust relative to stature indicates values ranging from 46 to 48%.

In cases where it was possible to carry out the research, it was shown that parents are also an anthropological typology that falls within the category of longilin disharmonic fracture, which is of great significance for the initial and secondary selections. From the researches carried out it results that the sum of the height of the genitor for the water samples should be between 340 -380 cm, with the sum of the spans between 360 -390 cm. For females, bieliac angle research revealed that it had to show values between 45-65 °, exceeding them being able to imply optimal typology. We appreciate that it is very important to test this parameter also on the maternal line, because it gives important information about the endocrine type, which, if it is hiperestrogen, is not favorable. It also results from the research that, in order to achieve the optimal anthropological type of watering, it is favorable, both for girls and for boys, that puberty will appear later one year, respectively, 13-15 years old girls and 14-16 years old Boys, which favors growth processes. Knowing the age of puberty in parents gives very important hereditary indications for initial and secondary selection.

The palmar dermatoglyphs indicate a number of seven whirlwinds, or two more than the average encountered in ordinary individuals. Planetary dermatoglyphs indicate plant length values, in girls, between 35-39, and in boys, between 41-44, the angles between the anatomical and functional axes are between 13-17 °. And this index should be investigated in parents because the degree of hereditary determination is high, indicating close correlations for the cases where we were able to study them. The active body index indicates that the body weight should be 14-15 years for girls, 84% for the girls, and for the group 16 21 for 81.8%. In boys, in group 13 16 years, between 85 and 89%, and in group 16 22 years, between 84 88%, the hereditary determination of this indicator is very important. In cases investigated by parents, a large correlation coefficient for active body mass has been observed, and this fact will be further specified in subsequent researches in order to establish values for the generators. Body conformative complexes for girls, and for boys to be better specified in future research, highlights the following preliminary values that may constitute selection parameters:

A=770 – 840,
B= 23,2- 24,5,
C= 13,5– 15,5.

The data presented justifies the value of the cited anthropological and genetic parameters determined by the sports subjects and their parents in order to achieve a sportive efficiency of the selection as process, thus enriching the existing national selection system with us.

It can be concluded that anthropology and genetics opens up a very high perspective of raising the sport efficiency by a higher targeting of the selection, thus diminishing the capping phenomenon, which leads to an increased efficiency of the activity, By avoiding investing labor and material capital in subjects lacking the anthropological and genetic qualities necessary to achieve great performances.

To these are added the following data on differentiation on swimming styles.

Representatives from the craft disciplines (free style and back craw) are larger than those of the back or dolphin style.

Mean lengths of swimmers over long distances are smaller than those of short swimmers.

Body weight is the same:

• Swimmers are the heaviest; Followers from behind, dolphin and brass;

• Body weight of long-distance swimmers (except for 200 m bras) is reduced.

These differences in body build-up are particularly accentuated to swimmers.

Regarding relative body weight, performance swimmers are the heaviest (exception, 200 m - back, 100 m - dolphin), so athletic expression of the body influences swim performance. Anthropometric values obtained (*Tittel*) indicate that a swim sharing is required depending on the swimming styles. Thus, the breasts approach (176.7 cm), in body size, in those of free styles and dolphins (179.6 cm - 179.0 cm) (p> 99.0%). Body weight is grouped in such a way that the high values of brass style (76.4 kg), compared to free styles (72.9 kg) and dolphin (73.5 kg) [p> 99.0 %], Values that are also highlighted by relative weight (*Quetelet index*) (406, 411,433).

These differentiated body heights correspond to length measures (sitting height, extremity length, distance of the distant arm), and the differences between absolute and relative weights correspond to trunk and extremity circumferences, as well as fat deposits. These tendencies of body construction correlate in particular with the width of the shoulders of the dolphin swimmers, and with the thoracal sagital diameter of the brass, so that complementary typological features can be extracted. Swimmers of 100m free style are the tallest (181.6cm). Corporal weight, width and circumference measures exceed the average. The 200 and 400 m free shooters are somewhat smaller (179.5 cm), which adds to the decrease in other lunges (sitting height, extremity length, extended arms), widths (chest width, shoulder width), and, To a lesser extent, with all the slightly increased body weight, and circumferential measures, the decrease being progressive from the group for 100 m to the 400 m. The body height of the 1 500 m free style is approximately equal to the height Of the above mentioned, the body weight decreases (1.0 kg). Therefore, the change in the ratio between the trunk (seating height - [1.5 cm]) and the length of the extremities (length of the arms [-j-2P2 cm], lower member length [+1.5 cm]) is emphasized, The circumference of the trunk (1.6 cm) and the extremes (-2.3 cm) decreased.

Dolphin swimmers of 100 m are larger and heavier than dolphin long distances (182.2 cm - 179.1 cm) (77.2 kg - 73.7 kg)]. Differences from other height measures result from differences in body height, and the difference in body weight results in a decrease in the circumference. On short distances, it seems that the force component is predominant in speed, as a determining factor for performance; Swimmers from 200 m inches have a slightly higher height (+1 cm) than 100 m inches. Therefore, the longer length of the extremity, the greater distance of the extended arms and the greater width of the shoulders of the 200 m bras are of particular importance.

At a proportional representation, the characteristics of each discipline of swimming remain. While swimmers from free styles and dolphins resemble, in terms of the length of the extremities, the extremities of the swimmers are shorter, and the height is longer. In terms of trunk width measures, swimmers of the free style exceed the others by 0.1%. The most noticeable differences are those of the circumference of the trunk and the extremities, the highest values being those of the brass style (up to + 2%), and the values of the dolphin style being higher than those of the Free style (up to + 0.8%). Free-style swimmers appear to be the least athletic, which is also reflected in the shoulder / width width ratio (index 53).

Performance swimmers (free styles, dolphins and suits) are in a limited area of body typology. The corporal type, after Conrad (1963), corresponds to the mezo leptomorphic type, which is not always expressed by extreme hyperplasia. Success, however, may also have swimmers with mezo picnomorphic conformation. The subcutaneous adipose tissue deposit is of interest to swimmers as well as sprinters (Kohlrauschi, 1927). But as these athletes do not differ in body weight at all, and as barely at the height of sprinters, jumps and runners from fence samples, there is hardly any difference in that. The body active substance corresponds to the values of sprinters and jumpers with the pole. She is so great. The shape of their body is an athletic form. Calculation of the AKS index indicates optimal values of 1.15 1.18 (Figure 43).

In terms of body height in women, literature data (Tittel) does not show the existence of differences between fins of different styles, although those of free style are smaller, correlated with increasing distance. The same is true of body weight (except for free style - long distances). Due to the small differences in height and body weight, the Quetelet index (relative weight) varied very little interdisciplinarily.

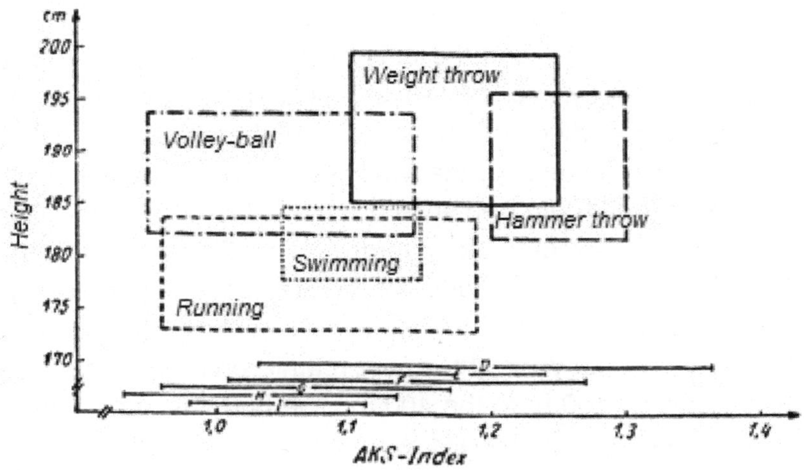

Fig. 44. Influence of the type of body construction (metric index) on the distribution of the AKS index (Active body / body height) and various groups of athletes (Tittel).

Bras style swimmers appear the smallest ones, and those in the back style as the highest (Tittel). Body weight has the same trend and only dolphin fins are heavier. The back-style swimmers have the closest performance, the bras have the circumference of the trunk and the lower extremities; Those of the dolphin, the largest ones, and in terms of length proportions, the small fins in the bras can be compared with the great fins in the back style. In this way, the two types of fins can form two polar groups among which are those of free styles and dolphins.

The highest percentage of adipose tissue reaches dolphin style (18.2%) and varies within this style by only 1.9% (16.3 18.2%). The value is high compared to the runners (7.3% [80 m fences] - 13.5% [80 m]), approaching that of the jumpers in height (15.3%), but does not reach the value of the throwers (19.4 25.1%), canoeing or other sports. The relative values of the active body (AKS index 1,05 1,09) are small, but the high percentage of young people (Tittel) must be considered. In the different types of swimming, body measures have a different action to stimulate performance. On the basis of the influence calculated by superior mathematical methods, it has been found that even in the style of suits the bodily characteristics influence decisively sport performance, while in the free, dolphin and back styles this influence is great but not the only decisive. In the back style cannot establish relationships between body construction and performance. Since in all disciplines a factor is eliminated, namely circumferential measures, but instead complexes of body characteristics and their corresponding indices accumulate, one can say that the influence of this group of characteristics is the greatest.

Factors analysis of free-style faces indicates that circumference, as well as the various corpo- rational complexes (Wuischerk, 1969) (body characteristics complex C and B), are the most important variables. Body height does not appear as a determining variable for performance (r-0.06). Favorable influence, performance, circumference, and weight should be understood as a pro-growth. Also, this style corresponds typologically to meso-leptomorphic body construction (after Conrad, 1963), with a particularly mesoplastic expression. (Figure 44)

For breed fins, factorial analysis extracts four factors that influence performance. The first factor has a relatively high load (0.66). Its most important variables are circumferences, body weight, and body characteristics complexes B and C. It is defined as a "weight factor and circumference." There are three other similar factors (value 0.35 0.40), the first of which is characterized mainly by the distance between the anterior anterosperioses (0.40), the other by length measures (0.35) and the last Through the "metric index", "sagital diameter of the chest" (0.36). Breast style is mostly influenced by large circumferences, increased body weight and complex B and C body characteristics, and to a lesser extent by body height, extremity length, basal width and type of body construction (Fig. 45-47).

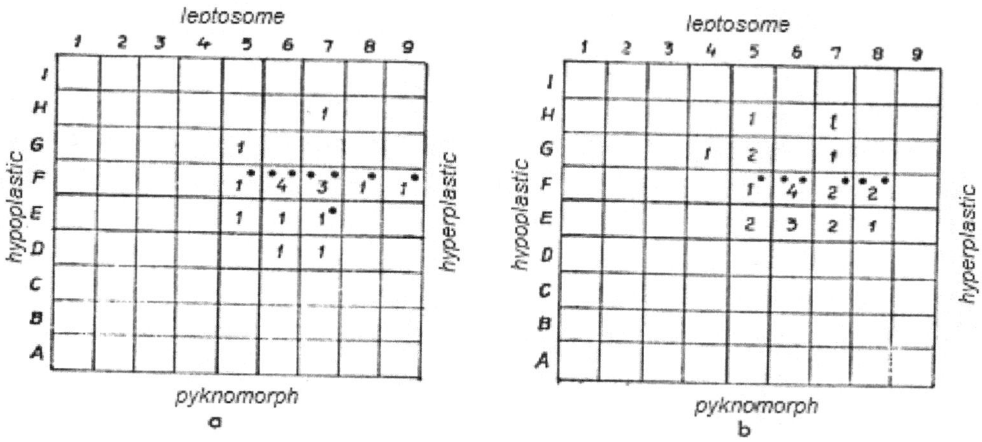

Fig. 45. The distribution of body types to swimmers in the Conrad coordinate system: a) Free style, b) Dolphin style (Tittel).

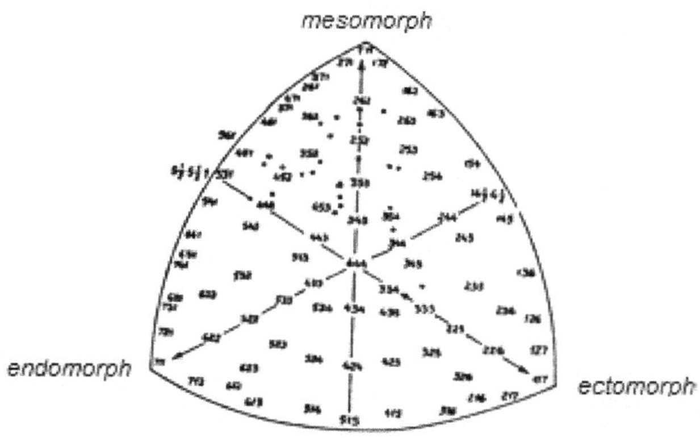

Fig. 46. The distribution of bodybuilding types to 24 performance swimmers (Sheldon).

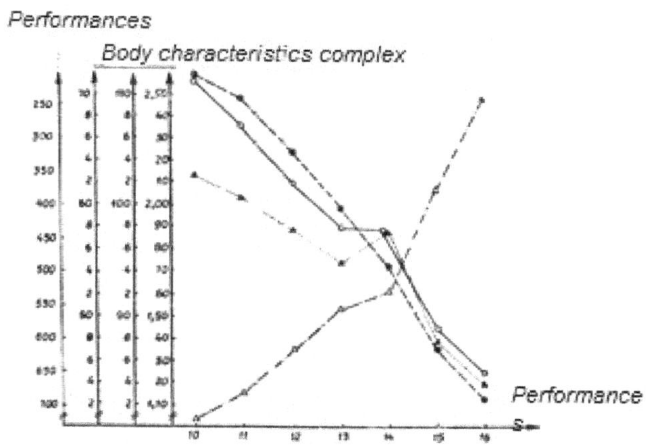

Fig. 47 Correlation between body conformation complexes A, B, C and performance level evolved in a swim point system.

Factorial analysis of dolphin fins resembles that of free style. For a sufficient representation of relationships, a single factorial load (0.49) occurs around the significant range (p = 95% Z oa = 0.60). Since the variables are ordered the same way (sum of the circumference of the extremities, the complex of body characteristics C, body weight) is the same factor that occurs in the other two styles, namely "circumference and weight factor".

Interesting are the measures that a second factor (unsignificant), namely, the width of the hand, the width of the foot, the circumference of the hand, not only because - by their growth - it negatively influences the performances, but also because they are expressive Of a bodily construction towards the mesomorph, and by the fact that the influence on performance becomes negative by increasing the circumferences and the weight (Tittel) (Figure 48).

Factor analysis calculations show that in the back-end fins, the "circumference and weight" factor is important for athletic body formation. The second factor shows that the trend toward picnomorphic conformation is favorable for sports performance, but swimmers remain the highest for all distances.

When looking at the typologically constitutional basis, in the water, we note the following:

The initial selection is at pre-school age of five seven years, the secondary one at 10 12 years and the final at 12-14 years in girls and 13-15 years in boys. The above-mentioned morphological anthropometric indices (height, biacromial diameter larger than the bitrochanterian diameter, height 3-4 cm above height, etc.), specific weight, body volume, hydrodynamic index - I = height / (Y x 100), where Y = (biacromial diameter + bitrochanterian diameters) / 2 - aerobic capacity (very good values), articular mobility, palmar and plantar surfaces, vital capacity (over 15 20% versus standard) Purdue Pegboard test, clues of strength, type of nervous system (Woodwarth Mathewes test), anaerobic capacity for sprinters.

The model of the performer is characterized by: hydrodynamic qualities (specific gravity 1.08 and average 1.02 g / cmc and less than 1), small hydrodynamic body void, maximum aerobic capacity 70 75 ml / kg in boys and 65 to 70 ml / kg in girls.

Height: 174 178 cm for women; 185 190 cm for men - sprint, and semi-finals slightly less; Joint mobility scapulo umeral, tarsus tibia and large spine; Higher vital capacity (compared to standard +15 - + 20%), 4,6 cm above height, long palm length (10,4% height); Very good balance; Very good respiratory and locomotricity neuromotricity coordination; Strength or speed strength according to the specificity of the sample, especially in the scapular belt muscles; Very good anaerobic capacity for sprinters.

These elements respond to the swimming effort characterized by: high O_2 consumption; A difficult thermoregulation, through loss of renal function due to lack of sweat; Soliciting the cardiorespirator; Nervous system request for perfect motion coordination; The necessity of the existence of higher skill parameters - depending on the sample - of the motricity skills of skill, force in speed or force in resistance mode, strength or speed (Figure 48).

Sports games

We will only stop on some of them, to illustrate the correlations between the constitutional type and the sport performance. (Figure 49-52)

A. *Football*

Soccer players are not a homogeneous population, but differ in body building depending on the position in the game. Especially porters are different from the rest of the players. With regard to the type of body construction, after Conrad, most footballers have a mesomorphic construction with hyperplasic expression. Young footballers tend to the leptomorphic and hypoplasic pole. A typical typological position has only porters and defenders who have the average position and thus partially deviate towards the picnomorphic pole.

Soccer players have a medium, normal, athletic (hyper-plastic) type of body construction, which corresponds to the qualities required for football play (strength, speed, strength, skill). The optimal anthropological type is characterized by a high height (over 176 cm), weighing 5 kg less than centimeters above 100, aerobic capacity 4800-5200 ml O2 / minute (65 ml / min / kg body), The total anaerobic capacity between 3000-3200 kgm (38-40 kgm / kg body), vital capacity 3800-5000 cmc (ie over 65 cmc / kg body), the lower train muscles having a force representing values above 200% Body weight, intelligence, skill, speed, strength, high-level force.

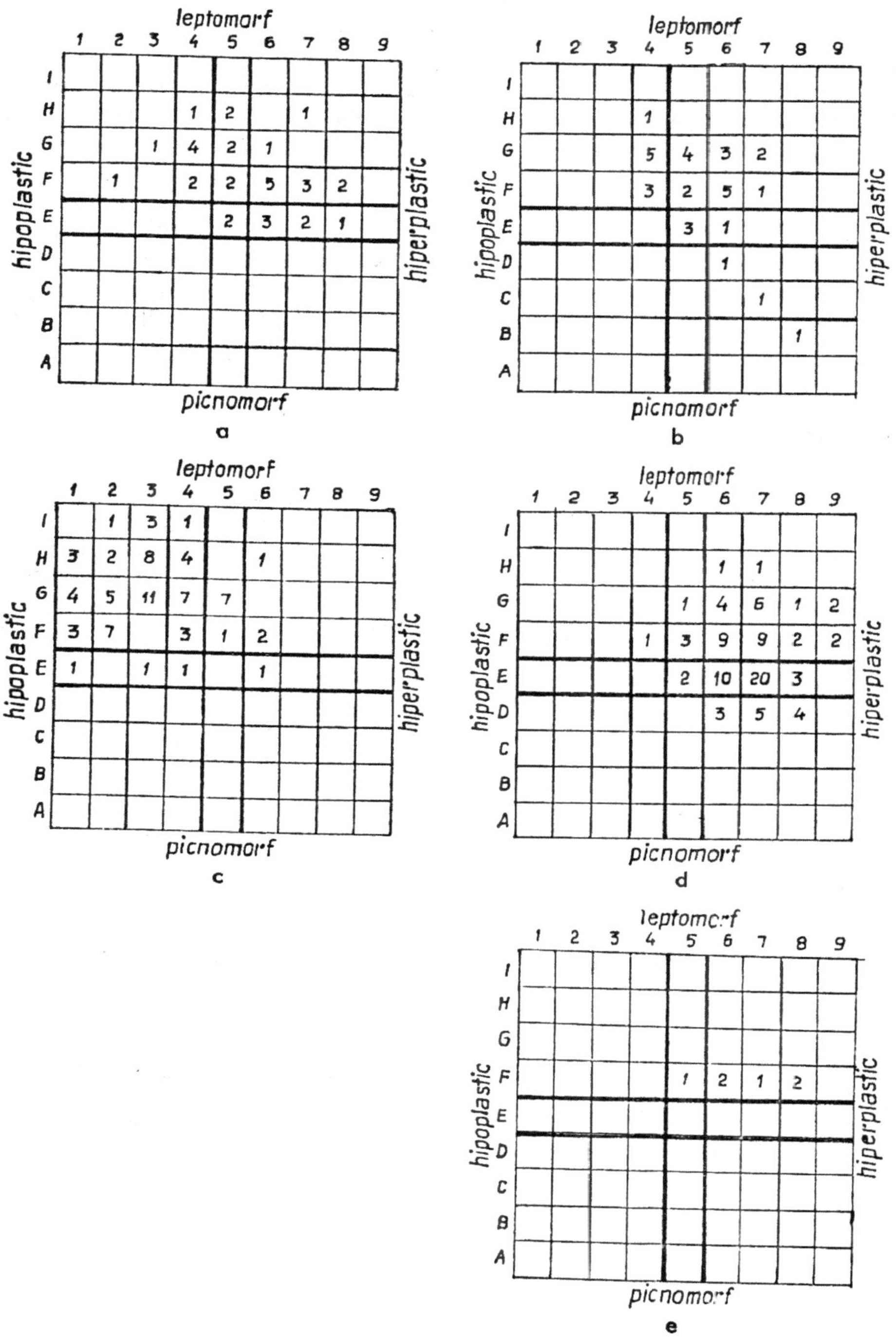

Fig. 48. Body Design Types of Conrad Performers
(A - free style swimmer, b - free-floating free style, c - junior footballers, d - senior footballers,e - finishers butterfly style swimmers).

The portrait is very high (over 185 cm), 107,108% in height, palm length 10-11% in height, with very high reactivity. Apart from the somatic-physiological type elements, football selection must take into account the typological parameters of motricity activity and psychic activity. The most important driving quality, given that it is a common denominator throughout the 90 minutes of play, is the psycho-biomechanical skill. This is all the more so since the conception of the game leader has changed, in the sense that the demands of modern tactics and techniques demand that, depending on the situation, any of the players can take on the role of game leader. There is also a requirement for a high concentration capability for both field and field players, as well as a perfect neuromotricity equilibrium and coordination, with a high anticipatory capacity (the highly developed rhinencefalus area) needed to anticipate and counteract the opponent's actions.

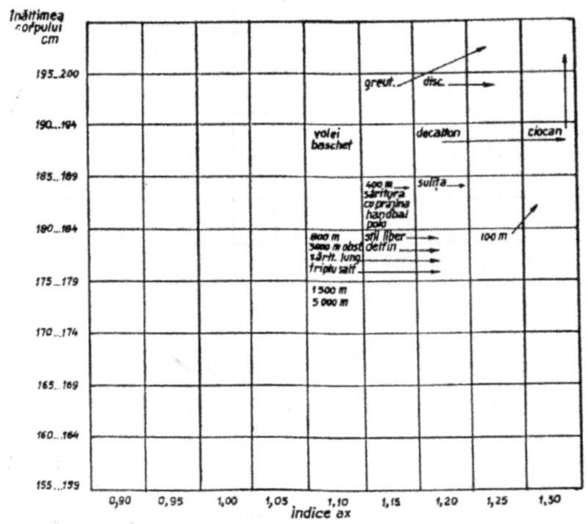

Fig. 49. The AKS index and body height at performers in sports games and some disciplines in male athletics (Tittel).

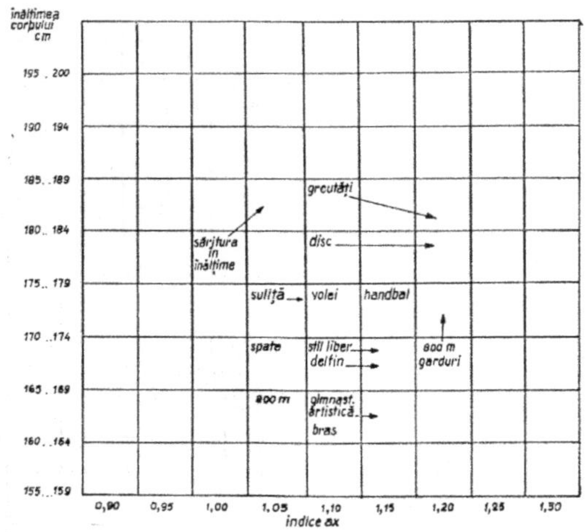

Fig. 50. The AKS index and body height at performers in sports games and some disciplines in female athletics (Tittel).

Under these conditions, the Purdue Pegboard intelligence tests, concentration and prediction tests, with rigorous observation of the skill test scores included in the national selection system, become mandatory. In soccer (as in other sports games), I can not get performance than intelligent players. In Germany, in order to play in Division C, secondary schools are compulsory and, for upper divisions, university studies completed or in progress. Along with skill, football, speed, resistance, strength and strength of the lower train, trunk, head and neck muscles are required. Samples of speed (100m running), strength (1500m and 3000m) and force are mandatory both in the selection and in the objectification of the progress in the training. The initial selection for football is at the age of 14.

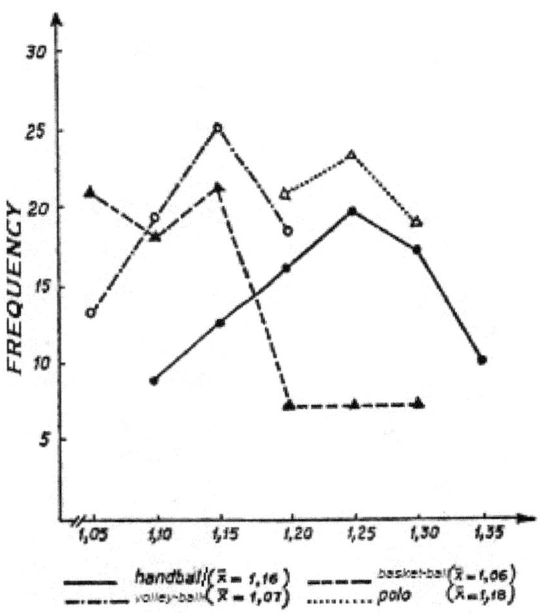

Fig. 51.
AKS index to a number of sports gaming teams (Tittel).

The secondary selection at 15-16 years (young juniors) should aim at the overall height above 15-20 cm, good aerobic and anaerobic capacities, lumbar force of 180-200% of body weight, vital capacity 50-55 cmc air / kg body, High intelligence, neuromotricity coordination and skill at elevated parameters, tested by the above mentioned methods. For the goalkeeper, we mention the height of 178-180 cm, the height 8 10 cm above the height, the high clearance (55-60 cm), the palm length 23-25 cm, plus the qualities mentioned to the players.

The final selection requires a waist above 176 cm, very good aerobic capacity – 60-65 ml O_2/min/kg -, anaerobic capacity 38-40 kgm/kg. high clearance (over 60 cm), lumbar force 200% versus 6, vital capacity 65 Cmc air / kg body, intelligence, skill, speed, strength, resistance to the highest parameters. At the wardrobe, the height reaches over 185 cm, the height 108-110% from the height, the palm length over 7% of the height, the very good reactivity, the intelligence and the double-speed skill at very high parameters.

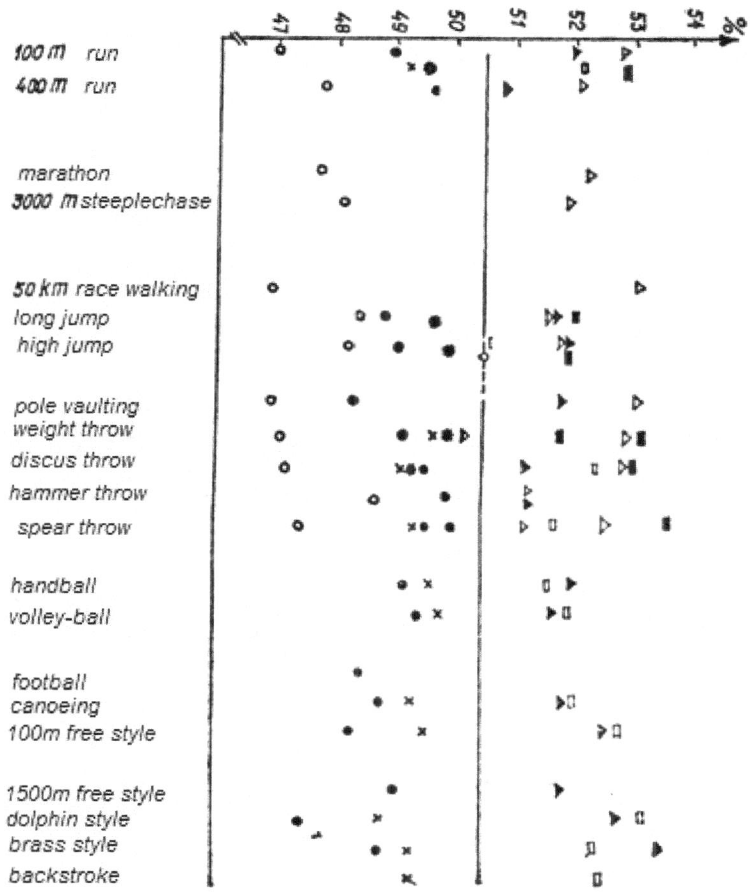

Fig. 52. Bodyweight at lightweight athletics, swimming, games, canoeing (T-203).

B. Basketball

The optimal anthropological type is characterized by a very high height (over 190 cm in boys, over 182 cm in girls, with variations between pivots, which are the highest, followed by extremes and defenders), very good aerobic capacity, good anaerobic capacity, Good general psychomotricity reactivity, good general intelligence (test over 60 points / 80 minutes maximum), good metric coordination (high Purdue Pegboard tests). The initial selection is eight to nine years, secondary to 14-15 years, following the height (in boys between 185,200 cm in 175-195 cm), good aerobic capacity, very good skill (Purdue Pegboard test with high values), intelligence Good overall (test I3 over 110 points), palm length 20-21 cm, 6-8 cm above waist, good vital capacity. (Table 17, 18) The final selection approaches, in terms of the performance requirements, the value of the anthropological optimal type.

Table 17

Standard values for the interpretation of maximum oxygen consumption in adult performance athletes (ml / kg) (after I. Dragan)

Weight (kg)	Weak	Medium	Good	Very Good	Excelent
50,1- 55	52	52-63	63-74	74-86	86
55, 1-60	50	50-62	62-73	73-84	84
60,1- 65	49	49-60	60-71	71-82	82
65, 1-70	48	48-59	59-69	69-80	80
70,1- 75	47	47-57	57-68	68-78	78
75, 1-80	46	46-56	56-66	66-76	76
80,1- 85	44	44-54	54-64	64-74	74
85, 1-90	43	43-53	53-62	62-72	72
90,1- 95	42	42-51	51-61	61-70	70

Table 18

Standard values for the interpretation of anaerobic capacity in adult performance athletes (based on the regression equation: TTR / kg (kgm / kg min 1) = 71.33 0.268 weight) (after I. Dragan)

Weight (kg)	Weak	Medium	Good	Very Good	Excelent
50,1- 55	34	34-42	42-50	50-57	57
55, 1-60	34	34-41	41-49	49-56	56
60,1- 65	33	33-40	40-47	47-55	55
65, 1-70	32	32-39	39-46	46-53	53
70,1- 75	31	31-38	38-45	45-52	52
75, 1-80	30	30-37	37-44	44-51	51
80,1- 85	30	30-36	36-43	43-49	49
85, 1-90	29	29-35	35-42	42-48	48
90,1- 95	28	28-34	34-10	40-47	47

The mass of subcutaneous fat in men is not different from other athletes. It has a value of 9.9% of body weight so that the active body generally has a value of 71.3 kg. A visible difference in these values occurs only after the body height compensation (AKS index), basketball players with a low AKS index (0.06), as well as volleyball players, so they turn out to be low-table athletes.

C. **Handball**

The optimal anthropological type is characterized in boys by height over 190 cm, range from +6 to +10 cm above waist, lumbar force over 200% by weight, palm length 26-28 cm boys, 20-22 cm in girls, High aerobic power (67-70 ml O_2/kg body in boys, 55-60 ml O_2 in girls), anaerobic capacity in boys 40-46 kgm / kg body, and in girls 28 32 kgm / kg body weight, O_2 (maximum pulse of 28-30 ml In boys and 18-20 ml / girls), general intelligence, skill, strength, speed, resistance to elevated parameters. The trunk is stronger for handball players (versus volleyball and basketball players, thorax width - 310 mm, chest circumference - 1006 mm) The advantages of a more athletic expression result from the following research: at repeated measurements it was noticed that, at average, body height (183, 3 cm) and slightly increased body weight (81.4 kg = + 16 kg), other measures increased (boom circumference = +1.0 cm, thigh circumference = 7 cm, girth circumference = +1.9 cm). Functionally, these changes lead to the improvement of the strength properties (jumping, throwing force) because the statistically determined correlation coefficients (p = 95%, 0.48) show the positive influence of the increase in the circumference of the arm (r = 0.48) (R = 0.55) on strength. If this is only partially valid for the calf (r = 0.22), it should not be forgotten that the tendency to bury the calf leads to an improvement in the jumping force. Subcutaneous adipose tissue has a distribution of about 10.3%. This value correlates with an active substance of 71.3 kg, as shown by the values of the AKS index (Handball 1.16, Polo-1.18). Players in which the game is determined by strong throws, compared to those in baseball or human to field combat, have higher values of the index. Handball therefore requires an athletic body. In recent years, the AKS index has increased in handball players. We also see the increase in body weight that indicates an increase in the active body.

Handbags have a relatively short trunk, opening arms less than body height (-19 mm), short extremities. As width and circumference values correspond to volleyball players. Adipose tissue resembles that of volleyball players with regard to the proportion of body fat, active body, index of AKS as well as the distribution of these values. The initial selection is 10-11 years. Secondary selection is 14-16 years in boys and 13-15 years in girls, taking into account the following parameters: high height, 5-6 cm above waist, palm length 1 / 8-1 / 9 waist, maximum pulse oxygen And good aerobic good capability, good anaerobic capability, very good neuromotricity coordination, skill and intelligence at high levels as well as speed, strength and strength. The final selection has parameters close to the ideal anthropological value for this sporting branch.

Applied technical sports

We make a special mention of these sports, because we believe that they should be developed because in the conditions of cooperation with the companies producing automobiles, motricitycycles and bicycles the winning of international races on vehicles produced in our country can be of considerable benefit Both industry and sport. Considering this, a good selection and knowledge of the optimal anthropological type for these sports disciplines is of major importance, being a national interest.

• *The anthropological type for motricitying.* The initial selection is around the age of 16. The somatic type, except for the proportionality of the organism, is not essential, having great variations in the morphological parameters. Essential is the neuropsychic type. Response and execution speed to the most elevated parameters. Visual driving coordination and stable sensory-motricity balancing, the 5-minute trace test should reveal a stack of at least 171 points (*I. Dragan*). Spatial representation to be correct - ("shape relationship" test 10.5 points) and well-developed distribution attention (*Ricossay* test 187 points). The temperament must be balanced (*Woodworth Mathewes* test, a score of 120 points for each of the eight personality traits studied). The final selection must reveal well-developed general psychic reactivity, very good visual coordination, concentration, very good attention (Kraepelin test duration 10 minutes execution speed 495 points and response accuracy 980 points), distributed distribution attention - Prague - 10 minutes - 39 points), good emotional stability, balanced temperament.

• *The somato-typological and motricity type*, as I said, remain in the secondary plane. First of all, it is the neuropsychic type and first of all the biopsychomotricity skill of skill, with the predominance of a perceptive driving and intelligent driving skill. The intelligence test must indicate high values, and the statochinezimetry will show a very good balance. Cycling selection differs as a velodrome sample, where the effort is predominantly anaerobic or a road test, where the effort is mainly aerobic.

• *The optimal anthropological type* which, in terms of age, in the high performance, is 22 26 years, is somatic for the speed samples 1.80 1.85 m and for the fund 1.70 1.75 m, with a weight With 5 7 kg less than the number of centimeters exceeding 100.

The lower limbs must be long, with the above-mentioned general center of gravity (L5 S1), with the triple flexion chains and well-developed inferior limb extensions, with a planar cavity, with the angle between the functional and anatomical axes between 5 7 degrees with very high chest elasticity. The anaerobic capacity at speeds should be 45 48 kgm / kg, and aerobic 60 70 ml / kg (maximum oxygen consumption 5200 5500 ml); Oxygen pulse, 25 28 ml; Cardiac / oxygen peak volume ratio below 42. Speed and strength motricity skills are at the forefront.

For background samples the maximum oxygen consumption should be 5500 5700 ml (75 85 ml / kg / with max. 30 ml pulse oxygen); Anaerobic capacity of 45 50 kgm / kg (3250 kgm globally). The strength of motricity strength, strength in strength and speed of the moment are the priority. Initial selection is made at eight 11 years, the sense of balance tested by statochimensional and velocity is very important; Somatically, body proportionality is important, with a higher center of gravity located (L5 S1). The secondary selection is 15 16 years and according to the heritability coefficients should be at those levels relative to the optimally described anthropological type. The same scores are given to the motricitying qualities as in the initial selection, and some particular qualities (will, tenacity) and psychobiomotricityity, such as skill, are being tested, with particular emphasis on neuromuscular coordination and equilibrium, in this sport being especially Imposed a proprioceptive and motricity sensorial skill.

In training it is necessary to know the effort structure in the sample, according to the model of canoeing, and to direct the training, consequently, in the annual and competitive cycles. Also, correlations between constitutional typology and sports performance have also been made for other sports. Among them, we quote that constitutional typological values for height, seated height, trunk length, upper and lower limbs, plants, biacromial and bicristal diameters, width of elbow, fist, knee, ankle and plant in different categories of judoans Of great interest for selection and for the correlation between the typology and the methods in which they yield optimal results (*M. Marchocka* et al.)

- Constitutional typology and biorhythm

The human organism, defined as somatic, motricity and psychological constitution (phenotype), genetically determined (genotype) and external environmental factors (paratip), presents a periodic variability of series of biological qualities, variability which constitutes the content of the biorhythm notion.

Human biorhythm, in turn, is made up of a series of such variations, some expressing global parameters (physical capacity - physical biorhythm, emotional capacity - emotional biorhythm, intellectual capacity - intellectual biorhythm), and others, parameters strictly limited to Certain hormonal constants (hormonal concentrations, concentration of adenosine triphosphate in the muscle, etc.). Knowledge of biorhythms is of particular importance for sports activity, giving us some indications of periods when the athlete is at the peak of his biological abilities or, on the contrary, at a lower level, which allows us to individualize both the training and the means of recovery that we Are available for maximum sporting performance. Bioperiodicity appears as a phenomenon of adaptation of the individual and species to the predictable variations of certain environmental factors. The quantitative study of biological rhythms shows that any biophysical or biochemical phenomenon varies periodically and predictably over time (*Aschoff*, 1963, *Bunning*, 1963, *Halberg, Reinberg*, 1967). It is known today that rhythmic activity is a fundamental property of living matter (Reinberg, Ghata, 1957). Biological rhythms have been highlighted in all living beings, from nucleic-nucleic forms to humans, and at all levels of organization: the individual as a whole, organ systems, organs, tissues, cells and subcellular substance. Biological rhythms possess similar fundamental properties to plants and animals:

- they have a genetic origin;
- they persist in the absence of time signals and information;
- they may be characterized for a given species (eg rat, mouse, man), but taking into account that interindividual differences have been highlighted (e.g. Differences between mouse genetic strains (*Halberg* et al., 1978); Differences between dizygotic and monozygotic twins in humans (*Barcal*, et al., 1968)];
- they may be influenced by cyclical variations of certain environmental factors called synchronizers or *Zeitgeber* ("time donors").

In other words, natural synchronizers provide signals for periods of approx. 24 hours or approx. A year that, by a sensible body, allows them to adapt these endogenous biophytic processes to cyclical variations in the environment.

Everything happens as if these biophytic changes resulted, at least in part, from phenomena adapting to predictable variations of a set of factors directly linked to the rotation of the earth around its axis (in about 24 hours) or around Sunshine (in about 365.25 days). In fact, the examples illustrating the temporal organization of the creatures relate, in particular (but not exclusively), to the circadian and circanaal domains of biological rhythms. Hormonal biophyroidal phenomena and other similar manifestations, with a period of approx. Seven days, approx. One month, etc., were highlighted in both women and men (*Halberg*, 1969; *Smolensky* et al., 1974), but to a lesser extent than circadian and circanaal rhythms.

When biological rhythm is regarded as a phenomenon of adaptation to predictable variations of environmental factors, two possibilities have to be considered. The former refers to a given species, to its survival over many generations and to its likely evolution. The second refers to a given individual of the conscious species, the subject being confronted with cyclic and non-cyclical manipulations of environmental factors, including synchronizers. Biological rhythms can be better understood if one compares the properties of rhythms to different species (*Edmunds*, 1978 and *Bunning*, 1978) and, on the other, if individual tolerance is studied for the effects of manipulation of synchronizers (*Halberg, Reinberg*, 1967, *Hayes*, 1976, *Aschoff*, 1978, *Reinberg*, 1979). The circadian organization of humans (and perhaps its circular and circanaal organizations) is the expression of a population of self-sustained oscillators that are interconnected (with a certain hierarchy) and influenced by a set of synchronizers.

Biophyroidal variation and its parameters. Regular cyclical change of any biological variable may be subject to approximation by a sinusoidal function. This can generally be done by reporting gross results by time (chronogram) or can be done with precision using the least squares method to obtain the cosine function, which gives the best approximation of the total gross results Is the temporal series: the cosinor. For the latter, Halberg et al. (1972) proposed the use of the classical equation:

$$Y(t)=M+A \cos (\omega>t+\Phi),$$

Where M is the mesh (system-adjusted mean), A is the amplitude of the rhythm, ω> is the angular frequency, t is the time and Φ, acrophas; The angular frequency ω> is equal to 2π / τ, where π is the period and 1 / τ frequency.

An example illustrating the characterization of a biological rhythm is given in Fig. 53. The study refers to nine young, healthy subjects, synchronized with a daytime activity at 7am in the morning at midnight and a night off. They automatically measure the muscular strength of the right hand by means of a dynamometer (Colin Centile, Paris) under standardized conditions, every four hours within 24 hours, except during sleep. The analysis of this transversal study of a circadian rhythm (t = approximately 24 hours) can be done in two ways:

1) Schedule. The averages of the values obtained, with their confidence limits (for a typical error, for example) are reported, depending on time. Under these conditions, muscle strength reaches its maximum value at about 15 o'clock and its minimum value at around 7 o'clock, the difference being statistically significant (p> 0.0005). It is also noticed that the variation takes over the approximate shape of a sinusoid within 24 hours.

Muscle strength of the right hand
time in hours

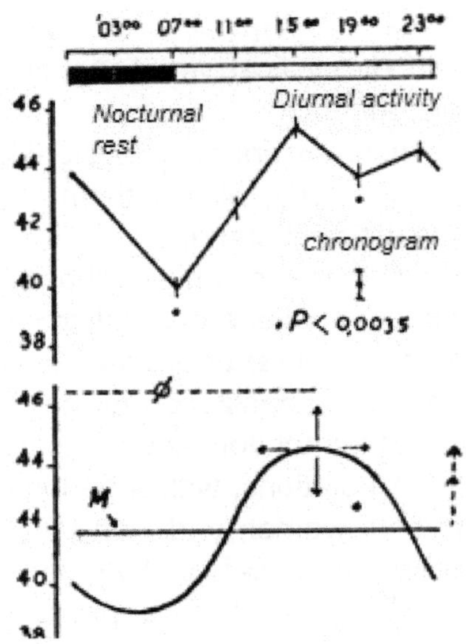

Path detection P> 0.005
τ (period) = 24h
M (mesh) = 16h
ϕ (acrophase) = 16h
A (amplitude) = 2.7kg force
Confidence limits of 95% for φ and A

Fig. 53. Example of a biological rhythm analysis, that of the right-hand muscle; Top timing method, low cosine method.

2) The cosinorm method. In the chosen example, the period is 24 hours, which corresponds to the synchronization of the subjects. The right hand muscle acrophysis is located in this case at 16,11 (16 and 11 minutes); If the confidence limits extend to 95% safety, this phase may be between 12 h 36 and 19 h 46. The amplitude is 2.7 kgf (between 1.1 and 4.2 kgf for 95% safety).

The gap is 41.8 kgf ± 1.8 kgf. This means that the muscular force can reach approximately 46 kgf at the time of acrophase and may be about 37 kgf 12 hours earlier or 12 hours later. The *period* γ is the duration of a complete cycle of a rhythmic variation. γ is usually expressed in a unit of time (seconds, minutes, hours, days, months, years). Amplitude A corresponds to the half of the total variation of the rhythm change over the considered γ period. A can be expressed in conventional units (Celsius for temperature, mg / h for 17 urinary OHCs, etc.) or in percent of M. The M-range is the adjusted average of the rhythm over the period considered or is the arithmetic mean (24 hours, one month, one year) when the measured measurements were performed at equal intervals. Acrophase Φ is the time location of the peak over the period considered, so Φ has to be given in relation to a starting point or a reference phase Φ = 0.

Cosinor and similar methods are widely used by chronobiologists. They can now be programmed for small office computers. The hypothesis of a non-zero amplitude A (P <0.05) can be verified by the cosine method, which allows to know if a rhythm is detected over a given time t.

Spectrum of biological rhythms. Logic, as well as the methodology, demand that the analysis of a detectable rhythm always begins by evaluating its period. Indeed, knowing the time of a biological rhythm is indispensable for assessing its amplitude and its acrophasis. Let's take the periodic changes of a physiological variable, for example temperature in humans. If the time series of measurements is long enough (several days, months or years) and measuring points made at short intervals (several seconds, minutes or hours), a rhythm with a γ of about one Minute (rhythm ultradiane), a rhythm with a γ of about 24 hours (circadian rhythm), a rhythm with a γ of about seven days, about 30 days, about one year, etc. (Infrared rhythms). In other words, for the same biological process, several cyclical variations can be highlighted, each of them having a different period. As shown in Table 19, ultradiane, circadian and infrared periods exist in the child, the healthy woman and the man for an ensemble of Biological variables. In the field of chronoendo-crinology, ultra short-wave oscillations (γ <24 hours) are sometimes called pulsatile secretions. The spectral analysis of pulsatile processes shows that their period can be quantified and therefore can find a precise place in the field of ultradiane rhythms (*Copinschi* et al., 1977).

Table 19

Spectral analysis of human biological rhythms

Examples of rhythms	Spectrum range		
	High or ultra radiant frequency (r<20 h)	Average or circadian frequency (r≈24 h)	Low or infaradian frequency
Radial pulse.....	≈ 1 S	≈ 24 h	1 an
Temperature (digital = dig.; Oral = or.; rectal = rec.)	≈ 1 mm (dig.)	≈ 24 h (dig., or., rec.)	30 j (F) 7 j et 1 an (F et H) (or., rec.)
Plasma cortisol	≈ 45 et	≈ 24 h	30 j (F)Â 1 an (H)
Plasma testosterone	≈ 90 mm	≈ 24 h	1 an
Sexual Behavior (H)	≈ 8 h	≈ 24 h	1 an
Eating behavior (E, F, H)	?	≈ 24 h	1 an

The period γ is often considered to be known. Let's take the example of a synchronized man through a steady alternation of daily activity and night rest (both related to the constraints of social life and ecological “niches”) with an average of 24 hours. It is therefore likely that, under these circumstances, circadian rhythms of this subject will have an average γ of 24 hours.

Time organization. For any species (including human species), knowing the rhythms of various biological variables allows a precise representation of its temporal organization for a given spectral domain. But even for the most studied species (human, mouse, rat, Acetabularia) we still have only an insufficient and very incomplete representation of this temporal organization.

To simplify the presentation of this temporal structure, for example, the aerophase relations of different rhythms (and amplitudes) can be shown for circadian, circular and circanaal periodicities. The schematic of some aspects of the human circadian temporal organization

(Figure 54) was performed based on the results obtained (Figure 55) under controlled and standardized experimental conditions. Figure 55 illustrates an aspect of the temporal circulatory structure of the young adult female, spontaneously menstruated. We emphasize that all the subjects studied were similarly synchronized in terms of circadian rhythms. This methodical necessity, however elementary it may seem, is sometimes neglected, although it is indispensable.

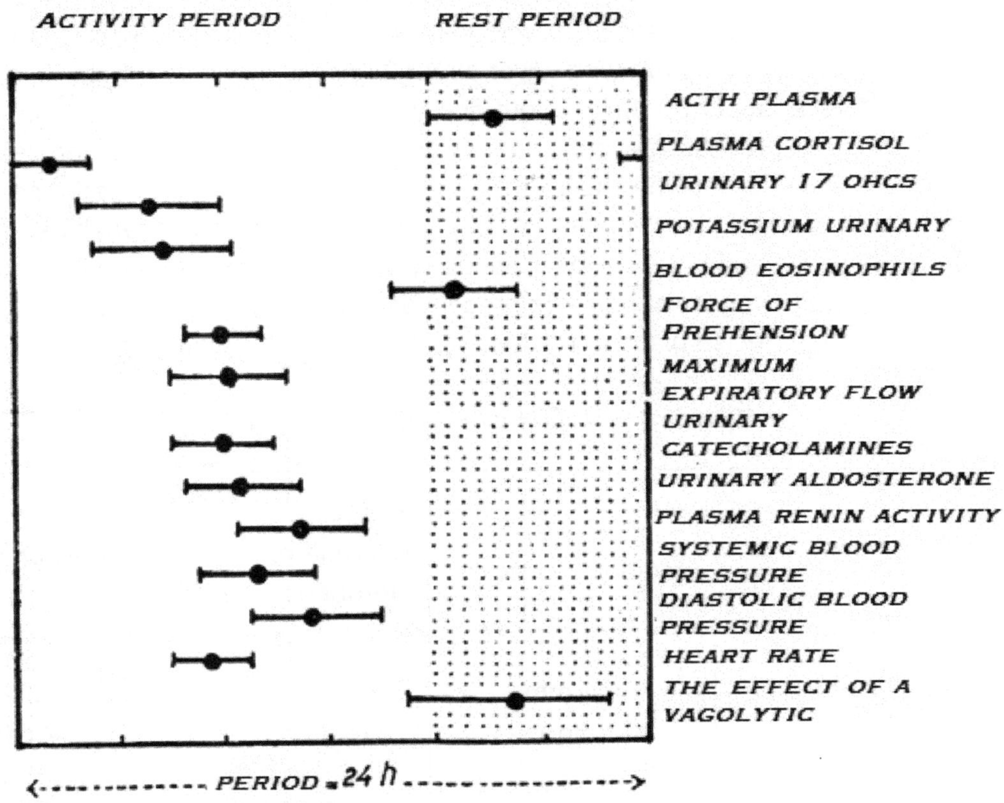

Fig. 54. Aspect of the day-long circadian organization of the healthy adult human. Acrophase Φ, peak of circadian variation, has its location represented by a point. The horizontal bar corresponds to the confidence limits of Φ for a 95% fuse. The daytime and night-time activity intervals are represented to allow knowledge of subject synchronization for a 24-hour period. Acrophases of different circadian rhythms in synchronized subjects are not randomly distributed on the 24-hour scale; On the contrary, this distribution, at all levels of organization, is a specific temporal structure. The classical causal relationship between various physiological functions must be supplemented with information on their temporal relationships. Phase relations between biophytic phenomena thus considered lead to the description of coherent circadian systems. Thus, plasma peak ACTH precedes in phase the plasma cortisol which, in its turn, precedes in phase the muscles of force (prehensive force), bronchial freedom (maximum expiratory flow) and urinary excretion of potassium and 17 OHCS, the peak of circulating eosinophils Corresponds to the minimum plasma cortisol and vice versa.

It is found that the acrophases of the different variables are not randomly distributed. Thus, the peak of plasma ACTH precedes, in phase, that of cortisol, which in turn precedes, in phase, urinary OHCS acrophases, muscle strength, bronchial freedom, etc. The peak of blood eosinophils corresponds to the minimum plasma cortisol and vice versa. (Figure 55) The possible interference of a circadian rhythm must be considered when studying a monthly rhythm and vice versa. This event was usually ignored or underestimated. In five spontaneously menopausal women with a good apparent health status, the monthly changes of several physiological variables were analyzed based on the results of the circadian rhythm of these variables measured every four hours on days 1 (first day of menstruation) 8, 15, 22 and 29 of a menstrual cycle.

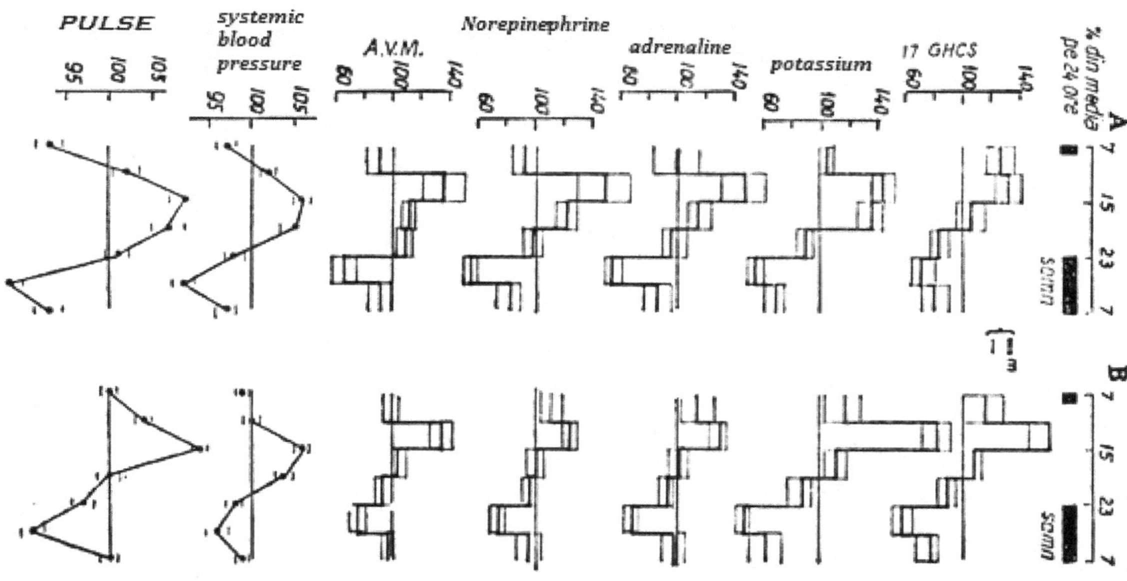

Fig. 55. The timing of circadian rhythms of physiological variables studied in seven healthy adults A: Normal activity and spontaneous regime. B: full bed rest (36 hours), hipocaloric regimen, meals at equal intervals (every 4 hours: water = 200 ml, K = 7 mEq, carbohydrate = 56). Circadian variation is expressed as a percentage of the 24-hour average (6 measurements) of each subject, then statistically controlled. Circadian rhythms persist under these conditions, with amplitude changes for some variables. After A. Reinberg, /. Ghata, F. Halberg, P. Gervais, Ch. Abulker, J. Dupont and Cl. Gandeau (1970) Ann. Endocrinol, (Paris), 31, 277, 287.

Taking as reference the median circadian level, the following monthly rhythms were validated and quantified (rectal temperature method) (Φ = day 23), cutaneous histamine reactivity (Φ = day 30), urinary excretion of water (Φ = day 21) Estrogen (Φ = 19), pregnanediol (Φ = day 20), 17 OHCS (Φ = 19), etc. Self-assessment of the mood and physical vigor shows that they also have circadian and circadian rhythms the latter being at the limit of statistical significance. (According to A. Reinberg, M. Smofensky, J. Ghata, A. and P. Gervais (1974) - Ann., Endocrinol (Paris), 35, 309-310) (Figure 56).

Besides, in humans, which is an animal with diurnal activity, the hours corresponding to the maximum values of cortisol, catecholamines, muscle strength, bronchial freedom, etc. Is within the day. On the contrary, in nocturnal animals such as rats and mice, nocturnal maxima of physiological variables occur in adaptation to the environment.

Social ecological synchronizers. We do not exaggerate when we say that we were born with a certain temporal structure exactly as we were born with a certain anatomy (spatial structure). A set of indirect arguments advocates the hereditary character of biological rhythms in humans. Direct arguments stem from experiments on plants and animals (*Bunning, 1963, Aschoff, 1963, Pittendrigh, 1960, Rensing, 1973, Hastings 1976, Van den Driessche 1971*). For example, biological rhythms persist during the isolation of man, thus living in the shelter of rhythmic variations of environmental factors (*Halberg, Reinberg, 1967, Aschoff, 1973, Reinberg, 1970, Mills, 1966*); Circadian variations are similar to monozygotic twins, but not to dizygotic twins (*Barcal* et al., 1968).

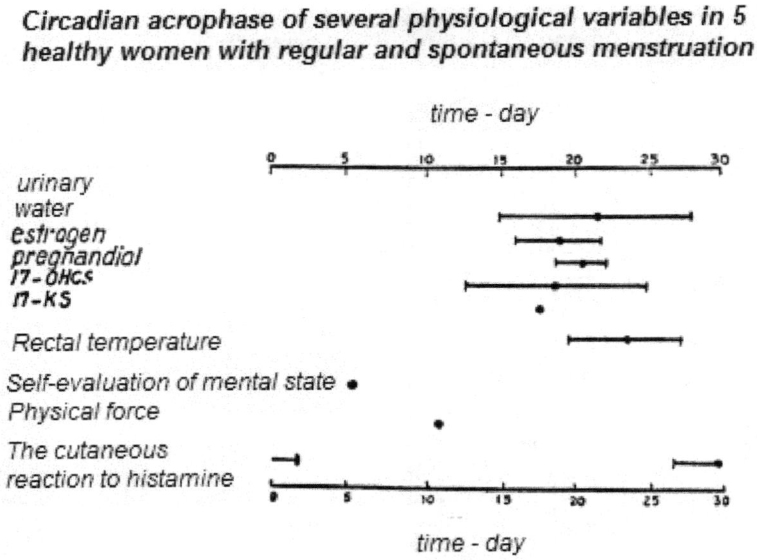

Fig. 56. Circumferential rhythms in five young women, spontaneously menstruated, Studied on a circadian basis.

However, biological rhythms are influenced by the periodic variations of a set of environmental factors: synchronizing or "time donors" or *Zeitgeber* (these are synonyms). The term "synchronizers" applies to any environmental factor that exhibits cyclic variations capable of modifying one or more of the parameters serving to characterize a biological rhythm (t, f, A, M). For many plant and animal species, the regular alternation of light and dark over a period of about 24 hours is one of the most powerful synchronizers. On the other hand, the regular alternation of noise and quiet, heat and cold, etc. Also acts as a circadian synchronizer for certain species and / or under certain experimental conditions. In humans, the most effective synchronizer is of ecological social nature (*Halberg et al., 1967, 1969; Aschoff et al., 1971; Apfel-baum et al., 1969*). This means that the alternation of the whole light-noise-heat activity and the rest-dark-quiet-cold ensemble, both of our social life and our ecological "niche", have a preponderant role in our synchronization.

Manipulation of a predominant synchronizer may refer to, for example, its period. It is possible - within certain narrow limits - to impose circular human rhythms for a period other than 24 hours, for example 23 or 25 hours (*Aschoff*, 1978 a and b). However, it was not possible to impose a period of 21 hours (*Simpson*, 1970) or 30 hours (*Gouars*, 1977) by manipulating the parameter t of ecological social synchronizers. When manipulation of a synchronizer is essentially focused on its phase, a movement of the circadian acrophase occurs. It is what happens, for example, after a six-hour Transmeridian flight between Paris and New York.

As far as the circanaal rhythms of man are concerned, there is probably a sin-crowning. Its nature is still unknown. It has been demonstrated by the experiences of the man-years: a) that the circana rhythms persist during isolation and b) that circana (seasonal) variations of the circadian photofrac- tion are capable of performing the role of a signal (Bunning, 1963; Benoit and Assenmacher, 1970; Pengelley, 1974; Assenmacher and Farner, 1978). In other words, the time of a 24-hour signal is interpreted by the sensitive body to carry out its circular function program. The latter is often a phenomenon related to reproduction: plant flowering, gonadal development in animals, certain migration processes in birds and mammals, periodic manifestation of secondary sexual processes (change of plumage, drowning, growth of cervids in cervids etc.). The signal can be given by light (the respective days and nights), but also by temperature or the process of an endocrine secretion. Observations regarding the study of the temporal and circanaal temporal organization in humans. Four observations may be useful:

Circadian, circamensul and circannual rhythms should be studied within the same experience. The fact that the bioperiodicity of a certain physiological variable can be expressed in several frequency domains has been verified in several animal species, especially in mice (Hans and Halberg, 1970), frog (Dupont et al., 1979) and man (Reinberg, 1974). When sampling takes place once a day, for example every two days, every week or every month, at different times or even at the same time, the values obtained may reflect a circadian variation rather than a circadian variation, or circanuală. In fact, not only the 24 hour average level, but also the time course of the circadian acrophase of a physiological variable may present a circadian or circular rhythm (Figure 57). The geographical situation (city, state) where the study was conducted should be indicated. In humans circular acrophase may depend on this situation, as shown for some variables by *Batschellet* et al. (1973), *Simpson* and *Bohlen* (1973), *Ghata* et al. (1977). Annual variations in daytime latitude appear to be one of the predominant factors (or signal) to be considered in various animal species. The results summarized in this paper have been obtained in subjects living in the northern hemisphere.

A temporal relationship between two variables does not, by itself, demonstrate a direct causal relationship. The latter may be presumed if, in addition to the temporal relationship, a number of other arguments can be presented (*Halberg*, *Reinberg*, 1967; *Reinberg*, 1974). Specifically, chronoendocrinology and reproductive phenomena must not be forgotten That several biophytic processes can play a role. Indeed, bioperiodicity (circadian, circulatory, circadian) may interest (among other things) on the one hand the production of a hormone and, on the other hand, the sensitivity of organs or target organisms to this hormone. In other words, we can not thank to study the biological rhythms of the plasma (or urine) values of a hormone. Periodic variations of systems capable of responding to their stimulation, including cellular hormone receptor systems (*Hughes* et al., 1976; *Spelsberg* et al., 1979), should also be studied.

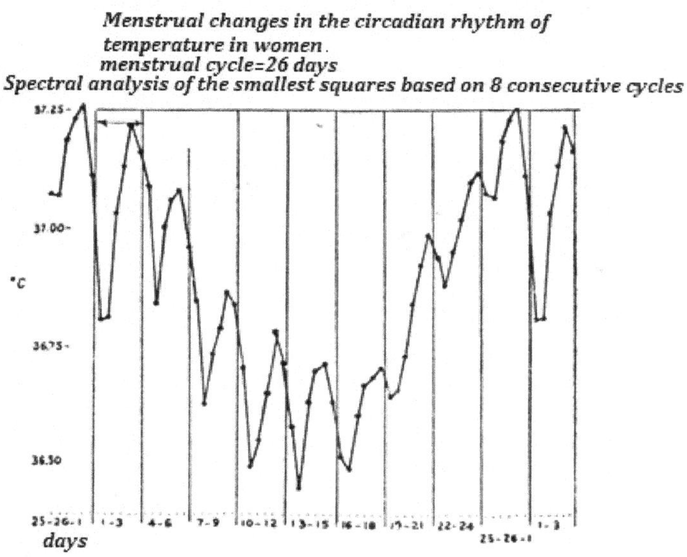

Fig. 57. Circumstances and circadian variations of oral temperature Of a spontaneously mistreated young woman.

The study covers eight cycles of 26 days. Circadian variations are studied on the three day averages (days 1- 3, 4- 6, etc.). The overlapping of the two periodicities (circadian and circadian) appears clearly on the chronograph. It is noted that the circadian tip is at 20.00 in the first part of the cycle (on days 1 and 15) and at 12 in the second part of the cycle. According to H. Simpson and E. Halberg in Biorhythms and Human Reproduction. John Wiley and Sons, New York, 1974, p. 552. We also mention that biorhythm is an anthropological parameter with a very high degree of individuality, being specific to every human organism. The correlation of global biorhythms (physical, emotional and intellectual) with the date of birth is explained, based on recent research, by the synthesis of genetically determined proteins. Thus, it has been shown that the moment of birth is achieved as a result of the growth in the fetus of the concentration of polypeptides synthesized by the genes of the conception product. This research explains scientifically both the materiality and the particular genetic component of biorhythms.

We will deal with global, physical, emotional and interelectric biorhythms, just to remember the other multiple biorhythms that are beginning to become more and more known. We mainly deal with these global biorhythms because they can be easily established by the coach, being of real use in his work, while the other biorhythms, although extremely important, in most cases require a meto- More complex dology of setting, where biochemistry is at the forefront and, corollary, the accessibility of use in ordinary sports practice is less.

The beginning of biorhythmology studies dates back to Hippocrates, indicating its disciples to write “good days”, “bad days” to both the sick and the healthy, and to consider their fluctuations in the treatment of patients.

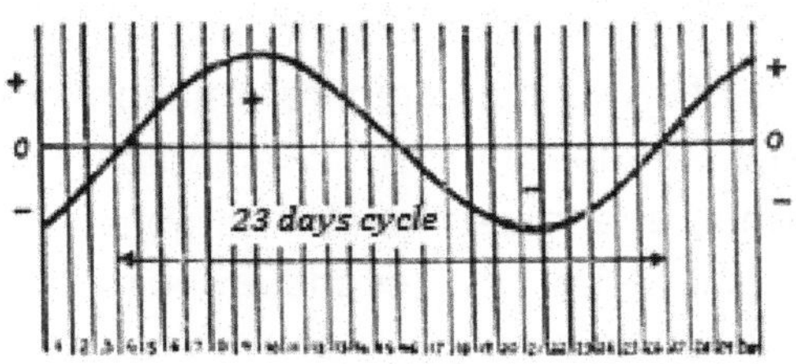

Fig. 58. On this graph, the physical cycle of 23 days begins a new period on the fourth day of the month and ends on 26th day. The first 11 days and a half correspond to a plus or a high period; The next 11 days and a half of a reheating or recovery period.

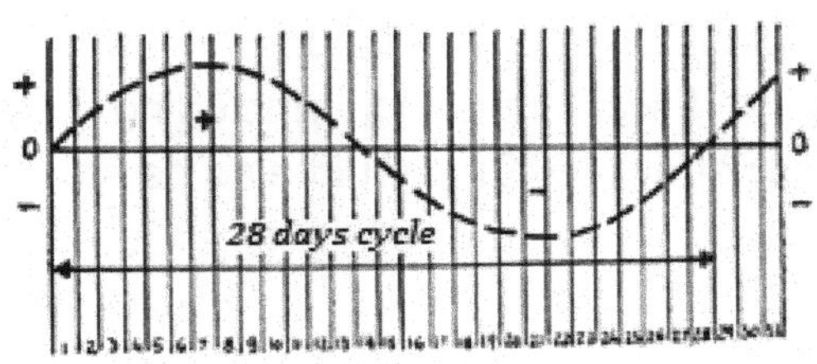

Fig. 59. The 28-day emotional cycle includes a “plus” period of 14 days and a period of” Minus” of 14 days, which can also be called recovery days.

At the end of the nineteenth century, *H. Swoboda* discovered two basic rhythms in man, one 23 days, physical and another 28 days, emotionally; Also shows that a series of biological manifestations in humans are periodically repeated, according to a genetic determination conditioned by the date of birth, by establishing a method of calculation for the detection of critical days according to the date of birth.

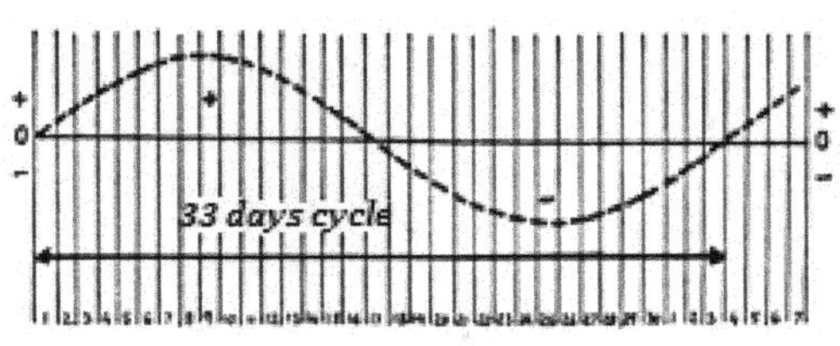

Fig. 60. Example of a 33-day intellectual cycle. This cycle comprises two periods of 16 and a half days, one. Plus and minus, as shown on this graph.

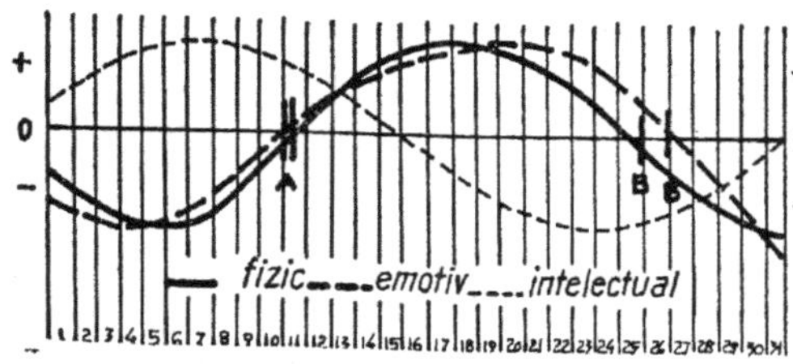

Fig. 61. Critical days are those days in which the cycle passes from the low phase to the high phase or vice versa, passing through the zero line. This graph shows a two-fold critical situation: the 11th of the month, in which the physical and emotional cycles (or emotional) are in their last day; 25th day of the month, the physical cycle goes down, day 26 - the emotional cycle goes down.

At the same time, Wilhem Fliess develops similar research to Swoboda's, confirming the existence of these biorhythms. He correlates biorhythms with the fact that the heredity of the human being is bisexual, each individual having both female and male characteristics, but some of them are predominant. Sigmund Freud, the founder of psychoanalysis, has also attested the existence of biorhythms of 23 and 28 days in humans.

Later, Alfred Teltsder in Innsbruck, through research on a large number of students, demonstrates the existence of an intellectual pace of 33 days, with successive regular intervals of maximum and minimum intellectual capacity among the investigated subjects.

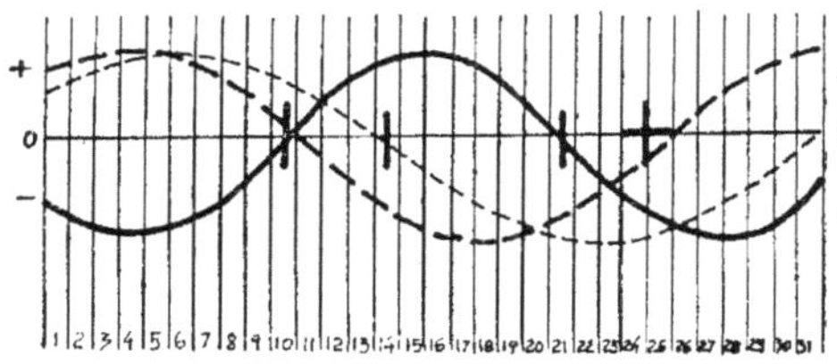

Fig. 62. Prime Minister Winston Churchill. On January 15, 1966, a medical bulletin from London announced that Sir Winston had an attack and was in a coma. It was a critical day in his intellectual cycle, which rarely corresponds to a heart attack. This enigma was resolved later when his doctor revealed that cardiac attack had been kept secret for four days and that Sir Winston had actually been shot down on January 11, which was a critical day in his emotional cycle and even a period Double criticism. His pulse continued to beat on Day 21, a critical day in his physical cycle, and death occurred on January 24, at the end of a period of his emotional cycle.

At the same time, *Rexford Hersey* in Pennsylvania, by doing a similar research, also discovers the existence of intellectual rhythm. The pleiad of researchers who have dealt with these three biorhythms (physical, emotional and intellectual) is numerous. We quote among them: Schawing, Bochaw, Tope, Pfeffer, W. Dements, Schlieper, Thomen, and others. All these researches and many others have provided biochemical, physiological, neurological, and psychological evidence of the existence of these biorhythms and the usefulness of their knowledge in conducting multiple human social activities, including sports. We will continue to present the three global, physical, emotional and intellectual cycles, showing their foundation on scientific data, the calculation of the three cycles and their applicability in different areas.

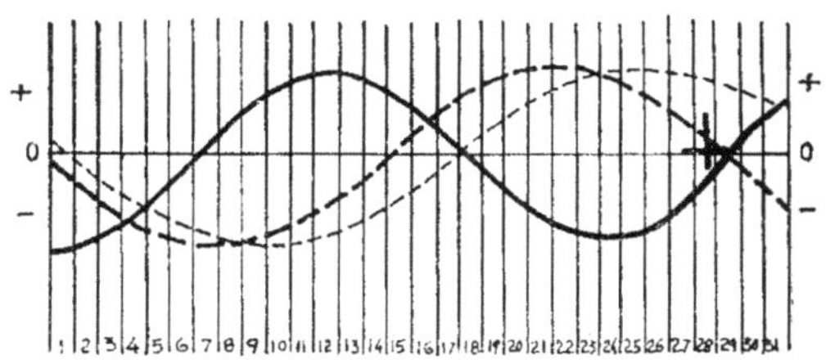

Fig. 63. Gamal Abdel Nasser succumbed to a heart attack on September 23, 1970. Nasser was born on January 15, 1918. At his death, his 28-day emotional cycle was in a critical position, going from high to low.

I. Physical Cycle. It has a span of 23 days (see Figure 58).

The first half of the cycle - lasting 11 and a half days - is the upward period. These are the days when man feels full and his vigor and resilience is at their maximum value, where physical work seems the easiest. Athletes generally - achieve their best performances during this positive period. The second half of the 23-day cycle is the descending period. Within 11 and a half days, a person tends to get tired more easily; For example, athletes are often in low form, have fewer physical reserves, less energy or resistance. Physicians consider descending periods as propitious for healing, because by temperament, during this period the patient is more willing to accept the rest.

The two important points in this cycle are the first day, when a new cycle begins (half way point) (11 days and a half) when the energy goes into the negative period.

We emphasize that the existence of this cyclicity has been based lately also on biochemical research on the various components that make up the substrate of muscle contraction. Thus, it has been shown that ATP, creatine phosphate, some enzymes that interfere with muscle contraction, etc. Have higher concentrations in the ascending period, which explains increased muscle strength and also aerobic and anaerobic capacity have higher values (Wiliams). These elements also allow us to use, in the negative phase, starting from the knowledge of this cycle, appropriate and more energetic means of refreshing, capable of avoiding physical, physiological decline and performance.

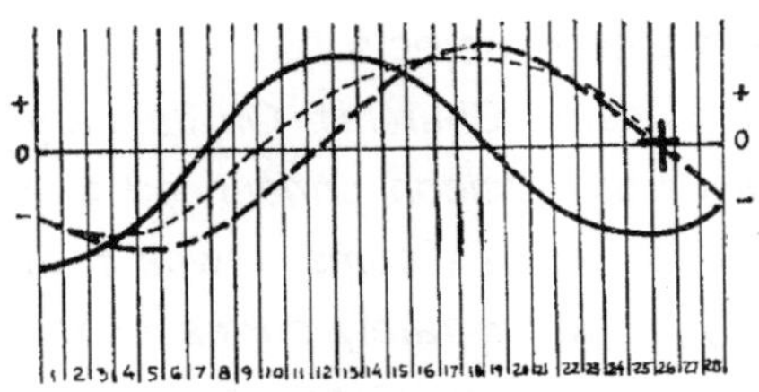

Fig. 64 "Fernandel". The great French actor Fernand Joseph Desiré Constantin, born on May 8, 1903, died of lung cancer on February 26, 1971, a double critical day.

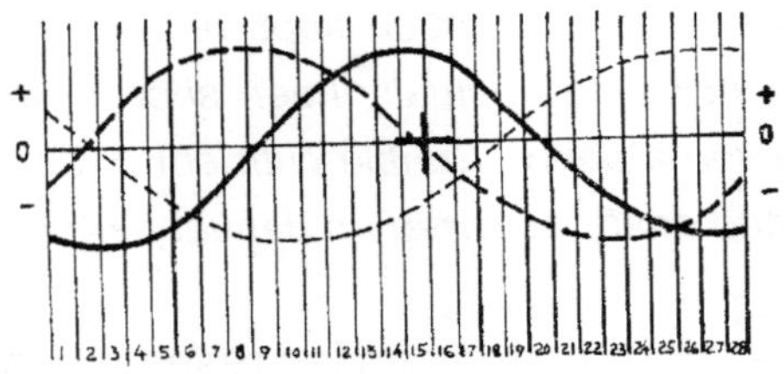

Fig. 65. Edgar Inow, born on 19 July 1905, a writer, died in Lausanne after having been operated on the night of 15 to 16 February 1972, which corresponds to a critical day in his emotional cycle.

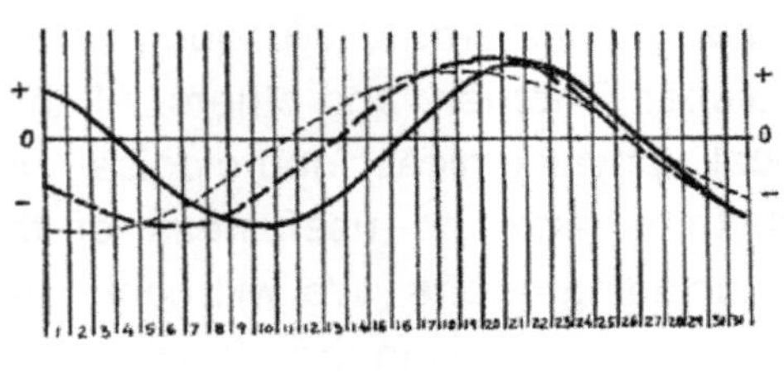

Fig. 66. The Duke of Windsor, born June 23, 1884, former King Edward VIII of England, died on May 28, 1972, a few days after a triple critical period.

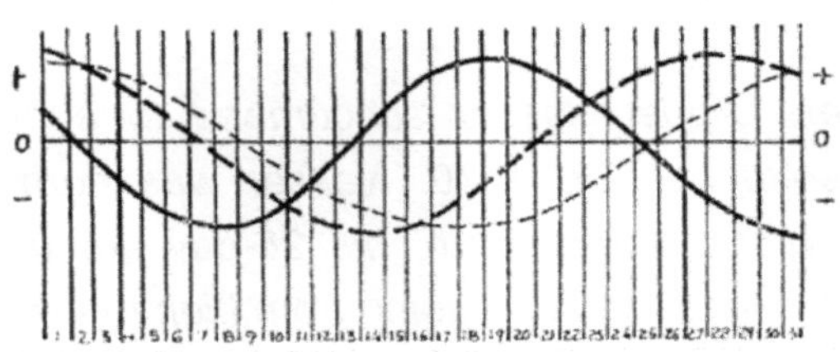

Fig. 67. Harry S. Truman, former US president, was born on 8 May 1884; After having had kidney and cardiac complications, died on a double critical day on December 26, 1972.

II. Emotional (emotional) cycle. It has a stretch of 28 days (see Figure 59)

This emotional cycle is divided into two equal periods. The first 14 days are the positive period, during which man is more inclined towards optimism. This period has a favorable influence on the creative spirit, the feelings, the activity of the nervous system. The second half, from day 14 through 28, is the negative period during which man is prone to irritation and negative attitude. Emotional people note that their sensitivity differences are more perceptible than in warm people. The 28-day emotional cycle involves critical days, which are the first day of the new cycle and the 15th day, after which the curve goes into a 14-day negation period. Careful days have to be taken care of, especially by the drivers of means of transport and all those who doubt their ability to react quickly and the safety of their judgments. The percentage of accidents, of personal origin, occurring on emotionally critical days, is additional and convincing proof of the influence of these cycles.

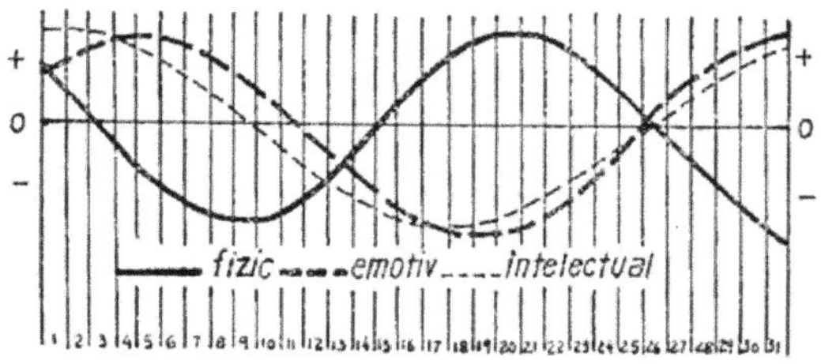

Fig. 68. This biorhythmic graph highlights a three-day critical of the well-known television star Arlene Francis on May 26, 1963. According to press reports, she lost control of her car, pulled down a barrier of separation and struck By another car. Calculated on the date of his birth (October 20, 1912), on May 26, 1963, his physical cycle alternated from a high phase to a low phase, and the emotional and intellectual cycles began a new period.

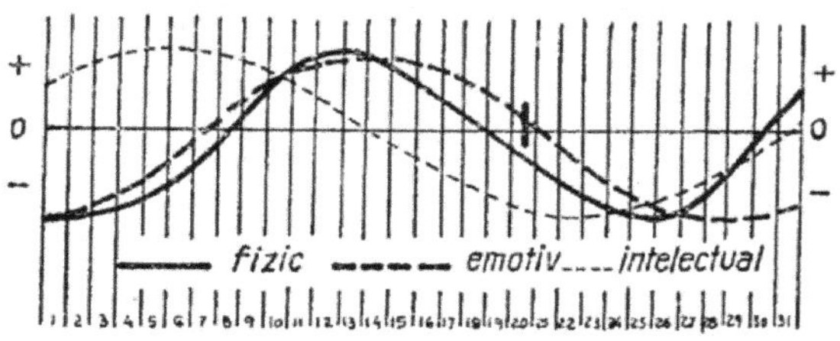

Fig. 69. Captain Virgil I. Grissom, born on April 3, 1926, described an orbit around the Earth on June 21, 1961. In the US, Saxon opened for unexplained reasons, causing the flood of the sinking capsule to flood. Grissom was about to drown. On this day, his biorhythmic mood was close to a critical situation in the emotional cycle, and his physical and intellectual cycle was both low-phase.

Convulsions of neurophysiology lately bring scientific evidence of the biochemical substrate of the existence of this cycle. Thus, Weiss, from the Rockefeller Institute in the U.S.A. Showed that in the positive period, the nervous cell contains an increased amount of glutamic acid and lecithin, its function being superior. Also, polarization and depolarization processes, which condition the transport of the nervous influx, are more intense. At the same time, the transconvulsive continuum voltage is greater, allowing a better balance between excitation and inhibition processes and irradiation and concentration processes (Secker, Ch. Bochman and H. Friedman, New York, U.S.A.).

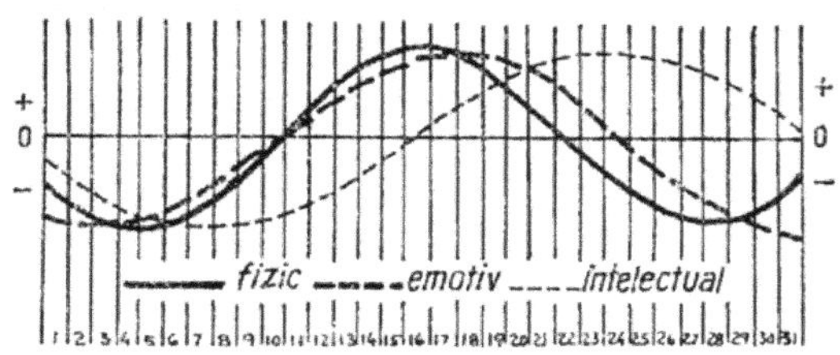

Fig. 70. Captain M. Scott Carpenter, born May 1, 1931, described three circumnavigating orbits on May 24, 1962. He exceeded his expected 250-mile america. The biorhythmic graph shows him close to a critical situation, both his emotional and physical cycle being in the low phases, and only his intellectual cycle being in the "plus".

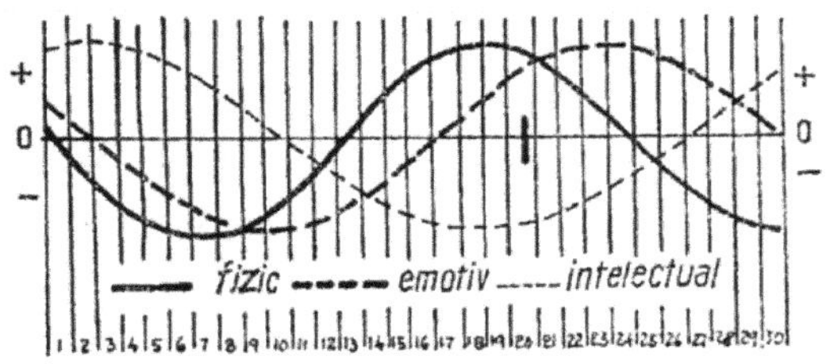

Fig. 71. When he won the title of world champion on the evening of June 20, 1960, Floyd Patterson, born on January 4, 1935, was in a high position in physical and emotional cycles.

III. Intellectual cycle. It has a stretch of 33 days (see Figures 60 and 61).

During the first half (16 days) of this cycle, man is able to think more clearly, memory works well and mental spontaneity is more vivid. This period is considered the optimal time for assimilation of new problems, for study and for creative thinking. The next 16 days and a half of cycle 33 constitute a period in which thinking capacity is reduced, in which new notions are difficult to assimilate, and in which the previously studied subject has to be revised and revised. Now is the best time to memorize (store) the knowledge in the subconscious and memory.

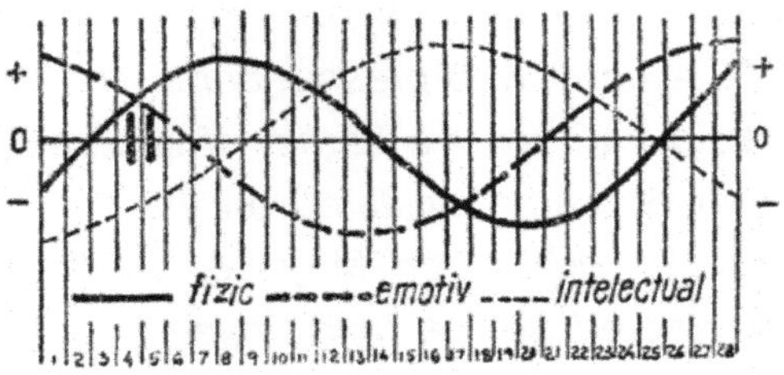

Fig. 72. Ingemar Johansson, born on 22 September 1932, was in a low position with his physical and emotional cycles when he lost the championship.

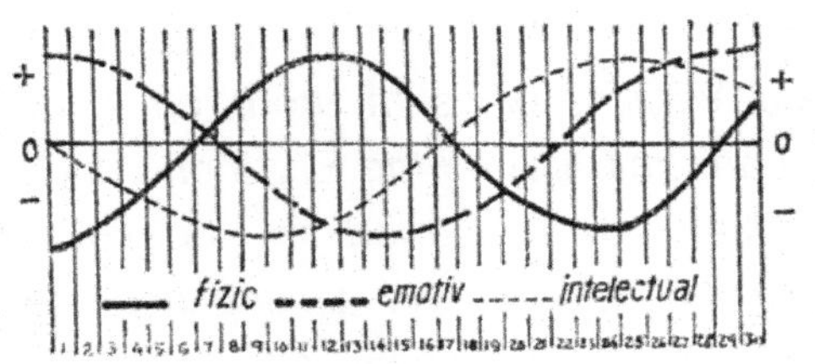

Fig. 73. John Uelses, born on July 14, 1937 in Germany, beat the world record of jumping with two successive evenings on February 4 and 5, 1962. With a 16-foot jump and a quarter of a finger: his physical and emotional cycles were both above. However, two weeks later, he could not even jump 14 feet, the two cycles being then down.

Here too, the critical days of the 33-day intellectual cycle are those that need to be supervised most rigorously. These are the 1st and the 17th day, being the beginning, respectively the half-cycle of the 33-day cycle. It is more prudent to know when these days occur, especially to those who have to make an important decision. If possible, decisions should be delayed for later, for more favorable days; But if this cannot be done, a maximum effort must be concentrated to think things well. We mention that the existence of this intellectual cycle was objectively based on neurological and psychological research. The presence of differences between electroence-phalographically recorded cerebral currents in positive and negative periods has been demonstrated; There were net differences in the performance of memory, verbal facility, logical thinking, based on negative and positive trials demonstrating superior intellectual capacity in the ascending phase, respectively in the first 16 days of this cycle.

As for the critical days of the three cycles, the first day of a new cycle and the one in which a cycle passes from positive to negative, they can be considered cycles switches, similar to electric phenomena related to lower intensity of some Light sources when switched to the network. These days man has to be more cautious, because it seems that the nervous system is the ground of frequent changes and has a very high degree of instability. Critical days, in themselves, are not dangerous. These are rather the days when the individual's reactions to the environment can lead to critical situations.The great advantage of biorhythm theory is that the critical day configuration scheme can be easily determined in advance. As these days account for less than 20% of an individual's life, protection and precautionary measures must be taken these days. The proverb “a man warned as two” is perfectly applicable to the person who makes his biorhythmic calculations.

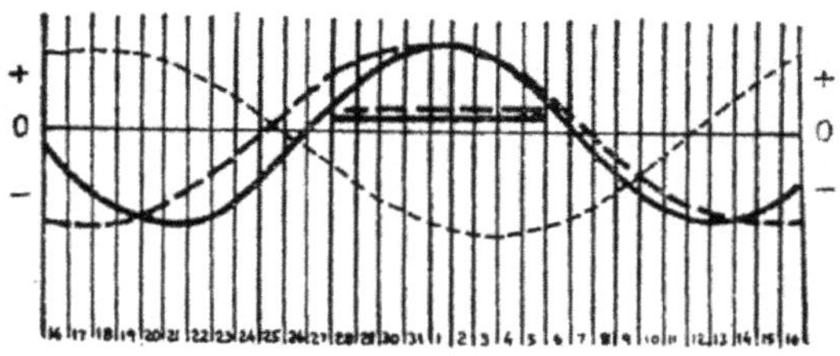

Fig. 74. Mark Spitz, born on February 10, 1950, a super Olympic champion, won seven gold medals and set new world records at the water. This one-week performance is unparalleled in the history of modern Olympics. At the end of August and the beginning of September in Munich, Mark Spitz was in a high period in both cycles, physically and emotionally.

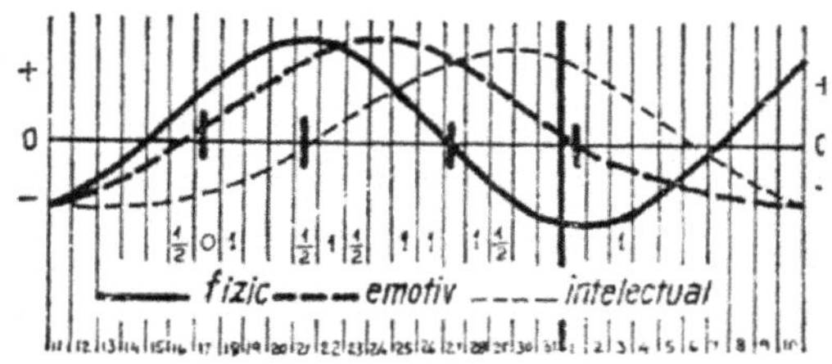

Fig. 75. Bobby Fischer, born March 9, 1943, lost only one game during the World Chess Championship in 1962 when he had a critical day In his emotional cycle - December 18, 1962.

It is estimated that the day or critical period has a duration of 24 hours. Since we have no compelling results of biological research, this estimation is empirically based on the analysis of accidents.

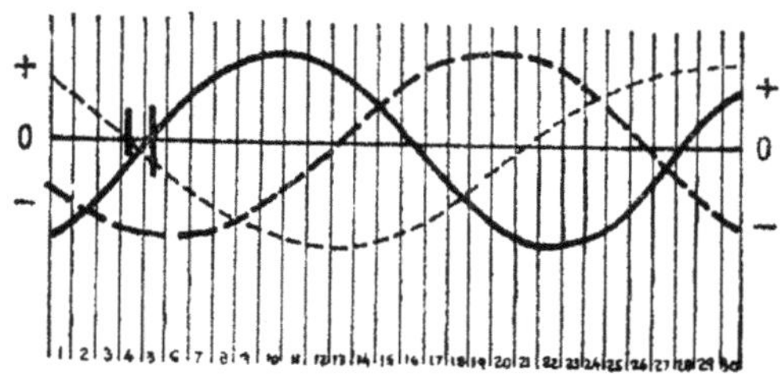

Fig. 76. Marilyn Monroe was born in June 1926. During the night of June 4 to June 5, 1961, the queen of stars and Hollywood stars swallowed too much a dose of sleeping pills.

Luckily the incident was discovered. Marilyn came back and could not be saved. His biorhythmic graph displays a critical position of his two cycles - intellectually and physically - combined with a depression of the emotional cycle. Experience shows that knowing the exact time of birth is of some importance. The subject that was born immediately after midnight or early morning will already be nearly a day old when another baby born in the last hours of the same day will make his first cry. Knowing the time of birth or at least the approximate moment of the day allows the biorhythmic plot to be drawn with more precision; in general, people born during the morning will have their critical days on the date of the chart that corresponds to the actual day of their birth and vice versa, People born late on the same day will find their biorhythmic graphical situation based on the day after birth.

Calculation of biorhythms

The biorhythmic mathematical method consists of counting the total number of days spent by an individual from his birth to the first day of the month we want to study. After determining this amount, it must be divided into 23, 28 and 33 days; The days remaining indicate the position of each cycle for the first day of the month to be shown on the graph. The process is simple but boring arithmetic, modern biorhythmic methods allow for avoidance of these calculations. However, it is good to review this biorhythmic computation method to understand the method as a whole. To give an example as clear as possible, let's take a clear example: a person born on August 10, 1940, and calculating the biorhythmic cycles for October 1, 1972.

From 10 August 1940 to 9 August 1972 are:

32 years of 365 days	→11,680 days
8 extra days for bite-years	→8 days

From 10 August 1972 to 1 October 1972 inclusive, there are also:

August	→22 days
September	→30 days
October	→1 Day
	53 days
Total	11,741 days

These are the base figures corresponding to the date of birth of August 10, 1940, chosen in this example. Numbers 4, 3 and 6 may be used for any period of this person's life in relation to any of the figures in Table C, as shown below. In other words, the basic figures obtained by combining Tables A and B are, in this calculation method, reliable assessments. By collecting the third figure, which will be found in Table C, it can obtain the exact position of each cycle at the beginning of each month to which it is chosen to be relayed. To finish with this example, we will use the October 1972 figures in Table C as follows (Table 21):

The final results - 11 for the physical cycle, 9 for the emotional cycle and 26 for the intellectual cycle - are the same as those obtained in the overall example of the mathematical calculations explained in the previous section. It is obvious that the use of tables allows not only time and effort, but also reduces the risk of errors.

Following our calculation, this person lived a total of 11741 days between the date of his birth, 10 August 1940 and 1 October 1972 inclusive. Now we divide this number of 11741 days with the units of the cycles, respectively, with 23, 28 and 33 days. The goal is to establish complete cycle units to obtain the exact position of each cycle on October 1, 1972. These divisions give the following results:

11741 divided by 23 = 510 complete units of 23 days and a plus of 11 days.

11741 divided by 28 = 419 complete units of 28 days and a plus of 9 days.

11 741 divided by 33 = 355 complete units of 33 days and a plus of 26 days.

The remaining figures, the 11, 9 and 26, indicate that the person on October 1, 1972 started the 11th day of a new physical cycle period (23 days). His emotional cycle (28 days) enters the 9th day, a new period beginning 8 days before, and his intellectual cycle (33 days) is at his 26th day, 7 days before his ending.

The interpretation of figures 11, 9 and 26 shows that on October 1, 1972, this person, born on August 10, 1940, approached the end of a high phase in his physical cycle (23 days), on October 2 being a critical half-day. The emotional cycle (28 days) reached the 9th day and is the same in high phase, during which the intellectual cycle (33 days) is in a low phase. An examination of the biorhythmic graph shows how a different compound scheme is formed each day (each cycle has a different length).

Interest in biorhythmic studies has been greatly amplified by introducing a series of spreadsheets, a triangulation calculation. Table A (Table 23) indicates a number for each day of the year and for each cycle the numbers are in line with all the possible birthdays in one year. Table B (Table 24) indicates a complementary number for each year from 1887 to 1990; These numbers are in reference to the year of birth.

By combining the numbers in Tables A and B for any given date, we can establish the base figures from the date of birth. Once set, these figures will not change for a particular person and will be used in all future calculations. To get the coordinates for a specific month, add the numbers in table C (table 25) to the base figures. Using the same birth date as in the previous example, proceed as follows (Table 20):

Table 20

	Physical cycle of 23 days	The emotional cycle of 28 days	The intellectual cycle of 33 days
Table A: August 10 Table B: 1940 If one of the totals is greater than 23, 28 or 33 respectively, then this figure is decreased.	9 +18 27 -23	3 +0 3 (28)	10 +29 39 -33
If it is smaller, make it appear as it is	4	3	6

These are the base figures corresponding to the date of birth of August 10, 1940, chosen in this example. Numbers 4, 3 and 6 may be used for any period of this person's life in relation to any of the figures in Table C, as shown below. In other words, the basic figures obtained by combining Tables A and B are, in this method of calculation, reliable assessments. By collecting the third figure, which will be found in Table C, the precise position of each cycle can be obtained at the beginning of each month to which it is chosen to be re-evaluated. To finish with this example, we will use the October 1972 figures in Table C as follows (Table 21):

These final results - 11 for the physical cycle, 9 for the emotional cycle and 26 for the intellectual cycle - are the same as those obtained in the example of the mathematical calculations explained in the previous section. It is obvious that the use of tables allows not only time and effort, but also reduces the risk of errors.

Table 21

	Physical cycle of 23 days	The emotional cycle of 28 days	The intellectual cycle of 33 days
The basic figures after the date of birth, as set out earlier Figures for October 1972 in Table C. Lower, respectively, 23, 28, or 33 when the totals are greater than 3 digits If they are smaller, leave them like that.	4 +7 11 (23)	3 +6 9 (28)	6 +20 26 (33)
Exactly precise figures for October 1972 chart	11	9	26

There is generally the tendency to look at the positive phase of biorhythm as good, and the negative one as bad. Japanese school research still shows that this is a simplistic and even erroneous vision. The investigations undertaken show that for those who tend to live in a high, excessive phase, the low phase is an excellent period in which they operate best.

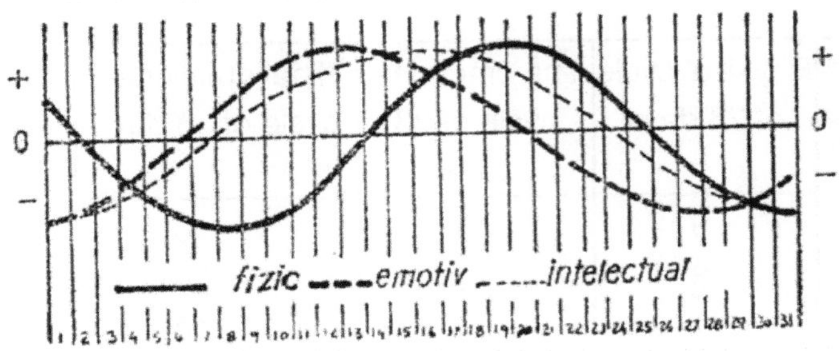

Fig. 77. William Faulkner, Nobel Prizewinner for Literature, born on 25 September 1897 and died on July 6, 1962, of a heart attack. His biorhythmic chart indicates a critical day in his emotional cycle.

For correct biorhythm interpretation, a test should be performed which resulted in optimal biorhythm timing. The Biorhythm Laboratory led by Professor Kichinosuke Tatai, the director of the Institute of Biorhythmology in Tokyo, has produced a test sheet for testing biorhythmic skills for physical, emotional and intellectual cycles.

In each cycle, the test characteristics that match the individual's individuality are revealed and the differences between positive and negative notations are seen. Depending on the number of positive or negative elements recorded and the differences between them, the biorhythm is interpreted according to a biorhythm self-training sheet indicating what conduct the person concerned should adopt in order to obtain an optimum return in both positive and negative phases. Biorhythm self-training record is a systematized model of planning the application of biorhythm to everyday life and finding the most fruitful way of self-training. The Japanese have also established psychological and working means to increase their individual potential according to the biorhythm phase.

To make good use of biorhythm in everyday life, the following test, developed by the Japanese biorhythmology school, should lead to the optimal application of the biorhythm calendar. The secret of success in this endeavor is to combine test results with the biorhythm calendar and knowledge of one's own personality (introverted or extrovert). You combine in each cycle the features that suit you. If there is a difference of more than three of the + / - rounded aspects in each cycle or if there is a difference of more than five between the circumscribed +/- total characteristics refer to the biorhythmic skills advice (s) that is in the self-.

CHICAGO VERIFICATION FILE - BIORITM

Made by the Japanese Biorhythm Laboratory

KICHINOSUKE TATAI

F (Physical Cycle)

+	Predisposed to cold Predisposed to constipation You suffer from liver Refuse to listen to the tips You like fat meals
-	Predisposed to diarrhea Predisposed to fatigue Rheumatic tendency Become thirsty slightly Tilted to simple, light dishes You can not fall asleep fast at night

I (Intellectual Cycle)

+	You often have brilliant ideas (good) You are often worried You are disturbed slightly Unhappy if your ideas Is not achieved Tilted to modern music
-	You like mystery novels Plan things well Good, skillful in manual work You have beautiful writing You enjoy listening to classical music Good grades at school

E (Emotional Cycle)

+	Speak frequently and easily at conferences You suffer from frequent migraines You have many friends You lose your calm and small issues You pay attention to money
-	Sensitive to mode Carefully put things to one side for storage You suffer from a lack of malleability You are easily deceived by people You are sentimental and romantic Perpetual poor physical condition You like cleanliness

BIORITHM AUTHORITY DOCUMENT

(Made by the Japanese Biorhythm Laboratory)

F (Physical Cycle)

• If you have surrounded more than six positive and negative elements on critical days 0, be cautious with speed, drink or other activities that may physically harm you.

• If you have surrounded more than three positive features, be careful not to do anything unhealthy or excessive during the positive (high) phases.

• If you have surrounded more than three negative features, be careful to have proper rest and eat consistently during the negative (low)

E (Emotional Cycle)

• If you encircled more than six positive and negative features on critical days 0, keep yourself safe: do not overtake other cars if you are driving and do not want to express your opinions.

• If you have surrounded more than three positive features in your phases. Positive, be moderate in all, and respect the feelings of others.

• If you have surrounded more than three negative features, you are struggling to be positive and not to inconvenience others in your phases. negative.

I (Intellectual Cycle)

• If you have surrounded more than six positive and negative features at critical times 0, be especially careful when checking the stops before crossing the street and avoiding losing things.

• If you have surrounded more than three positive features in your phases. Positive, do not be hasty or greedy; Work carefully with the piece.

• If you have surrounded more than three negative features in your phases. Negative, sleep long enough and plan your work especially in the morning.

It also follows that there are no absolute values in biorhythm, and it produces wobbling movements and fluctuations that, due to their low value, involve difficulties in their individual assessment compared to circadian cycles. Considering this, American scientist Wilder formulated the law of the initial value of biorhythm. Thus, for example, a hereditary intelligent child, even in its low phases, is brighter than an unintelligent child, even when it is in its high phase. Similarly, a strong physical person, even in its low phases, is superior to a weak man in its best form.

On the basis of this law we have established graphs that indicate the value of the positivity or the negativity of the biorhythmic phases. We emphasize that biorhythm does not have to be looked at fatalistically. His knowledge can lead to self-training and proper self-education associated with the directed action of external environmental factors that ultimately lead to a substantial optimization of sports activity. This is all the more evident as Japanese research demonstrates the marked participation of hormones in the biorhythm determination by the variations in concentrations that they record during the different biorhythmic phases, variations which, as they are known, can be corrected in the course of time depending on the requirements of the activity sportive.

The applicative aspects of biorhythms are multiple (Figure 62-75).

Thus, between biorhythms and the performance of some cosmonauts have established obvious correlations.

The flight of Lieutenant Commander M. Scott Carpenter on May 24, 1962, which described three circumferential orbits, was about to have a tragic ending. On the day of his adventurous flight, Carpenter was emotionally critical, in a top position intellectually and physically depressed. As noted before, peak and depression positions do not have such a strong influence as critical day. This is especially true if two of the cycles are in opposition to one another - one is at the top, the other in the depression - because an adjustment or compensation element comes into play - in Carpenter's case it is A critical period of the emotional cycle that could come into question. After his reports, he mistakenly used too much fuel, leaving the automatic control system running, so he also used fuel for manual maneuvers to determine the capsule during its orbital flight. From the return, the space ship n was tilted to the right angle, so that for several minutes he thought the pilot was lost. His mistakes made him overcome the 250-mile-long amphibious point. Later, in an interview with a newspaper, Carpenter has excused himself for his “monumental gaffe.”

Carpenter's biorhythmic graphs clearly show the possibilities of human error for the period May 24, 1962. (Figure 70) Reporting on aviation accidents by the US Air Force Center. To find that in 80% of cases, the catastrophe coincided with at least a critical day of the pilot (Wooham).

In the medical field, we can refer to *Dr. F. Wehrli's* exposure in Lucarno, Switzerland, in the preface of the book "Bioritm", where he certifies that he has used biorhythmic mathematics in his hospital over a period of more than 15 years, To determine the most favorable days for surgery, where delays could be made. He practiced more than 10 000 operations without any failure or smallest complication. Statistics show that 30% to 60% of the cases of complication are not considered when biorhythmic cycles are not taken into account. Similar data are provided by *Wehrli* and *U.S.A.* In Japan, biorhythm graphs and their application to road, rail and air transport are in the field of current practice and have led to a marked decrease in the number of accidents. Thus, we quote the Naga Hama Transport Division, Seibu Transport Company and IMO Railways, which, by applying biorhythms to transport managers, have reduced accidents by 35 40%. We mention that in Tokyo there is a biorhythmology institute with 5000 researchers.

There is also a series of data on the links between biorhythm and sports performance.

The reason that explains the abundance of material about sport and biorhythm is the broad way in which biorhythm methods were used by German team coaches at the Munich Olympics to improve performance. For a long time, coaches and leaders of Professional teams have formed biorhythmic maps that they used to train the members of those teams to make them able to evolve to the maximum during the meetings. Coaches and managers continue to use biorhythm.

We quote a few significant examples.

The complex interpretation of the biorhythmic phases based on the above-mentioned sheet attests to the validity of the biorhythms for sport performance.

Thus, *Nobunon Taguchi*, who set a new world brass record and won Japan's first gold medal in swimming, adopted a calm attitude. He said he would win in the second half of the race and did it. This attitude, supported by the three low negative phases of the three cycles of biorhythm, played an important role in his victory.

Winners of major horse racing games in Japan often had a similar biorhythm condition, demonstrating the erroneous character of simplistic belief that the positive phase is always good and the bad one is always bad. Research into studying the careers of famous swimmers, such as Taiho and Kashiwado, revealed that the two were strongly influenced by biorhythm conditions and that the influence is stronger for experienced swimmers. Biorhythm conditions can create the difference between two people of equal power.

Boxing requirements, different from those of swimming, make it possible to predict a biorithm of gain or defeat easier. The observation of various sporting performances reveals how much change in biorhythmic position can lead to Profound and significant influence on victory, defeat, and death. This was the boxing series between Floyd Patterson and Ingemar Johansson, who made a big deal in the newspapers. From a biorhythmic point of view, the two men were almost inversely. In the three cycles, when Floyd was "up," Ingemar was "down" and the other days. Otherwise, they were equal in strength, skill and training, so only the biorhythmic position, we can say, is a decisive factor, which has been shown successively in important matches. At the first match in Stockholm, Sweden, Ingemar received the title of champion, his emotional and intellectual cycles being both "up", while the emotional cycle was at the end of the recovery period. For Floyd only the emotional cycle was "up" (fig. 71, 72)

When Ingemar went back on the ring for the return match against Floyd in New York, on June 20, 1960, all the bets were for him. At him the physical and emotional cycles were "down," while these cycles were "upstairs" at Floyd. Victory was Floyd's. Further their encounters have demonstrated the correlation between cycles and performance.

Benny Paret and his death is a demonstrative example of a boxer entering the ring when his bio chances were triple critically. Such a situation is particularly difficult to overcome, especially for someone who should have come back into shape after a great effort and after a particularly hard fight. After it was made K.O. by a brave opponent, the chances of making it right were very small. The records tell us that Paret never came to his senses and died on the next critical day; As indicated by its biorhythmic graph, its biorhythmic "batteries" could not be loaded again so quickly.

The case of John Uelses - the rookie - demonstrates very well the connection between the sudden change in the shape of an athlete and the fluctuations of his biorhythmic graph. On February 3, 1962, Madison Square Garden, an unknown - Uelses - established a new record in the world, with a 16-foot leg jump and a quarter-finger (old-ness). No one before, either in the hall or in the open air, has jumped sixteen feet to the jump.

This tremendous performance was somewhat spoiled by a very zealous photographer who, after the Uelses jump, accidentally hit the pillars that held the bar making him fall. Without being distracted by this unpleasant adventure, Uelses repeated his performance the following night in Boston during the "Atletic Association" games.

However, two weeks later at Louisville, when he had expected another star performer from Uelses, he was unable to jump fourteen feet. The setting of the chart highlights Uelses' favorable biorhythmic position when he had his record of jumping and his subsequent negative position on February 17, 1962. (Figure 73) His three cycles - physically, emotionally, intellectually - were all three up almost all the time, and two of his "virtual" critical days were "relach" days. It would have been interesting to ask what score he would have done if the contests were held two weeks earlier. When his three cycles were in the low position, to the maximum.

Chess being rather an examination of mental dexterity than physical tension, it can be considered that the emotional cycle of 28 days and the intellectual cycle of 33 days are the most important. The first game, which took place on December 17th, ended in a null match on the eve of Fischer's first critical day and lost on December 18, a critical day in his emotional cycle. It had to be a deceptive debut, but it was the only match lost by Fischer throughout the championship and also the only critical day he played. (Figure 75)

On December 20, he won, but the next day had some stress again, with only a nil, his intellectual cycle being in a critical time. A winning game, another null and two other games followed on December 26 and 27. On day 28, he criticizes in his physical cycle, the commissioners commissioned to schedule him favored without knowing, giving no game to play on that day. On January 1, the New Year's Day, again "relache"; He finished the championship by a victory on January 3rd.

The scheme of victories, null parties, and Fischer's victories shows that biorhythms can predict "performance whims". Applying biorhythmic mathematics to the field of games is therefore as logical as possible. However, it does not mean that a player who knows his biorhythmic position is not favorable, must give up a match. The spirit and the body of man are quite malleable because, knowing the contrary conditions, they can remedy them. Also, the means of rehabilitation and psychological training, correctly conducted in a negative biorhythmic phase, can balance this disability. Recent research reveals the existence of correlations between mother's biorhythmic periods and the sex of the conception product.

The sex of a child is determined at the moment of conception. The decisive factor is the male body, because it depends on the fertilization of the egg - the exclusive X chromosome - by a sperm cell possessing either a X (female) chromosome or a Y chromosome (male). There is also another factor that must be taken into account in establishing the relationship between biorhythms and the determination of the sex of a child. Biologists say that, in general, only the event decides whether it is an X cell or a Y cell that will first reach the egg and fertilize it. Another theory claims that the egg is at times more prone to accept an X cell, and at other times, a Y cell. Therefore, if the first seeded cell that reaches the ovum and produces fertilization is accepted by this egg, would depend on certain female physical factors present at that time.

From a biorhythmic point of view, this assumes that when the mother's physical cycle is positive at the time of conception, the egg is prone to accept the Y cells, which will give birth to a male child. Also, if the emotional cycle is positive for the mother, at the moment of conception, the researchers have the belief that a girl will be born. What makes these hypotheses grounded is that the high physical cycle (of 23 days) carries an alkaline composition in the blood, while an emotional cycle (28 days) tends to create an acidic environment. Also, the biorhythm study provides sociologically important data on the compatibility of some people. There is thus a high level of compatibility between couples that have similar or similar biorhythmic characteristics. Comments: The percentages corresponding to the 28-day and 33-day cycle calculations have been rounded to the nearest whole numbers.

Hugo Max Cross in his book "Biorhytmik. Das Auf und Ab Unserer Lebenskraft "(Theory of Biorhythms, High and Low Phases in our Life) devotes several chapters to explaining cyclical correspondence within marriages, associations, teamwork, and other sociological situations. Having the same date of birth would mean a 100% biorhythmic compatibility for all three cycles. There are, however, many fluctuations that allow the three cycles to be close to each other; For the 23-day physical and emotional cycles of 28 days, they are harmonized over the full with each multiple of 644 days (Table 22). The calculations that make it possible to find biorhythmical compatibility between two people are really simple. It starts by comparing "base figures by birth date" (totals of tables A and B) or figures for the current month. The idea is to determine by how many days each person's cycle departs from the corresponding cycle of another person. Once the difference days gap has been established, we can know the appropriate percentage on the "Compatibility Table". For example, D.J., born 6.1.1926 and D.M. Born 16.XI.1928 will calculate their biorhythmic compatibility as follows:

DJ	DM
Born January 6, 1926	Born November 16, 1928
Table A 19 24 29	Table A 4 18 12
Table B 2 17 27	Table B 7 14 22
21 41 56	11 32 34

To decrease each complete cycle; If it is smaller, it does so:

23 28 33	23 28 33
21 13 23	11 4 1

The figures based on the birth date of D. J.:21 13 23
The figures based on the birth date of D.M.: 11 4 1
The lowest of the highest figures are subtracted 10 9 22
To find the number of days
Consult the "Compatibility Table" to know the amount of the corresponding percentage:
10 day difference in the 23 day cycle = 12% compatibility
9 day difference in the 28 day cycle = 36% compatibility
22 days difference in the 33-day cycle = 33% compatibility
Total =82%

Table 22

Compatibility table

The 23-day cycle		The 28-day cycle		The 33-day cycle	
No. of days away	Percentage %	No. of days away	Percentage %	No. of days away	Percentage %
1	2	3	2	5	6
0	10	0	10	0	10
1	91	1	9	1	9
2	82.6	2	8	2	8
3	73.9	3	7	3	8
4	65.2	4	7	4	7
5	56.5	5	6	5	7
6	47.8	6	5	6	6
7	39.1	7	5	7	5
8	30	8	4	8	5
9	21	9	3	9	4
10	1	1	2	1	3
1	4	1	2	1	3
1	0	1	1	1	2
11.5	4	1	7	1	2
1	1	1	0	1	1
1	21	1	7	1	9
1	30	1	1	1	3
1	39.1	1	2	16 1/2	0
1	47.8	1	2	1	3
1	56.5	1	3	1	9
1	65.2	2	4	1	1
2	73.9	2	5	2	2
2	82.6	2	5	2	2
2	91	2	6	2	3
2	10	2	7	2	3
3	0	2	7	2	4
		2	8	2	5
		2	9	2	5
		2	10	2	6
		8	0	2	7
				2	7
				3	8
				3	8
				3	9
				3	10

To find the average compatibility of D.J. And D.M., divide the total of the three percent by three (82: 3); The average compatibility is therefore 27.3%. The 27.3% compatibility percentage of this couple is a relatively low average, and their reactions and feelings will often be contradictory, but their personality counts too much. To study the theory of biorhythmic compatibility, it is important to evaluate separately the percentage of each cycle. A high 23-day physical cycle compatibility is very important for those who are part of a sports team or for those who have a very active physical life. In fact, their peak and depression times will occur approximately in the same days. In Europe, some soccer teams use these guidelines and make up their front lines in such a way as to obtain the best results. There is little appeal to key players during their vacation days, so that their forces are put on hold. The 28-day cycle that looks at nerve reactions and emotion is the one that demands the most attention for a couple and in family life. Given that the 33-day intellectual cycle indicates the fluctuations of the intellect (the ability of a man to assimilate new subjects and to remember them), this cycle only has a minor influence on the ability to understand with the neighbor. Lately, apart from these physical, emotional and intellectual biorhythms, the biological rhythms of some homeostatic constants of the body and their correlations with the global biorhythms we have presented are being investigated more and more.

The role of hormones in biorhythm

From the point of view of the balance of the human being, the autonomic nervous system and the endocrine system, which is controlled by the first one, are of the greatest importance. The center of endocrine regulation is the hypothalamic pituitary system. It is particularly interesting from the point of view of biorhythm that C.I. Parhon reported the efficacy of thyroid hormones in the treatment of cyclical diseases.

The study of the connection between the nervous and endocrine systems is physiologically correlative. Pro-fault in this study has influenced biorhythmic research. Cyclical action of biorhythm is activated by hormones. The menstrual cycle seems to be one of the conclusive factors of this hypothesis. Unfortunately, even the most sophisticated modern scientific knowledge is not able to define why the menstrual cycle is on average 29 days. All that can be said is that experience demonstrates this. Also, we can not explain why the biorhythmic cycles are 23, 28 and 33 days.

It is known that the menstrual cycle results from the dynamic balance of operations of more than five hormones: three products of the anterior lobe of the pituitary gland, plus ovaries produced by the extrogenes and progesterone. Moreover, the balanced process of these hormones influences the nervous state and innumerable other factors.

The adrenocorticotropic hormone produced by the anterior lobe of the hypophysis stimulates the adrenal cortex to secrete corticoid hormones. These and the catecholamine group (adrenaline and noradrenaline) provide important energy sources for circadian cycles.

Richter shows that not only human beings, but also animals, there are many data that indicate the significant participation of thyroid hormones: thyroxine and triiodothyronine. However, there is a dynamic balance in the amounts of these hormones produced by thyroid stimulation by pituitary-secreted pituitary hormone. Reducing thyroid function aggravates those diseases described by Richter as cyclic. Conversely, stimulation of the thyroid can lead to ameliorations in such diseases, both in humans and animals. From the data presented, it is possible to deduce the following: pituitary and hormone adrenal system, acting together or separately, determine the biorhythm. Also, acad works. Stefan M. Milcu proves that there is an individual biorhythm of hormonal secretions that reach a maximum of 24 hours for each individual. Investigating the rhythm of the secretion of the main hormones involved in the exercise, cortisol, catecholamines and thyroid hormones by immunological radioactivity, concludes that a maximum yield in the sporty sample is obtained when the maximum concentration in organisms is reached by these hormones.

Hence the possibility of managing them strictly individualized, without harming the organism and being dopping, so that we can positively influence the sporting result obtained in competitions. We conclude that biorhythms are the biologically determined genetic parameters that define globally the constitutional type, their knowledge being of particular importance both for the attainment of the sport form and for the individualized training of the training and the adequate use of the means of rehabilitation and of the psychological training. Biorhythmic negative phases can be offset. Thus, the negative physical cycle benefits from all the biochemical and rehabilitation methods; Emotional and intellectual intellectual cycles can be balanced both by administering tonic substances to the nervous system and through adequate psychological training. Without being a universal panacea, the knowledge of physical, emotional and intellectual and homeostatic global rhythms (hormonal, energetic, sexual, etc.) allows, by adequate balancing of the organism, in accordance with the physiological situation created by the biorhythmic moment, to lead to Enhancing physical, emotional, intellectual, biochemical, energetic capacity, etc. Of the body, to give the possibility of achieving greater performances in different fields of activity, including sports.

The biological rhythms, as I have already pointed out, reflect only the reaction of organisms to some periodicities of the environment, which are probably periodically fixed genetic responses such as the electrical waves produced by the encephalic activity (the electroencephalogram), the pulse, the menstrual cycle but which are influenced By the environment, such as the geophysical cycles, the astronomical night, the success of the seasons, etc., and these biological rhythms reflecting, in fact, the interference between genotype and paratip. Valuable research in this area of chronobiology was undertaken in our country at the Institute of Endocrinology (Ştefan M. Milcu and then Grazziela Nicolaie) in collaboration with the University of Minesota (USA), demonstrating the circular and circulatory frequency of endocrine and Of the biochemical parameters of special clinical importance, which characterize the age groups of the Romanian population. It has been shown that each hormonal or biochemical homeostatic component has a characteristic synchronicity. These include ACTH, insulin, progesterone, testosterone, Ca, cholesterol, glucose, serum proteins, immunoglobulins, gastric acid, etc. The same applies to the blood components: hemoglobin, red blood cells, leucocytes, reticulocytes, etc. Interestingly, diurnal blood pressure variations are also interesting. Thus, in day-time staff, tension increases in the afternoon and evening. It decreases in the first hours of sleep and increases in the last hours and in the early hours of the morning. Associated with hormonal rhythms, it has been shown that the maximum tension value coincides with the maximum level of aldosterone concentration, while the diastolic maximum is related to the maximum concentration of plasma renin. This is important both for the pathology and therapy of hypertensive disease and for the programming of sports training at the time of day when the tension values are minimal and the adaptation can be done in better conditions. Similar rhythms are known to be characterized by a very strict individualization for hematopoiesis, pulse, antibody production, all of which are of particular importance in the prophylaxis of some diseases, in pathology, in therapy, and in the scientific periodization of sports training.

An important area of applicability of these biological rhythms is cronophar-macology, which has as objective the study of the effects of the drugs according to the temporal biological synchronization, as well as the deciphering of the effects of the drug agents on the very biorhythms themselves. On this basis the principle of chronotherapy was based. Clench showed for indomethacin that the fastest rate of disappearance and the shortest time to obtain maximum plasma concentration is obtained by administering between 7-11 in the morning and the opposite effect when administered between 19-23. The highest effect of acetylsalicylic acid (aspirin) is in the morning and caffeine around 15.00 hours, of course, there are individual variations, with the stability of each biologically determined, genetically determined rhythm that characterizes each human subject. The deciphering of these rhythms opens up special perspectives in the most efficient, strictly individualized administration of the supporters of the athletes' effort, and as I have emphasized, both in terms of the value and intensity of the sports training and in its daily, weekly and annual, so that its effectiveness is maximal for sport performance and craftsmanship.

A circadian rhythm of great importance for sports is that discovered by Winker. Body temperature variations are measured as follows: one hour after scaling (1) then 4 to 4 hours (II, III, IV, V). Thus, five values are obtained, resulting in a sixth (VI) by the following calculation (I + II + V) - (II + IV) = VI which is considered night temperature. Then a representation graph is made. By correlating this graph with physical and intellectual capacity, it was found that the temperature rises phases represent circadian periods in which the receptivity of the structures and the yield in the physical effort is maximum, while the phases of the temperature decrease are characterized by the maximum capacity of intellectual activity and Smart driving learning.

This element is of particular importance in training sessions over the course of a day, so that efficiency is maximized in the formation of motricity skills or in the development of the necessary motricitying skills in the sporting field where training is done.

Table 23

Table A

Day	January			February			March			April		
	F	E	I	F	E	I	F	E	I	F	E	I
1		00	0		25	0		2	0		22	09
2	0	27	0	1	24	2	1	5	7	0	21	08
3	0	26	32	5	23	01	0	04	06	2	20	07
4	2	25	31	1	22	00	0	23	05	0	19	06
5	2	24	30	4	21	32	9	22	04	1	18	05
	2		29	1		31	0	21	03	0		
6	1	23		3	20		8			0	17	04
7	2	22	28	1	19	30	0	20	02	2	16	03
8	0	21	27	2	18	29	7	19	01	2	15	02
9	1	20	26	1	17	28	0	18	00	2	14	01
10	9	19	25	1	16	27	6	17	32	1	13	00
			24			26		16	31	2	12	32
11	1	18		1	15		0			0	11	31
12	8	17	23	0	14	25	5	15	30	1	10	30
13	1	16	22	0	13	24	0	14	29	9	09	29
14	7	15	21	9	12	23	4	13	28	1	08	28
15	1	14	20	0	11	22	0	12	27	8		
	6		19	8		21	3	11	26	01	07	27
16	1	13		0	10		0			7	06	26
17	5	12	18	7	09	20	2	10	25	1	05	25
18	1	11	17	0	03	19	0	09	24	6		
19	4	10	16	6	06	18	1	03	23		04	24
20		09	15		07	16		07	22		03	23
	1		14	0		17	0	06	21	1		
21	3	03		5	05		0			5	02	22
22	1	07	13	0	04	15	2	05	20	1	01	21
23	2	06	12	4	03	14	2	04	19	4	00	20
24	1	05	11	0	02	13	2	03	18	1	27	19
25	1	04	10	3	01	12	1	02	17	3	26	18
	1		09	0		11	2	01	16	1		
26	0	03		2	00		0			2	25	17
27	0	02	03	0	27	10	1	00	15	1	24	16
28	9	01	07	1	26	09	9	27	14	1	23	15
29		00	06		25	08		26	13		22	14
30	0	27	05	0		07	1	25	12	1	21	13

Day	May	June	July	August
	F E I	F E I	F E I	F E I
1	18 20 12	10 17 14	03 15 17	18 12 19
2	17 19 11	09 16 13	02 14 16	17 11 18
3	16 18 10	08 15 12	01 13 15	16 10 17
4	15 17 09	07 14 11	00 12 14	15 09 16
5	14 16 08	06 13 10	22 11 13	14 08 15
6	13 15 07	05 12 09	21 10 12	13 07 14
7	12 14 06	04 11 08	20 09 11	12 06 13
8	11 13 05	03 10 07	19 08 10	11 05 12
9	10 12 04	02 09 06	18 07 09	10 04 11
10	09 11 03	01 08 05	17 06 08	09 03 10
11	08 10 02	00 07 04	16 05 07	08 02 09
12	07 09 01	22 06 03	15 04 06	07 01 08
13	06 08 00	21 05 02	14 03 05	06 00 07
14	05 07 32	20 04 01	13 02 04	05 27 06
15	04 06 31	19 03 00	12 01 03	04 26 05
16	03 05 30	18 02 32	11 03 02	03 25 04
17	02 04 29	17 01 31	10 27 01	02 04 03
18	01 03 28	16 00 30	09 26 00	01 23 02
19	00 02 27	15 27 29	08 25 32	00 22 01
20	22 01 26	14 26 28	07 24 31	22 21 00
21	21 00 25	13 25 27	06 23 30	21 20 32
22	20 27 24	12 24 26	05 22 29	20 19 31
23	19 26 23	11 23 25	04 21 28	19 18 30
24	18 25 22	10 22 24	03 20 27	18 17 29
25	17 24 21	09 21 23	02 19 26	17 16 28
26	16 23 20	08 20 22	01 18 25	16 15 27
27	15 22 19	07 19 21	00 17 24	15 14 26
28	14 21 18	06 18 20	22 16 23	14 13 25
29	13 20 17	05 17 19	21 15 22	13 12 24
30	12 19 16	04 16 18	20 14 21	12 11 23
31	11 18 15			19 13 20

Day	September	Octomber	November	December
	F E I	F E I	F E I	F E I
1	10 09	03 07 24	18 04 26	11 02 29
2	09 08	02 06 23	17 03 25	10 01 28
3	08 07	01 05 22	16 02 24	09 00 27
4	07 06	00 04 21	15 01 23	08 27 26
5	06 05	22 03 20	14 00 22	07 26 25
	17			
6	05 04	21 02 19	13 27 21	06 25 24
7	04 03	20 01 18	12 26 20	05 24 23
8	03 02	19 00 17	11 25 19	04 23 22
9	02 01	18 27 16	10 24 18	03 22 21
10	01 00	17 26 15	09 23 17	02 21 20
	12			
11	00 27	16 25 14	08 22 16	01 20 19
12	22 26	15 24 13	07 21 15	00 19 18
13	21 25	14 23 12	06 20 14	22 18 17
14	20 24	13 22 11	05 19 13	21 17 16
15	19 23	12 21 10	04 18 12	20 16 15
	07			
16	18 22	11 20 09	03 17 11	19 15 14
17	17 21	10 19 08	02 16 10	18 14 13
18	16 20	09 18 07	01 15 09	17 13 12
19	15 19	08 17 06	00 14 08	16 12 11
20	14 18	07 16 05	22 13 07	15 11 10
	02			
21	13 17	06 15 04	21 12 06	14 10 09
22	12 16	05 14 03	20 10 05	13 09 08
23	11 15	04 13 02	19 09 04	12 08 07
24	10 14	03 12 01	18 08 03	11 07 06
25	09 13	02 11 00	17 07 02	10 06 05
	30			
26	08 12	01 10 32	16 06 01	09 05 04
27	07 11	00 09 31	15 05 00	08 04 03
28	06 10	22 08 30	14 04 32	07 03 02
29	05 09	21 07 29	13 03 31	06 02 01
30	04 08	20 06 28	12 02 30	05 01 00
31	03 07	19 05 27	11 01 29	04 00 32

Table 24

Table B

Months of birth	year	FEI	Months of birth	Year	F E I
	1873	17 27 14		1909	02 11 00
	74	20 26 12		10	05 10 31
January–February	75	00 25 10	January–February	11	08 09 29
March–December	76	03 24 08	March–December	12	11 08 27
	76	02 23 07		12	10 07 26
	1877	05 22 05		1913	13 06 24
	78	08 21 03		14	16 05 22
January—February	79	11 20 01	January—February	15	19 04 20
March–December	80	14 19 32	March–December	16	22 03 18
	80	13 18 31		16	21 02 17
	1881	16 17 29		1917	01 01 15
	82	19 16 27		18	04 00 13
January–February	83	22 15 25	January–February	19	07 27 11
March–December	84	02 14 23	March–December	20	09 25 08
	84	01 13 22		20	10 26 09
	1885	04 12 20		1921	12 24 06
	86	07 11 18		22	15 23 04
January—February	87	10 10 16	January—February	23	18 22 02
March–December	88	14 09 14	March–December	24	21 21 00
	88	12 08 13		24	20 20 32
	1889	15 07 11		1925	00 19 30
	90	18 06 09		26	03 18 28
January—February	91	21 05 07	January—February	27	06 17 26
March–December	92	01 04 05	March–December	28	09 16 24
	92	00 03 04		28	08 15 23
	1893	03 02 02		1929	11 14 21
	94	06 01 00		30	14 13 19
January–February	95	09 00 31	January–February	31	17 12 17
March–December	96	12 27 29	March–December	32	20 11 15
	96	11 26 28		32	19 10 14
	1897	14 25 26		1933	22 09 12
	98	17 24 24		34	02 08 10
	99	20 23 22		35	05 07 03
	1900	00 22 20	January-February	36	08 06 05
			March-December	36	07 05 05
	1901	03 21 18		1937	19 04 03
	02	06 20 16		38	13 03 01
	03	09 19 14	January–February	39	16 02 32
January–February	04	12 18 12	March–December	40	19 01 30
March–December	04	11 17 11		40	18 00 29
	1905	17 15 07		1941	21 27 27
	06	14 16 09		42	01 26 25
January–February	07	20 14 05	January–February	43	04 25 23
March-December	08	22 12 02	March-December	44	07 24 21
	08	00 13 03		44	06 23 20

Table 24 - continuation

Months of birth	year	F E I	Months of birth	year	F E I
	1945	09 22 18		80	14 07 06
	46	12 21 16		80	13 06 05
	47	16 20 14	January–February	1981	16 05 03
	48	18 19 12	March–December	82	19 04 01
January–February	48	17 13 11		83	22 03 32
March–December	1949	20 17 09		84	02 02 30
	50	00 16 07		84	04 01 29
	51	03 15 05	January—February	1985	04 00 27
	52	06 14 03	March–December	86	07 27 25
January—February	52	05 13 02		87	10 26 23
March–December	1953	08 12 00		88	13 25 21
	54	11 11 31		88	12 24 20
	55	14 10 29	January–February	1989	15 23 18
	56	17 09 27	March–December	90	18 22 16
January–February	56	16 08 26		91	21 21 14
March–December	1957	19 07 24		92	01 20 12
	58	22 06 22		92	00 19 11
	59	02 05 20	January—February		03 18 09
	60	05 04 18	March–December	94	06 17 07
January—February	60	04 03 17		95	09 16 05
March–December	1961	07 02 15		96	12 15 03
	62	10 01 13		96	11 14 02
	63	13 00 11	January—February	1997	14 13 00
	64	16 27 09	March–December	98	17 12 31
January—February	64	15 25 08		99	20 11 29
March–December	1965	18 25 06		00	00 10 27
	66	21 24 04		00	22 09 26
	67	01 23 02	January–February	2001	02 08 24
	68	04 22 00	March–December	02	05 07 22
January–February	68	03 21 32		03	08 06 20
March–December	1969	06 20 30		04	11 05 18
	70	09 19 28		04	13 03 15
	71	12 18 26	January–February	2005	10 04 17
	72	15 17 24	March–December	06	16 02 13
January–February	72	14 16 23		07	19 01 11
March–December	1973	17 15 21		08	22 00 09
	74	20 14 19		08	21 27 08
	75	00 13 17	Januarv-February	2009	01 26 06
	76	03 12 15	March–December	10	04 25 04
January–February	76	02 11 14		11	07 24 02
March–December	1977	05 10 12		12	10 23 00
	78	08 09 10	JanuaryvFebruary	12	09 22 32
	79	11 03 08	March–December	2013	12 21 39

Table 25

Table C

Month	1961	1962	1963	1964
	F E I	F E I	F E I	F E I
1	16 26 18	13 27 20	10 00 22	07 01 24
2	01 01 16	21 03 18	18 03 20	15 04 22
3	06 01 11	03 02 13	00 03 15	21 05 18
4	14 04 09	11 05 11	08 06 13	06 08 16
5	21 06 06	18 07 08	15 03 10	13 10 13
6	06 09 04	03 10 06	00 11 08	21 13 11
7	13 11 01	10 12 03	07 13 05	05 15 08
8	21 14 32	18 15 01	15 16 03	13 18 06
9	06 17 30	03 18 32	00 19 01	21 21 04
10	13 19 27	10 20 29	07 21 31	05 23 01
11	21 22 25	18 23 27	15 24 29	13 26 32
12	0 24 22	02 25 24	22 26 26	20 00 29

Table 25 *continuation*

Month	1965	1966	1967	1968
	F E I	F E I	F E I	F E I
1	05 03 27	02 04 29	22 05 31	19 06 00
2	13 06 25	10 07 27	07 08 29	04 09 31
3	18 06 20	15 07 22	12 08 24	10 10 27
4	03 09 18	00 10 20	20 11 22	18 13 25
5	10 11 15	07 12 17	04 13 19	02 15 22
6	18 14 13	15 15 15	12 16 17	10 18 20
7	02 16 10	22 17 12	19 18 14	17 20 17
8	10 19 08	07 20 10	04 21 12	02 23 10
9	18 22 06	15 23 08	12 24 10	10 26 13
10	02 24 03	22 25 05	19 26 07	17 00 10
11	10 27 01	07 00 03	04 01 05	02 03 08
12	17 01 31	14 02 00	11 03 02	09 05 05

Table 25 *continuation*

Month	1969	1970	1971	1972
	F E I	F E I	F E I	F E I
1	17 08 03	14 09 05	11 10 07	08 11 09
2	02 11 01	22 12 03	19 13 05	16 14 07
3	07 11 29	14 12 31	01 13 00	22 15 03
4	15 14 27	12 15 29	09 16 31	07 18 01
5	22 16 24	19 17 26	16 18 28	14 20 31
6	07 19 22	04 20 24	01 21 26	22 23 29
7	14 21 19	11 22 21	08 23 23	06 25 26
8	22 24 17	19 25 19	16 26 21	14 00 24
9	07 27 15	04 00 17	01 01 19	22 03 22
10	14 01 12	11 02 14	08 03 16	06 05 19
11	22 04 10	19 05 12	16 06 14	14 08 17
12	06 06 07	03 07 09	00 08 11	21 10 14

Table 25 *continuation*

Month	1973	1974	1975	1976
	F E I	F E I	F E I	F E I
1	06 13 12	03 14 14	00 15 16	20 16 18
2	14 16 10	11 17 12	08 18 14	05 19 16
3	19 16 05	16 17 07	13 18 09	11 20 12
4	04 19 03	01 20 05	21 21 07	19 23 10
5	11 21 00	08 22 02	05 23 04	03 25 07
6	19 24 31	16 25 00	13 26 02	11 00 05
7	03 26 28	00 27 30	20 00 32	18 02 02
8	11 01 26	08 02 28	05 03 30	03 05 00
9	19 04 24	16 05 26	13 06 28	11 08 31
10	03 06 21	00 07 23	20 08 25	18 10 28
11	11 09 19	08 10 21	05 11 23	03 13 26
12	18 11 16	15 12 18	12 13 20	10 15 23

Table 25 *continuation*

Month	1969	1970	1971	1972
	F E I	F E I	F E I	F E I
1	17 08 03	14 09 05	11 10 07	08 11 09
2	02 11 01	22 12 03	19 13 05	16 14 07
3	07 11 29	14 12 31	01 13 00	22 15 03
4	15 14 27	12 15 29	09 16 31	07 18 01
5	22 16 24	19 17 26	16 18 28	14 20 31
6	07 19 22	04 20 24	01 21 26	22 23 29
7	14 21 19	11 22 21	08 23 23	06 25 26
8	22 24 17	19 25 19	16 26 21	14 00 24
9	07 27 15	04 00 17	01 01 19	22 03 22
10	14 01 12	11 02 14	08 03 16	06 05 19
11	22 04 10	19 05 12	16 06 14	14 08 17
12	06 06 07	03 07 09	00 08 11	21 10 14

Table 25 *continuation*

Month	1973	1974	1975	1976
	F E I	F E I	F E I	F E I
1	06 13 12	03 14 14	00 15 16	20 16 18
2	14 16 10	11 17 12	08 18 14	05 19 16
3	19 16 05	16 17 07	13 18 09	11 20 12
4	04 19 03	01 20 05	21 21 07	19 23 10
5	11 21 00	08 22 02	05 23 04	03 25 07
6	19 24 31	16 25 00	13 26 02	11 00 05
7	03 26 28	00 27 30	20 00 32	18 02 02
8	11 01 26	08 02 28	05 03 30	03 05 00
9	19 04 24	16 05 26	13 06 28	11 08 31
10	03 06 21	00 07 23	20 08 25	18 10 28
11	11 09 19	08 10 21	05 11 23	03 13 26
12	18 11 16	15 12 18	12 13 20	10 15 23

Table 25 *continuation*

Month	1977	1978	1979	1980
	F E I	F E I	F E I	F E I
1	18 18 21	15 19 23	12 20 25	09 21 27
2	03 21 19	00 22 21	20 23 23	17 24 25
3	18 21 14	05 22 16	02 23 18	00 25 21
4	16 24 12	13 25 14	10 26 16	08 00 19
5	00 26 09	20 27 11	17 00 13	15 02 16
6	08 01 07	05 02 09	02 03 11	00 05 14
7	15 03 04	12 04 06	09 05 08	07 07 11
8	00 06 02	20 07 04	17 08 06	15 10 09
9	08 09 00	05 10 02	02 11 04	00 13 07
10	15 11 30	12 12 32	09 13 01	07 15 04
11	00 14 28	20 15 30	17 16 32	15 18 02
12	07 16 25	04 17 27	01 18 29	22 20 32

Table 25 *continuation*

Month	1981	1982	1983	1984
	F E I	F E I	F E I	F E I
1	07 23 30	04 24 32	01 25 01	21 26 03
2	15 26 28	12 27 30	09 00 32	06 01 01
3	20 26 23	17 27 25	14 00 27	12 02 30
4	05 01 21	02 02 23	22 03 25	20 05 28
5	12 03 18	09 04 20	06 05 22	04 07 25
6	20 06 16	17 07 18	14 03 20	12 10 23
7	04 08 13	01 09 15	21 10 17	19 12 20
8	12 11 11	09 12 13	06 13 15	04 15 18
9	20 14 09	17 15 11	14 16 13	12 18 16
10	04 16 06	01 17 03	21 18 10	19 20 13
11	12 19 04	09 20 06	06 21 08	04 23 11
12	19 21 01	16 22 03	13 23 05	11 25 08

Table 25 *continuation*

Month	1985	1986	1987	1983
	F E I	F E I	F E I	F E I
1	19 00 06	16 01 03	13 02 10	10 03 12
2	04 03 04	01 04 06	21 05 08	18 06 10
3	09 03 32	06 04 01	03 05 03	01 07 06
4	17 06 30	14 07 32	11 08 01	09 10 04
5	01 08 27	21 09 29	18 10 31	16 12 01
6	09 11 25	06 12 27	03 13 29	01 15 32
7	16 13 22	13 14 24	10 15 26	08 17 29
8	01 16 20	21 17 22	18 13 24	16 20 27
9	09 19 18	06 20 20	03 21 22	01 23 25
10	16 21 15	13 22 17	10 23 19	08 25 22
11	01 24 13	21 25 15	18 26 17	16 00 20
12	08 26 10	05 27 12	02 00 14	00 02 17

Table 25 *continuation*

Month	1989	1990	1991	1992
	F E I	F E I	F E I	F E I
1	08 05 15	05 06 17	02 07 19	22 08 21
2	16 08 13	13 09 15	10 10 17	07 11 19
3	21 08 08	18 09 10	15 10 12	13 12 15
4	06 11 06	03 12 08	00 13 10	21 15 13
5	13 13 03	10 14 05	07 15 07	05 17 10
6	21 16 01	18 17 03	15 18 05	13 20 08
7	05 18 31	02 19 00	22 20 02	20 22 05
8	13 21 29	10 22 31	07 23 00	05 25 03
9	21 24 27	18 25 29	15 26 31	13 00 01
10	05 26 24	02 27 26	22 00 28	20 02 31
11	13 01 22	10 02 24	07 03 26	05 05 29
12	20 03 19	17 04 21	14 05 23	12 07 26

Table 25 *continuation*

Month	1993	1994	1995	1996
	F E I	F E I	F E I	F E I
1	20 10 24	17 11 26	14 12 28	11 13 30
2	05 13 22	02 14 24	22 15 26	19 16 28
3	10 13 17	07 14 19	04 15 21	02 17 24
4	18 16 15	15 17 17	12 18 19	10 20 22
5	02 18 12	22 19 14	19 20 16	17 22 19
6	10 21 10	07 22 12	04 23 14	02 25 17
7	17 23 07	14 24 09	11 25 11	09 27 14
8	02 26 05	22 27 07	19 00 09	17 02 12
9	10 01 03	07 02 05	04 03 07	02 05 10
10	17 03 00	14 04 02	11 05 04	09 07 07
11	02 06 31	22 07 00	19 08 02	17 10 05
12	09 08 28	06 09 30	03 10 32	01 12 02

Table 25 *continuation*

Month	1997	1998	1999	2000
	F E I	F E I	F E I	F E I
1	09 15 00	06 16 02	03 17 04	00 18 06
2	17 18 31	14 19 00	11 20 02	08 21 04
3	22 18 26	19 19 28	16 20 30	14 22 00
4	07 21 24	04 22 26	01 23 28	22 25 31
5	14 23 21	11 24 23	08 25 25	06 27 28
6	22 26 19	19 27 21	16 00 23	14 02 26
7	06 00 16	03 01 18	00 02 20	21 04 23
8	14 03 14	11 04 16	08 05 18	06 07 21
9	22 06 12	19 07 14	16 03 16	14 10 19
10	06 08 09	03 09 11	00 10 13	21 12 16
11	14 11 07	11 12 09	08 13 11	06 15 14
12	21 13 04	13 14 06	15 15 08	13 17 11

Table 25 *continuation*

Month	2001	2002	2003	2004
	F E I	F E I	F E I	F E I
1	21 20 09	18 21 11	15 22 13	12 23 15
2	06 23 07	03 24 09	00 25 11	20 26 13
3	11 23 02	08 24 04	05 25 06	03 27 09
4	19 26 00	16 27 02	13 00 04	11 02 07
5	03 00 30	08 04 30	20 02 01	18 04 04
6	11 03 28	00 01 32	05 05 32	03 07 02
7	18 05 25	15 06 27	12 07 29	10 09 32
8	03 08 23	08 12 23	20 10 27	18 12 30
9	11 11 21	00 09 25	05 13 25	03 15 28
10	18 13 18	15 14 20	12 15 22	10 17 25
11	03 16 16	00 17 18	20 13 20	18 20 23
12	10 18 13	07 19 15	04 20 17	02 22 20

– Immunoglobulins important conditioning on the completeness of constitutional type

The generally known integration apparatus of the human body are the imuno-endocrin system, the circulatory system and the osteo-articular apparatus (as seen by osteopathic medicine which grows increasingly as a distinct medical specialty). Lately, more and more attention is given to the immune system regarding the body's functioning as a whole.

Immunoglobulins (Ig), still called antibodies (Ab) constitute a significant fraction of serum proteins. They form a large family of molecules, displaying a huge diversity of sequences of amino acids not found in other families of protein molecules. In fact, the immunoglobulin makes up a super family of protein molecules.

Immunoglobulins may be separated from other serum proteins by electrophoresis. Albumin molecules move fastest in the electric field, while gamma molecules (most of which act as antibodies) move the slowest. Achieving electrophoretic separation of serum proteins - from rabbits heavily immunized with a vaccine based on the use of pneumococci killed by boiling - highlights an abundance of gamma globulins that occur as a large band of electrophoretic. The other serum proteins exhibit greater homogeneity of physico-chemical parameters. Immunoglobulins are effectors of the immune system (IS) that appear either as a molecule secreted by mature B lymphocytes, representing the free antibodies, or receptors of the cell surface for expression of cell designated as cell receptor B (BCR), consisting of a tetrameric immunoglobulin molecule, associated with LGA and LGF1transmembraneproteins.These are components of signaling that trigger intracellular pathways in response to the antigen binding to the antibody. BCR activation is influenced by interactions with other receptors, to be mediated by antigen-activated B cells interacting with the helper T cells.

Crystallographic studies allowed deciphering the structure of immunoglobulinsand the development of their shaped “Y” tetracatenara structure model. The immunoglobulin molecules prototype is that of the G IgGimmunoglobulin produced by derived (mature cells, plasma), secreting B lymphocytes. The IgG tetracatenara molecule has two polypeptide chains of 214 amino acids, called light chains and denoted by L and two polypeptide chains of 446 amino acids, called heavy chains and denoted by H. Therefore, the immunoglobulin molecule is a heterotetramer (2L + 2H). Assigning an L chain with an H chain by disulfide inter-chain bonds (S-S) between cysteine residues of chain H and chain L causes the formation of an H-L heterodimer. The union also two heterodimers, by conducting disulfide bonds (S S) between the heavy chains of heterodimers leads to formation ofa functional immunoglobulin heterotetramers 2(H-L).

The first 109 amino acids from the N-terminus of both chains make up the variable region of such chains designated Vl or Vh.The name derives from the fact that the amino acid sequence of this region is variable from one type of immunoglobulin to another.

Immunoglobulin chains are divided into doMayns. Each area extends over a length of a chain, corresponding to about 110 amino acids. Light chains have two such domains, one corresponding to the variable Vlregion, the second corresponding to the constant CL region;IgG heavy chains have one variable region of about 110 amino acids and a constant region with three doMayns designated CH1, CH2 and CH3.The immunoglobulin IgM H chain, there are four fields designated CH1 CH4, corresponding to its constant region.The amino acid sequence of the IgG doMayns are identical, representing the result of gene duplications.

Two types of light chains designated λ and κ five basic types of heavy chains designated α, δ, ε, γ and μ have been identified. The type of heavy chain determines the classification of immunoglobulin in the five classes that have been correspondingly designated asIgA, IgD, IgE, IgG, IgM. Within the immunoglobulin heterotetramer there is only one type of L-chain (either kappa or lambda; it's never a kappa chain and lambda chain), and one type of H chain. The two L chains of the heterotetramerare identical to each other, as the two H chains are, in turn, identical. The most abundant immunoglobulin class within human blood is IgG.In the initial stages of the immune response to an antigen that has not been previously interfered with the body's immune system, the Mayn role is played by IgM.

The N-terminal of L and H chainshave a remarkable variability in their amino acid sequence and contribute to the formation of the antigen binding site. The amino acid sequence of the CL light chain's constant region and the CH heavy chain's constant region, belonging to the heterotetrameric immunoglobulin presents a constant in their amino acid sequence. The variations that occur in the constantCH region as a result of point genetic mutation, have allowed the classification of heavy chains into types of immunoglobulin, as listed above.

The joint region of CH1 and CH2 is called hinge, joint or hinge region and confers to the heavy chain, and therefore to the heterotetrameric immunoglobulin, some flexibility. H and L chains have intrachain disulfide bridges (S-S) between the cysteine residues within the tetramerand in turn, the heavy chains are engaged through intrachainsulphide bridges, just as the light chains are bound to the heavy chains through molecular bridges.

The hinge allows the two branches of the immunoglobulin tetramerchainobtained by its position, to move, which facilitates the firm binding of both arms of the antibody to the same antigen (virus, for example).It is also possible for each arm to be bound to a specific antigen. This crosslinking of immunoglobulin molecules in solution helps make an efficient inactivation of infectious agents, in an optimal timeframe. The hinge region increases the effectiveness of their antigen binding and crosslinking reactions by allowing a change in the distance between the two antigen-binding sites.

The VL and VH region of theheterotetrameric immunoglobulin a particular area, which is the antigen-binding site, is differentiated. In this field there are three areas in which the amino acid sequence is the most variable so the sectors were called hypervariable. They constitute complementarity determining regions - CDR (the Complementary Determining Regions). Within the CDR the complementary combination of antigen antibody takes place according to the key lock mechanism. The antibody molecule joins complementary, not with all the antigen, but only a part of its molecule, which was called epitope.

The sectors of the hypervariable chains of the variable region of the L and H chains of the immunoglobulin tetramer L-H-H-L were designated CDR1, CDR2 and CDR3.

These sectors fold in a coordinated manner forming the epitope binding site. The complete sequencing of the human immunoglobulin chains has revealed the existence of invariant positions in the N and C thirds of heavy chains. Such structural restrictions have been conserved during evolution, molecular hybridization data highlights the absence of immunoglobulin sequences in the genes in question but support the involvement of the gene duplications phenomenon.

The amino acid sequence of the L and H chains of the immunoglobulin tetramer have regularities in the position of cysteine residues where disulfide bridges may occur, which leads to the formation of folded chain doMayns designated VL, VH, CL, CH, CH2, CH3. Between the CH and CH2 areas there is the hinge region of the H chains, this being where the junction of the two LH heterodimers of the immunoglobulin tetramer takes place.

The amino acid sequence of the carboxy terminal half of the L chain of about 110 amino acids constitutes the constant region (CL) of these light chains. The amino acid sequence of this CL region determinates the type of light chain - kappa or lambda. The nature of the amino acid sequence of the heavy chain determines the type of the heavy chain (CH) immunoglobulin - mu, epsilon, gamma, alpha and delta - and consequently the IgM, IgE, IgG, IgA, IgD imuglobuline class.

CHAPTER VI.
THE ANTHROPOLOGICAL AND GENETIC INVESTIGATION METHODOLOGY AND TECHNOLOGY

In what follows, we will address the anthropological, morphological, physiological, functional and genetic techniques meant to provide the data necessary to establish rules for selection of sports and sports training individualization in relation to anthropological particularities of the body. The conditions which must be met are related to the need to be unified, they need to be used based on a methodology for measuring and complex evaluation and to be handled by individuals possessing a high degree of technicality.

It is the merit of *Martin* to have established measuring tools and internationally recognized guidelines that, upon a careful examination and use, removes subjectivity and personal interpretation and creates the possibility to compare the performances of various researchers, while providing premises for generalizations (which would allow new, quality, knowledge in order to obtain regulations and systematizations).

- Anthropological methods

I. Instrumentation for morphological measurements

1. The stadiometer (Martin) allows projective body measurements and is great for length and height.
2. The mobile compass (Martin), such as a caliper, is formed by a 25 cm long metal line that is divided into millimeters on both sides. At point 0 (zero) there is a fixed arm, 12 cm long with a sharp point and a blunt point. On the metal line a second arm is fixed, mobile on the line, so the whole structure is transformed into a rectangular projection tool.
3. The head measuring compass (Martin), also used for measuring diameters with the maximum reading distance not exceeding 30 cm. It consists of two steel arms folded on top, equipped with a metal arm, joined together by a hinge. The left arm supports the torque of a line that the other arm slides on; and it is equipped with a screw which may be fixed on the line, for reading accurate measurement data. It can also be used for measuring small lengths.

Measurement of larger diameters (shoulders, pelvis, etc.) is done with the pelvis Martin compass, which is built simple and practical, like the gynecological compass, with the difference that it does not have a scale divided into centimeters but into millimeters.

4. The toolkit for measuring angles consists the Mollison type contact goniometer, the V.Torok type **gnatometer**, the Hambruchstype **mandibuloductor** (Enhanced by Black) and for sports anthropometry, especially where it requires measurements of motion in various joints of the arms or angles of the cubital angle, it seems that the best tool is the measurer of angles (type Moltgen).
5. Measuring tape, with a minimum length of 150-200 cm for perimeter or curve length.
6. Verified scales for determining weight with a weighing capacity of 200 kg. The accuracy of the scales must be checked after moving it by using a control weight of 20 kg. Before weighing the scales should be placed horizontally and the person being weighed should stand middle
7. To find indicators of sports medicine applicable in swimming it is useful to

determine specific body weight, which requires a diving pool full of water (according to Stadler) which basically would be a cylinder of soft metal with a height of 140 cm, diameter of 70 cm and wall thickness of 1 mm. The floor and walls are strengthened every 30 cm with metal rings. The measurement is made during the dive (during the inhalation, and during forced inhaling and exhaling), through a glass tube satiated in the upper third of the device, which communicates with the pool. The tube has a mobile measuring scale, 25 cm long with 1000engraved marks a quarter millimeter apart. Instead of these entire installations, Drobny (1958) imagined the following: he fixed, on a 1 m long and 40 cm wide board, on the edge of a pool, a scale. The plate that the individuals had to stand on was tied, through 2 chains, to a trapeze that, for adults, would hang 240 cm under water.

8. The ratio between "active bodily substance" and "fat deposits" has been, lately, given, increasingly higher importance, in different sports categories. Subcutaneous adipose tissue contributes not only to the external shape of the body, but establishes its correlation to the bodily active substance - that is specific for each athlete - a bond more or less important with sports performance ability. Measurement of subcutaneous fat in a fold of skin - which Richer did first, in 1890, with a "thickness compass" and he also gave the idea for caliper –which proved very interesting, currently different compasses being called caliper.

II Anthropological instruments for functional measurements

1. To determine the force, we usually use dynamometers based on the principle that muscle strength is opposed by a resistance that can be measured. For other assessments of muscle strength new types of dynamometers have lately been proposed.

The basic problem in such devices is the standardization of the body's position during the measurement to various muscle groups, which is very important as the research subject influences the outcome of a particular muscle group study by putting into action other muscles. Also, avoiding the occurrence of the phenomenon of adaptation - which affects all human experience, the tested subject playing an active part - is important. Of major concern is the knowledge of the tested action of every muscle or functional groups on a biomechanical basis (See Vol. I, Human Anatomy Atlas, coordinator MirceaIfrim).

2. The ergografs provide us with valuable information regarding the timing when fatigue appears in certain muscle groups. We quote in this regard Mosso - measuring finger strength - of Treves - recording capacity of the upper limb muscle performance - and that of Klerr - the forearm muscle testing.
3. In the field of anthropometric research a special role is held by functional tests: establishing the vital capacity, by which we mean the amount of air that the subject is able to mobilize - through a deep inspiration and deep expiration - in and out of a special device called spirometer that, in turn, can be a dry or wet spirometer.The height of the metal line exiting the spirometer (graded from 0 to 6600 cm3, up to 8500 cm3 in some devices) shows the volume change of a rubber balloon that is inside the dry spirometer.Dried spirometers do not usually work, as accurately as the wet ones, but instead are easier to transport.There is a correlation between calculating the vital capacity

and the median and maximum lung capacity, which are graphically rendered.Body height and body weight, as well as current methodical training are reflected in increased average lung capacity.Vital capacity size is determined by its relation to with body height, body weight, the possibility of increasing the diameters of the chest, and to a great degree, of development of normal and accessories respiratory muscles.(By strengthening the respiratory and accessories muscles we have found that after only three months of training, for beginners, vital capacity has increased by 300 to 500 cm3.)

We note that, given the correlations above, Beckert has researched during 1961-1968, a total of 3140 people (1230 men and 1910 women) aged 18 to 40, students from the Pedagogical Institute in Leipzig, who had their origins throughout the former Democratic Germany; *Querg (1957)* and he also brought his contribution to the tables of standards by developing some formulas for calculating normal breathing capacity, for young men, according to the following formula: (body height (cm) 100) / 20 = vital capacity in liters. The values for girls, Querg, placed them 10% below. Since these formulas do not prove valid in adults, Beckert has developed the following formulas (which after his evaluations were good):

- For people between 18 and 40 (men):

(Body height (cm) 100) / 20 = vital capacity in liters

- Women 18 to 40 years:

(Body height (cm) - 100) / 20 = vital capacity in liters

To this anthropological toolkit other devices and anthropological means of investigation have been added, that are not exclusive to these disciplines and we will detail them along with the exhibition of geneticanthropological investigative technology.

III Actual body measurements

Tangible measurements that determine Maynly the somatic type or body segments proportions, the interrelations between them, the basic elements in defining constitutional typology, is fundamental in anthropological investigations, which is why we give them special attention.

A. We, initially, present craniometry elements.

1. Basion (Ba) is the point on the midline of the anterior edge of the occipitalhole.
2. Bregma (B) represents the meeting point of the sagittal coronary suture.
3. Eurion (I) designates the point on the side of the external wall of the skull.
4. Glabella (G) is the most prominent point of the skull, above the nazofrontale suture between the two superciliary arches.
5. Lambda (L) is located at the intersection point between the sagittal suture and the lambdaticsuture. When there arewormienebone the route of the sutures is extended until they intersect on the middle line.
6. Inion (I) marks the point where the nuchal line overlays the mediosagital plan.
7. Opisthokranion (Op) is located in farthest posterior point on the sagittal plane of the skull.
8. Opisthion (O) is the point on the medial edge of the foramen magnum of the occipital.
9. Asterion (Ast) is the meeting point of lambdoid, occipitalo-mastoidiene and parietal-mastoid sutures.
10. Auricular (Au) designate a point at the root of the zygomatic temporal mastoidbone, above the middleedge of the ear.
11. *Porion (Po) is located mid-point upper limit auditory processing region, a point which is always lower than the previous.*

12. fronto temporal (Ft) marks the point on the edge of the frontal temporal fossa, ranked the largest narrowing of the upper region of the external orbital frontal apophyses.

13. Metopion (M) designates the point at the intersection front lines comprising projections mediosagital plan.

14. Vertex (V) is the highest point on the height of the skull horizontally oriented Frankfurt.

15. Nasional (N) designates the point at the meeting point of the suture line nazofrontalemediosagitală.

16. Nasospinale (Ns) marks the point on the anterior nasal spine, ie at the bottom of the pear-shaped aperture.

17. Prosthion (Pr) is a point in the median sagittal plane, the alveolar edge of the upper jaw, between the two medial incisors.

18. Rhinion (Rhi) designates the point situated in the region most prominent nasal bones at the terminal end of the suture internazale.

19. Zygion (Zy) marks the farthest side of the zygomatic arch.

20. Ektoconchion (Ek) is a point on the outer edge of the orbit, to where it intersects the transverse line parallel to the upper edge of the orbit, and the orbit divided into two halves.

21. Maxilofrontale (Mf) is located at the intersection point edge orbit internal suture maxilofrontală.

22. Dakryon (D) marks the point on the inner wall of the orbit, the meeting place of sutures between the bones frontal, lacrimal and epiphysis front of the jawbone.

23. Orbital (Or), points located in the lower portion of the lower edge of the orbit, points that serve to guide the skull horizontally in Frankfurt.

24. Zygomaxilare (Zm) is the lowest point on maxillary suture.

25. Zygomaxilare 1 (Zm1) marks the point somewhat higher than Zm and the resulting zigomaxilare suture junction with the upper border of the masseter muscle insertion malar bone.

26. Frontomalare time (FMT) designates the point at external suture malarofrontală shore.

27. Frontomalare orbital (FMO) marks the point on the outer edge of the orbit, at its intersection with suture malarofrontală.

28. Oral (Ol) indicates the point in the anterior portion of the palate bone, mediosagitale line at the intersection with the line joining the posterior edge of the medial incisors alveoli.

29. Staphylion (Sta) is a palace located in the back of the bone at the junction mediosagitale line with assembling the deepest points of the rear edges of incisors palate.

30. Infradentale (Id) designate a point above the upper edge of the mandibular alveolar processus between the two medial incisors.

31. Gnathion (Gn) is the point on the center line of the lower edge of the mandible.

32. gonion (Go) marks the point at the angle of the mandible.

With these benchmarks cranial and facial diameters can be measured

1. The anterior posterior diameter is the maximum distance between glabella and opisthokranion. According to the values we found, skulls are divided into:

	Male	Female
Very short	169 x	x 161
Short 170-177	162	169
Medium 178-185	170	176

2. The maximum transverse diameter measures the distance between the two eurioanes. According to the values we found, skulls are divided into:

	Male	*Fem*
Very	x-139	x-13

narrow	140-1	135-
Average	148-1	142-
Wide	156-1	150-
Very	164-x	158-

3. The basilobregmatic diameter is the distance between the basion and the bregma.

4. The minimum frontal diameter is the distance between the two frontotemporals.

5. The total face height is the distance between the nasion and gnathion. According to the values we found, faces are divided into:

6. The upper height of the face corresponds to the nasion-prosthion. According to this, faces are divided into:

	Male	*Fem*
Low	x-68	x-64
Average	69-73	
Tall	74-78	
Very tall	79-x	75-x

7. The bizygomatic diameter is the distance between the two zigioans.

8. The maximum width of the piriform aperture is the width of the nasal alarhole.

9. The nose height is measured from nasion to nasospinal. Based on these diameters two indices can be calculated:

1. The cranial index, which characterizes the general shape of the skull seen upright and is the centesimal ratio of width to length of the skull:

(eu-eux100)/(g-op).

By this index, skulls are dolico, meso and brahicranethe indices category scale is as follows:

Dolicocrane	– Ultradolicran -64,9; – Dolicocran 65-69,9; – Hiperdolicocran 70-74,9; – Mezocran 75-79,9;
Brahicrane	– Brahicran 80-84,9; –Hiperbrahicran85-89,9; – Ultrabrahicran 90-x;

2. Vertico longitudinal Index characterizes the development of the skull height relative to its length. The formula is:

(ba bx100)/(g op).

This index reflects the overall shape of the skull seen in Profile and divides skulls into:

Camecran	x-69,9;
Ortocran	70,0-74,9;
Hipsicran	75, 0-x.

B. *Somatic elements*

To enable comparison with data obtained before or with those that appeared at the same time, we recommend a single unified and methodical measurement, each measurement must be done accurately and conscientiously. Sufficient time is required for the anthropometric research of an athlete and it must be compared, at intervals, with data accurately obtained from other subjects. It is advisable to first seek every skeleton point and to practice measurement here, before moving to the living man, to minimize as much as possible the opportunities to make mistakes.

All measurements are made with body stripped naked and only in some circumstances, medical situations, the subject can wear a bathing suit. The examined person must stand at attention with feet together, arms straight at the sides and palms inward. It is very important that this position should not be changed during the measurement because otherwise the measurements can be wrong. The order in the measurements are taken must be set practically so that, for example, after length the diameters are immediately measured, thus we avoid the frequent change of measuring tools and so we don't waste time.

These measurements are usually made on the right side of the body, with the exception of left handed people; to measure both sides (mentioning which arm is used for throwing or pushing) means easting too much time, even though, the differences between the left and the right, in athletes, raise very interesting questions.

All results will be dictated by the researcher to their aids, who repeats them out loud and then carefully writes them in a spread sheet (which aloe for later recalculation, All results will be dictated by the researcher). If we want to make an observation sheet, then we must take care that the sheets for the two sexes differ in terms of the column, which will greatly facilitate subsequent work. There are different observation sheets: the somatological observation sheet for the type and the constitution of the body (*Martin*), the somatological observation sheet for school investigation (Martin), the skull observation sheet (*Martin*), the paternity observation sheet (*Saller*) and anthropological tests (*Eickstedt*).

A measurement includes three essential elements:

1. The age, rounded to full years or to the nearest decimal corresponding to the nearest month. Also, we estimate, if possible, the developmental stage or "biological age". Thus, Tittel, observes, during an investigation performed on 13 year old children, regardless of sex, a biological dvelopent that corresponds to the age of 10 or 15. Based on the relationship between the general development of the body and the separate development of the parts, it is possible to calculate the "biological age" judging by ossification criteria, sexual maturity criteria or anthropometric values.
2. Body weight (in kg with decimals) is measured, scientifically, in the nude. Care must be taken so that the weighing is performed in the same conditions (the time of day - there are differences in weight at different times of the day - food, bowel and bladder emptying), and the person being weighed should be positioned in the center of the scale.
3. Height, width and depth (*Martin Saller*)

We will present the main anthropometric body points in order to understand the measurements that need to be made. (fig. 78)

1. Suprasternal (sst), the midpoint located on the upper edge of the sternum.
2. Symphizion (FMIS), the midpoint of the upper edge of the symphysis pubis.
3. Iliocristale (ic), the highest point of the iliac crest side.
4. Iliospinale (is), the highest point on the anterior superior iliac spine lower.
5. Acromion (a), which corresponds to point our skin-side scapula.

6. Radials (ra), the highest point of the upper edge of the radial head.

7. Dactylion (yes), point located at a distal finger environment.

8. Stylion (sty), at the lowest point of the radial styloid process.

9. The epigastric point is located at the crossing of the midline of the body with the horizontal passing the lower edge of the rib X.

10. Sphyrion (sphy), corresponding peak point tibial malleolus.

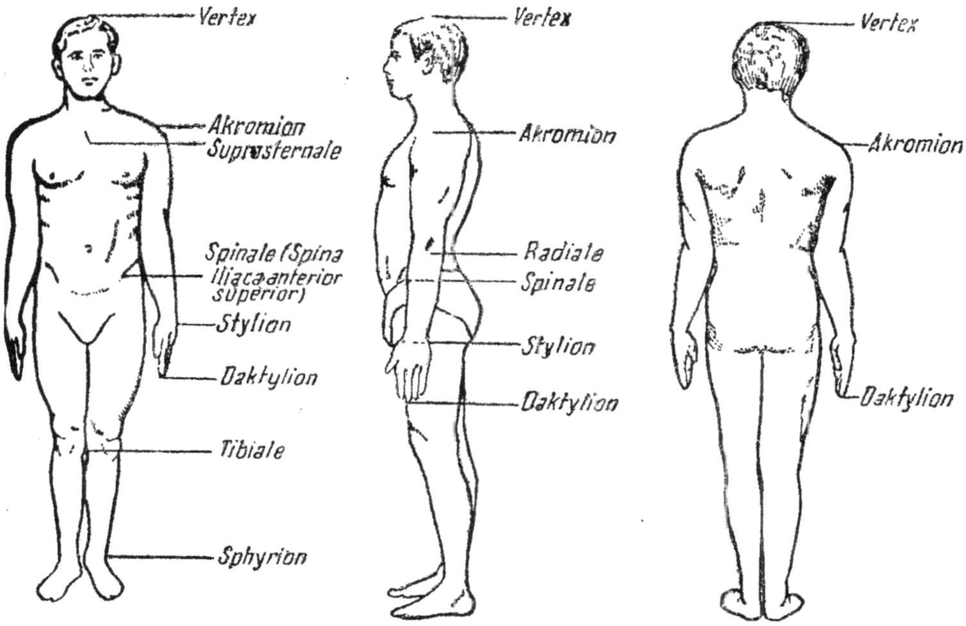

Fig.78 The main anthropometric body points

Next, we present the technique through which we perform measurements of key importance in the world of sport.

- Body height is represented by the distance from the vertex (top of the head) to the plane of the lower limbs.

It must be measures accurately because it correlates to other body measurements (the height from the shoulders, the distance between the hands with the upper limns apart, etc). *Saller* (1950) puts forward the idea that comparing heights between individuals would not be possible as correlation due to differences of height, that in turn influence other body measurements, disappear. The subject who is standing at attention, next to a wall, beside a measuring board which they touch with the heals, the backside and the back, while the head is in a flexed position and does not touch the board. The researcher stands to the right of the subject, places the anthropometerin the median plane of the subject, places their right on the anthropometric vertex line and with the left hand makes sure that it does not slide (girls must be careful so that they don't have tails or hair buns that must be set aside).The differences noted in body weight and in terms of time of day appear in height as well, between morning and evening is a difference of about 3 cm. Weight and height values are used to calculate body surface area, for which we use the nomogram (*Hannoh*).

- - Shoulder height- the vertical distance between the right acromion and the floor. The anthropometr will be placed at the right upper end of the subject, the right hand brings the line to shoulder height, while the left hand without touching the extremity, highlights the acromion. The left hand pushes the line until the tip touches the acromion. During measurement, the subject should not raise or lower the shoulder.

- -The upper edge of the radial head height -the vertical distance of the radial head straight to the floor (radial - ground). With his left-hand examiner highlights that the upper edge of the radial bone which is in a well defined foseta behind brachioradialis.
- - Calculating the length of the arm is done by decreasing the height at the shoulder towards the top of radial body.
- - The height of radial styloid process - the vertical distance from the styloid process of the radius (stilion) from the floor. The anthropometer is in the same position. Palpate with thumb the stilion, which is situated between the long abductor muscle tendons of the extensor muscle of the thumb one side and the tendon of the long extensor muscle on the other side, where the tip of the anthropometer should be placed.
- Forearm length calculation is made by subtracting the height from the top of the body radial styloid, process radial height.
- The iliac antero-superior height – the vertical space from the antero-superior iliac spine to the measuring board. The antropometer is in the same position as it is when measuring the upper member. With the left hand the researcher palpates the spine thusly: with the 4 fingers they palpate the anterior edge of the canal, and with the thumb they palpate until the measured point is highlighted
- For calculating the length of the lower member there are two ways (*Martin* 1924):
  a) The length of the lower member – the height of the antero-superior iliac spine from which we subtract a correlation index which is, according to body height:

     Height over/up to 190 cm-15mm
     Height over/up to130 cm – 20mm
     Height over/up to 131-150 cm – 30mm
     Height over/up to 151 – 165 cm – 40mm
     Height over/up to 166 - 175 cm – 50mm
     Height over/up to 176 – 189 cm – 60mm

  b) The length of the lower member –body height minus the height while sitting.
- The knee height. The vertical space from the upper median edge of the tibia to the measuring board. The researcher, or an assistant take the antropometer, which must be held as before. The thumb and the index finger grip the patellar ligament. The index finger pushes the skin upwards and inwards until the upper and median edges of the tibia can be palpated. The maneuver is easier if the lower limb is bent slightly.
- Calculating the height of the thigh. The height from the antero-superior iliac spine minus the height of the knee plus the correction mentioned above. (Martin)
- The height of the tibialmalleolus. The vertical space from the right tibial malleolus to the measuring board
- Calculating the length of the calf. The height from the knee minus the height of the tibial
- The height while sitting. The vertical space from the vertex to the sitting plane, with the spine extended. The subject sits on a 40 cm high chair with a horizontal sitting plane, legs pressed together and knees bent at 90 degrees. The antropometer is placed at the back of the subject and the sitting plane, making sure that the line of the member is horizontal thus the body is straight.

The sitting height is, relative to the body height, 52% for males and 53% in females, the larger percentage in females being probably due to a more developed torso.(*Saller,* 1959). Overall, the sitting height is not a special measurement because it's very little comparable to body height

(especially if we take into account the physiological curvature of the spine while sitting)

- The length of the hand. The line between the head of the second metacarpal and the fifth, with fingers spread.
- The length of the foot. The line between the most posterior point of the heel to the most anterior point of the hallux, with the foot of the floor.
- The width of the foot. The line from the head of the first metatarsal to the fifth, on the right foot, with the foot flat on the floor
- The orbital angle (the angle formed by the arm and the forearm, with a radial opening). The measurement is done with the upper member completely stretched, with the forearm in suspination, with Moltgen's angle measurer, which will be placed on the anterior surface of the arm so as the graded half of the arc blade (180 degrees), which corresponds to the axis of rotation of the two metal arms is to be placed at the elbow. The cubital angle has an average value of about 170 ° and 168 ° in men, women.
- The length between the open arms is comprised of the length of the two arms and the width of the chest. It's represented by the distance between the medius peaks while the arms are stretched out horizontally. The subject sits with arms in abduction at shoulder height, with the back to the wall with arms glued to the wall. The simples method is marking on the wall the place of the two peaks of mediuses and then measuring the distance between the two points.
- Shoulder width (biacromial width). The distance,in a straight line between the two acromions, measured so that the peaks of the compass sit in the middle of the outside edge of the acromion (the examiner's thumb is placed between the front third and the median third of the deltoid muscle).Care should be taken so as the subject to Mayntain the normal position of the shoulders, as a position with the shoulders towards thefrontwould lead to a lower value.
- Bispinal width. The distance, in a straight line, between the two antero-superior iliac spines. The researcher must use their finger to correctly establish the lower edge of the antero-superior iliac bone.

Establishing the bispinal width is much more accurate and more scientific than measuring the width of the pelvis or measuring the distance between the ridges of the iliac bone. The difficulty lies in the precise determination of the external edge of the iliac bone.

- The transverse thoracic diameter. The distance, in a straight line, between the side points locates furthest away, measured by the pelvic compass, in a median position, between inhaling and exhaling, at the level of the fourth costernal joint. The tips of the compass must be situates on the rib and not the muscle.
- Thoracic sagittal diameter. The distance, in a straight line, between the lower part of the sternum and the spinous process. We measure the intermediate position between inhaling and exhaling, keeping the measuring device horizontal
- Thoracic circumference (in intermediate respiratory position). A measuring tape is placed under inferior angle of the scapula, then the armpits (risingthe armsslightly) and then the circle closes over nipples. In women with more developed mammary gland, the measuring tape sits slightly above (the mammary gland).

Then measuring the absolute thoracic circumference, the development of the subcutaneous fat layer, especially in women, must be held into account, since part of it is measured on the breast. This is why, the thoracic perimeter cannot be compared between men and women.

- Thoracic circumference (after maximal inhaling). The subject is standing, with arms loosely by their side and breaths deeply in. Meanwhile the measuring tape is held so as to allow the expansion of the chest.

- Thoracic circumference (after maximal exhaling). The subject is standing, with arms loosely by their side and exhales forcefully. Meanwhile the measuring tape is held a little tight for it to mold to the chest
- Area of respiratory movements (the distance of thoracic excursion). It is functional-structural measurement for breathing, calculated through the difference between the thoracic perimeter when at maximum inhaling and at maximum exhaling.
- Abdominal circumference. The measuring tape is placed around the abdomen at navel level
- Upper abdominal arch. The arch shaped space between the lower edge of the lower xifoid appendix and the middle of the navel, measured with the measuring tape
- Lower abdominal arch. The arch shaped space between the middle of the navel and the upper edge of the symphysispubis, measured with the measuring tape. The difference between the last two measurements can serve as orientation point for an eventual weakening of the of the supporting tissue, which can manifest itself as a deformation or a bulging of the abdominal wall; *Akaltin*(1952) established three levels: over 7 cm, between 5 and 7 cm, and between 3 and 5 cm
- The circumference of the waist. The measuring tape is places in the center of the distance between the costal arcs and the coxal bone, at the same height as where the abdomen, while being looked at from the front, has the smallest width. During the measuring, the subject will only take shallow breaths since a deep breath can lead to erroneous values.
- The great brachial circumference (with arm stretched out). The right arm hangs by the trunk, the measuring tape is placed on the spot where the brachial muscle is most developed. Care must be had that the flexor muscles of the forearm are contracted.

Also, the measurement is taken with the arm bent at a 90 degree angle as well. The measurement is taken with the upper limb bent at the joint of the elbow and held horizontally during the maximum contractions of the forearm's flexor muscles. The differences between the two measurements paint a picture about the development of the flexor muscles of the arm

- The great circumference of the forearm. The measuring tape is placed horizontally at the point where the brachioradial muscle is biggest, just under the joint of the elbow, while the upper limb hangs freely by the trunk
- The circumference of the hand
- The circumference of the thigh. The researcher measures the point of maximum medial musculature development (*Martin*). Tittel, however, recommends, for a better comparability between the two sexes, that the measurement be made 20 cm above the upper edge of the kneecap, on the right leg, while sitting. This prevents the appearance of differences that are too big between the two sexes due to the differences of subcutaneous fat deposits.
- The great circumference of the calf. The measuring tape is placed on the calf after measuring the perimeter of the thigh, without removing it, the measurement is done at the point of the greatest musculature development.
- Measuring the thickness of skin folds is done using standardized caliper and are currently as follows:

  1. The head: on the cheek at the height of the tragus;
  2. On the chest wall: the edge of the great pectoral axillary border;
  3. On the chest wall: on the 10th rib on the anterior axillary line;

4. On the chest wall: on the 10th rib on the axillary line, joining the anterior superior iliac spine to the umbilicus;

5. The pelvis: the top of the anterior superior iliac spine;

6. On the back: under the lower angle of the scapula;

7. On the arm: the brachial triceps, shoulder height and between the olecranon;

8. On the thigh: superior patella with the knee slightly bent;

9. On the leg: the lower limit of the popliteal fossa

All measurements will be made on the right half of the body with the subject standing. The skin fold will be caught between the thumb and index finger of his left hand, will be away from the muscle and fascia will be measured with a caliper.

- It was stated that the ratio of "tangible substance" to the fat deposits has special importance for the motricity ability of athletes. It will be recorded as the logarithm value of the amounts of all thickness of skin folds according to the formula by Parizkova (1963), in a regressive execution after hydrostatic weighing results:
    - $Y = 39{,}572 \lg x_1 \ldots\ I_a - 61{,}25\ I_a$
    - $Y = 22{,}32 \lg x_1 \ldots\ I_a - 29{,}\ 20\ I_a$

From this value (which gives the fat percentage of the total body weight) can be calculated - kg - and subtracted from the total weight - the weight of the "active body substance"

- Vital capacity. The measurement is done with wet or dry spirometer.
- The force of pressure, or traction of the hand. The Collin dynamometer will be used. For children and some women this device is too big (to grip) so a smaller model must be used. Before the measurements are to be taken, both the hand and the device are to be thoroughly wiped with a piece of cloth. During the measurement, which is being done standing up; with the right arm away from the body (in right handed people) the indicator will be pointing outwards. Usually, during a one minute interval two measurements are done with the dynamometer, using all the strength of the subject, the biggest value being taken into consideration.

When determining the tractive force of the vertebral extensor muscles, the device is used (scale-oriented floor) in an oblique position to the subject. This device latches to the ends of the dynamometer, and is pulled with the greatest force. Of course, dynamometry is very complex, comprising muscle growth that we will not describe in detail, since there is greater detail in Vol. I of Atlas of Human Anatomy.

The techniques are standardized according to the muscles groups, and there are also different prototypes of dynamometers

IV. Evaluation of anthropometric measurements

Body measurements, which were made on different groups of people, are often incomparable directly since their correlative relationship establishes as real and absolute size. Thus, body height and body weight vary in both young and older populations and in selected adult groups. Because of this only the comparison is not possible until after finding a relationship between various measures (index of proportionality). This relationship is achieved, usually following this formula

(the small size x 100) / (the large size).

In this way all body size measurements can be expressed as a percentage of body height. As a common term, we have "relative measure", while for other reports of body measurements such as

(Arm length x 100) / (Length of upper limb)

or

(Shoulder width) / (width of the pelvis);

The term "index" is better suited.

Examples of indexes:

Kaup index = (body weight) / (body height) (body building index);

Rohrer Index = (body weight) / (body height) (corpulence index);

Livi Index *(F)* = $\sqrt{\frac{\text{body weight}}{\text{body height}}}$

These indexes led to the establishment of normal body weight (Broca - minimum height - 100) (Brugsch - up to 165 cm height - 100, from 166 up to 175 cm height - 105; over 175 cm height - 100). There are further proposals to specify these formulas (Beckert, 1966) who still take into account, to a small extent, the characteristics of body typology, age or sex.

Jones (1947) took into account when determining normal weight and age:

6- 14 years = (body height 100) (body height 125) / 2;

15-18. years = (body height 100) (body height 125) / 2;

Over 18 years = (body height 100) (body height 150) / 2.

The assessments and calculations of sports anthropometry indices have more practical significance.

1. Relationship between shoulder width - anterior superior iliac spines width - Index SB = width between spinals / shoulder width.
2. SBE Index = Index SB x (sum) circumferences (extremities) (mm) / 100.
3. The active relative body substance - AKS Index = body active substance (kg) X100 / body height (cm 3).
4. The circumference length perimeter = sum of extremity circumference 2 / sum of the length of extremities.
5. The relative length of extremities - AB Index = amount extremity length x 100 / body height.
6. The relative length of the foot = leg length x 100 / body height
7. Pignet constitutional index (or robusticity) = body height (cm) - Chest circumference (cm) + body weight (kg).
8. Lorenz constitutional index = (body height (cm) body weight (kg)) (body weight 150) X0,25) abdominal skin-fold thickness.

Also, very important are the complexes body features A, B, C. (see following pages).

Abundance of morphological indices had little significance in terms of practical guidance for choosing and guiding athletes.Because of this, lately we have resorted to comparing each separate body feature with athletic performance, taking into account the fact that relations between the characteristics statistically acquired can not be guaranteed, even if correlations are based on average values obtained in groups.

Efficient indications are obtained, for the relationship between body characteristics and athletic performance, using the so-called "complex features body" (Srimis 1958 1960 b, 1961; Kretschmer, 1967), by which we can recognize the action of the feature in relationship with a larger group of features. Factor analysis calculations (Tanner, 1964 b; Tittel, 1967; Wutscherk 1968, 1969) have shown that the shape of the body can be expressed by several "factors" - a factor which contains a measure of length (Tanner - 'trend increase in length "; Wutscherk -"

factor of length ") and a factor which contains special measures circumference and weight (Tanner -" growing trend nonlinear "Wutscherk -" factor circumference weight "Tiitel -" factor circumferential width ").

In the athletic anthropometric assessment it has been proven that a new differentiation for youth (Wutscherk, 1969), in which the measures of length, circumference and weight are concentrated in a dimensional factor, which gives special guidance on the degree of body development (biological age), and relative measures, in a proportional factor that summarizes the linear and nonlinear growth trends mentioned above, namely measurements of length and circumference (in relation to the state of the body). The makers that have been summed identical features, such as the length of the extremities (the length of the upper extremity [arm + forearm + hand] + length leg [thigh + calf]), respectively perimeters limb (arm + forearm + thigh + shank) have been shown to be representative.

This is how complexes of features A, B, C are:

- Complex of body features (extremity features) A

  (arm length x arm circumference) + (thigh length x thigh circumference) (dm 2);

- Complex body features (torso features) B:

$$\frac{\text{Shoulder height + pelvis width } \times \text{ body height}}{2 \times \text{body height}} \qquad \frac{cm2}{kg}$$

- Complex body features C ("total features" Wutscher, 1966, 1968, 1970; Tittel and Wutscherk 1968)

$$\frac{0{,}5 \times (\text{shoulder width + width of the iliac spines} \times \text{body height})}{(\text{arm length} \times \text{arm circumference}) + (\text{length of lower limb} \times \text{thigh circumference})} \qquad \frac{m^2}{dm^2 kg}$$

For these characteristics closer relations with the ability to benefit, rather than separate features, could be established (*Tittel,* 1963, 1965, 1967, *Tittel* and *Wutscherk,* 1968, *Wutscherk*, 1966, 1968, 1969). Limitations to these complex bodily features are that their internal determination can be increased by multitude of variables that they contain and also by adding or multiplying the measured errors. The C structure of complex body features, which, in men, is normal between 0.80 -1.20 and between 1.10 and 1.40 in women, could be clarified by *Wutscherk* factor analysis, (1968, 1968 b, 1968 c, 1969), it was concluded that it is mainly:

1 - dimensional sizes to juveniles;

2 - degree of body development (biological age);

3 - specific body typology

In assessing the efficiency of heavy physical work or a long-term intensive sports training, the human body structure two indicators were showed to be expressive:

1. Thoracic index $= \dfrac{\text{sagittal thoracic diameter} \times 100}{\text{transverse thoracic diameter}}$

2. Muscle index $= \dfrac{\text{The difference between the circumference of the contracted muscles of the arm while the arn is bent and the same with the arm stretched out } \times 100}{\text{circumference of the contracted muscle of the stretched arm}}$

Example of calculation for muscular index:

- Maximum circumference of the contracted right arm, bent = 33cm;
- Maximum circumference of the contracted right arm, stretched = 28, 5 cm;
- The difference between them = 4, 5 cm. It follows that:

Muscle index=(4,5x100)/28, 5=14,3.

Experience has shown that:

- Values under 5 – characterize an underdeveloped musculature;
- Values 5-12 - normal for people with mild physical performance capacity;
- Values 12 - characterize a very well-developed forearm flexor muscles

In a higher stage, these data are required to be processed by mathematical statistical methods. As prerequisites for the introduction of mathematical statistical methods are needed:

- the existence of measurement values and, in sufficient numbers, obtained by diagonal evaluation and length;
- the assurance that the processing parameters were obtained through a methodical and accurate measurement technique. Experience has shown that the "measurement error" factor and its role is not given enough attention.

Measurement errors arise through:

- Imprecise measuring instruments, in the absolute or relative sense;
- Imprecise methods (in anthropometry, measurement of small or large surfaces instead of measuring points).
- Incorrect or imprecise measurement (subjective error).

It is desirable that subjective errors approach 0 (zero), which can be achieved through practice. Only thus can errors due to apparatus and method be eliminated, or their value be close to 0 (zero). However, objective measurement errors are not to be ignored, but should be determined quantitatively, in order not to characterize the field as being un-interpretable. Objective error measurement calculation becomes very important especially when working with groups, or collective assessment is made.

A proper preparation of data groups, achieved through measurement, imposes, depending on the number if individuals, the calculation of median values. It is usually a mathematical average, though it can never offer a characterization of the population when looked at alone. In order to characterize this more comprehensively, we have graphical and computing devices.

Without special calculations we can find the variation limit (minimum... maximum), which should be only a minimal factor for the spread of individual values, because it is characterized by extreme values. The square spread (S2), necessary for the comparison of averages or other methods of correction (eg., Analysis of variance) is called variant.

Other possibilities for statistical processing provide comparison of the means or spread. This is because the average value may be equal to an uneven spread and unequal average values may have a same spreading. From statistical methods so far used to study assessing anthropometric and differences that arise, the more expressive one seems to be that of Bravais, complemented by Pearson, ie, the coefficient of correlation necessary to prove a relationship between several features tangible and sports performance.

The many tables of correlation data can be used successfully in multifactorial analysis, in order to concentrate the characteristics and properties of these complexes. With their help it is possible that the correlation coefficients between the multitude of variables, number and type of basic factors (Petersen, 1961) conclusions being reached, ie: "extracting factors" of which characterizes a factor of length (L), a width (B) and the third weight or circumference. Factors should be used for the extraction of the centroid method of Thurstone, because it is simpler and more straightforward than the methods hitherto, requiring electronic computers in the main axes method, and the method of maximum Likelihood. Such calculations are required to be made in data centers that have necessary equipment.

Given that the relationship between sports performance and various measures of body resulting linear calculation will perform linear regression coefficients and then they will be translated into diagrams regression, in order to make a quantitative assessment. Interested in sports activities also influence the performance characteristics in common body, for which we will assess multiple regression up to 12 variables. Solving such a system of equality with so many unknowns involves many calculations that can be made on the computer. Coefficients obtained multifunctional regression in this way have the advantage that enables us to objectify the relationship between physical and performance characteristics influence, provided that all other characteristics (which also influences performance) to be constant. While the simple regression possibility sporting measurable (expressed numerically), it is regarded as a function of body features to take into account the multiple regression mathematical dependence of all bodily characteristics; and here is based on the premise that the report is straightforward: all variations occur only at power 1. Finally, it can investigate the extent to which each characteristic body participates in multiple regression.

Statistical and mathematical formulas used are:

1. Normal distribution $\varphi(x) = \frac{1}{s\sqrt{2\pi}} \bullet e - \frac{(x_i - \bar{x})^2}{2s^2}$ (I)
   π = 3,14159
   e = 2,71828
2. Parity with 3 parts $f_i = \frac{f_{i-1} + f_i + f_{i+1}}{3}$ (II)
3. The arithmetic average $x = \frac{\sum_{i=1}^{n} x_i}{n}$ (III)
4. Average square deviation $s = \pm\sqrt{\frac{\sum_{i=1}^{n} (x_i - x^2}{n-1}}$ (IV)
5. Distribution of averages $s_x = \pm\frac{s}{\sqrt{n}}$ (V)
6. The width variation $V = x_{max} \ldots x_{min}$ (VI)
7. Variation coefficient $v = \frac{w \bullet 100}{x}$ (VIII)
8. Research averages for large collective differences $I = \frac{\bar{x}_1 - \bar{x}_2}{\sqrt{\frac{s_1^2}{n_1} + \frac{s_2^2}{n_2}}}$ (VII)
9. Regression coefficient $b = \frac{\sum x_i y_i - \frac{\sum x_i \sum y_i}{n}}{\sum x_i^2 - \frac{(\sum x_i)}{n}}$ (IX)

10. Equal regression y = b x + a

a = y – b x (X)

11. Total linear correction coefficient $r = \dfrac{\sum x_i y_i - \dfrac{\sum x_i \sum y_i}{n}}{\sqrt{(\sum x_i^2 - \dfrac{(\sum x_i)^2}{n})(\sum y_i^2 - \dfrac{(\sum y_i)^2}{n})}}$ (XI)

12. Factor Theory (basic equation) $r_{ij} = \sum_{i=z}^{p} a_{iz} a_{jz} = a_{i_1} a_{j_1} + a_{i_2} a_{j_2} + .. a_{i_p} a_{jp}$ (XII)

We also stress the importance of graphical representation possibility of obtained values. For graphical representation, which is known to be more expressive than a plurality of digits, curves that indicate density and distribution (variation lanes, spread lanes or spread ellipsis) columns of charts, diagrams of deviation, Profile diagrams (eg., subcutaneous fat sequencing to characterize the two sexes at different ages *Parizkova*, 1962, 1963) and proportional figures are better suited.

Measuring skin folds (Caliperometry) after Parizkova, 1962. (Table 30 32)

1. Definition

Thickness of the skin at fixed body regions.

2. Description of measuring points

(1) - head - projection located in front of the ear canal (tragus)

(2) - on the floor of the mouth, upper hyoid bone.

(3) - on the side of the armpit on the edge of the pectoralis major.

(4) - on the chest - the height coast 10 per anterior axillary line.

(5) - abdomen - obliquely under physiological navel scar after the first quarter on the line joining the anterior superior iliac spine to the navel.

(6) - the hip, directly above the iliac crest.

(7) - back - in the lower angle of the scapula.

(8) - arm - on the back at her, over the brachial triceps muscle.

(9) - thigh – above the upper edge of the patella, at the level crossing rectus femoris in the patellar ligament.

(10) on the shank - over gastrocnemius muscle on the front of the popliteal

3. Calculation of percentage of subcutaneous fat

Once measurements of the thickness of skin folds were taken in the ten places mentioned before, the sum of ten values is calculated. Between that amount and the percentage of subcutaneous fat deposit there are regression relationships that are expressed as follows:

17-40 years	y=22,32	logx-29,20
17-40 years	y=39,57	logx-61,25

These equalities were tabulated (tab. 30)

Under the heading for age and sex, we are looking for the sum of the ten measurements of the skin folds (mm), and under the next heading we read the subcutaneous fat percentage.

The body fat mass deposit (kg) is evidenced from:

(body mass x subcutaneous fat percentage kg %)/ 100

After decreasing the body fat mass from the total body mass (kg) we are left with the so-called active body substance (AKS) which is more accurately called thusly than body mass without fatty tissue (essential body mass, lean body mass). From the body mass substance we have the AKS index, thorough which we evaluate the, muscle expression (tab 31):

[active body substance kg / body height 3x10 m]

Specific body weight

1. Definition

The specific weight gives us data about the alteration of proportions of different body tissues to the overall body mass (eg., bone and connecting tissue, muscle and adipose tissue) (Table 32)

The specific gravity is defined by GY wherein:

G = n x g (kg × m/s^2= 1N) and 9,806 N = 1 kg.

For G we can approximately use m. Specific weight thus corresponds to the body mass (kg) body volume (cm3), which, usually is known under the name of body weight.

This suggests several possibilities for calculating the specific weight

2. Forms of calculation.

According to the equality above:

- Assessment of body mass;
- Evaluation of the body volume;
- Calculating the equality above body weight / body volume (kg / cm3).

Hydrostatic weighing (Archimedes' principle)

Measurement technology using a people scale placed at the edge of a pool was devised by Drobny (1958). The method is complicated by the fact that the person must spend more time under water; it can be accelerated by using a balance with a steel spring.

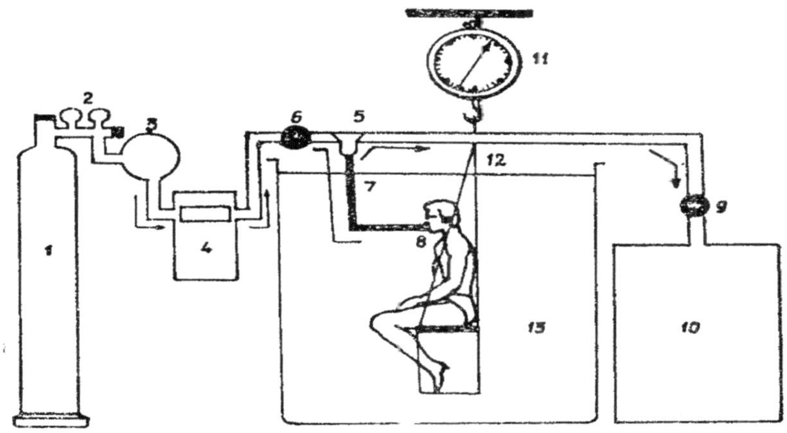

Fig. 79. The apparatus for determining the specific weight

1. oxygen cylinder; 2. gas reducer; 3. The oxygen inhaler; 4. gas meter; 5, 6, 9. valves for breathing apparatus; 7. oxygen hose; 10. Douglas to capture air bag; 11. scale; 12. Hook; 13. water tank.

Regression subcutaneous adipose tissue (skin fold measurements) equalities.

Parizkova (1962) established by comparison with hydrostatic weighing results, regression equalities of the sum of skin folds (10 points) size and specific weight. Thus:

Y=specific body weight,	X= the sum of the 10 skin folds,
Young men=9-12 years	y=1,180-0,069 logx,
13-16 years;	y=1,205-0,078 logx,
Young women=9-12 years;	y=1,60-0,061 logx,
13-16 years;	y=1,205-0,078 logx.

Nomogram - When calculating specific body weight, the above data is given by the author in nomograms, which shows that the specific weight can be determined on the basis of only two places measured.

Establishing body surface and body volume

A. Stabilirea body surface

Methods of determining the body surface will be harder to find in specialty literature. However, this process would be able to be expanded in the future. A geometric experience, carried out by Pfaundler (1916) represents the human body as the sum of the different geometric shapes such as cylinders and truncated cones. From this point of view, the human body can be decomposed into various geometric forms, surfaces calculated for each and the results summed. A more detailed description of this process gives Grimm (1966). The simplest way is to determine body size based on height and weight. In this respect, we performed Tittel tables and Wutscherk (1972), according to calculations by Du Bois and Hannon's nomograms (Table 35). For these assessments are only required height and weight.

B. Establishing body volume

1. The process of the submerged tank: The measurement principle is based on the compression exerted on submerged water in a tank. The amount of water compared will be contracted in interconnecting pipe, which has a scale engraved or painted by the passage of water and lifting them up to a certain level or by passing it into the measuring vessel (Grimm, 1966).

2. Anthropometric Measure: The body volume varies according to the degree of filling of the lung (vital capacity, residual volume). For comparison we give the following calculations after the Bugyi (1973).

1) Chest circumference at the level of the diaphragm (BU)

(2) The length of the sternum (ST)

Thoracic volume (VB) is calculated as follows:

$$\left(\frac{BU}{2\pi}\right)^2 \times \pi \times ST$$

If VB is known, then it appears:

- Vital capacity VB + 820 = 057 (ml);
- Residual Volume = 0.213 VB 324 (ml);
- Total capacity VB = 0.80. + 400 (ml).

In establishing body volume, the person measured should be investigated below the water surface. Both plenitude and interconnecting pipe with a diameter relatively narrow, so equalizing the two surfaces of water occurs slowly. Both plenitude and interconnecting pipe have a diameter that is relatively narrow, so equalizing the two surfaces of water occurs slowly. In this regard the person being investigated must sink slowly into the basin so that, when sinking only the volume of the body will be displaced. Of course, the tank should be filled with water at body temperature and to comply with hygienic norms (fig. 79).

3. The assessment method: The body volume can be measured by equalities which comprise the “body height” and “body weight” variables. It's known as the Cowgill (1957) formula corrected by Wittig (1964) for sports physiology.

V. Determining the type of body build

The morphological picture of human expression is varied (possibility same combination of genes is [after Bach (1965)] 1 / 7X1012). However, the basic features of the human form (size and proportions of length, width and depth) are relatively few. Attempts to classify growth trends and types of body build go as far back as antiquity (Hipokrates - 460 377 BCE). Many of these experiences have in common that they all start from appearances (externalization). The concept of "type" is methodologically defined by common characteristics of a type, other features may be different. However, such communities (similarities and identities) must refer to the basic characteristics of the individual. Properties are arising only from the interplay of two objects ie invariable properties, only by treating them with defined structural systems. Illustrating the body shapes of the athletes using anthropological methods, which refer verbally or metricly growth trend is purely descriptive and reMayns dependent on chance as the average values of each body features (Table 26).

Table 26

Construction characteristics of the constitutional types of body

	Men			Female		
	leptosome	athletic	picnic	leptosome	athletic	picnic
1. Height (cm)	168, 4	170,0	167, 8	153, 8	163, 1	156, 5
2. Body mass (kg)	50,5	62, 9	68, 0	44, 4	61,7	56, 3
3. Shoulder length (cm)	35, 5	39, 1	36, 9	32, 8	37, 4	34, 3
4. Thoracic circumference (cm)	84, 1	91,7	94, 5	77, 7	83, 0	86, 0
5. Abdominal circumference(cm)	74, 1	79, 6	88, 8	67, 7	75, 1	78, 7
6. Pelvic circumference (cm)	84, 7	91,5	92, 0	82, 2	95, 8	94, 2
7. Inferior limb length. (cm)	80,4	90,9	87, 4	79, 2	85, 0	80,5

Therefore, the body typology of the athlete must start from the structural and functional relationships, relationships determined by general laws, relations between body construction and performance skills, ie to build on purpose. Since this failed so far, sports anthropometry still uses descriptive methods, which, theoretically, are subject to the laws of the above, and the methodical point of view is based on objectivity and may be reproduced for the purpose of subsequent sampling. It is therefore necessary that we to reproduce the first three methods whose results can still be found in the sports literature (Kretschmer)

1. Determining the type of body build according to Kretschmer: This method has spread rapidly since the author tried to combine the morphological form with the special characteristics and predispositions to disease.

Table 27

Characteristics of types of body according to Kretschmer

Type	– Trunk proportions	Relief de suprafaţă	Extremitate
Picnic	– short, concave chest, obtuse rib angle	rotunde, forme moi, datcrită ţesutului adipos bine format	moi, relativ scurte, mâini şi picioare osoase, scurte şi late
Athletic	– Broad shoulders, strong trunk trapezoid-shaped with a relatively narrow abdomen	relief muscular puternic, plastic	membre, palme şi plante puternice, acrocianoză
Leptosom	– Long chest, flat, sharp rib angle, relatively wide abdomen	slab, cu puţin ţesut adipos subcutanat	extremităţi lungi, subţiri, cu mâini şi picioare lungi şi subţiri

Classification and three types (leptosom, athletic and picnomorf) is based on subjective representations (Table 27). Establishing metric differences of the body characteristics that these groups have is something achieved only in part (*Tittel and Wuscherk*, 1972).

2. Determining the type of body build according *Sheldon*.

The author had a hard time trying to fit 4,000 American students in the three groups above.

Altogether emerged:

- 9% - leptosomi
- 12% - athletic
- 7% - ***Picnic***

72 of those surveyed could not be put into any category because of the mixture of ***picnic leptosome and athletic*** features.

Sheldon sees the body shape as a result of the sharp development of one of the three embryonic skins (endoderm, mesoderm and ectoderm) and shares the basic types as all three Kretschmer extreme (endomorph, mesomorphic, ectomorph). The assessment was made according to subjective impressions obtained by full body photography. Features include seven degrees on a scale. The number seven corresponds to a total expression of a type, the number one corresponds to the zero (0) identity (non - identity). The average values of characteristics assessed for the expression of endo meso and ectomorph body type given us three figures:

7.1.1. Clear endomorph type

1.7.1. Clear mesomorphous type,

1.1.7. Clear ectomorph type.

Within the system there are positions for intermediary values (eg., 3.5.3.)as well, which is an advantage for the researcher. Meaning that the 70% of cases that could not be included in the Kretschmer scale were classified as morphological phenomena and understood and differentiated as legitimate mixtures and variations by Klaus (1953).

3. Determining the type of body build according Heath Carter.

This method corresponds to the basic principles of the Sheldon method. She completes on this because the authors try to eliminate some criticisms that relate in particular to grading on the scale (1-7) and their representation in the population and also trying to eliminate the subjectivity of the author (Meredith, 1940). The authors give corrections to the degrees on the scale that, according to Parnell's method (1954, 1957) can be researched and metric.

According to this point of view:

- As a measure for expressing endomorph we have thick skin folds on the arm over the triceps muscle(8), inferior to the angle of the scapula (7), superior to the iliac crest (6) (F scale; f = fat);

- As a measure for expressing mesomorph we have the ratio of the fours measurements of width and circumference (***epicondyle*** width of the humerus and the femur arm and leg circumferences corrected by measurements of skin folds) to body height (Scale M; m = muscularity);

- As a measure for expressing ectomorph we have the ratio of body height and body weight (body height / body weight = in / Lb) (Scale L; Ilinearity)

Body type of construction is calculated in the following manner: the position on the measured value size scale is passes onto the F and L scales. For calculating values on the M scale we need to calculate the "midpoint" of the four measuring spots. Their deviation from the value of body height is transformed to the same value on the M scale (Table 28).

Table 28

Heath-Carter evaluation form body type design

Name: Ocupation: Project:	Age:												Data: Researcher:												
Skin fold mm: triceps brahialis	Superior limits	1_2	14.9	18.9	22.9	26.9	31.2	35.8	40.7	46.2	52.2	58.7	65.7	73.2	81.2	89.7	98.9	108.9	119.7	131.2	143.7	157.2	171.9	187.9	204.0
scapula	Average value	9.0	13.0	17.0	21.0	25.0	29.0	33.5	38.0	43.5	49.0	55.5	62.0	69.5	77.0	85.5	94.0	104.0	114.0	125.5	137.0	150.5	164.0	180.0	196.0
Iliac crest = 9.9	Inferior limits	7.8	11.0	15.0	19.0	23.0	27.0	31.3	35.9	40.8	46.3	52.3	58.0	65.8	73.3	81.3	89.8	99.0	109.0	119.8	131.3	143.8	157.3	172.0	188.0
total	1.first component F Scale	10.9	1	1'2	2	2'2	3	3'2	4	4'2	5	5'2	6	6'2	7	7'2	8	8'2	9	9'2	10	10'2	11	11'2	12

Height (In)	55.0	66.5	58.0	59.5	61.0	62.5	64.0	65.5	64.0	68.5	70.0	71.5	73.0	74.5	76.0	77.5	79.0	80.5	82.0	83.5	85.0	86.5	88.0	89.5
widh (cm)	5.19	5.34	5.49	5.64	5.78	5.93	6.07	6.22	6.37	6.51	6.65	6.80	6.95	7.09	7.24	7.38	7.53	7.67	7.82	7.97	8.11	8.25	8.40	8.55
Humerus femur	7.41	7.62	7.83	8.04	8.24	8.45	8.66	8.87	9.08	9.28	9.49	9.70	9.91	10.12	10.33	10.53	10.74	10.95	11.16	11.37	11.58	11.79	12.00	12.21
Arm circumference skin fold	23.7	24.4	25.0	25.7	26.3	27.0	27.7	28.3	29.0	29.7	30.3	31.0	31.6	32.2	33.0	33.6	34.3	35.0	35.6	36.3	37.1	37.8	38.5	39.3

1.3 = 31.7 Shank circumference skin fold (95)= 34.1	27.7	28.5	29.3	30.1	30.8	31.6	32.4	33.2	33.9	34.7	35.5	36.3	37.1	37.8	38.6	39.4	40.2	41.0	41.8	42.6	43.4	44.2	45.0	45.8
1. a 2-a M componets	1_2	1_2	1	1'2	2	2'2	3	3'2				4	4'2	5	5'2	6	6'2	7	7'2	8	8'2	9		

Body mass Lb = 147.0	Superior limits	11.99	12.32	12.53	12.74	12.95	13.15	13.36	13.56	13.77	13.98	14.19	14.39	14.59	14.80	15.01	15.22	15.42	15.63
	Average value		12.16	12.43	12.64	12.85	13.05	13.26	13.46	13.67	13.88	14.01	14.29	14.50	14.70	14.91	15.12	15.33	15.53
Height In = 12.76	Inferior limits	und weniger	12.00	12.33	12.54	12.75	12.96	13.16	13.37	13.56	13.78	13.99	14.20	14.40	14.60	14.81	15.02	15.23	15.43
	a 3-a L Scale component	I_2	1	1'2	2	2'2	3	3'2	4	4'2	5	5'2	6	6'2	7	7'2	8	8'2	9

Constitutional type	1st component	2-nd component	3-rd component
Corporal anthropometrical	4	5	2 ½
Filled by photographic evaluations			

Signature:

....

....

4. **Determining the type of body build according Conrad.**

After using Kretschmer's typology (*Tittel*, 1963 *Wutscherk*, 1966) currently we use the Conrad method (1944, 1963) (*Wutscherk*, 1968). This change is motivated by the advantages of the method. Characteristic for this method is:

- The types of body build are not seen as polar types, meaning extreme types, but as logical appearances within the normal relationship of characteristics. The average is therefore the most common is normal;
- All normal distributions have mutually exclusive poles. In Conrad's chart these types are leptomorfe and picnomorfe. That's why the athletic type cannot be identical to the average. This type deviates, as far as the characteristics of the tendenciesare concerned, from the limits of the characteristics reappearance, versus the leptomorfe and picnomorfe types
- The "athletic" body shape must be understood as a specific form of expressing body construction. leptomorfe and picnomorfe body constructions can be expressed as athletic but, also within normal limits, with an inverse tendency (non-athletic). Conrad uses the term hyperplasia athletic expression, to contrast the term hypoplasia;
- Conrad typology is based on two distinct planes called variation 1 and 2;
- The characteristic order within the plane of variation based on the metric sizes of the body characteristics are:

• The first plan of variation: body height, width and depth of chest. These measures are brought together in the metric's index (*Stormgren*, 1937) in a single module design incorporates value and proportion;

• The second level of variation includes: shoulder width, forearm circumference, idem hand. They appear in the plastic index and incorporates the dimensional conception;

- metric and plastic index values will be converted by tables (Table 29) and listed in a coordination scheme consisting of 81 fields. This requires us to divide the spectrum of distribution of the two indices in nine classes. The metric classes index will be denoted by uppercase letters (A - picnomorf, E - mesomorphous, L - leptomorf) and the plastic index of Arabic numerals (1 - hypoplasia; 5 - mezoplazic; 9 - hyperplastic). An athlete who matches the terms of normal body construction, of the average will be placed in the scheme coordinated by the "E5" and verbally, as mesomorphous mezoplazic;
- establishing the body typology is based on the normal distribution of body characteristics in the population. Therefore, by this method we can evaluate types of bodies in women, children and youth

Morphological properties will show in researches to come, how much this method contributes to the representation of athletes. Typological differences in the body construction of athletes from various disciplines should, however, be showed with priority (*Wutscherk* 1968; *Tittel* and *Wutscherk*, 1972).

Conrad himself shows that it is impossible to fit the wide variability of the human body construction in two or three types of forms. It is also difficult to prove that through metric index, ie the ratio of body height, width and depth of chest, we can reveal morphological structural elements; here, the levers and forces of the extremities and body mass ratios and all those concepts have a decisive role and must be included in phenomenology. (See Table 33).

It is however certain that using this method of typology of subjective corporal construction became objective, from being previously subjective, and thus becoming comparative.

Table 29

Changes in body construction characteristics in different types of body constitutions in 100 female students (Tittel)

characteristics	3 - 19			2. 17-18 years			1. 16		
	2	A	P	L	A	P	L	A	P
Body height (cm)	164.9	161.3	162.3	165.4	162.2	162.9	165.6	162.4	163.1
Body weight (kg)	54.1	58.1	68.9	53.7	58.0	67.3	54.8	57.6	69.2
Active body substance (kg)	45.5	47.7	51.8	44.6	47.3	52.1	45.9	46.9	52.1
AKS index	1.04	1.13	1.21	0.96	1.11	1.20	1.01	1.10	1.20
Fatty tissue %	8.2	11.1	16.6	8.9	10.9	16.9	9.7	11.4	17.2
Body build complex: A	59.7	62.7	68.5	59.7	63.4	70.1	62.0	63.5	70.5
B	85.9	80.4	70.4	88.9	81.7	72.3	86.1	81.5	72.0
C	1.49	1.31	1.04	1.50	1.31	1.06	1.39	1.29	1.02
Relative body weight	328	360	424	325	358	413	331	355	424

L = leptospom, A = atletic, P = picnic

Data for determining the type of body construction according to *Conrad's* method. The procedure was as follows:

a. The measurement

- body height
- transverse diameter of the thorax,
- Sagittal diameter of the chest,
- Shoulder width,
- forearm Circumference
- hand Circumference

b. Calculating the metric index. The best way to calculate this using Stormgren and Thooris chart and a pointed compass. On the vertical we search for the value of the body size and on the horizontal the value of the diameter of the thorax. The place where the two lines intersect we place one tip of the compass. We search for the shorter diagonal line that corresponds to the sagittal thorax diameter; if it is above the first point, than the value receives a negative sign on the scale; if it is situated below that point it receives a positive sign. These indices will form nine classes, which give the position A to L of the abscissa (fig. 81).

Respective index values will be included in the tables with 5 and 9 classes and will be marked with letters from A (picnomorf) to L (leptomorf) (Table 33)

c. Calculationg the plastic index. The plastic index is easier to calculate. It is the sum of values - shoulder width, forearm and hand circumference - which then are then transformed according to the tables. (Table 34).

d. The formulation of the type of body construction. For determining the position we use a diagram consisting of 81 fields.

Metric and plastic index values, which have been transformed in accordance with the table in the 9 classes, give us the crossing point of the coordinates, ie the position of general distribution within the body construction. Corresponding to the basic tenets of coordinates, the types of body construction will be defined verbally, for example:

- B5 – picnomorf-mezoplazic,

- E8 – mezomorf-hiperplazic,
- I2 – leptomorf-hipoplazic.

And the forms of transition can be finalized, for example.:

- F 6 – mezoleptomorf - mezohiperplazic,
- H 6 – leptomorf - mezo-hiperplazic,
- C 3 – picnomezomorf – hipo-mezoplazic.

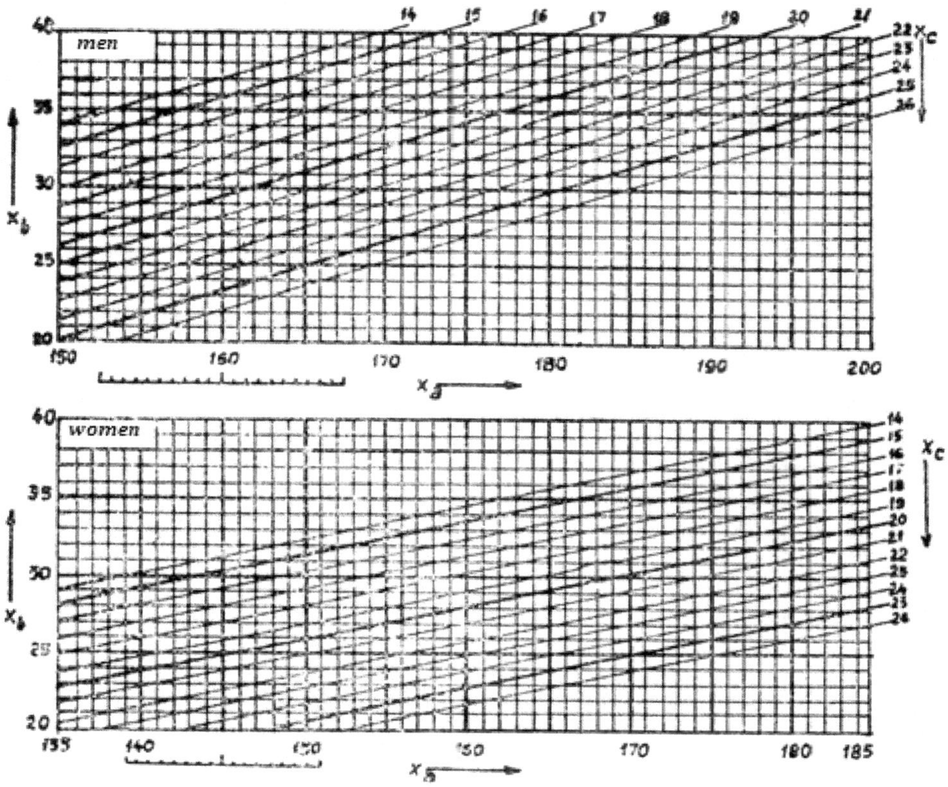

Fig. 80 metric index calculation chart.

Antropometrografică method of establishing constitutional type (Briant) applicable in sport.

With the techniques that we remember very quickly, it may be appropriate, first, to emphasize fundamental concepts underlying the method presented (and other similar methods).

- the normal distribution curve law has great significance for each ample and uniform sample but has no value for the individual, who must almost always be considered as a mosaic of different "tendencies".
- The deviations of each subject from the average normality are evaluated through measurements chosen so as to the three fundamental dimensions of space is well represented. Thus, the correlations of individual morphology with physiology appear more obvious.
- The individual is a unique reality that the constitutional concept we have to address it and fit it as clearly as possible, with the precision and simplicity of mathematics elementary, especially the geometrical representation, which gives us the perception of immediate absolute measures and relative to the individual himself, against the medium of the corresponding part of the population (fig. 80 82).
- Formulas and diagnostics guidance, but especially genetic definitions of typology

proposed by many other authors more or less remove from the reality that individual antropometrogramele are most clearly close; the latter represent the fundamentals of the antropometrografice method (Amf).

Thus, the advantages that this method has for its subjects of a certain age, from childhood to old age appear. Constructions start with a general chart (GG) for every sex and age, built with data on very large samples, in no case less than 60 individuals each.

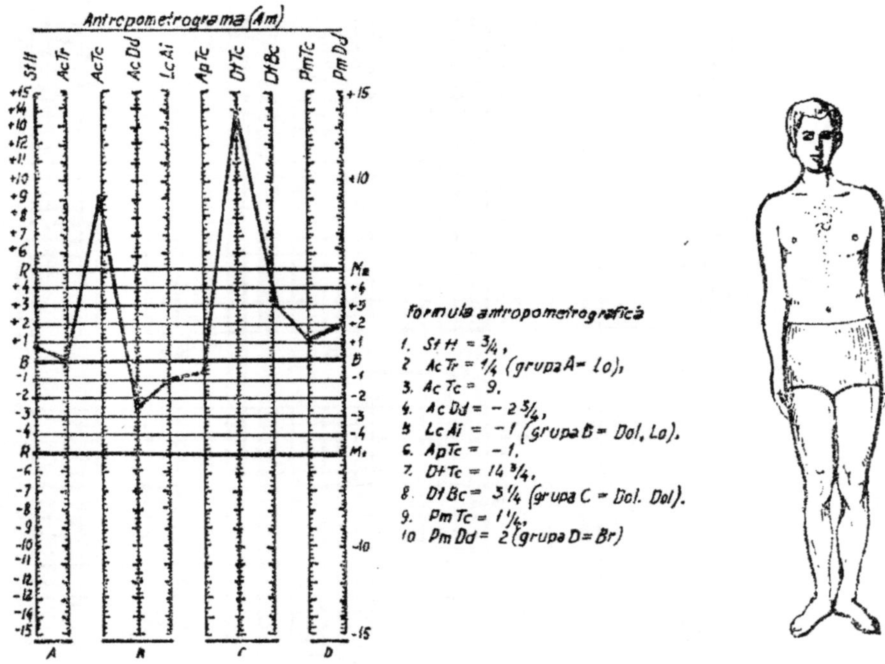

Fig. 81 fractomegamorf dizarmonic type

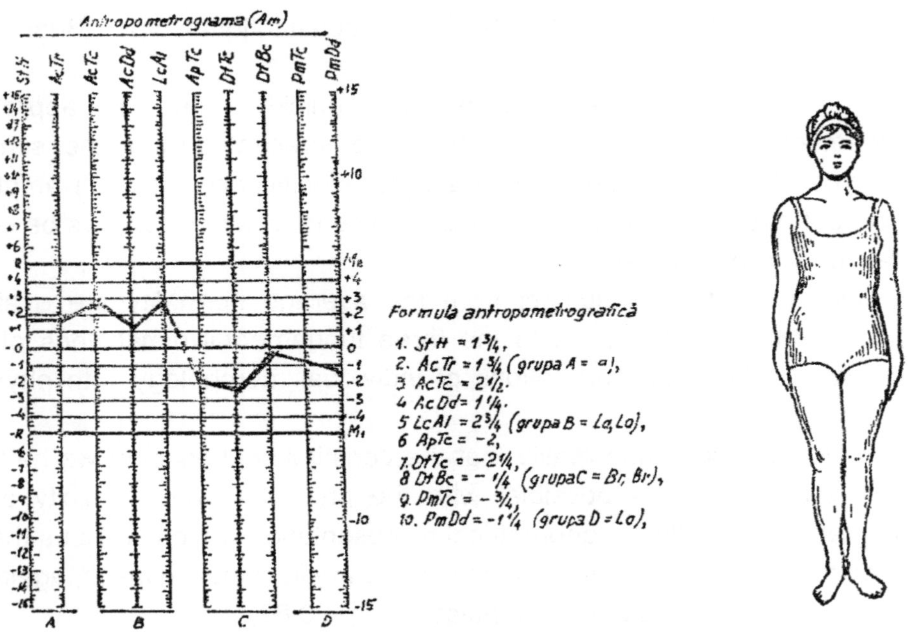

Fig. 82 fractomediomorf paralongilin armonic type

We present here first, the antropometrografic sheet. The new form is a simple sheet of paper folded in the middle (so there are four pages). The first page contains, marital status and medical history of the subject, the second and third have the size list (10 in the AMF system) with the AMF formula and the Antropometrograma (Amm) under the shape of a broken line on the standard GG grid; on the fourth page there is place for the subject's photo and the diagnosis.

The fundamental theoretical reference or rectoform types, for each sample are the bazomorf type (*BB*), which is the expression of median ideal normality, the major rectomegamorf *(RMa) and the minor* rectomegamorf (*RMi*); the corresponding measurements are on the central abscissa and on the two external parallels of the relative GG consisting of the standard grid mentioned before, involving several other measures, relative to 10 decimal degrees (Gd) - which lead to eight rectomorfe types (+ 1, + 2, + 3, + 4), whose action is recorded on the intermediate horizontal lines.

Antropometrograms can be made:

- Short time and with maximum precision, using appropriate facilities;

- Provided immediately by dividing into four equal parts, standard grid, each vertical segment, represents the size of the decimal degree to which it relates.

In the latter case, which we present here, we must record the GG, with Gd values (-5 to +5 at appropriate vertical intersections with 11 horizontal parallel, one for each degree, including the degree zero of BB) the middle points of the segments corresponding to the above-mentioned vertical.

After individual, irreplaceable Amm was constructed, it's very easy to reach the Amf formulas in which the symbol for every size is followed by a number that shows decimal degrees corresponding to the measurement of each subject.

Diagnoses guidance, similar to those proposed by other authors, reveal, with improvements and always based graphical overview of each individual constitutional physiognomy. Real subjects are named in diagnoses "fractomorfi", which are divided into harmonic and disharmonic, the latter with evidently more pronounced deviations.

The table for automatically establishing the guidance diagnoses for a subject refers to the following 10 dimensions of the reduced Amf system.

Group A: 1) stature (St. Tt), 2) Conventional trunk height (AcTr);

Group B: 3) Conventional chest height *(AcTe);* 4) Conventional abdominal height *(AcDd);* 5) Conventional leg length *(LeAi);*

Group C: 6) anterior-posterior diameter of the chest (ApTc); 7transverse diameter of the chest (DtTc); 8) transverse diameter of the pelvis (DtBe);

Group D: 9) thoracic perimeter (PmTc); 10) abdominal perimeter (PmDd). other symbols: Br=**parabrevilin (armonic), Bra=brahitip (dizarmonic), Dol=Dolicotip (Dizarmonic), Lo=paralongilin (armonic).**

Partial diagnoses: Lo or Br the predominance of a measure over another in the same group, the orientation of less than 2, 5 Gd (Gd / 2 is the addition of the largest possible errors); Dol or Bra = predominance as above, more than 2.5 Gd.

Figures 82 and 83 represent Amm, Amf formulas and diagnostic guidance on two adults subjects, male and female. On the same figures, it should be noted that thin vertical lines on the grid indicate standard dimensions whose measures are higher in subjects Lo to Dol and thick lines show dimensions that are greater in subjects measures Bra to Br. We must also observe on the figures mentioned above, the vertical segments that emerge from the standard central grid (including between + 5 Gd), segments used for extrapolation.

As far as the time needed to establish individual Amm, hence the possibility of applications even in the largest samples, we have noticed a few things. After a reference GG has been developed, for every sex and age that we are interested in, the measurements of the subjects, which have been established with the aid of instruments mentioned on the chart, can be written on the chars itself, than reported to the corresponding points on the standard grid in approximately 6-**10 minutes,** consequently a comprehensive evaluation of 6 to 10 subjects can be done in an hour. Of course, very adequate results may be obtained, if we have a specialized staff, at least two people and good work management. In addition, instead of performing all measurements, one after another on the same subject, it is indicated, for the same size, to find the corresponding measures of small groups of subjects in a same sample that is studied (repeating each measurement at least twice). In order for the process to become almost automatical it is preferable that the conditions, very simple, which relate to the immediate construction of Amm, must always be applied by the same technicians.

It can be concluded that the above organization of labor is still able to provide, very easily and in minimal time, the most accurate Amm or formulas and diagnostics guidance for the larger samples. The proposed method helps, as many authors have recognized, the most diverse research, applied to lots of athletes who require or may start from a clear constitutional assessment. The method is completed in the report by performing it on parents and children, and we can conclude on some aspects of the hereditary fund.

Table 30

Subcutaneous fat deposit as a percentage of body weight, based on measurement of 10 points (Parizkova, 1962)

60	male	female	13-16 years girls and boys	9-12 years youths	9-12 years girls
30	1.5		3.9	8.1	11.2
31	1.9		4.4	8.5	11.5
32	2.3		4.8	8.9	11.8
33	2.7		5.2	9.2	12.1
34	3.1		5.6	9.6	12.5
35	3.5		6.0	9.9	12.7
36	3.8	0.4	6.3	10.2	13.0
37	4.1	0.8	6.7	10.6	13.3
38	4.5	1.3	7.1	10.9	13.6
39	4.8	1.7	7.4	11.2	13.9
40	5.1	2.1	7.7	11.5	14.1
41	5.4	2.6	8.0	11.8	14.4
42	5.7	3.0	8.4	12.0	14.6
43	6.0	3.4	8.7	12.3	14.9
44	6.3	3.8	9.0	12.6	15.1
45	6.6	4.2	9.3	12.8	15.3
46	6.9	4.5	9.6	13.1	15.6
47	7.1	4.9	10.0	13.3	15.8
48	7.4	5.3	10.1	13.6	16.0
49	7.7	5.6	10.3	13.8	16.2
50	8.1	6.0	10.7	14.0	16.4
51	8.2	6.3	10.9	14.3	16.6
52	8.4	6.6	11.1	14.5	16.8

60	male	female	13-16 years girls and boys	9-12 years youths	9-12 years girls
53	8.7	7.0	11,4	14.7	17.0
54	8.9	7.3	11,7	14.9	17.2
55	9.1	7.6	11,9	15.1	17.4
56	9.4	7.9	12.1	15.4	17.6
57	9.5	8.2	12.4	15.6	17.8
58	9.8	8.5	12.6	15.8	17.9
59	10.0	8.8	12.8	16.0	18.1
60	10.2	9.1	13.0	16.2	18.3
61	10.4	9.4	13.3	16.3	18.5
62	10.6	9.7	13.5	16.5	18.6
63	10.8	9.9	13.7	16.7	18.8
64	11.0	10.2	13.9	16.9	18.9
65	11.2	10.5	14.1	17.1	19.1
66	11.4	10.7	14.3	17.3	19.3
67	11.6	11.0	14.5	17.4	19.4
68	11.8	11.2	14.7	17.6	19.6
69	12.0	11.5	14.9	17.8	19.7
70	12.2	11.8	15.1	17.9	19.9
71	12.3	12.0	15.2	18.1	20.0
72	12.5	12.2	15.4	18.3	20.2
73	12.7	12.5	15.6	18.4	20.3
74	12.9	12.7	15.8	18.6	20.4
75	13.0	12.9	16.0	18.7	20.6
76	13.2	13.1	16.1	18.9	20.7
77	13.3	13.4	16.3	19.0	20.8
78	13.5	13.6	16.5	19.2	21.0
79	13.7	13.8	16.6	19.3	21.1
80	13.8	14.0	16.8	19.5	21.2
81	14.0	14.2	17.0	19.6	21.4
82	14.2	14.5	17.1	19.8	21.5
83	14.3	14.7	17.3	19.9	21.6
84	14.5	14.9	17.5	20.0	21.7
85	14.6	15.1	17.6	20.2	21.9
86	14.8	15.3	17.8	20.3	22.0
87	14.9	15.5	17.9	20.4	22.1
88	15.0	15.7	18.1	20.6	22.2
89	15.2	15.9	18.2	20.7	22.3
90	15.3	16.1	18.4	20.8	22.4
91	15.5	16.3	18.5	21.0	22.6
92	15.6	16.4	18.6	21.1	22.7
93	15.7	16.6	18.8	21.2	22.8
94	15.9	16.8	18.9	21.3	22.9
95	16.0	17.0	19.1	21.5	23.0

60	male	female	13-16 years girls and boys	9-12 years youths	9-12 years girls
96	16.01	17.2	19.2	21.6	23.1
97	16.3	17.3	19.3	21.7	23.2
98	16.4	17.5	19.5	21.8	23.3
99	16.5	17.7	19.6	21.9	23.4
100	16.7	17.9	19.7	22.1	23.5
102	16.8	18.1	19.9	22.2	23.6
101	16.9	18.2	20.0	22.3	23.7
103	17.0	18.4	20.1	22.4	23.8
104	17.1	18.6	20.3	22.5	23.9
105	17.3	18.7	20.4	22.6	24.0
106	17.4	18.9	20.5	22.7	24.1
107	17.5	19.0	20.6	22.8	24.2
108	17.6	19.2	20.7	22.9	24.3
109	17.7	19.4	20.8	23.1	24.4
110	17.9	19.5	20.9	23.2	24.5
111	18.0	19.7	21.1	23.3	24.6
112	18.1	19.8	21.2	23.4	24.7
113	18.2	20.0	21.3	23.5	24.8
114	18.3	20.1	21.5	23.6	24.9
115	18.4	20.3	21.6	23.7	25.0
116	18.5	20.4	21.7	23.8	25.0
117	18.6	20.6	21.8	23.9	25.1
118	18.7	20.7	21.9	24.0	25.2
119	18.8	20.9	22..0	24.1	25.3
120	18.9	21.0	22.1	24.2	25.4
121	19.2	21.1	22.2	24.3	25.5
122	19.0	21.3	22.3	24.4	25.6
123	19.1	21.4	22.5	24.5	25.7
124	19.4	21.6	22.6	24.5	25.7
125	19.5	21.7	22.7	24.6	25.8
126	19.6	21.8	22.8	24.7	25.9
127	19.7	22.0	22.9	24.8	26.0
128	19.8	22.1	23.0	24.9	26.1
129	19.9	22.2	23.1	25.0	26.1
130	20.0	22.4	23.2	25.1	26.2
131	20.1	22.5	23.3	25.2	26.3
132	20.1	22.6	23.4	25.3	26.4
133	20.2	22.8	23.5	25.4	26.5
134	20.4	22.9	23.6	25.4	26.5
135	20.4	23.0	23.7	25.5	26.6
136	20.5	23.2	23.8	25.6	26.7
137	20.6	23.3	23.9	25.7	26.8
138	20.7	23.5	24.0	25.8	26.8

60	male	female	13-16 years girls and boys	9-12 years youths	9-12 years girls
139	20.8	23.6	24.1	25.9	26.9
140	20.9	23.7	24.2	25.9	27.0
141	21.0	23.8	24.3	26.0	27.1
142	21.1	24.0	24.4	26.1	27.1
143	21.2	24.1	24.5	26.2	27.2
144	21.3	24.2	24.6	26.3	27.3
145	21.3	24.3	24.7	26.4	27.3
146	21.4	24.5	fete	26.4	27.4
147	21.5	24.6	24.8	26.5	27.5
148	21.6	24.7	24.9	26.6	27.6
149	21.7	24.8	25.0	26.7	27.6
150	21.8	24.9	25.1	26.7	27.7
151	21.8	25.0	25.1	26.8	27.8
152	21.9	25.1	25.2	26.9	27.8
153	22.0	25.2	25.3	27.0	27.9
154	22.1	25.3	25.4	27.0	28.0
155	22.2	25.4	25.5	27.1	28.0
160	22.6	26.0	25.9	27.5	28.4
165	23.0	26.5	26.3	27.8	28.7
170	23.3	27.0	26.7	28.2	29.0
175	23.7	27.5	27.1	2S.5	.29.3
130	24.1	28.0	27.4	28.9	29.6
185	24.4	28.5	28.0	29.2	29.8
190	24.7	28.9	28.1	29.5	30.1
195	25.1	29.4	28.5	29.8	30.4
200	25.4	29.3	28.8	30.1	30.6
205	25.7	30.2	29.1		
210	26.0	30.6	29.5		
215	26.3	31.0	29.8		
220	26.6	31.4	30.1		
225	26.9	31.8	30.4		
230	27.1	32.2	30.7		
235	27.4	32.5	30.9		
240	27.7	32.9	31.2		
245	27.9	33.2	31.5		
250	28.2	33.6	31.7		
255	28.4	33.9	32.0		
260	28.7	34.3	32.3		
265	28.9	34.7	32.5		
270	29.1	35.0	32.8		
275	29.4	35.3	33.0		
280	29.6	35.6	33.2		
285	29.8	35.9	33.5		

60	male	female	13-16 years girls and boys	9-12 years youths	9-12 years girls
290	30.0	36.2	33.7		
295	30.3	36.5	33.9		
300	30.5	36.8	34.1		
305	30.7		34.4		
310	30.9		34.7		
315	31.1		34.8		
320	31.3		34.9		
325	31.5		35.2		
330	31.7		35.4		
335	31.9		35.6		
340	32.0		35.8		
345	32.2		36.0		
350	32.4		36.2		

Table 31

Calculating the AKS index (active body substance)

Body height (m)	**active body substance** (kg)												
	35	40	45	50	55	60	65	70	75	80	85	90	95
1	2	3	4	5	6	7	8	9	10	11	12	13	14
1.50	1.04	1.18	1.33	1.48	1.63	1.78	1.93	2.07	2.22	2.37	2.52	2.66	2.81
1.51	1.02	1.16	1.31	1.45	1.60	1.74	1.89	2.03	2.18	2.32	2.47	2.61	2.76
1.52	1.00	1.14	1.28	1.42	1.57	1.71	1.85	1.99	2.13	2.28	2.37	2.56	2.71
1.53	0.98	1.12	1.26	1.39	1.54	1.68	1.81	1.95	2.09	2.19	2.42	2.51	2.65
1.54	0.96	1.10	1.23	1.37	1.51	1.64	1.78	1.92	2.05	2.23	2.33	2.46	2.60
1.55	0.94	1.07	1.21	1.34	1.48	1.61	1.75	1.88	2.01	2.15	2.28	2.42	2.55
1.56	0.92	1.05	1.19	1.32	1.45	1.58	1.71	1.84	1.98	2.11	2.24	2.37	2.50
1.57	0.90	1.03	1.16	1.29	1.42	1.55	1.68	1.81	1.94	2.07	2.20	2.33	2.45
1.58	0.89	1.01	1.14	1.27	1.39	1.52	1.65	1.77	1.90	2.03	2.16	2.28	2.41
1.59	0.87	1.00	1.12	1.24	1.37	1.49	1.62	1.74	1.87	1.99	2.11	2.24	2.36
1.60	0.85	0.98	1.10	1.22	1.34	1.46	1.58	1.71	1.83	1.95	2.08	2.20	2.32
1.61	0.84	0.96	1.08	1.20	1.32	1.44	1.56	1.68	1.80	1.92	2.04	2.16	2.28
1.62	0.82	0.94	1.06	1.18	1.29	1.41	1.53	1.65	1.76	1.88	2.00	2.12	2.23
1.63	0.81	0.92	1.02	1.15	1.27	1.39	1.50	1.62	1.73	1.85	1.96	2.08	2.19
1.64	0.79	0.89	1.04	1.13	1.25	1.36	1.47	1.59	1.70	1.81	1.93	2.04	2.11
1.65	0.78	0.91	1.00	1.11	1.22	1.34	1.45	1.56	1.67	1.78	1.89	2.00	2.15
1.66	0.76	0.87	0.98	1.09	1.20	1.31	1.42	1.53	1.64	1.75	1.86	1.97	2.08
1.67	0.75	0.86	0.97	1.07	1.18	1.29	1.40	1.50	1.61	1.72	1.83	1.93	2.04
1.68	0.74	0.84	0.95	1.05	1.16	1.27	1.37	1.48	1.58	1.69	1.79	1.90	1.97
1.69	0.72	0.83	0.93	1.04	1.14	1.22	1.35	1.45	1.55	1.66	1.76	1.86	2.00
1.70	0.71	0.81	0.91	1.02	1.12	1.24	1.32	1.42	1.53	1.63	1.73	1.83	1.93

1.71	0.70	0.80	0.90	1.00	1.10	1.20	1.30	1.40	1.50	1.60	1.67	1.80	1.90
1.72	0.69	0.79	0.88	0.98	1.08	1.18	1.28	1.35	1.47	1.57	1.70	1.77	1.87
1.73	0.68	0.77	0.87	0.97	1.06	1.16	1.25	1.38	1.45	1.54	1.64	1.74	1.83
1.74	0.66	0.76	0.85	0.95	1.04	1.14	1.23	1.33	1.42	1.52	1.61	1.71	1.80
1.75	0.65	0.75	0.84	0.93	1.03	1.12	1.21	1.31	1.40	1.49	1.59	1.68	1.77
1.76	0.64	0.73	0.83	0.92	1.01	1.10	1.19	1.28	1.38	1.47	1.56	1.65	1.74
1.77	0.63	0.72	0.81	0.90	0.99	1.08	1.17	1.26	1.35	1.44	1.53	1.62	1.71
1.78	0.62	0.71	0.80	0.89	0.98	1.06	1.15	1.24	1.33	1.42	1.51	1.60	1.68
1.79	0.61	0.70	0.78	0.87	0.96	1.05	1.13	1,22	1.31	1.39	1.48	1.54	1.66
1.80	0.60	0.69	0.77	0.86	0.94	1.03	1.11	1.20	1.29	1.37	1.46	1.57	1.63
1.81	0.59	0.67	0.76	0.84	0.93	1.01	1.10	1.18	1.26	1.35	1.43	1.52	1.60
1.82	0.58	0.66	0.75	0.83	0.91	1.00	1.08	1.16	1.24	1.33	1.41	1.49	1.58
1.83	0.57	0.65	0.73	0.82	0.90	0.98	1.06	1.14	1.22	1.31	1.39	1.47	1.55
1.84	0.56	0.64	0.72	0.80	0.88	0.96	1.04	1.12	1.20	1.28	1.36	1.44	1.52
1.85	0.55	0.63	0.71	0.79	0.87	0.95	1.03	1.11	1.18	1.26	1.34	1.42	1.50
1.86	0.54	0.62	0.70	0.78	0.85	0.93	1.01	1.09	1.17	1.24	1.32	1.40	1.48
1.87	0.53	0.61	0.69	0.76	0.84	0.91	0.99	1.07	1.15	1.22	1.30	1.38	1.45
1.88		0.60	0.63	0.75	0.83	0.90	0.98	1.05	1.13	1.20	1.28	1.35	1.43
1.89	0.52	0.59	0.67	0.74	0.81	0.89	0.96	1.04	1.11	1.19	1.26	1.33	1.41
1.90	0.51	0.58	0.66	0.73	0.80	0.87	0.95	1.02	1.09	1.17	1.24	1.31	1.39
1.91	0.50	0.57	0.65	0.72	0.79	0.86	0.93	1.00	1.08	1.15	1.22	1.29	1.36
1.92	0.49	0.56	0.64	0.71	0.78	0.85	0.92	0.99	1.06	1.13	1.20	1.27	1.34
1.93	0.49	0.55	0.63	0.70	0.77	0.83	0.90	0.97	1.04	1.11	1.18	1.25	1.32
1.94	0.48	0.54	0.62	0.68	0.75	0.82	0.89	0.96	1.03	1.10	1.16	1.23	1.30
1.95	0.47	0.53	0.61	0.67	0.74	0.81	0.88	0.94	1.01	1.08	1.15	1.21	1.28
1.96	0.46	0.53	0.60	0.66	0.73	0.80	0.86	0.93	1.00	1.06	1.13	1.20	1.26
1.97	0.46	0.52	0.59	0.65	0.72	0.78	0.85	0.92	0.98	1.05	1.11	1.18	1.24
1.98	0.45	0.52	0.58	0.64	0.71	0.77	0.84	0.90	0.97	1.03	1.10	1.16	1.22
1.99	0.44	0.51	0.57	0.63	0.70	0.76	0.82	0.89	0.95	1.01	1.08	1.14	1.21
2.00	0.44	0.50	0.56	0.63	0.69	0.75	0.81	0.88	0.94	1.00	1.07	1.13	1.19

Table 32

Specific weight – calculated on the base of the measurements of the skin folds in the 10 points (Parizkova.1962)

Fat (mm)	youths 9-12 years	girls 9-12years	Girls and boys 13-16 years	fat (mm)	youths 9-12 years	girls 9-12 years	Girls and boys 13-16 years
10	1.111	1.099	1.127	55	1.060	1.054	1.069
11	1.108	1.096	1.124	56	1.059	1.053	1.069
12	1.106	1.094	1.121	57	1.059	1.053	1.063
13	1.103	1.092	1.118	58	1.058	1.052	1.067
14	1.101	1.090	1.116	59	1.058	1.052	1.067
15	1.099	1.088	1.113	60	1.057	1.052	1.066
16	1.097	1.087	1.111	61	1.057	1.051	1.066
17	1.095	1.085	1.109	62	1.056	1.051	1.065
18	1.093	1.083	1.107	63	1.056	1.050	1.065
19	1.092	1.082	1.105	64	1.055	1.050	1.064
20	1.090	1.081	1.104	65	1.055	1.049	1.064
21	1.089	1.079	1.102	66	1.054	1.049	1.063
22	1.087	1.073	1.000	67	1.054	1.049	1.062
23	1.086	1.077	1.099	68	1.054	1.048	1.062
24	1.035	1.076	1.097	69	1.053	1.048	1.061
25	1.084	1.075	1.096	70	1.053	1.047	1.061
26	1.082	1.074	1.095	71	1.052	1.047	1.060
27	1.081	1.073	1.093	72	1.052	1.047	1.060
28	1.080	1.072	1.092	73	1.051	1.046	1.060
29	1.079	1.071	1.091	74	1.051	1.046	1.059
30	1.078	1.070	1.090	75	1.051	1.046	1.059
31	1.077	1.069	1.089	76	1.050	1.045	1.058
32	1.076	1.063	1.088	77	1.050	1.045	1.053
33	1.075	1.067	1.087	78	1.049	1.045	1.057
34	1.074	1.067	1.086	79	1.049	1.044	1.057
35	1.073	1.066	1.035	80	1.049	1.044	1.057
36	1.073	1.065	1.034	81	1.048	1.044	1.056
37	1.072	1.064	1.083	82	1.048	1.043	1.056
33	1.071	1.063	1.082	83	1.048	1.043	1.056
39	1.070	1.063	1.081	84	1.047	1.043	1.055
40	1.069	1.062	1.080	85	1.047	1.042	1.055
41	1.069	1.062	1.079	86	1.047	1.042	1.054
42	1.063	1.061	1.078	87	1.046	1.042	1.054
43	1.067	1.060	1.077	88	1.046	1.041	1.054
44	1.067	1.060	1.076	89	1.045	1.041	1.053
45	1.066	1.059	1.076	90	1.045	1.041	1.053
46	1.065	1.059	1.075	91	1.045	1.040	1.052
47	1.065	1.058	1.074	92	1.044	1.040	1.052
48	1.064	1.057	1.074	93	1.044	1.040	1.052
49	1.064	1.057	1.073	94	1.044	1.040	1.051
50	1.063	1.056	1.073	95	1.044	1.039	1.051
51	1.062	1.056	1.072	96	1.043	1.039	1.050
52	1.062	1.055	1.072	97	1.043	1.039	1.050
53	1.061	1.055	1.071	98	1.043	1.039	1.050
54	1.060	1.054	1.070	99	1.042	1.038	1.049

Table 32 - continuation

Fat (mm)	youths 9-12 years	girls 9-12 years	Girls and boys 13-16 years	fat	youths 9-12 years	girls 9-12 years	Girls and boys 13-16 years
100	1.042	1.038	1.049	151	1.030	1.027	1.035
101	1.042	1.038	1.048	152	1.029	1.027	1.035
102	1.041	1.037	1.048	153	1.029	1.027	1.035
103	1.041	1.037	1.048	154	1.029	1.027	1.034
104	1.041	1.037	1.047	155	1.029	1.026	1.034
105	1.041	1.037	1.047	156	1.029	1.026	1.034
106	1.040	1.036	1.047	157	1.028	1.026	1.034
107	1.040	1.036	1.046	158	1.028	1.026	1.034
108	1.040	1.036	1.046	159	1.028	1.026	1.033
109	1.039	1.036	1.046	160	1.028	1.026	1.033
110	1.039	1.035	1.046	161	1.028	1.025	1.033
111	1.039	1.035	1.045	162	1.028	1.025	1.033
112	1.039	1.035	1.045	163	1.027	1.025	1.033
113	1.038	1.035	1.045	164	1.027	1.025	1.032
114	1.038	1.035	1.045	165	1.027	1.025	1.032
115	1.038	1.034	1.044	166	1.027	1.025	1.032
116	1.038	1.034	1.044	167	1.025	1.024	1.032
117	1.037	1.034	1.044	168	1.026	1.024	1.032
118	1.037	1.034	1.044	169	1.026	1.024	1.032
119	1.037	1.033	1.043	170	1.026	1.024	1.031
120	1.037	1.033	1.043	171	1.026	1.024	1.031
121	1.036	1.033	1.043	172	1.026	1.024	1.031
122	1.036	1.033	1.042	173	1.026	1.023	1.031
123	1.036	1.033	1.042	174	1.025	1.023	1.030
124	1.036	1.032	1.042	175	1.025	1.023	1.030
125	1.035	1.032	1.041	176	1.025	1.023	1.030
126	1.035	1.032	1.041	177	1.025	1.023	1.030
127	1.035	1.032	1.041	178	1.025	1.023	1.030
128	1.035	1.031	1.041	179	1.025	1.023	1.029
129	1.034	1.031	1.041	180	1.024	1.022	1.029
130	1.034	1.031	1.040	181	1.024	1.022	1.029
131	1.034	1.031	1.040	182	1.024	1.022	1.029
132	1.034	1.031	1.040	183	1.024	1.022	1.029
133	1.033	1.030	1.040	184	1.024	1.022	1.028
134	1.033	1.030	1.039	185	1.024	1.022	1.028
135	1.033	1.030	1.039	186	1.023	1.022	1.028
136	1.033	1.030	1.039	187	1.023	1.021	1.028
137	1.033	1.030	1.039	188	1.023	1.021	1.028
138	1.032	1.029	1.038	189	1.023	1.021	1.028
139	1.032	1.029	1.033	190	1.023	1.021	1.027
140	1.032	1.029	1.038	191	1.023	1.021	1.027
141	1.032	1.029	1.038	192	1.022	1.021	1.027
142	1.031	1.029	1.037	193	1.022	1.021	1.027
143	1.031	1.029	1.037	194	1.022	1.020	1.027
144	1.031	1.028	1.037	195	1.022	1.020	1.027
145	1.031	1.028	1.036	196	1.022	1.020	1.026
146	1.030	1.028	1.036	197	1.022	1.020	1.026
147	1.030	1.028	1.036	198	1.022	1.020	1.026
148	1.031	1.028	1.036	199	1.021	1.020	1.026
149	1.030	1.027	1.035	200	1.021	1.020	1.026
150	1.030	1.027	1.035				

Table 33

Metric index (Conrad, 1963)

boys	group	girls	group
+1.1 and higher	Ultra	+0.9 and higher	Ultra
+ 1.0+0.9+0.8	A	+0.8+0.7+0.6	A
+0.7+0.6+0.5	B	+0.5+0.4+0.3	B
+0.4+0.3+0.2	C	+0.2+0.1+0.0	C
+0.1+0.0—0.1	D	—0.1—0.2—0.3	D
—0.2—0.3—0.4	E	—0.4—0.5—0.6	E
—0.5—0.6—0.7	F	—0.7—0.8—0.9	F
—0.8—0.9—1.0	G	—1.0—1.1—1.2	G
—1.1—1.2—1.3	H	—1.3—1.4—1.5	H
—1.4—1.5—1.6	I	—1.6—1.7—1.8	I
—1.7 and lower	Ultra 1	—1.9 and lower	Ultra 1

Table 34

Plastic index (Conrad, 1963)

boys AB + HU + UU	group	girls AB + HU + UU	group
Up to 73.3	Ultra 1	< 66.8	Ultra 1
73.4...75.9	1	66.9...69.2	1
76.0...78.5	2	69.3...71.6	2
78.6... 81.1	3	71.7...74.0	3
81.2... 83.7	4	74.1...76.4	4
83.8...86.3	5	76.5...78.8	5
86.4...88.9	6	78.9...81.2	6
89.0...91.5	7	81.3.... 83.6	7
91.6...94.1	8	83.7...86.0	8
94.2...96.7	9	86.1...88.4	9
96.8 and higher	Ultra 9	88.5 and higher	Ultra 9

Table 35

Body surface (m2) in relation to body length and body weight

Body height (cm)	weight									
	25	30	35	40	45	50	55	60	65	70
210							1.90	1.98	2.04	2.11
205							1.87	1.94	2.01	2.07
200							1.84	1.91	1.97	2.03
195						1.73	1.80	1.87	1.93	1.99
190				1.56	1.63	1.70	1.77	1.84	1.90	1.96
185				1.53	1.60	1.67	1.74	1.80	1.86	1.92
180				1.49	1.57	1.64	1.71	1.77	1.83	1.89
175	1.19	1.28	1.36	1.46	1.53	1.60	1.67	1.73	1.79	1.85
170	1.17	1.26	1.34	1.43	1.50	1.57	1.63	1.69	1.75	1.81
165	1.14	1.23	1.31	1.40	1.47	1.54	1.60	1.66	1.72	1.78
160	1.12	1.21	1.29	1.37	1.44	1.50	1.56	1.62	1.68	1.73
155	1.09	1.18	1.26	1.33	1.40	1.46	1.52	1.58	1.64	1.69
150	1.06	1.15	1.23	1.30	1.36	1.42	1.48	1.54	1.60	1.65
145	1.03	1.12	1.20	1.27	1.33	1.39	1.45	1.51	1.56	1.61
140	1.00	1.09	1.17	1.24	1.30	1.36	1.42	1.47	1.52	1.57
135	0.97	1.06	1.14	1.20	1.26	1.32	1.38	1.43	1.48	
130	0.95	1.04	1.11	1.17	1.23	1.29	1.35	1.40		
125	0.93	1.01	1.08	1.14	1.20	1.26	1.31	1.36		
120	0.91	0.98	1.04	1.10	1.16	1.22	1.27			

Table 35 – continuation

Body height (cm)	weight											
	75	80	85	90	95	100	105	110	115	120	125	130
210												
205												
200												
195	2.17	2.23	2.29									
190	2.13	2.19	2.25	2.35	2.40							
185	2.09	2.15	2.21	2.31	2.36	2.45						
180	2.05	2.11	2.17	2.26	2.31	2.41	2.51	2.56	2.60	2.65	2.70	2.74
175	2.02	2.08	2.13	2.22	2.37	2.36	2.46	2.51	2.56	2.61	2.65	2.70
170	1.98	2.04	2.09	2.18	2.23	2.32	2.41	2.47	2.51	2.56	2.60	2.65
165	1.95	2.00	2.05	2.14	2.19	2.28	2.37	2.42	2.47	2.51	2.56	2.60
160	1.91	1.96	2.01	2.10	2.15	2.24	2.33	2.38	2.42	2.47	2.51	2.55
155	'1.86	1.91	1.96	2.06	2.11	2.20	2.29	2.33	2.38	2.42	2.46	2.50
150	1.83	1.88	1.93	2.01	2.06	2.16	2.25	2.29	2.33	2.37	2.41	2.45
145	'1.78	1.83	1.88	1.98	2.03	2.11	2.21	2.24	2.28	2.37		
140	1.74	1.79	1.84	1.93	1.98	2.07						
135	1.70	1.75	1.80	1.89								
130	1.66	1.71										
125												
120												

- Genetic methods of analyzing the constitutional body type

When we studied the influence of heredity and environment on quantitative characters variability, we are able to investigate the phenotype, but we cannot exclusively investigate genotype.

The result of our research is constituted by data representing phenotypic values of a character (noted by P). In a research mass, these values have a certain variant called phenotypic variation (Vp). Underlying all methods used to analyze genetic data is an effort to assess the extent to which heredity and environment participate to this phenotypic variation. In other words, the solution is analyzed in terms of a genetic component (G) and a non-genetic component (E).

The term "non-genetic component "is synonymous with environmental influences, so the symbol is E ("environment"), while the genetic component is denoted by G. Other signs also come from the English terminology, variant - V, phenotype - P.

Applying the symbols mentioned we have the formula

$$P = G + E \quad (1);$$

Regarding the level of dispersion of values:

$$V_P = V_G + V_E \quad (2).$$

Where Vp is the total phenotype variant of a character, VG is the genotype conditioned variant – the genetic variant- and VE is the environment conditioned variant – non genetic variant.

Such a formulation gives us the classic notion of the so-called additive model of the influence of heredity and environment. It is based on the concern that while creating the character there a simple summoning of the two factors. The notion is enough for us, but, in reality this is a matter of hyper-simplification, because, on a series of characters, especially with those tied to various behavioural manifestations (and thus, motricity manifestations), we cannot ignore the fact that there are certain connections between the influences coming from heredity and those coming from the environment. It is more accurate to use any of the models that take into account this fact, and for the equation to use other components.

An example of this could be comparison between two children of the same sex, same weight, same body size and are absolutely identical in terms of nutrition, care etc. Despite this, after some time these children will be different, both in weight and size, as the effects dependent on environmental influences their susceptibility genotyping. The same is true for a group of individuals subject to a specific training effort - the effect will be visible effort differently. Examples cited in support of the argument concerning the phenotypic variance variant genotype dependence, which in our simplified equation would represent another component of variance (Vg / G). The example can not be excluded oppositely shows the dependency of the variant Phenotypic genotypic variation. Besides these unilateral links may not exist any dependence between the two factors expressed by their common variant. Another component, the co-variant (COVGe) can thus be included in the education.

The links mentioned between genetic and non genetic influences certainly exist, as in the example, but humans still have the possibility to define and describe them. The majority of statistical processes that are used to analyze genetic data is based on simple sumation and assuming there is no link between the influence of hereditary and environmental factors. Some of the results should be evaluated from this point of view because, for the reasons given, they do not always correspond to reality.

So far we have considered the variant genotype to equation (2) as a whole and we have noted as such(VG). In reality within these genotype variants other components that must be taken into account differ. They are the result of connections that form between genes and as such they can influence the manifestation of a character. In connection with this talk about the so-called genetic variation adder (additive), subject to the dominant version (dominant version) and subject to epistasis version (epistatic version).

Additive genetic variant (Va) is a part of the total genotypic variation caused by the difference in the additive effect of a particular gene locus. It is passed from one generation to another (from parents to children), and it is the Mayn factor of similarity. Dominant variant (VD) version is produced by deviations on the manifestation of dominance and recesivităţii. Therefore it depends on the ratio between the recessive alleles dominant and that will decide what would the resultant manifestation of character. Epistatic version (VE) allele express the mutual influence between different loci.Given the data above, we can further specify our occupation (2), regarding both the phenotypic version and genotypic one. The resulting equation for a simplified model additive will be:

$$V_P=V_A+V_D+V_I+V_E \text{ (3);}$$

or:

$$V_P=V_G+V_E.$$

An analogous equation for a complicated model may also include other components. The correct application of this model must take into account other solution as well. It is caused by incorrect or inaccurate measurements performed test. It is included in the so-called error variation (V). Because this type of variation is manifested as a component of total phenotypic variance, it can distort information on the contribution of the genetic component or non-genetic. This should not be forgotten, especially when we evaluate heritability component.

Heritability. One of the most important factors of quantitative genetics is without doubt the so-called heritability (h2being its symbol). It expresses the extent to which heredity (or more precisely genotypic variability) participates in total phenotypic variability of a particular character of a population. The term "heritability" is relatively old and is often tied to the so-called index of heritability suggested Holzinger (1929), for analyzing genetic data from the twins. In his recent form however, heritability has been established and defined by Lash (1945), especially in relation to animal husbandry practice needs. In this area it is used as a selection factor for determining the effectiveness and usefulness of selected generation. A further specification of the method is due to Falconer (1960). Statistical genetic determination is quite simple and yet sometimes is incorrectly understood and interpreted. One reason is the confusion between the narrow and broad sense of the term heritability and application of the various processes numerical determination.

Heritability in the narrow sense (symbol h_n^2) is the contribution of additive genetic variance (VA) and total phenotypic variance (VP), which may be expressed as follows:

$$h_n^2 = \frac{V_A}{V_P} (4)$$

In other words, it is part of the total phenotypic variant, which is an important result of the influence of genes with additive effect. Not included is the variant caused by the interaction of genes, dominant and epistatic. Regarding the fact that the genetic variant additive is transmitted to offspring and the Mayn factor of similarity, heritability as understood and defined is a very important feature, especially for selection purposes in the practice of livestock (allowing assessment of whether the offspring will inherit properties of their parents). Usually we establish it based on regression analysis and correlation of the results to parents and their children.

Heritability in the broad sense, h_b^2 expresses total phenotypic variance contribution. Applying symbols, we have:

$$\mathrm{h}_\mathrm{b}^2 = \frac{\mathrm{V}_\mathrm{G}}{\mathrm{V}_\mathrm{P}} (5)$$

which shows that in addition to additive genetic variant included are component and component dominant epistatic (VG = VA + VP + V1). Heritability broadly defined in this way, therefore consistent with the general conception about heritability for the purposes specified by us initially. It reflects the total effect of genotypic variability resulting manifestation of a certain character of a population and is therefore more perfect feature appropriate to assess the role of heredity in differences between individuals (variability). Therefore, the coefficient obtained based on this, instead of heritability coefficient, coefficient of determination is called a gene. In the study conditioning genetic different properties and capabilities of man, this coefficient is of fundamental importance and his research is the subject of numerous studies which we will discuss later, most often in connection with the research method twins.

Heritability coefficient. The quantitative evaluation measure of heritability of a particular character is actually the so-called coefficient of heritability. Symbol is usually or sometimes h2 H.

It varies between 0-1 (similar correlation coefficient) or expressed in percentage, between zero and 100. The value is higher, the effect is more pronounced phenotypic and vice versa. For example, a zero-limit value, the whole variability of nature as the result of "the ability to modify" influence of environmental factors, while the other alternative - value 1 - would conditioning absolute deviations of character variability genotypic effect. Heritability coefficients used to assess sense heritability in narrow or wide are based on various theoretical assumptions and therefore can not be compared with each other. They are, for example, similarity coefficients calculated based on the assessment of parents and their children and coefficients set by twin studies. There are differences even within a same method, for example in studies on twins, because there are several methods for determining heritability coefficient and, as the results show, the respective coefficients frequently differ among themselves. Therefore such a manner research can not be recommended.

Interpretation of heritability coefficient. Information on the extent to which heredity participating in inter-individual variability of properties and human capacity information obtained heritability coefficient, are very welcome. On the other hand, sometimes they lead us to make incorrect statements and draw conclusions. Several authors emphasize this (Lewontin, 1974; Jensen, 1972) and therefore may be useful to present some general suggestions regarding the interpretation of heritability coefficient.

a) genetic and non-genetic factors are not opposed to each other but are in interaction, complementing each other. From this point of view, the heritability coefficient of variability tells us how much of a population's character of is caused by genetic variability (ie h2) and what part is due to the non-genetic variability; This means that differences in the effect of the environment and the environment (1-h2).

b) Heritability is a characteristic of population that determines the genetic component of the character of the population and thus has no relationship with the individual. Therefore it can not be argued that, for example, a property of a particular individual is 70% heritable.

c) The heritability is not a biological constant, but an empirically determined amount, which is a function of genetic and non genetic variant of a character of the population. It will be higher if environmental variability (ie on the character) is reduced and, conversely, would be lower if the differences influence the environmental conditions are great. Also, when genetic variant is relatively low population and environmental conditions are not optimal for character development, heritability will be reduced.

d) The heritability determined by a calculation of heritability component feature is only a sample and, as such, is accompanied by a certain sampling error and is limited "confidence interval". It is merely an evaluation (more or less accurate) and refers only to that part of the population has been established. Parallel to increased variance determined by measuring decreases the coefficient of error or inaccuracy, despite the fact that the contribution of the genetic component and non genetical reMayns the same. This is true for the reverse situation (why heritability component can not exceed the trust factor).

e) The component of heritability can be linked only to the character (ownership, capacity) for which valid measurement or test question. Therefore it is not generally applicable.

Previous suggestions are closely linked to the general principles for the application of statistical and mathematical methods and are very important. Regarding the application of heritability coefficient, calculated for different properties and capabilities, which is linked to the alleged efficiency or motricity sports, and its application to concrete practice, there are several possibilities Let us assume that properties and capabilities with a relatively high heritability (h2> 0.50), ie entailing an important influence or genotypic differences inter-individual variability will be more heavily influenced by heredity than those with a heritability low (h2 <0.30). Based on the finding earlier can be determined (quite accurately qualitatively, meaning "more or less") which one possesses a higher degree or less conditioning genetic and they can be differentiated and evaluated from this point of view.

Let us assume then that the properties and capabilities with a higher degree of genetic conditioning are greater disturbances, and environmental conditions than those whose genetic conditioning is reduced. Their development opportunities will be limited evident even in the best conditions they will not exceed the individual reaction norms (genetically determined). This applies also to different means of conditioning intentional process of physical education and sports training. On the other hand, if the properties and capabilities with low heritability are expected, there is a relatively high possibility of influencing and adapting (both positively and negatively). From this point of view, the heritability coefficient can serve as a measure for assessing the ability to influence certain predispositions of motricity efficiency and sports.

The conditioning gene is expressed not only by individual differences, but at the same time, the intra-subject variability, during adolescence. In terms of individual development of various efficiency predispositions during a lengthy training session, properties and capabilities with a higher heritability seem to be less changeable and relatively stable (issue to be dealt with in detail later). In terms of individual development of various predispositions efficiency during a lengthy drives, properties and capabilities with a higher heritability seem to be less changeable and relatively stable (issue to be dealt with in detail later). The final level of their development depends to a considerable extent by their original level and therefore allows them to make a prediction (prognosis) more accurate. This can apply to evaluating individual development and the selection of subjects for a sporting activity performance (talent selection). It also can be applied to the development of various criteria (tests) for selecting and evaluating their predictive validity (prognostic value), because accurate information is expected only if the factors having a high degree of heritability.

Mutual relations between relatives. Genetic continuity between consanguineous individuals of the present generation and that of descendants, is a complex of mutual relations reflecting both genotypic resemblance and on the phenotype. Description and quantitative expression of these relations is very important for us because we can evaluate them based on, for example, a character heritability, and thus indirectly to the degree of genetic conditioning.

The most appropriate measure for evaluating the relationship between related persons mentioned is the correlation coefficient. In this sense we can speak of phenotypic or genotypic correlation, the degree of genotypic correlation coefficient is determined by so-called kinship.

In connection with the fact that genotype is inaccessible to our observation, we can only infer based on phenotypic values of a character, so genotypic correlation established solely as a measure of dependency is linked to certain prerequisites. Among these there is the fact that the parents are an ideal chance of a panmictice population (marriage was coincidental, there is no relationship between parents and they resemble one another in terms of given character) and the effect of genes on interim results of the event (no manifestations of dominance or recessive). Also, transmission of genetic information is carried out in such a way that one half of the corresponding genes of the parents of the child, while the other half is different. Only then we can consider the correlation coefficient values.

Monozygotic twins, for example, are the only case in which two individuals have a genotype absolutely equal and therefore their kinship coefficient is 1. The coefficient of relatedness between dizygotic twins, siblings and between parents and children is 0.50, between a grandfather and child is 0.71 (which is the square root approximate value 0.50). If it is considered a more distant relationship, the correlation decreases until it becomes negligible. Degree of relatedness thus depends on the component variant, which is common to both subjects related, which means that it depends on covariance. It can be seen that only if monozygotic twins and to a lesser extent the twins dizygotic twins and brothers (sisters) both parents there, besides genetic variant additive (VA), and a variant conditional dominance (VD), the resemblance between parents and therefore children rely on the transmission of genes with additive effect, so heritability derived from this relationship is always a heritability in the narrow sense (h_n^2). So far we have talked about the Genotypic variation correlation that is common to related subjects. We will now explain the relationship between genotype correlation (rG) and phenotypic (rp), on the one hand, and the heritability (h2) on the other. The following relationships are valid:

$r_P = r_G h^2$ (6),

or:

$h^2 = r_P / r_G$ (7).

From the above equations we show that the phenotype correlation coefficient may increase as a result of either a high genotype (kinship closest) or by a high heritability, which means a conditioning gene with a more intense character. If heritability it is equal to 1 (one character is subjected to a variability of genotypic effects), then phenotypic correlation value is equal to the expected (theoretical) genotype given to kinship. This principle is based on the method of assessing the similarity between parents and children and consequent appreciation of diverse genetic conditioning properties (attributes) and skills. When the value calculated phenotypic correlation (seen) approaches genotypic value is expected a relatively high degree of genetic conditioning of a character, and vice versa.

In addition to general equations, we can deduce other findings that are applicable in practice. This concerns in particular the link between heritability coefficient (in the narrow sense, h^2) and phenotypic correlation (r) or regression (b).

We also noted that the assessment of interlinkages parents - children, regression coefficient that is more appropriate than the correlation coefficient. He may refer to regression of a son or daughter to a father, as a son or daughter to the mother, so in reality there are four possible alternatives (BSF, BDF, BSM, BDM).More there two alternative because sometimes parents evaluate and get through such a mean regression of a son or daughter to grandfather.

Relations mentioned can be applied to calculate the heritability coefficient in practice and to assess the genetic conditioning of a character. But some of them are not appropriate, for example, usually are not recommended to children values correlate with parents' values (though we often encounter this type of evaluation).

The cause is that some characters are connected to sex (or controlled by sex) and in the grandfather these links are deformed. Another distortion may occur in the evaluation of the mother- daughter relationship or mother-son relationship, as a result of so-called “maternal effect”, by which is meant the possible effects of maternal influence on a character body. In a number of cases we find that partner selection is not random (as assumed), but there is some similarity in terms of character (and this may be just the character we're investigating). The term is called assortative mating (e.g. when a tall man is looking for a tall partner). In sport there are plenty of examples regarding other characters. One such couple (right) increase homozigots (genotypic resemblance), which is manifested by the fact that between partners there is some degree of dependence, which can be assessed by phenotypic correlation. After Spuhler (1968), for example, the dependence of the partners is approximately 0.20 in terms of height and weight and in terms of value IQ and found a high correlation of 0.40. This is often overlooked in practice, which is not correct, because - as the results (*Susaune*, 1977) - there is a dependency between partners often leads to higher values of heritability coefficient in assessing the relationship parents children. Another problem that distorts the results of research of mutual relations between parents and children is the influence of non-genetic factors. This concerns in particular the influence of family environment (same skills, the same daily regime, education and other factors), causing a family resemblance individual in terms of a series of events. The similarity may not be caused only by their genotype, but can be largely caused by environmental influences and conditions specified family. In such cases there is a considerable increase heritability coefficient values, overstating the influence of heredity and environmental factor understatement. This can be seen particularly in assessing the similarities between brothers, that dependence it is usually higher than the dependence between parents and children, although the theoretical values are equal kinship coefficient (0.50).

Monozygotic and dizygotic twins comparison method. The method consists of comparing the phenotype of the investigated character in a group of pairs of monozygotic (MZ) and dizygotic (DZ) who were reared together and subjected to the same stimuli. If the character is unequivocally investigated under the influence of the environment, the differences within pairs (differences "between the pairs') MZ and DZ twins should be the same. On the other hand, if a character is genetically determined, without influence of the environment, the individuals in the MZ twins pair must correspond in terms of their phenotype, while DZ pairs must be different. This is the basis of most methods for calculating heritability coefficient into practice and evaluating the influence of heredity. One possibility is the amount of similarity in individuals within an MZ and DZ twin pairs using intraclass correlation coefficient (RMZ and RDZ). Heritability coefficient can thus be calculated using the formula's classic Holzinger (the index of heritability and with the symbol H) as follows:

$$\mathrm{H} = \frac{\mathrm{r}_{\mathrm{MZ}} - \mathrm{r}_{\mathrm{DZ}}}{1 + \mathrm{r}_{\mathrm{DZ}}} \quad (8).$$

Another possibility is to implement an adaptation recommended by Falconet (1960), where:

$$h^2 = 2\left(r_{MZ} - r_{DZ}\right) \quad (9).$$

There are also other formulas in addition to the two mentioned above, for example, the Jensen (1967) and Nichols (1965) formulas.

Comparison, relatively the most objective, of an MZ and DZ pairs group and a specific calculation of the heritability coefficient is achieved by testing the significance of the difference between variants. This is based on the fact that the medium variant within a pair (pair inside - VW) is, if a big factor heritability influence on MZ twins (VMZW), less from them than DZ twins (VDZw). If environmental influences prevail, then the increase to VDZw VMZW variant and the difference between the two types of twin pairs decreases. This problem is tested using F ratio test, where:

$$F = \frac{V_{DZW}}{V_{MZW}} \quad (10).$$

This hypothesis's test is the consistency variant between pairs (between different Vb pairs) in a group of monozygotic (VMZb) and dizygotic (VDZb) which is again tested by statistical test F (the variance is always larger numerator). Some authors recommend assessing the significance of heredity influence only in this way (Vandenberg, 1965), without calculating the heritability coefficient. Another argument in support of the genetic factor is significant statistical difference between the differences within pairs of MZ and DZ groan, calculated according to the equation (10), and that the report Vmzc / Vdzc is above par, while the report:

$$F = \frac{V_{MZb}}{V_{DZb}} \quad (11)$$

is considerably less than unity. If there is a match between the pairs of twins version MZ and DZ then coefficient of heritability (h2) can be applied to determining the role of heredity. It is well known fundamental adaptation without decreasing the variation caused by an error of measurement, that:

$$h^2 = \frac{V_{DZW} - V_{MZW}}{V_{DZW}} \quad (12).$$

This calculated heritability coefficient is the most appropriate measure for evaluating heritability broadly. The "intra-pair" comparison method of monozygotic twins. Besides the aforementioned comparison between MZ and DZ twins there is another interesting method of investigation of monozygotic twins by controlling "co twin" (different environmental conditions). This method is based on the identity of the genotype of the two individuals in the pair, and implies that there are differences in respect of phenotypic influences of the environment. If despite different environmental conditions in the pair (eg., After the birth of twins each family living in different under different conditions etc.), both twins are similar in terms of phenotype, then, according to the degree that similarities can be assessed conditioning investigated the genetic character. The same applies for the reverse situation. If different environmental conditions, large phenotypic differences are found, it means that the influence of heredity factor seems to be decisive for the given character.

The measurement of expressing similarity between the twins is an intra-class correlation coefficient, but only if the monozygotic group investigated is sufficiently large. Its value can serve as a rough assessment of heritability coefficient.

Regarding likeness of monozygotic twins with "co twins" control (ie raised separately), we have at our disposal and the test results of the same character to twins kept equal environmental conditions (grown together). Thus, the so-called coefficient is calculated, which is a measure for assessing the influence of the environment (in this case one h2). Its calculation is based on knowledge of intra-class correlation coefficients to twins raised apart (rMZa) twins raised together (rMZt) or a variant thereof (rMZa and rMZt) so:

$$E = \frac{r_{MZt} - r_{MZa}}{1 - r_{MZa}} \quad (13),$$

or:

$$E = \frac{V_{MZa}}{V_{MZa} - V_{MZt}} \quad (14).$$

The possibilities offered by the study of monozygotic twins are very precious and interesting methodological point of view, but realization of this type of research is very difficult. This is because the existence of twins held in different environmental conditions intra-pair is very rare, most often it is isolated, with no possibility of further analysis of statistical data. But even such type of results is instructive and can serve for further research.

Twin studies until now have been considered a method that provides value and is among the most widely applied methods. Like any method, however, and it has its weaknesses.

One of the complaints against it is the problem of accurate assessment of the type zygote, ie assessing whether a given pair of twins is monozygotic or dizygotic. Although the complaint is largely unfounded and anthropological examination allows an accurate assessment of the character extremely zygote, however, a number of earlier research did not contain an accurate verification of zygotes. Other objections relate to alleged environmental conditions. Sometimes it is hard to verify that the environment is in fact identical, and as regards the conditions of prenatal development, it is basically a non-verifiable phenomenon. Regarding another assumption, namely additive influence of heredity and environment and lack of a relationship between the two factors, this is only a hypothesis unchecked. Therefore, the question arises to what extent is true that model. There is another important fact to be taken into consideration: the occurrence of twins in a population is very rare (less than 1%) and that most research is carried out on a limited number of subjects and very heterogeneous group. As a result, the heritability coefficients calculated error involves a relatively large selection and wide confidence interval.

Other objections are brought up, ie disregarding the variant as a result of measurement error, inaccuracy test etc. We must consider all the objections mentioned above and the results we have to be evaluated from this point of view. These objections do not decrease the value of studies on twins, but they reveal some important facts observance of which leads to a more objective and drawing conclusions most plausible.

Assessing the relationship between parents and their offspring. This type of method is based on the existence of a reciprocal relationship between individuals related generation of parents and children and the quantitative assessment of these relations.

The starting point for assessing the influence of heredity is the principles formulated above, transmission of genetic information on quantitative characters, generally expressed by a certain degree of correlation Genotypic and by a coefficient of kinship, in the simplest case, these theoretical values can be compared with phenotypic correlation values, ie once the calculated relationship between relatives (the expected) and based on these facts to assess whether they are approaching it or not. Naturally, we must consider all the conditions related to them, because, as mentioned above, the degree of phenotypic correlation is determined by a number of factors (eg., The so-called mating appropriate, the influence of family environment, sexual relations etc..).

Another important rule is the rule of Galton's "subsidiary regression", according to which the average values of character progeny lies midway between the average value of both parents and the average population. But even in this case are valid statements and objections mentioned above, so often there are large deviations in individual cases.

The method most frequently applied for the expression of conditioning character investigated is the calculation of regression coefficients (b) regression offspring to parents or the calculation of correlation coefficients (r) between individuals in different relationships and heritability coefficient deduced from they (in this case it the heritability in the narrow sense).

For these purposes applied following simplified transmission relationships can be:

$$\left.\begin{matrix} Father - son \\ Father - daughter \\ Mother - son \\ Mother - daughter \end{matrix}\right\} \frac{h^2}{2c} = 2r$$

$$\left.\begin{matrix} mid - parent - daughter \\ mid - parent - son \end{matrix}\right\} h^2 = b = \sqrt{2r}$$

$$brothers\ (sisters)\ \ h^2 \leq 2r$$

If a character (ownership, capacity) is the relationship between parents and children, a relatively high degree of correlation and regression coefficient allows an assessment relatively exact value of character in children based on knowledge of those values of their parents, it is possible practical application and a longitudinal prognosis. On this principle we based, for example, some nomograms or prediction equations for assessing the child's height (the first is due to all of Galton). As experience shows, however, even on this character that is among the strongest genetically caused, such predictions are sometimes misleading and inaccurate. Therefore, the following question arises: to what extent the investigation method of interdependence children parents can be applied to evaluate different properties and capabilities that compared to body height, have a considerably reduced genetic conditioning? This applies to various motricity skills or physiological functions, on the possibilities of this type of prediction would be very interesting and useful. The method is to investigate interdependence parents' children (which, in our opinion, is the most important relationship) in terms of capabilities that depend on motricity manifestations of human (and therefore its effectiveness and motricity sports) is impeded by another fact important in some specific measure. Most of these capabilities, unlike, for example, the height of the body or other body dimensions (or other characteristics of personality) are subject to adulthood, a considerable individual variability. They are relatively stable because it does not depend only on genotypic predisposition, but at the same time and environmental influences. In addition, while the size of the body to a large extent reached its final form in adulthood (with the exception of body weight), motricity skills are constantly influenced by the environment. Therefore they depend on age, health status, type of occupation (ie., There is a big difference between the situation where a parent runs mostly manual labor and where the parent performs a so-called sedentary work), physical activity and sports. All items mentioned above soft interdependence parents and children do research very difficult in these cases. As such method is not applied too broadly.

Analysis of genealogy (pedigree). Analyses of genealogy are among the classical methods of human genetics because they are the most common and most easily accessible. These methods are focused mostly on genetic analysis of characters, in terms phenotype manifests as some characters quality, and therefore are applied especially in areas where such an assessment method is common. They are most commonly used in medical conditions and pathological deviations as they occur or not occur or to an individual and frequency of their occurrence can be easily recorded. Sometimes we refer to family genealogical charts in which a large number of individuals with a special aptitude for certain activities, eg music, painting, mathematics etc have appeared. For this are ultimately related characters even books of eminent athletes, artists etc.

The current analysis of the genealogy consists of a thorough research of all the members pursued generations, research carried out according to certain rules and principles. The result of such research is usually expressed through a genealogical chart, using standard symbols. In a mass research, the appearance of a character can be expressed as a percentage, the occurrence probability values etc.

We showed that pedigree analysis refers specifically to qualitative characters. It is used for evaluating the type of inheritance (eg., A certain type of inheritance is related to the sex), the evaluation of the penetrant or the expressiveness of a character; particularly important is assessing the likelihood that one might expect, for example, disease in the offspring.

On the other hand, the possibilities for applying the method genealogical quantitative characters are very limited. Since phenotypic manifestation is always conditioned by the interaction of hereditary and environmental factors, it is impossible to determine which of the factors is important. One such character is manifested in reality all subjects related, but there is a level difference (value) character. From this point of view, the method for quantitative evaluation of recessive behavior between relatives is more appropriate and objective.

Despite this, some genealogical charts of specific families are very interesting sport, contributing to the usual arguments genetic mastery sports conditioning. In addition, these arguments have had a stimulating role, which led to the application of methods and conducting a more detailed study of the whole problem.

Longitudinal investigation of the stability of individual development. Besides genetic methods classics as, for example, twin study, evaluating the similarity between parents and their offspring or analysis genealogy, valuable information can be obtained also by using so-called investigation longitudinal (long), with the objective of assessing changes in the course of development of the individual. The method is based on developing ties investigate a particular character (ownership, quality, suitability) the same individual or group investigation carried out in several successive intervals and over a relatively long period (sometimes 10 years or more).

From our point of view, longitudinal research is especially effective because it can be accompanied by an experiment. There is the possibility of stimulating an individual intentionally (say, through some effort to drive) and to observe how this manifests experimental factor and what causes changes. This is particularly important in that it allows the investigation of the dynamics and character development of various properties and skills in terms of a different degree of physical exertion, or on other factors controllable and observable (eg., material conditions and social, nutrition, education, etc.).

Thus, we evaluate the real extent and ability to adapt phenotypic about predispositions genotyping of an individual, which allows us to appreciate (assuming optimum conditions in terms of environmental influences) the highest level of adaptability possible, that the highest standard of responsiveness. It is assumed that this aspect may be investigated in humans only in this way and, therefore, longitudinal investigation results on the development of the individual, in combination with a controlled experiment, has a high gnoseological value.

In connection with the study of various genetic conditioning qualities often mentioned so-called stability (constancy).

This means that the characters (properties, capabilities), which involves a considerable contribution in terms of the influence of heredity, are relatively stable, and the changes it undergoes these characters are under the most part, within the limits of variability ontogenetic intra (as a result of natural changes in the development of an individual). Such characters are relatively unstable even under optimal stimulation and conditioning because environmental conditions influence them only to a limited extent. On the other hand, properties and skills with a lower degree of genetic conditioning have only a low stability. They are less conservative measure, are highly variable, not only in terms of intra-individual variability, but also within the interindividual variability, which results in the group that individuals often change their positions.

The problem of stability are closely related forecasting possibilities. Properties and capabilities that are relatively stable, allowing a forecast accurate and, therefore, for example, based on the knowledge level of their childhood (so-called properties and skills juvenile), we can assess relatively well, though only with a certain probability, values adulthood (final value). This offers various possibilities, especially, for example, efficiency prognosis sports for selecting individuals for performance sports etc. But again we can see that in individual cases, such an outcome is not always right, even for some features such as body weight. The probability assessment increases especially in repeated investigations and assess a larger number of factors. The problems mentioned above relates to various methods and applying mathematical statistics, which are prepared thoroughly for these purposes. Besides the usual correlation calculation, we find in this area, simple and multiple regression, various methods of analysis of trends, some of factor analysis techniques etc.

Plausibility and value through a longitudinal study results are related to certain assumptions and are accompanied by certain deficiencies. Thus, for example, any investigation of this kind should be made on the long term and should include the entire period that is important for character development. The longitudinal study, however, is difficult, it involves big problems designing research. The results are known only after many years and it is not easy for a group of subjects (a representative, homogeneous and relatively large) to be kept unchanged for so long, in addition, under the influence of experimental. Environmental conditions and some changes intentionally set must be controllable and comparable for all subjects in the selection. It must take into account the individual characteristics in terms of biological age, especially during adolescence, because just at that age, developing a series of qualities and skills are progressing the most. The elements mentioned and others make longitudinal research results to be less numerous, especially in relation to research various manifestations and functional capabilities.

Analogies between test methods and those of quantitative genetics.

Evaluating different predispositions efficiency and motricity sports is closely related measurements and tests. Thus, for example, some sports results, different functional characteristics of the body, the body size, weight, and other factors are measurable. Testing applies to motricity skills tests evaluating motricity diagnosis physical functions etc. Therefore, the theoretical basis of measurement and testing are given considerable attention and terms of validity, accuracy or objectivity are very usual. It would be interesting highlighted some links between the theory test and the theory of quantitative genetics, as shown, for example, by De Vries, Vandenberg and McClearn (1976) and in connection with the issue of us, especially by Weiss (1978).

In the classical test and measurement theory the following is frequently presented:

$$X = T + E \qquad (15),$$

where X is the observed result, EC is the actual outcome, and E is the error of measurement. A very similar pattern exists in quantitative genetics theory:

$$P = G + E \qquad (16),$$

where P is the observed phenotypic, genotypic value G, and E is the variant as a result of environmental influences. Environmental factors include, on the one hand, the influence to the environment and, on the other hand, influences random error related to testing (measurements).

S proved also to the theory of the test, the two tests are equivalent to the (parallel) if the actual give equal results, and if errors are not correlated with each other. A similar situation occurs in quantitative genetic studies of twins, monozygotic twins if they had equal environmental conditions intra-pair (in the pair). Both subjects in the pair have the same genotype and supposedly there is no relationship between genotype and environmental influences.

If the previous model theory test is expressed by those variations, we get the following equation:

$$V_x = V_r + V_E \qquad (17).$$

This brings us to a very important factor in terms of the theory test, namely, the accuracy of a test. This is defined as the quotient between the observed results and outcomes variant true and can also be expressed by a correlation coefficient or regression:

$$\frac{V_T}{V_X}=\frac{r^2}{x_T}=b_{XTt}=r_{XX} \quad (18),$$

where r2 / xT is the correlation between the actual values and the observed BXT expressed regression real values than those observed, and is the correlation between the results equivalent to or, more frequently, between the results obtained repeatedly by the same test (so-called test method retest to assess the stability coefficient, which is the most frequently used to assess the accuracy of a test).

A term that is exactly equivalent in quantitative genetics theory, the term The heritability. If we start from a known equation, with which we describe the basic model of the influence of heredity and environment:

$$\text{accuracy} = V_P = V_G + V_E \quad (19),$$

then heritability, like accuracy, is expressed by the following relationship:

$$\text{heritability} = V_G / V_P = b_{GP} = r_{pp^1} \quad (20),$$

where p and p1 is seen in monozygotic goals kept under environmental conditions equal to the pair. For the practical application of theory test data validity, it is important to always be lower than the square root of its accuracy or, at most, equal to it. If accuracy is evaluated by a factor of stability, it will not exceed its value. In the context of quantitative genetics there is a similar situation, for example in analyzing animal selection.

We are talking about the so-called coefficient of repeatability, which is the highest possible character heritability investigated. It is obtained as a coefficient of determination (r2), in dependence on the values, the correlation values calculated between the observed phenotypic repeatedly. Above analogies are not only interesting but also instructive because based on them can be inferred that the heritability derived and calculated through mathematical and statistical methods are not to exceed the coefficient of stability.

If there is a longer interval between repeated test results, we will not talk about testing the accuracy of retesting, but the so-called longitudinal correlation (or longitudinal stability), which was mentioned in connection with investigations of individual development. Another important finding may be deducted from the links above. Longitudinal correlation and heritability (broadly) are to some extent in terms equivalent for the expression of long-term forecast accuracy and stability studied character assessment (property, ability). The only difference is that the heritability can be calculated relatively easily and earlier (Weiss, 1973).

Determination global anthropological constitutional hereditary type. The degree of heritability of construction plant and equipment (anthropological) Sheldon somatotipul show that presents a high heritability index. Skibinska, studying monozygotic and 22 dizygotic twins 29, recording the Sheldon and Milicerova, working with natural indices confirms this data. Using the method of Heath and Carter, Skibinska bring the following items on the type constitutional hereditary determinism. Typology Heath and Carter I, II and III can be compared with the types endomorph, ectomorph's mesomorphous and Sheldon. Genetic dependence was assessed with body construction method for determining

$$h^2 = \frac{V_{Dz} - V_{mz}}{V_{Dz}},$$

where *V* defines the variant: $(S^2) = \frac{(X_1 - X_2)^2}{2K}$

and are two values for each pair of twins received the qualities that define the typology Heath Carter, and K is the number of pairs of twins (Table 36, 37). He also used the F test (*Clark*).

The heritability of body building components that define typological shows a high genetic stability of somatotipului. The influence of environmental factors on the quantitative level of body fat is higher in women where the number of adipocytes is higher than in males, which allows greater variations in the amounts of fat. Regarding muscle (mesomorph) environmental action is reduced in both sexes. It is estimated that in defining constitutional type, and genetic factors play a major role sexual determinism. After Osborn, the genetic element is more urgent ectomorfism and sexual differentiation endomorph and mesomorph is expressed. The common denominator of these works is striking finding of genetic determination of constitutional typology, which allows, based on knowledge of anthropological type of parents to estimate what will become child initially selected at age maximum sports performance, the final selection stage.

Table 36

Variant values ((S2), F test, body building components h^2 valued using the Heath Carter method (According to Skibinska and Sklad)

Twins			boys		girls	
			MZ	DZ	MZ	DZ
Number of pairs			13	12	9	12
years	average		15.06	14.44	13.93	14,66
			12.50-19.42	12.25-17.92	12.16-16.50	12,25-18,92
Component (endomorf)	I	S^2	0.067	0.656	0,236	0,385
		F	9.750**		1.632	
		h^2	0.897		0.387	
Component (mesomorf)	II	S^2	0.058	0.223	0.028	0.625
		F	3.863*		22.563**	
		h^2	0.741		0.955	
Component (ectomorf)	III	S^2	0.058	0.49	0.097	0.771
		F	8.485**		7.930**	
		h^2	0.882		0.874	
Whole somatotype		S^2	0.356	3.135	0.653	4.261
		F	8.812**		6.558**	
		h^2	0.886		0.848	

*significant from 0.05. ** significant from 0.01.

Table 37

H2 values estimated by different authors and typological methods (According to Skibinska and Sklad)

Somatotipical method	Sheldon	Sheldon	Parnell	Natural Indiexes	Heath and Carter
Author	Osborn and George	Skibinska andSklad	Orczykowska- Swia tkowska and al.	Milicerova and al.	Skibinska andSklad
Sex	M F	M F	M F	M F	M F
number	32 55	28 23	63 57	28 26	25 21
Endomorfic (F)	484 444	838** 670*	770** 852**	870** 711**	897** 387
Mezomorfic (M)	333 240	917** 936**	762** 765**	392 947**	741** 956**
Ectomorfic (L)	182 745**	904** 911**	797** 745**	928** 761**	882** 874**
global Somatotype (FML)	365 609*	893** 942**	727 793**	- -	886** 848**

* significant from 0.05 ** significant from 0.01

- Methods for evaluating the body's tissue components

The anthropological morphological characteristics of the human body are based on the analysis of a whole range of anthropometric features, among which the most commonly diagnosed are the height and weight of the body.

Direct methods. We can undertake a quantitative analysis of the human body's tissue through the methods of anatomical and chemical analysis performed on the corpses.

The ease of doing such an analysis is only apparent, due to the low accessibility of the severed material, unchanged before death by the processes of illness.

Because of this, there are few works that make known the results of such percentage analyzes of their body mass.

Indirect methods. The development of indirect methods of assessing body parts began 50 years ago by the works of Czech anthropologist J. Matiegki. This researcher, based on anatomical body weight and somatic data, proposed a quantitative method of defining skeletal, epidermal mass along with adipose tissue under the skin and skeletal muscles.

This method has not aroused the interest of researchers, yet it has become an incentive for future searches.

An important contribution to the development of indirect methods has been the experimental work on animals. These papers have provided theoretical models, helping search and processing of research methods on the human body. The work of American researchers in the Minnesota group has contributed to the further development of indirect methods and, in particular, has strengthened the methodical and methodological part of body component research.

There are now many ways to define the various components of the body. In close connection with the method we use, we can hold information about the formation of a component or more. These methods are characterized by complexity and accessibility, as some of them have been presented very thoroughly, others are only signaled.

The roentgenographic method. This is a highly appreciated method, which allows for the correct assessment of the amount of fat, muscle and bone tissue. Thanks to a special technique for the execution of photographic images, so-called radiograms are obtained, in which the shadows of the three layers of layers are seen. Photographs are performed under special technical conditions and at predetermined points, shoulder, thigh and under thigh. The basic element of this method is the measurements made with an accuracy of 0.1 mm (the lengths of the shadows of the main tissues on the radiogram). For the purpose of subsuming the measurements, the length of these shadows is measured at strict, well established points of the extremities, for example: 1/0 of the length of the shoulder and 1/2 of the length of the thigh, as in the upper point (the highest) of the length of the area under thigh. The tissues are also measured perpendicularly to the long extremity axis, instead, the length of the bones is measured perpendicularly to the long axis of the bone. With all its indisputable attributes, the roentgenographic method can not be used on a large scale because of its low accessibility and the harmful effects of Roentgen rays.

Densimetric method. This is a classic laboratory method which helps us make precise, quantitative measurements:

1 – Weight of all the layers of fat in the body

2 – Weight of the body without those layers. It measures the so-called active tissue which participates in the processes which transform material and energy into movement.

The starting point for the densimetric method varies, but the known density of adipose tissue comes to 0.9007 g/cm³ and that of active tissue is 1.100 g/cm³.

With this method, Fat and active tissue create together a structure in which the density of both elements is known as well as the density of the whole structure, defining the proportion of the weight of the two elements becomes possible:

$$D = \frac{M_1 + M_2}{\frac{M_1}{d_1} + \frac{M_2}{d_2}};$$

M_1= weight of fat,
M_2=weight of active tissue,
d_1=density of fat,
d_2=density of active tissue,
D_2=body density – empirically defined
If $M_1+M_2=M=1$ then also:

$$D = \frac{1}{\frac{M_1}{d_1} + \frac{M_2}{d_2}}$$

.

From here:

$$M_1 = \frac{1}{D} \cdot \frac{d_1 \cdot d_2}{d_2 - d_1} - \frac{d_1}{d_2 - d_1}$$

$$M_2 = \frac{1}{D} \cdot \frac{d_1 \cdot d_2}{d_1 - d_2} - \frac{d_1}{d_1 - d_2}$$

.

Body density can be empirically defined, in accordance with existent ratio of body mass compared to its volume:

$$D = \frac{M}{V},$$

where: D=body density, M=body weight, V=body volume.

Body weight can be easily measured with the help of a set of medical scales. Body volume can be determined using Archimedes law, by submerging the body in water and using techniques to measure the volume of water displaced or gasometrical techniques. Using the first technique to measure volume and then density of the body we can calculate that:

$$V = \frac{M_A - M_W}{D_W}$$

,

Where: V – body volume,
M_A – weight of body in air,
M_W– weight of body in water,
Dw – density of the water at the given temperature

On the basis of this equation regarding body volume (V) against the equation for the density of the body we obtain:

$$D = \frac{M_A}{\frac{M_A - M_W}{D_W}}$$

Two factors which influence the body density (D) should be taken into consideration: volume of air which is present in the lungs and airway at the point of hydrostatic measurement as well as the density of the gases in the digestive track. The first of these measurements is worth taking into consideration, whereas the second one may be negligible. It's well known that the volume of gases in the digestive is relatively unchanged provided the research is carried out on an empty stomach. So, the density of the body can be determined by the equation:

$$D = \frac{M_A}{\frac{M_A - M_W}{D_W}} - R_V\,(volum\ respirator).$$

This equation may also be presented in this way:

$$D = \frac{M_A - D_W}{M_A - M_W - R_V - D_W}$$

	Anticipated equations	Standard error
1	D=1.124 358 – 0.000 120 logx_2 – 0.000 175 logx_3 – 0.000 075 logx_4	0.006 013
2	D=1.125 180 – 0.000 176 logx_2 – 0.000 185 logx_5	0.006 054
3	D=1.165 474 – 0.000 126 logx_2 – 0.000 125 logx_3 – 0.000 008 logx_4 + 0.000 282 logx_5	0.005 758
4	G.P.$_{kg}$=–114.301 898 + 0.402 288x_5 + 0.300 042x_8 +0.614 360x_9 + 0.485 907x_{10} + 0.648 468x_1 +0.328 230x_{12}	1.977
5	G.P.$_{kg}$= –103.854 058 + 0.443 921x_6 +0.133430x_7 +0.458056x_8 +0.838 395x_9	2.315

x_2 – layer over shoulder
x_3 – layer on the thoracic cage
x_4 – layer on the knee
x_5 – layer on the abdomen
x_6 – height of the body
x_7 – hip circumference
x_8 mean thoracic cage circumference.
x_9 – knee circumference
x_{10} – neck circumference
x_{11} – forearm circumference
x_{12} – shoulder breadth
D – anticipated body density
G.R.– anticipated weight of active fibre

Fig. 82. Table with anticipated equations of development of some components of the human organism.

Empirical definition of body density is summarized by the estimated volume of body fat percentage, from which the weight of the fat and the active tissue can be calculated, as well as the active tissue percentage.

Calculating the body fat percentage can be done using Keysu and Brozka's method, F%=100(4, 201/D=3, 813), where F% represents the weight of the fat layer of the body as a percentage and D-the density of the body; 4,201 and 3,813 are numbers, unchanging values.

Similar techniques worked out:

Siri: F%=100 · (D/4,950) · 4,950;

Brochen: F%=100 · (4,172/D) – 4,142.

The weight of fat is calculated with the equation:

$$F_{Kg} = \frac{greut.corp. - F\%}{100},$$

Whereas the weight of the active tissue is the difference between the body weight and the fat weight. The active tissue percentage is represented by the difference: 100-F%

Hydrometric method. Almost 2/3 of the body's mass is made up of water. The entire water quantity from the body's composition may be divided into intracellular water (55%) and extracellular water (45%). Both of the components of the body water are defined the technique of dilution. This constitutes the introduction of some substances into the patient's body using well dissolved powders, which are unabsorbed by certain tissue components.

The whole water mass of the body is measured with the help of heavy water (deuterium), radioactive water (tritium), anti-pirins, urea etc. Water outside the cells is measured with the help of other substances (non-penetrating to cellular plasma) such as thiocyanate. So, the difference between the whole quantity of body water and the extracellular water is calculated as intracellular water. The hydrometric method allows us to establish the total of fatty structures in the body and body mass without the fatty structures.

It's well known that water represents a proportion of 73.2% of the body's mass without fat and that adipose tissue does not contain water.

Percent of body fat F% can be calculated with the equation:

$$F\% = \frac{\text{cantitatea integrala de apă în procente greut.corp}}{0{,}732}$$

The weight of the fatty tissue and the active tissue is similar to the densiometric method and we calculate from the value F%

Radiometric method. This is similar to the hydrometric method. It's based upon the principle that the entire quantity of potassium in the body is a stable indicator of body weight without adipose tissue. The ratio of the whole potassium content expressed in milliequivalents (mEq) against the body weight without adipose tissue is expressed by the number 68.1. From this we obtain the body weight without adipose tissue:

$$Ff_{Kg} = \frac{\text{cantit. integr.de potasiu/ în m/g}}{68{,}1},$$

While the weight of adipose tissue is calculated as the difference between the body weight and the body weight without adipose tissue (FfKg). Calculation of both components can be expressed as a percentage of body weight. The entire potassium quantity can be measured using radiobiological method determining the quantity of the isotope or natural K^{40}, which represents 0.012% of the potassium existing in the organism.

Creatinine elimination. An important part of whole body weight is represented by muscle fiber. Energetico-phosphoric reactions (ATP, Phosphocreatine) which furnish indispensible energy for muscle activity, influence biochemical transformations which lead to creatinine formation. These substances being muscular metabolites are eliminated from the body together with urea. The quantity of creatinine eliminated is proportionally higher in people with well-developed musculature and respectively, lower in people with smaller muscle mass. Thus the quantity of creatinine is dependent on the existing muscular tissue. The proportion of creatinine+uree, eliminated from the body, oscillated between 1.5 g-2 g in men and 0.8-1.5 in women. In practice measuring the quantity of creatinine is done by using the creatinine index expressed as milligrams eliminated over 24 hours. Talbot affirmed that 1g of creatinine eliminated over a period of 24 hours corresponded to 17.9kg of muscular mass, but according to Chcek – 20kg. For practical reasons some scientists used the mean value between the two indicators – 18.95kg. The methods offer an approximate evaluation of the body's components.

The Willoughby method. With its help the grade of proportionality, symmetry of segments and some tissular components of the organism are determined.

It is well known that in order to succeed in performance sports, a proportionality between the body's segments and tissular components is imposed (bone tissue, muscular etc.) and at the same time existence, in various measures, of symmetry, something which will be discussed further in the next chapter. Willoughby's typological constitutional method allows bodily harmony, proportionality of the segments and tissular components to be established in an ideal ratio, evaluation the grade of symmetry, the maximum limits which can be reached by certain organic components (bones, muscle), the level of sexualisation, on the basis of certain morphological parameters. One of the principles of the method is body harmony being expressed by the level of efficiency of exercise, determining ideal weight and dimensions according to the general structure of the body as a goal. In fact the Willoughby's standard includes the evaluation of the ideal body structure in relation to its height. This offers conclusions referring to the optimal skeletal parameters (the joints of the hand, knees and ankles) and skeletal diameters (of the shoulders, pelvis and hips) in relationship to stature. In other words, this indicates an optimum range for given height with regard to general size as well as skeletal proportions. As long as his recommendations about ideal parameters are based fully on the general dimensions of the skeleton, Willoughby's standard indirectly prescribes a canon for all ideal muscular dimensions and ideal bodyweight in relation to height. This ideal height of Willoughby's, for example, in men aims toward an anthropometric description of the skeleton and musculature, which would equip a man with a greater variety of possibilities for motricity skills and is "ideal": speed, strength, skills, stamina, and presentability.

Willoughby's optimal measurements indicate all muscular parameters and diameters based on a coefficient of the general thickness of the bones, composed of a number of the bones dimensions; each expressing the structural size of a region of the skeleton. Respective measurements, taken where the bones are closest to the surface of the skin, at the wrists the knees and the ankles, the biacromial, biilliac and bitrochantarian diameters.

Now what remains is to describe how we find the coefficient of skeletal thickness, using the seven skeletal measurements which we mentioned. Simplified, the procedure is as follows: the different bone measurements are convertible, into a single representative value, through the intermediary of typical or optimal skeletal symmetry. First, each of the skeletal measurements is converted into a value corresponding to this dimension using the same skeletal symmetry coefficient. Any of the six bone measurements can be used as a base from which all other measurements are converted. The perimeter of the ankle was chosen as a base. Therefore it's taken as it is and measured, while all the other skeletal values are converted into their implicit values. After this, the mean of these values is taken as a coefficient, denoting the general thickness of the skeleton. This small measurement was named, arbitrarily, due to the necessity for a better expression, the "corrected ankle". This lone value, the "corrected ankle" is all that is required with regards to calculating the ideal parameters for each segment of the body: forearm, arm, neck, chest, waist, hips, thighs and calves and also the breadth of the shoulders. This, in relation to the personal height, gives us the ideal body weight. Optimum coefficients of skeletal symmetry are shown in table 38, ankle perimeter being the standard unit.

Table 38

Ideal relationships between the measurements of skeletal thickness

Men		Women	
100	Ankle perimeter	1.000	
.667	Knee perimeter	1.690	
.811	Poignet perimeter	0.733	
1.715+0.83	(2.23) inch Biacromial	1.376−2.51	(6.350) inch
1.146+1.09	(2.540) inch Biiliac	1.182+1.13	(2.858) inch
1.312+1.24	(3.175) inch Bitrohanterian	1.364−1.13	(2.858) inch

Inversely, the corrected ankle is obtained by applying the following formula for the derivation of the proportional perimeter of the ankle from the other skeletal dimensions (table 39) for a male subject.

Wrist (mean of both right and left) divided by 0,811;
Knee (mean of both) divided by 1,667;
(Biacromial minus 0,83 (2,223) inches) multiplied by 0,5831;
(Biiliac minus 1,09 (2,540) inches) multiplied by 0,8726;
(Bitrohanterian minus 1,24 (3,175) inches) multiplied by 0,7622.

Table 39

Ideal relationships between the muscular measurements and corrected ankle.

Men		Women
1.000	Corrected ankle	1.000
1.433	Right forearm perimeter	1.1525
1.405	Left forearm perimeter	1.1295
1.720	Right biceps perimeter	1.338
1.686	Left biceps perimeter	1.312
1.813	Neck perimeter	1.511
2. 071+1.06(2. 540) inch	Bideltoid diameter	1.642+2. 51(6. 350) inch.
4. 732	Normal chest perimeter	3. 986
–	Bust perimeter	4. 110
3. 549	Waist perimeter	3. 114
4. 259	Hip perimeter	4. 475
2. 555	Thigh perimeter	2. 625
1.703	Calve perimeter	1.625

For female subjects:
Wrist (mean of both) divided by 0.733;
Knee (mean of both) divided by 1.690;
(Biacromial minus 2. 51 (6. 350) inches) multiplied by 0.7269;
(Biiliac minus 1.13 (2.858) inches) multiplied by 0.8460;
(Bitrochanteric minus 1.13 (2.858) inches) multiplied by 0.7331.

Optimum male weight in pounds per inches in height is 0.02966 times the "corrected ankle" squared plus 0.140. Optimum female weight in pounds per inches in height is 0.02610 times the "corrected ankle" squared plus 0.119.

By Willoughby's standards optimum range can be expressed by saying the values of the soft tissues and body weight of any individual must be within the values given by their own "corrected ankle" plus or minus 0.25 (0.635) of an inch. In other words, if the "corrected ankle" is 8.05 (20.32 inches), the optimum range includes the measurements and body weights described for a corrected ankle between 7.80 (19.869) and 8.30 inches.

The skeletal symmetry coefficients were listed in table 38.

The character of actual skeletal proportions is, largely, hereditary. However, it is possible to modify this heredity through special intensive training throughout the growth period. Exercises on gymnastic apparatus may increase the bone width of the shoulders if they are too narrow, exercised for the forearm can increase the size of the wrist if it is too small; and so on.

The coefficient for perfect muscular symmetry is presented in table 39.

Perfect masculine symmetry

Forearm should be 0.833 times the biceps.
Forearms (mean of both) should be 0.300 time the chest.
Biceps should be 1.200 times the forearm.
Biceps (mean of both) should be 0.36 times the chest.
Biceps (mean of both) should be equal to the calf.
Outstretched arm should be 0.962 times the biceps minus 0.81 inch.
Neck should be 0.383 times the chest.
Chest should be 1.333 times the waist.
Chest should be 1.111 times the hips.
Waist should be 0.750 times the chest.
Waist should be 0.833 times the hips.
Hips should be 1.200 times the waist.
Hips should be 1.667 times the thighs.
Hips should be 0.900 times the chest.
Thighs should be 0.600 times the hips.
Thighs should be 1.500 times the calf.
Calf should be 0.667 times the thigh.
Calf should be equal to the biceps (mean of both).

Perfect female symmetry

Forearm should be 0.86 times the biceps.
Forearms (mean of both) should be 0.286 times the chest.
Biceps should be 1.161 times the forearm.
Biceps (mean of both) should be 0.332 times the chest.
Biceps (mean of both) should be 0.815 times the calf.
Outstretched arm should be 0.975 times the biceps minus 0,72 inches.
Neck should be 0.379 times the chest.
Chest should be 1.280 times the waist (middle).
Chest should be 0.891 times the hips.
Bust should be 1.031 times the chest.
Bust should be 1.320 times the waist.
Bust should be 0.918 times the hips.
Waist should be 0.781 times the chest.
Waist should be 0.758 times the bust.
Waist should be 0.696 times the hips.
Hips should be 1.123 times the chest.
Hips should be 1.089 times the bust.
Hips should be 1.437 times the waist.
Hips should be 1.705 times thigh.
Thigh should be 0.587 times the hips.
Thigh should be 1.615 times the calf.
Calf should be 0.619 times the thigh.
Calf should be 1.226 time the biceps (mean of both).

Like when determining the optimal muscular values in relation to the bone size, it is necessary that there be a range of tolerance within which deviations from the median will still represent proportional symmetry of the body segments. The physical examiner gives a procentual estimate by which we describe general symmetry, relative muscular development and reaching ideal proportions.

Evaluation of the masculine physique. First of all the body structure is evaluated. To obtain the bone thickness relative to height you simply divide the corrected ankle by the height in inches, then the result is divided by 0.12846. The final number is multiplied by 100 in order to obtain a procentual value. Classification of the structural build is determined by referring to the following numbers from table 40.

Table 40

Minimum	80
Very tall	87.4 and less
Tall	87.5-92.4
Medium tall	92.5-97.4
Medium(ideal)	97.5-102.4
Medium-short	102.5-107.5
Short	107.5-112.4
Very short	112.5 and over
Maximum	120

For the muscular proportions evaluation of the general symmetry is the mean of the six estimations of regional symmetry. They are determined as follows, all limb measurements used are the mean between leg or arm on both left and right:

1. Divide forearm by bicep and multiply by 1.2;
2. Divide calf by thigh and multiple by 1.5;
3. Divide the neck by the chest and multiply by 2.609;
4. Divide (biceps plus forearm) by (thigh plus calf) and multiply by 1.3636;
5. Divide the chest by the hips and multiply by 0.9;
6. Divide the waist by the hips and multiply by 1.2.

If the evaluations from above will be greater than 100%, the reciprocal will be used (so 1.045 will be 0.957). These six measurements are added together and divided by six. Then the value is multiplied to the power of three. This final number is multiplied by 100 and will obtain a procentual evaluation of general symmetry. Evaluation of relative muscular development is determined as follows, all the limb measurements used being the mean value between arms and legs both left and right. We obtain a sum from (forearm × 0.1174) plus (biceps × 0.0978) plus (neck × 0.092) plus (chest × 0.0352) plus (thigh × 0.0652) plus (calf × 0.0978). Divide this by the corrected ankle. Then multiply to the power of three. In the end it is multiplied by 100 in order to obtain a procentual evaluation of relative muscular development.

Evaluation of the feminine physique. With regards to body structure, to obtain a bone thickness relative to height, simply divide the corrected ankle by height in inches, after which the result is divided by 0.1305. The final value is multiplied by 100 in order to obtain a procentual evaluation. Classification of the body type is determined by referring to table 41.

Table 41

Minimum	84
Very tall	89.9 and less
Tall	90.0-93.9
Medium tall	94.0-97.9
Medium(ideal)	98.0-101.9
Medium-short	102.0-105.9
Short	106.0-109.9
Very short	110.0-and over
Maximum	116

For the muscular proportions evaluation of the general symmetry is the mean of the six estimations of regional symmetry. They are determined as follows. all limb measurements used are the mean between leg or arm on both left and right:

1. Divide forearm by bicep and multiply by 1.161;
2. Divide calf by thigh and multiple by 1.615;
3. Divide the neck by the chest and multiply by 2.637;
4. Divide (biceps plus forearm) by (thigh plus calf) and multiply by 1.724;
5. Divide the chest by the hips and multiply by 1.123;
6. Divide the waist by the hips and multiply by 1.437.

If the evaluations from above will be greater than 100%, the reciprocal will be used (so 1.045 will be 0.957). These six measurements are added together and divided by six. Then the value is multiplied to the power of three. This final number is multiplied by 100 and will obtain a procentual evaluation of general symmetry.

Evaluation of relative muscular development is determined as follows, all the limb measurements used being the mean value between arms and legs both left and right. We obtain a sum from (forearm × 0.146) plus (biceps × 0.126) plus (neck × 0.11) plus (chest × 0.042) plus (thigh × 0.063) plus (calf × 0.102). Divide this by the corrected ankle. Then multiply to the power of three. In the end it is multiplied by 100 in order to obtain a procentual evaluation of relative muscular development.

The evaluation for reaching ideal proportions is simply the mean of the evaluations of general symmetry and relative muscular development. They are both added together and divided by two, with these corrections if the evaluation of the relative muscular development is higher than 100% then the reciprocal value must be used (so, 102, 4% will become 97.6). In other words, as long as overdevelopment represents a deviation from idea proportions, like underdevelopment, it must be calculated the same.

Likewise, there is an absolute limit of muscular dimensions, over which it is not possible to cross regardless of weight or length of the bones. These absolute maximum muscular parameters are: forearm, 16 inch (40.64); biceps, 19 inch (48.26); neck 20.5, inch (52.07); shoulder breadth, 24.1 inch (61.28); normal chest, 52 inch (132.1); waist, 38.5 inch (97.79); 47 inch (119.4); thigh, 28.2 inch (71.76); calf, 19.3 inch (48.90). For this reason, maximum muscular body weight possible is estimated at being 3.776 pounds per inch in height. Height over which the strict continued growth of muscle dimension is not possible is presumed to be 72.5 (6 feet, 0.5 inches) (184.2). In other words, it is not possible for a human with the height of 76 inches (193.0) to possess muscular perimeters which are over the calculated limits for a man with the height 72.5 inches (184.2).

In reference to the sexual determination of these characteristics we mention the following:

In ideal male physique, the perimeter of the biceps (mean between both arms) is equal to the perimeter of the calf, while in the ideal female physique, the biceps are no more than 81.5 of the calf perimeter. Again, in male ideal the chest measures 11% more than the thighs, while in the female ideal the thighs are 12% larger than the chest.

When a strong sportswoman has arms with an inch or larger than calves, this is an exaggeration of the masculine characteristics, while a man who has arms two inches smaller than his thighs tends to suggest female body constitution.

Willoughby's indicator for sexual grades (sexometer) is a fitting method for evaluating the general proportions of a body under the differential sexual ratios of 81.5% of the perimeter of the calf. Once again in the masculine ideal the chest measures 11% more than the thighs whereas in the female ideal the thighs are 12% larger than the chest.

CHAPTER VII.
THE HUMAN BODY VIEWED AS AN ANTHROPOLOGICAL, MOTRICITY, BIOMECHANICAL SYSTEM, BASIS OF OSTEOPATHIC MEDICINE

Basis of osteopathic medicine

In this chapter we present the human body as a biomechanical motricity system.

It's well known that the regulation of internal organ functionality is carried out by the neuroendocrine system, blood and lymphatic circulatory system and the immune system. Together, through complex mechanisms these elements constitute regulation of the entire homeostasis of the organism.

Regulatory system outlines were first tied together by the scientists *Ferdinand Hoff*, a German and *Daniel Danielopolu*, a Romanian.

Recently, the American medical school added to these, the osteoarticular and muscular system, the support structure for the entire organism, of which, an essential feature are the various forms of connective tissue. From this, it was established that action upon the osteoarticular and muscular system can influence various components of homeostasis within the body, resulting in a beneficial therapeutic effect in various illnesses. This vision was applied by osteopathic and chiropractic medicine. While osteopathic medicine uses only manoeuvres on the osteoarticular and muscular system, chiropractic medicine is even more limited, manipulating only the spine and acting only on pathology at that level. For example, herniated discs, on well balanced manoeuvre can lead to healing without having to appeal – as is usually the case- to surgical treatment. Osteopathy, through a complex of individual actions used upon a patient, may lead to a series of healings starting with the attenuation of stress-related tiredness and having a continued benefit even in certain metabolic disorders such as diabetes etc.

In the USA there are medical universities which offer the title of osteopathic doctor, universities in which, as well as the classic western medicine, osteopathy is also taught, which forms a part of a successful therapeutic arsenal. We cite as such the Lomalinda University of Medicine, Phoenix etc. In Europe this speciality gained terrain especially in recent years with the European Society of Osteopathy being established. In fact, osteopathy and chiropraxy along with homeopathy, herbal therapies etc. are recognised by the WHO under the generic of alternative medicine. Adopted terminology is widely discussed, proposing and arguing over names such as complimentary medicine or traditional medicine, because the majority of these specialities, like acupuncture, have their origins in the Far East. As such the International Society for Alternative Medicine has its headquarters in Tokyo.

In the USA the country most open to new things, the notion of integrative medicine appeared which has two components, a western one, efficient in surgical problems and infectious diseases etc. and oriental medicine (alternative or complimentary) with maximum efficiency in metabolic diseases and even oncological maladies, respectively where the homeostatic equilibrium of the organism is disturbed and needs realigned. In the Orient we find universities of western medicine with course duration of four to six years, universities of traditional medicine with the same course duration as well as universities of both traditional and western medicine with course duration of eight years. Coming back to osteopathic medicine which is taught in the US though specialist universities, while in Europe it is a masters degree lasting 3 years after graduation from the faculty of medicine, we will present (in order to understand osteopathy) the human body in all its motricity and biomechanical complexities, the substrate of which is the osteoarticular and muscular system.

The aim of this chapter is tied to the individuality of human biomechanics and we hope that in the future in Romania that there will be masters in osteopathics and other specialities in the domain of alternative medicine which are recognised by the WHO, anthropology having an essential role in this regard. If up until the end of the last century the understanding of the structures of the human organism was based on analytical studies of the morphological aspects, then the beginning of this century has laid its foundation for the scientific study of functions on the integrated synthetic concept.

Researching the organised substrate of life through to the leptonic structures, using the most modern techniques (electron microscopy, histochemistry, enzymology) deepen the knowledge regarding live organisms, but only integrative synthesis gives the possibility to discover differentiated organic realities.

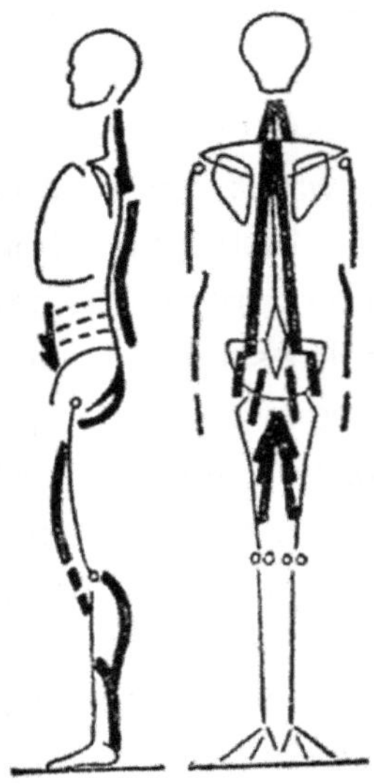

Fig. 83. Groups and muscular chains which allow normal standing position (Profile and dorsal view)

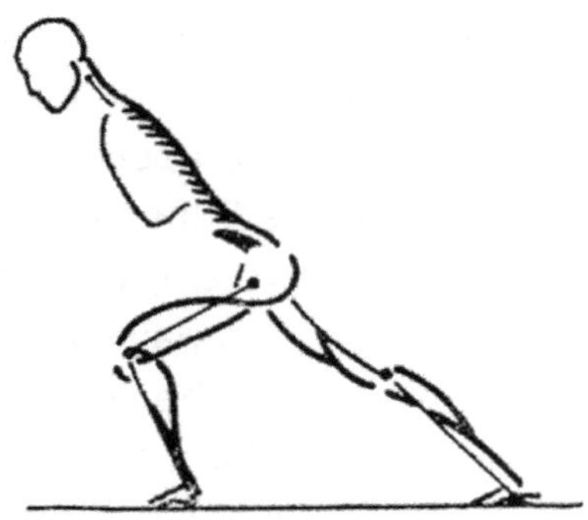

Fig. 84. Standing position with the left calf flexed forward

In the current concept, the human organism represents a biological unit (organism and environment in which they appear and develop) and ontogenetic unit (individual organism, a product of reciprocal harmony between component cells- evaluated, for an adult as an astronomical 100 catrillion, representing 1/3 of the body mass- and of intracellular formations constituting the other 2/3). Homeostasis, respectively the totality of morphophysiological constants which condition normal organism functionality, is the dynamic expression, in dialectic movement, of these ecotropic interrelations (from the external medium) and idiotropic (from the internal medium).

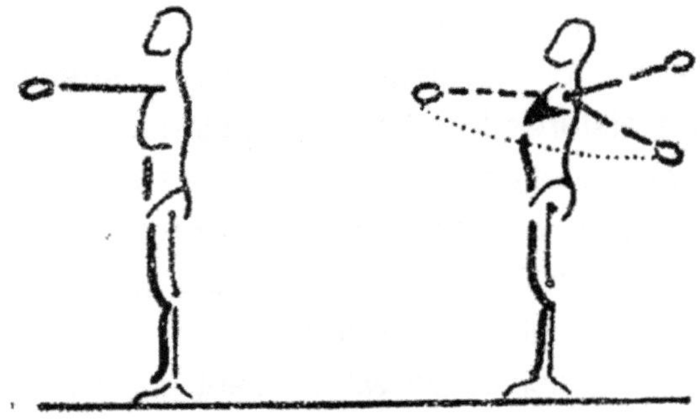

Fig. 85. Outstretching of arms via extension

The nervous system constitutes an entity which is irrefutably tied to the external environment, the source for the import of matter and energy, and the internal environment, where the chemical regulator of its function is homeostasis. Its subdivision into the nervous system of relational life (ecotropic) and its vegetative life (idiotropic) is schematic. Its interrelations with the endocrine system imply its involvement in a correlative apparatus.

Regarding this, the human organism presents itself as a whole entity, its different systems and apparatus being in close functional correlation, integrated by the nervous system as much between themselves as with the external environment. Any change in one part of the organism immediately attracts changes in the functionality of all the components of the living being. (To understand the content of this chapter, follow the explanatory images from fig. 83 to fig. 108).

In this integrative vision, the organism can be considered a biomechanical system. Within the system, we can identify schematically 3 principle components:

a) The locomotricity apparatus, formed from the bones, muscles and articulations, at which level modifications materialise in the movement of different areas of the body.
b) Neuroendocrine system, which coordinates the motricity function, through the functional correlation of the other systems and an apparatus (digestive, respiratory, cardiovascular, urinary) assure a metabolic level necessary to carry out motricity functions.
c) Metabolic apparatus: for the import of material (digestive and respiratory) and export (urinary) for transport (cardiovascular), which, acting adaptively, assures the optimum function of anabolic and catabolic processes carried out by motricity demand.

The human organism, a complex biomechanical system, may carry out sporting activities at optimum levels, at such time as all three components are in functional harmony, by their nature they confer corresponding adaptations to effort by maintaining a dynamic equilibrium of morphological constants, respectively of homeostasis. Thus, is achieved, as a total of physiological, physiopathological, organic, nervous, humoral, biophysical and biochemical processes, conditioned by the modification of the anatomical substrate, assuring adaptive reactions of the organism to motricity demand.

We can add to this concept of integrative systems, respectively the reproductive, circulatory and immune, as well as the osteoarticular and muscular systems. Osteopathic medicine was developed on the basis of this, which, through the manipulation of the osteoarticular system has a beneficial effect on various illnesses. Osteopathy has developed impetuously, in such a way that in the USA there are universities of osteopathic medicine with courses lasting 6 years and in Europe there are master's degrees in osteopathic medicine for those who have completed medicine. The human body, when viewed as a biological, biomechanical system, requires integration into its external environment which reacts with a proportional mechanics through the following factors: 1) external forces; 2) weight; 3) inertia

1. External forces which oppose the action of the biomechanical biological system. These are governed by the laws of physics and can be systematised as follows:
    a. External resistance which materialises in different apparatus for physical exercise (halters, traction, weights etc.), in strength training equipment. These external forces are exerted vertically, horizontally, obliquely, eccentrically or concentrically
    b. Configuration and measurement of the bodily segments involved in physical exercise. The value of this factor, in the context of accomplishing certain sporting activities depends on: the number of

bodily segments mobilised; volume, length, density and form of the segments, orientation in space.

2. Weight of the bodily segments, as a result of gravitational force, depends on the centre of movement, angle of the axis, the segments involved in the movement, the angle formed by the axis of progression against the vertical and the speed of progression.
3. Inertia, the tendency of the body to maintain itself at rest or in movement. Conditions required for movement are determined in particular by external factors, and can be summarised as three principle elements:
    a. Equilibrium, which can be with or without point of support and in the study of which we must consider the centre of gravity, the particular conditions of the execution of movement (incidences)
    b. Making levers which can be first, second or third degree
    c. Rhythm, by which we understand the alternation between action and reaction and which is conditional to the constitutional type of the individual, exterior forces and duration of exercise.

The laws by which govern the motricity actions of the biomechanic biological human, integrated into its external environment, can be synthesised as follows: 1)law of useful effort; 2)law of maximum voluntary force. Law of useful effort refers to obtaining a maximum output while reducing to a minimum the principle motricity requirements (selection of movement, elimination of useless gestures, distribution of effort throughout the entire body, adjusting the intensity of effort in ratio the resistance, seeking favourable compensatory movements).

Law of maximum voluntary effort applies especially to static exercises for developing different muscle groups. In general, the intensity of the motricity action is superior to exterior forces which need to be overcome; movements are established after their effect on the organism and the compensations are avoided. From this law, exercise programs are guided and graded to accomplish speed as well as improving the physical condition and correcting somatic deficiencies.

In this integrative vision, physical exercise can be an analogue to a cybernetically controlled system, where the controlled subsystem is made up of components from the locomotricity system which carry out the movement. The informational subsystem is represented by different levels of the central nervous system, which prepares the information in order to elaborate commands for the motricity execution, while the conductive subsytem is made up of efferent pathways of the central nervous system, which transmit nervous impulses to the musculature.

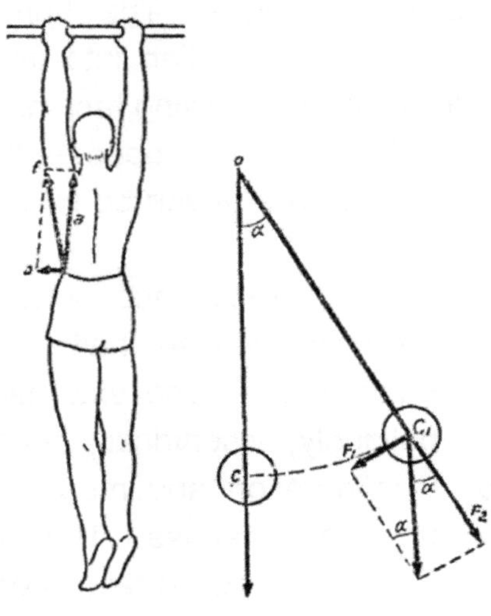

Fig. 86. Stable balance.

The informational system, made up of from structure and content of information, respectively from the entire problem of physical education and sport, penetrates in these complex cybernetics system via receptors and afferent pathways of the central nervous system. Coordinated movements are achieved within the framework of these complex cybernetics, the essential role falling back upon the central nervous system, analogued with an cybernetic informatic subsystem. Nervous coordination is achieved through a dynamic stereotype, be it through constant adaptation which leads to the perfection of the movement.

Outside of nervous coordination, movements know muscular coordination as much regarding external resistance as well as motricity coordination, which results in a correlation of movements with a motricity task being carried out, in a concrete external environment and in accordance with the functionality of the sportsman. Within this framework, numerous feedback mechanisms are at work regulating and harmonising the different components of the system.

We mention only that within the framework of these complex connections we set apart the connection channels from the external environment to the system and the connections between subsystems. The reversed pathways can be positive, leading to the amplification of movement or negative with an attenuating effect. Cycles of interaction and coordination are either peripheral, between the mobile rings of internal and external locomotricity force or central between the mobile rings and the central nervous system The external environment plays a role in this complex of executing movement, functionality and prior experience.

Physical exercise, viewed as a cybernetic system of conduction, performs on the basis of its programming. As such it requires programming through preparation, through choice (choosing the optimum option), through follow-up (when experimental deviations from the optimum program are carried out) and amplification. In these conditions, computers on larger and larger scales are used, analogical and hybrid, giving us the possibility to direct the optimum conditions for sports with the aim of achieving maximum output as much in the performance sport as in the mass.

-Biomechanical type of muscular activity.

Scientific training imposes other requirements, in which biomechanics can make an especially precious input. Recent research has shown that the activity carried out by the body's musculature is not that simple and that assuring position and movement are particular aspects of the muscular activity. It is well known that movement is carried out by dynamic muscular effort, which develops mechanics while position is achieved through the static-isometric muscular effort. Detailed studies have shown that in carrying out movements, as well as the isotonic dynamic component there is also a a component of static muscular effort, while the proportion between the dynamic and the static varies in accordance with the specifics of the movement. Likewise, studies of dynamic effort have allowed the distinction between several biomechanical particularities, which are essential for the scientific coordination of physical preparation.

-Biomechanical types of dynamic activity

Isotonic contraction of the muscles produces movement, or mobilisation of the bony segments; during contraction, the muscle shortens and lengthens, it changes dorm, while the volume remains the same. Bony segments where the muscles are inserted are moved closer together while the tension developed during contraction remains the same (isotone).

More Profound studies of movement have shown that it is produced when a muscle contracts and shortens its length slowly, it's still isotonic but through a reverse mechanism.

Today it is accepted in biomechanics that muscle can be developed through two active dynamics, one of "overcoming" and the other "releasing".

Overcoming dynamic activity means the movement produced through the shortening of the muscle which draws the bony segments together. For this reason, is still holds the name concentric action. Releasing dynamic activity by progressive shortening. The bony segments move away from one another slowly, for which reason this movement was called eccentric action. It is important to underline that dynamic activity of releasing should not be confused with relaxation: during release, the muscle is lengthened progressively, which in turn progressively releases the muscular shortening. Outlining the two types of dynamic muscular activity determined the change of some of the old functional anatomy which referred to the action of somatic muscles, which were divided – according to their action- to be flexors, extensors, abductors etc.

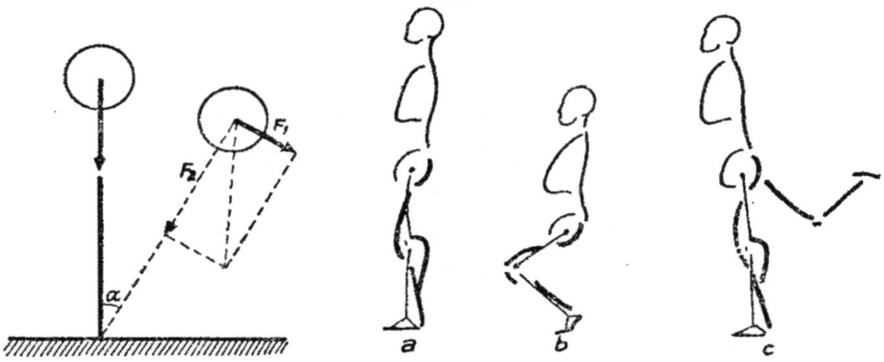

Fig. 87. Example of unstable balance

Nowadays it is known that one and the same muscle can both have a classic action as well as the antagonistic thereof. In this way, in classic anatomy, muscles of the vertebral column are known as the extensors of the vertebral column, assuring the upright position of the body through their "overcoming" dynamic contraction. At the same time, the same muscles of the vertebral column allow for flexion, inclining the body forward creating the "releasing" dynamic activity of the muscles. Biceps brachii is the flexor of the elbow through the dynamic activity of the muscles to "overcome" and is also the extensor of the arm by the dynamic activity of the muscle to "release".

In this way we demonstrate for every muscle in turn the two types of dynamic muscular activity. So the classic model of flexors and extensors etc. has become a relative idea, expressing only one aspect of their motricity skills. In a similar way, the muscles of the abdominal wall assure a supine position, flexion of the trunk through the dynamic of "overcoming" and extension through dynamic "release" of the muscles. The notions of "overcoming" and "release" have a great practical importance. Several examples will be edified through their practical application.

In this, squats, with weights – an exercise used extensively in strength training – is a movement composed of two phases: lifting and lowering. In the lifting phase extension is produced in the coxofemural articulation, the knees and plantar flexion in the talocrural articulation. The muscular chain which assures the lifting phase is triple extension in the lower limb through the active muscular dynamic of "overcoming". In the lowering phase, flexion in the articulations of the lower limb, obviously, are carried out by the flexor muscle groups of these articulations. In reality the lowering phase is still carried out by the chain of triple extensors but through their dynamic action of "releasing".

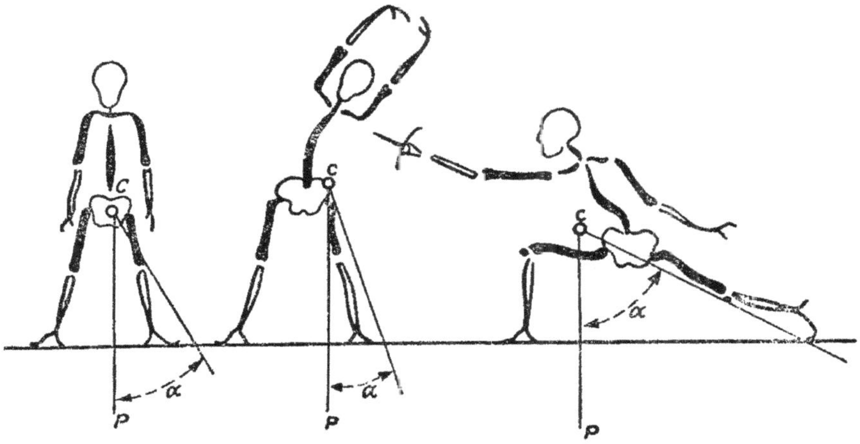

Fig. 88. Angle of stability -centre of gravity; P – Vertical BCG.;α – angle of Stability.

In conclusion, we see that the muscular effort that assures genuflexion with weights is fulfilled by a chain of triple flexion. This is why in certain movements we need to increase the force of the triple flexion chain, we need to find another exercise for example laying down and pulling weights with our legs. Traction movement, pull ups, in the arms on a fixed bar is composed of two phases: traction (lifting) and lowering. In the pull up phase, traction phase, the long muscle chain formed of the flexors of the hand, the elbow the retroductors and the adductors of the arm, the muscles which move the scapula lower and medially. The activity created by this chain is the dynamic of "overcoming". In the lowering phase, the same muscular chain is involved but in the action of "releasing".

As we see in a pull up- exercise on a regular basis increases the strength of the upper limb- we don't train anything but the aforementioned chain of muscles. For the rest of the muscular groups and chains we have to find other exercises. From the biometric analysis of this exercise we can draw important practical conclusions. There indications and contraindications for its application therefor it is only using in certain branches and sporting tests. It is useful in rowing, gymnastics, swimming, volleyball, handball, - where the muscular chain, trained through traction on the pull up bar, acts in the principle movements of these sports.

Pull ups are contraindicated in all throwing styles (to a lesser extent the hammer) in boxing, etc., since these sports have other principle muscle chains. In the long jump, in all variations thereof, the dynamic activities of "overcoming" and "releasing" contribute in various phases to increase the output. So, the battle is between the triple chain of extensors through "overcoming" and the same chain of muscles through their "releasing" action. When preparing for the long jump, the biochemical analysis and preparation of the athlete must be considered, exercises involving training the triple extension as much in the activity of dynamic overcoming as much as the releasing.

Types of static activity biomechanics

From a biometric point of view, the static activity involved in posture is complex. It is strictly linked to types of equilibrium found in the human body, either in stable or instable equilibrium. Analysed in this way, static activity is of three kinds: consolidation, fixation or equilibrium and maintenance.

- Static activity of consolidation is met in all cases when a body or its segments, taken separately, are in stable equilibrium. A body finds itself in stable equilibrium when the centre of gravity is found below the basis of support, such as all the suspended positions of the various apparatus. The principle mechanical characteristics are that if a force acts upon a body held in stable equilibrium it will pendulate until it returns to its point of origin.

In these situations, the body's musculature contracts isometrically with the purpose of protection, of consolidating the articulations against forces which would stretch or break ligaments. Static contraction of this type is called consolidation and is fulfilled by the participation of all antagonistic muscular groups and chains. The value of the force of consolidating static contraction is greatest closest to the base of support (rings, bars etc.) and decreases towards the hanging extremities; in rotative movements the entire body (gigantic) on a fixed bar, the force of consolidation is a maximum of 180 °, when the body passes under the bar, managing to increase two-three times the body weight of the athlete.

Static activity of consolidation may be used with success for the global increase of muscle strength, even in children and students, since, as shown, it statically solicits all muscle groups while the value of the solicitation is no more than in a hanging position. Diverse hanging positions, especially those on a fixed scale, are used is therapeutic gymnastics for the correction of certain physical deficiencies.

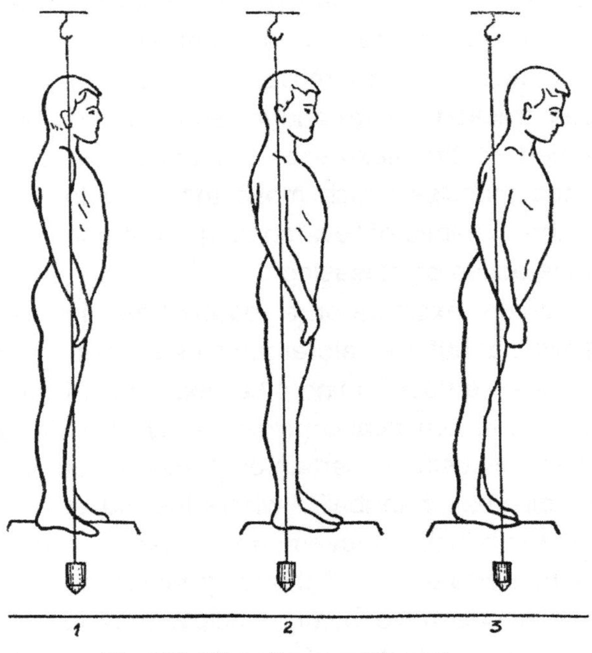

Fig. 89. Standing position.

- **Static activity of fixation (balance)** is met in all cases in which the body or segments therefore are in an instable equilibrium.

A body is in unstable equilibrium when the centre of gravity is situated above the base of support, standing, sitting etc. The vast majority of exercise is carried out in a position of unstable equilibrium. Even during exercise, as shown above, beside the dynamic activity there is also a component of static effort of varying amounts, according to the particularities of the movement. So, there are an infinite number of situations in which the body or segments thereof find themselves in unstable equilibrium, through the static activity of fixation, otherwise known as equilibrium, thus is the role of static effort in the muscles.

Static activity of fixation (equilibrium) is fulfilled by the antagonistic groups and chains of muscles, while their greatest value is closest to the base of support (floor, apparatus). The value of static effort of equilibrium is increased in vertical positions of the body where the BCG (body's centre of gravity) is not in the central base of support but towards the periphery or even outside of it (balancing on one leg with your body flexed)In contrast to inanimate objects, living things and human beings can maintain their balance to an extent even when vertical, when the BCG does not lie within the perimeter of the central base of support. In living things and humans this is possible due to static muscle contractions for balance, the more the vertical centre of gravity is outside the perimeter of the base of support, the greater the effort required maintaining balance.

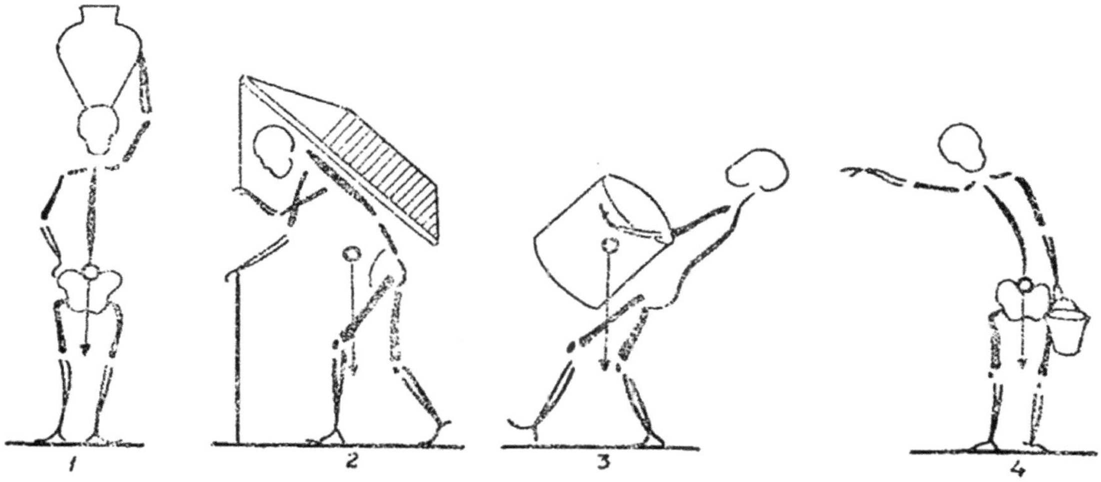

Fig. 90. Asymmetrical positions (with weights).

The value of effort for static equilibrium varies according to mechanical factors such as the angle of stability. This angle is formed from the vertical BCG and a straight line which joins the BCG with the margin of the base of support. The grade of stability is reduced in as much as the angle of stability is reduced, while the static activity of fixation (equilibrium) is greater.

There is, within the framework of unstable equilibrium, a great variety in the grade of stability within the parameters shown above. It's for this reason that biometric analysis of these positions, requires that you know the BCG height, surface area of the base of support and the area of the vertical BCG in order to appreciate correctly the value of effort of muscular static. In practice, static activity of equilibrium is used in the framework of general physical preparation, in the correction of certain physical deficiencies, particularly with the vertebral column and in the framework of several movements and positions with the purpose of increasing the capacity for equilibrium.

- **Static activity of maintenance** is the second type of static effort, which is seen as much in positions of stable equilibrium as much as in those which are unstable, as many times as the legs and arms are extended out from the vertical BCG of the body. Thus, the upper limb while it hangs in a free position beside the body is in stable equilibrium, supported in the scapulo-humeral joint, with consolidated static activity. If we lift that arm in straight anteduction, the muscular activity which holds this position is one of "maintenance" fulfilled by the anteductors or abductors, without the participation of the antagonists.

Likewise, in standing position, with the trunk bent forward, static activity for the trunk is maintenance, carried out by the muscles of the vertebral column. In the hanging forward position, the static maintenance activity is performed by a chain of muscles composed of the flexors of the thigh on the pelvis, extensors of the calves and plantar flexors. The importance of this kind of static muscular activity for the practice of physical education and sport comes from the fact that only certain groups and muscle chains are involved, without the participation of antagonists. In this way, certain muscle groups and chains which interest us can be selectively trained in order to increase their force through isometric effort.

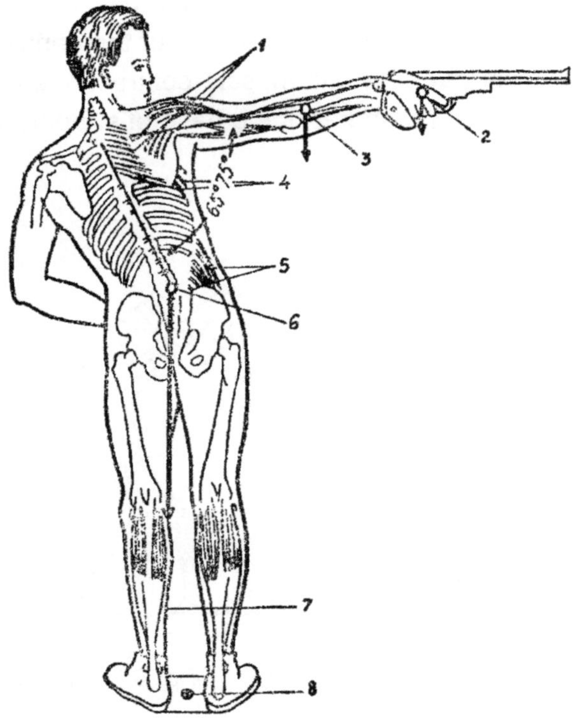

Fig. 91. Deviation of BCG. of the body when holding a pistol.
1 – Abductors and anteductors of the arm;
2 – centre of gravity of the hands with a pistol;
3 –Center of gravity of the forearm;
4 – greater serratus muscles;
5 – abdominal muscles;
6 – Center of gravity of the body;
7 – vertical deviation of BCG.;
8 – Normal vertical projection of BCG.

- Notions of muscular mechanics

Static and dynamic activity of somatic musculature is harmonious, after the specifics and needs of the movement or when assuring a position be it simple or complex. It can be confirmed that in order to execute any movement there is a dynamic component on which it is superimposed and a static component of variable importance.

In motricity activities with a high mobility, such as those from sporting games- skating, skiing, modern and sporting gymnastics- the component of static effort is smaller but not absent, in as much as the body needs balancing whilst carrying out various movements. In these cases the static component of effort is for stability or equilibrium.

There as, as such, cases in which the motricity activity is part of a large dynamism but in reality the muscular activity is predominantly static. Some examples of this appear in the gigantic movements at the fixed bar and in swinging a hammer.

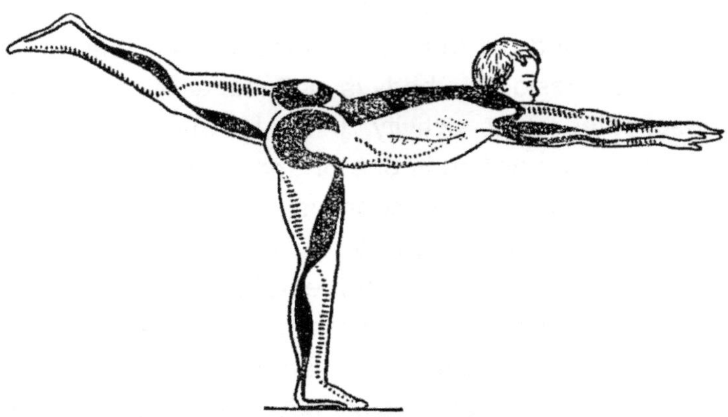

Fig. 92. On one foot with arms outstretched and torso flexed along with the muscular chains which hold it.

In the first case, rotation of the body around the bar assures a gravitational acceleration, to which is added over the course of the movement, as in between 180° (position below the bar) and 270°, a small dynamic component of the body's musculature, which executes a slight flexion on the trunk and inferior limbs. This shortening of the length of the body, reduced the ray of rotation and through this, the value of the break at the moment of inertia, it is through this that the body has the ability to rotate a complete 360° around the fixed bar. At the same time, in the course of rotating around the bar, a centrifugal force appears and develops which reaches its peak as the body passes 180°, under the bar and when, due to the gravitational acceleration, the weight of the body is increased two or three times. It is this which determines the appearance and development of a centripetal force, which is assured through the static effort of "consolidation" of the musculature of the body. The value of this type of static effort is several times greater than the value of the dynamic effort of this particular exercise. The same thing happens with the swing of a hammer, where the static effort during the pirouette is more complex.in a similar way, the static effort for the upper limbs is that of "consolidation", muscles opposing the disruptive force given by the powerful traction of the hammer. For the torso and inferior limbs, the static effort is that of "fixation" or balance, ensuring the stability of the body which will tend to be unbalanced due to the traction exerted by the hammer during the circular acceleration.

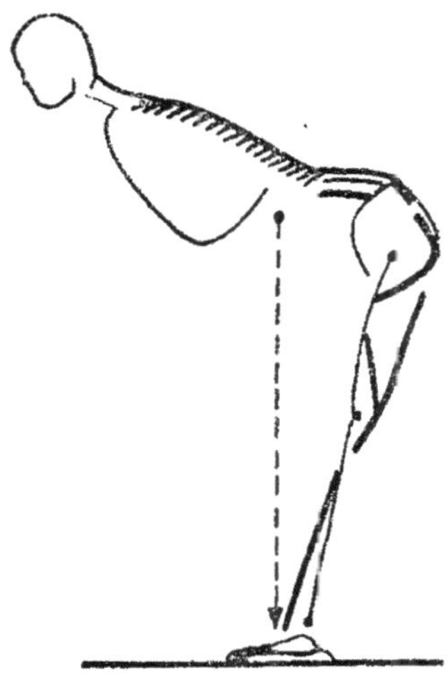

Fig. 93. Muscle chains which maintain a flexed position

Examples of the bond between dynamic and static activity of the muscles can be found in any motricity activity. As such, throwing a ball through a hoop, the motricity activity of the throw itself is grafted onto a fine and perfectly coordinated static activity "of balance", ensuring the most favourable position of the body for a successful throw. The same as when kicking a football, the support foot, trunk and upper limbs play a distinct role in maintaining balance, creating optimum conditions for the strike.

All of these examples and many others demonstrate that in motricity activities, there is a bond of various proportions between the dynamic and static muscular effort. The practical conclusion imposed is that any physical training should consider values of static and dynamic effort, and that in physical and technical training, new exercises, methods and apparatus is introduced correspondingly.

Muscles, motricity factors and bone levers

The human skeleton is composed of numerous bony parts of different forms and sizes. Through articulations between them they form kinematic couples and chains.

Kinematic couples and chains are articulations between two bony structures. Depending of the form at the end of the bones which participate in the articulation the movements possible may be more complex or simpler. When the bones are cylindrical, the articulation has only one grade of liberty – flexion and extension at the elbow, between phalanges, between the axis and atlas etc. If the bones form ellipsoidal shapes (condyles), the articulation has two grades of freedom and 2 axes of movement; flexion and extensions as well as lateral inclination of the hand against the forearm, or the occipital condyles with the atlas etc. In the case of spherical articulations there are three grades of liberty, around three axes of movement, as seen in the scapulo-humeral joint and the coxo-femural joint: flexion-extension, abduction-adduction, internal and external rotation.

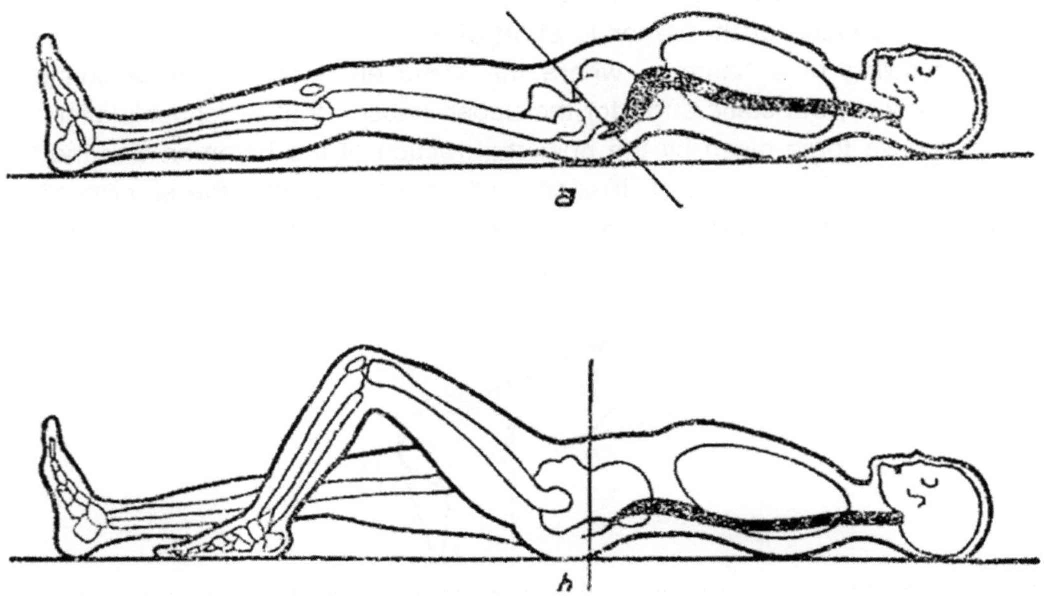

Fig. 94 Supine position:
a) when the lower limbs are extended, the lumbar curve is accentuated;
b) when one of the lower limbs is flexed, the lumbar curve reduces

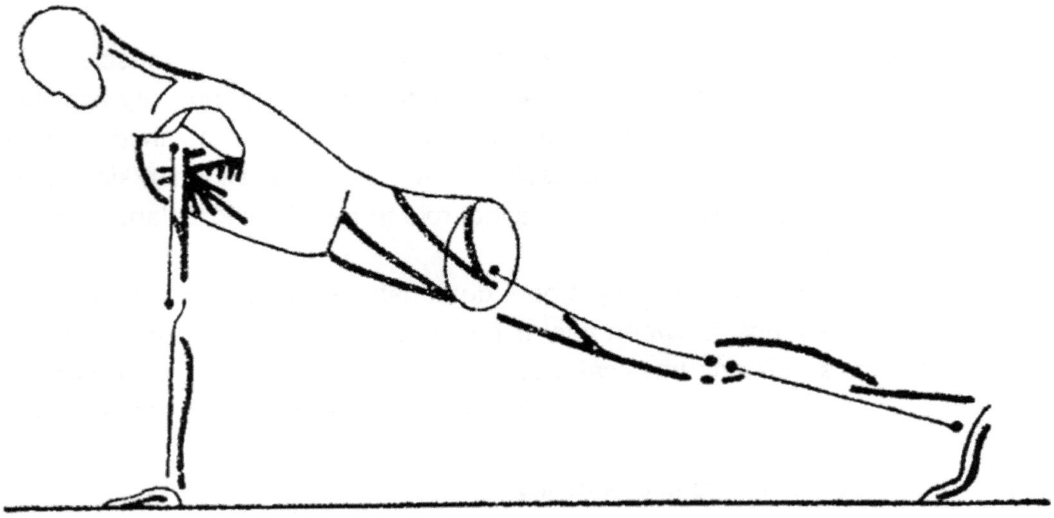

Fig. 95. Support anterior outstretched position with the kinematic chains involved

In the human body there are various types of articulations, through the chains of multiple kinematic couplings. It is this that allows the possibility of greater and more diversified movement. Kinematic chains are an articulated succession of kinematic couplings as seen for example in the upper and lower limb. In the case of the free upper limb the kinematic chain is known as open, however when the extremity of the chain is fixed, for example, the lower limb being supported on the floor or the upper limb being supported on an apparatus, the chain is known as closed. The difference between these two types lies in the fact that the open kinematic chain is capable of executing numerous movements which are, in fact, the sum of the grades of freedom of all articulations of which it is composed. Open kinematic chains can only perform partial moves, as in while some couples are fixed, the rest remain mobile.

The closed kinematic chain is characterised by the restricted number of movements and the fact that any movement carried out by a couple in the composition will require movement of the entire chain. Movements in articulations, in their respective kinematic chains, are carried out by somatic musculature, which are available around the joints, forming, from the biomechanical point of view, muscular groups and chains. One muscle group produces a movement, in one direction, other in the opposite or other directions according to the grades of movement possible. According to how they are grouped, muscles are agonists, as in the carry out the same movement, such as the flexors of the elbow, the calf, the fingers, or antagonists, as in the carry out the opposite movement such as the extensors of the same articulations. Muscles can also be synergic, as in at the level of one articulation produce one type of movement but are capable of executing other moves too. In this way the pectoralis major muscle is synergic with the deltoid in the movement of autoduction of the arm but can also perform adduction. The latissimus dorsi is synergic with the trapezius in the dorsomedial displacement of the shoulder but can also carry out the lowering of such. In order to carry out more movements, muscles need to have multidirectional fibres, which allow different tractional directions. Thus, the deltoid, the trapezius, the latissimus dorsi have 3 directions the fibres can move, carrying out three directions of movement. For this reason, as a group, their functional actions are similar. This assumes that there is a special innervation for each muscle which allows it to contract totally or partially as is necessary.

The play of synergism and antagonism allow for precise and fine movements which are established gradually over time as the movements are repeated.

Muscular force depends on the number of fibres which it contains and not the length thereof, it can be calculated by the multiplication of the surface area of the physiological section of the muscle with a constant of 10.

$$F = S \times 10$$

The surface area of the physiological section of the muscle is the cumulative surface of the section cut perpendicular to the directions of the muscular fibre. It is bigger than the anatomical section which was made perpendicular in the general direction of the muscle. In muscles with paralleled fibres and those which are fusiform, the two surfaces are equal, however the muscles that have multidirectional fibres, the fan shaped ones like the deltoid, the trapezius and the uni- and bipennate muscles always have a physiological section larger than the anatomical one.

In practice, on a man, calculating the muscular force is done globally with movements of flexion, extension, those which –as we know- have more muscles involved. The force of each muscle cannot be determined except on animals in experimental circumstances. In humans, the global force of a muscle group is calculated with special apparatus called dynamometer, constructed adequately for each principal movement. The constant from 10 of the formulas described above represents, in principle, the force per centimetre squared of anatomical section of a muscle: as is calculated for a young adult. For women and children, the value is much smaller whereas for well-trained athletes it can be as much as 12-14kg per centimetre squared of anatomical section.

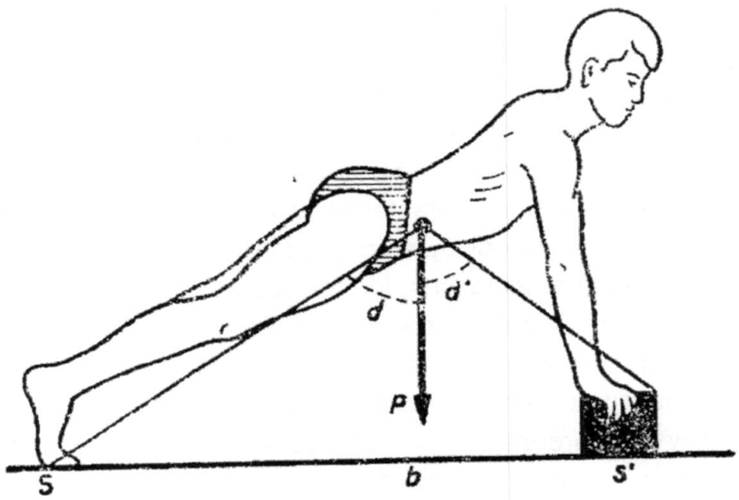

Fig. 96. raised plank position
P– vertical C.G.C.; S-S' – support surface; d-d – angles of stability.

Another method for determining muscular force is the disruptive (martin) method which is done by balancing out the force with gradual addition of weights. This does not satisfy all aspects wither, in fact, the total force of a muscle can only be determined when the lever of weights is done at 90°. Otherwise, or rather, as happens in the vast majority of cases, the traction is done by the muscles obliquely and so force is lost for the movement. In the case when muscular force acts obliquely on a bone lever, the lever is broken down into two parts namely:

- movement component which carries out the bony lever
- articular component, pressure or traction on the bones which form that particular articulation.

As we see global muscular force is not reduced for the movement, they also perform other roles, such as protection of the joint through its articular components. Essential to strength training is to develop strength greater than that necessary overcome the resistance, while executing a correct sporting technique. For this reason other causes of loss of useful force are considered during sport performance. Muscular antagonism causes a loss of useful force in movement when the athlete's nervous system doesn't conduct well or they are poorly coordinated such as is seen in beginners. Likewise, muscular force is distributed according to the nervous control which can produce global contraction of all the muscle fibres or just a portion thereof. In this way the muscular force can be distributed according to the requirements of the specific task.

In conclusion we can say from the information above that it is difficult to determine the "absolute force" of a muscle or group of muscles; practically it's important to determine the useful force required to fulfil any given motricity activity. This useful force also varies according to the phases and moments within the movement. Mechanical work or muscular labour is another useful biomechanical parameter for practice. Its determined by multiplying the force by the shortened length of the muscles, resulting in the equation: Lm=FxDisplacement (shortening in cm).

The unit of measurement for mechanical labour is a kilogram-metre, as in the force needed to lift a weight of 1kgf to a height of 1 metre. Mechanical labour is a complex parameter resulting from the directly proportional relationship between force and length of shortening. Often, in practice, mechanical labour is confused with force which is a mistake as to determine the mechanical labour, it is necessary to first calculate both factors and then multiply them. Regarding muscle shortening, we known that the muscle can shorten between 1/3 and ½ from its position at rest to maximum contraction. If the muscle is stretched beforehand, the length with which the muscle shortens will be greater according to the amount it was stretched. Consequently, the value of the mechanical labour will increase which in sport translates to output and performance. For example, in the release phase of throwing a javelin, before the final effort, a maximum extension of the muscle chain involved in the throw is produced. In this way, by stretching the muscles, they will shorten with as much as they were stretched. The result will be an increased mechanical labour, which in other words is increased performance.

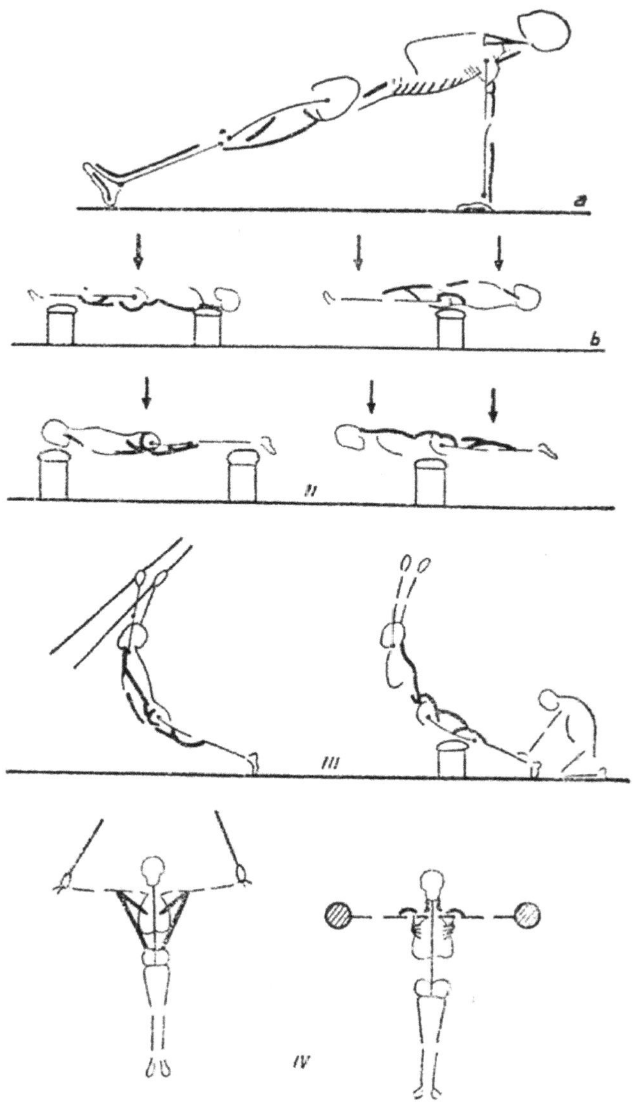

Fig. 97. Different positions: a – laid down with posterior support; muscular chains which maintain this position; b – muscular groups and chains which assure different supported positions on a training bench.: I – laid down with double dorsal support in simple dorsal support; II – laid down with double ventral support and laid down with simple ventral support.; III – inclined ventral supported position of extension with support on knees and toes.; IV – lateral supported position on the rings and standing position with superior limbs in abduction (with weights)

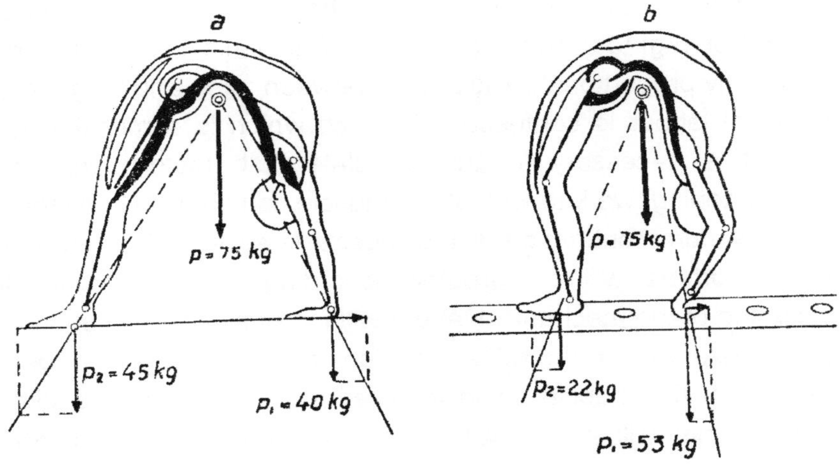

Fig. 98. "bridge" position. Distribution of force of weight over the limbs according to the angle formed between the BCG and the points of support on the floor.

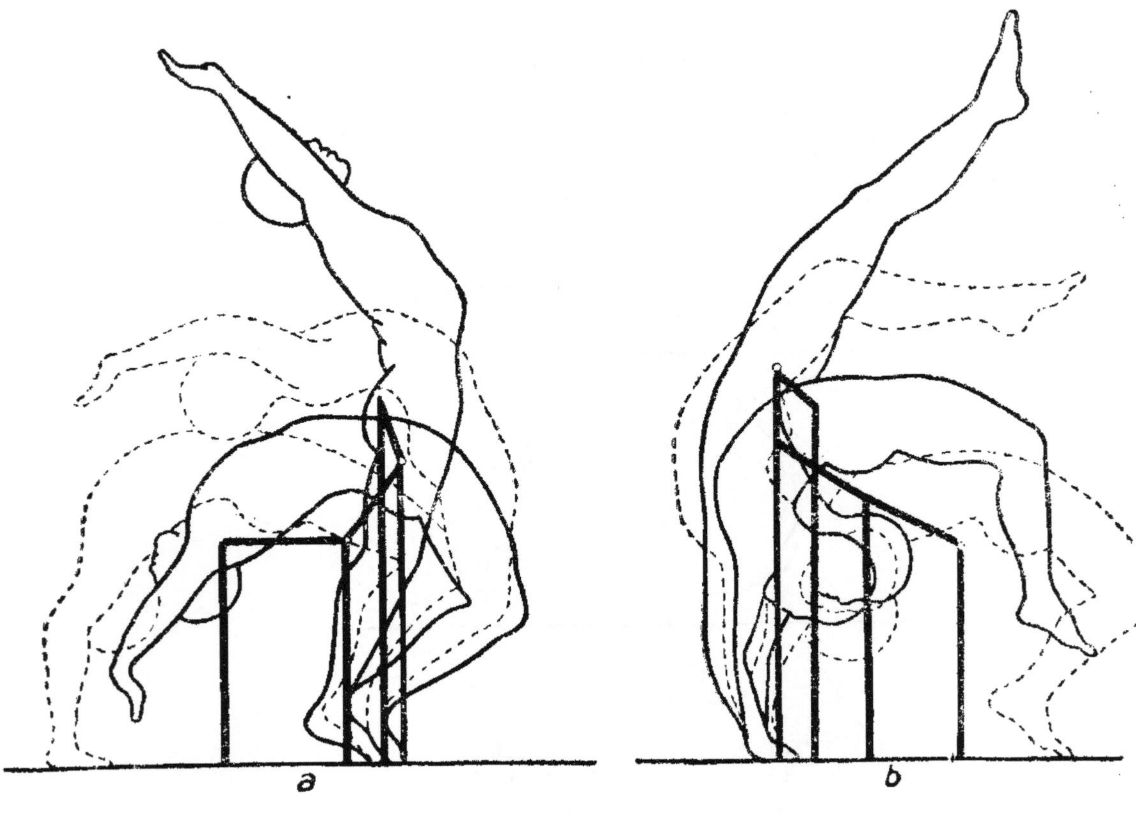

Fig. 99. Trajectory of transition into the bridge position:
a) – from normal standing position; b) – from standing on hands

This data is greatly important for the methodology of sport training, where the two factors which determine the value of mechanical labour must be taken into account- force and muscle shortening. It's not sufficient to only work on the force of the muscles involved in throwing, you also need to assure a high capacity of extension. For this you need to introduce exercises which increase the amplitude of movement in the scapulohumeral joint and the scapular belt, as well as exercises for flexibility of the vertebral column, especially for the extension.

- Muscular mechanics applied through levers

The bones of the body form levers, which are mobilised by muscles according to all the mechanical lever rules of First, second and third degree.

In our body, most of the levers are third degree. However, there are some particularities which result from the specific biological structures and functions of the human organism, which is capable of executing movements of great precision and amplitude. In this category of levers, we use "the golden rule of mechanics", through which we describe what is lost through force is gained in amplitude. Some writers contest the second degree levers; however the majority of specialists admit that there is a single example: when standing on the tips of your toes, where the point of support is the tip of the foot which is supported on the floor by the toes on the end of the metatarsian bones, the impact point of the force being on the calcaneus where the gastrocnemius is inserted via the Achilles tendon while the point where the resistance, represented by the body weight, is applied on the talocrural articulation.

First degree levers, while not numerous, are found in different segments of the body. Such as the articulation of the cranium with the vertebral column where the active force is represented by muscles of the neck and the resistance force by the weight of the cranium. Due to the fact that the centre of gravity of the skull is found at the level of the sela turcica, in front of the point of support (atlanto-occipital joint), the two arms of the lever are unequal. First degree lever conditions are created in other joints such as the coxofemural and talocrural joints in vertical position supported on the ground with the whole plantar surface.

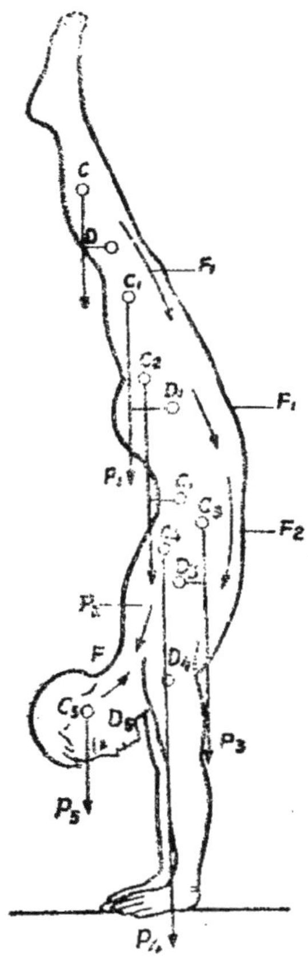

Fig. 100. "Standing on the hands" position. The arrows indicate the action of the gravitational force on the body segments.

The most important biological particularity of levers of the human body is that the degree of the lever may change according to the position of the body or its segments. For example, in standing position at the level of the coxofemural joint there is a first-degree lever relationship; but if we flex the thigh on the pelvis, the femur becomes a third-degree lever and responds to all the mechanical necessities as such. Likewise, in standing position at the level of the scapulohumeral joint with body hanging from the upper limbs, a first-degree lever is created but when we carry out abduction, autoduction etc, the lever relationship within the framework cannot be changed.

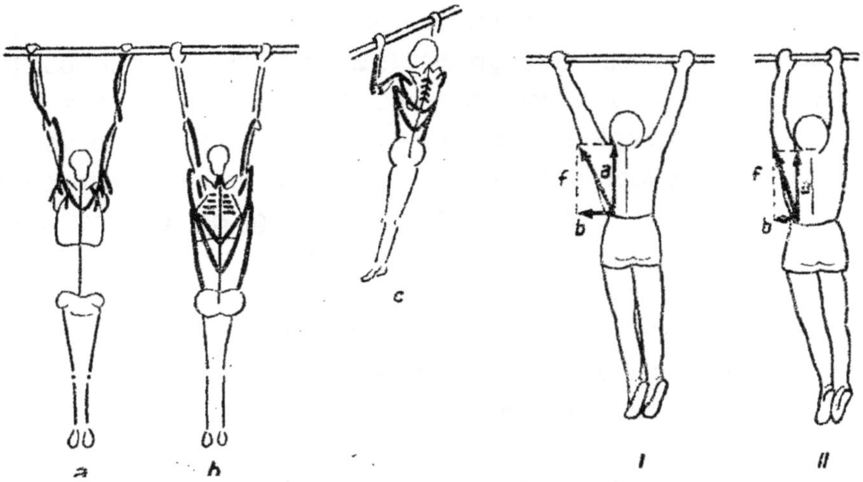

Fig. 101. Hanging position

a – muscular chains which assure hanging position (central view); b – dorsal view; c – muscular chains which create traction of the arms to the bar.; I – with arms apart; II – with arms together

There are many biomechanical particularities in third degree levers which are the most commonly found in the body. They are a result of the position which they have in relation to the direction of movement which is also the support point of the lever, the point where the active force mobilises the lever. With more force, or muscle, acting on a lever of smaller force, there will be a greater loss of force which, according to the "golden rule of biomechanics" will be compensated for by a larger displacement and the reverse is also true.

Another biomechanical particularity, and the most important is that within the human body there are third degree levers which are mobilised by many forces and third-degree levers which are mobilised by only one force. It's clear that a lever mobilised by one force will work under harder mechanical conditions than those with mobilised by many forces. Thus, the abduction of the arm is carried out by a single force, the deltoid muscle, who's point of insertion on the humerus is close to the axis of movement. Abduction is a difficult movement carry out, especially when carried out with weights because the single force which acts mobilises a small armed lever. The amplitude of the abduction movement compensates for the loss of force.

* * *

Activity of muscles in the framework of kinematic chains is even more complex due to the interplay of forces which appear while executing certain complex movements and to which the muscle needs to respond in a coordinated and efficient way. It's well-known that kinematic chains are mobilised by muscular chains, in the framework of this, muscular groups are interconnected as is necessary to carry out the movement. To achieve greater efficiency of the movement each muscle group must have a perfectly coordinated contraction or relaxation. In the light of this, Prof. K. Hochmuth (Leipzig) released a paper called the principle of the biomechanics of "partially coordinated impulses", on the basis of which – through electromyographic recording – he shows precisely the moment each muscle group of a muscle chain is engaged. Any precedence or delay of contraction creates within the muscular chain a breaking reaction which not only reduces the efficiency of the outcome but also can produce accidents (sprains or tears in the muscles).

As we have seen, maintaining movement and posture are the results of the activity of the body's musculature. The specificity of human movement is the great variety, finesse and precision it possesses. Due to open cinematic chains, movement can take place in many planes and axes not just that of each articulation in turn.

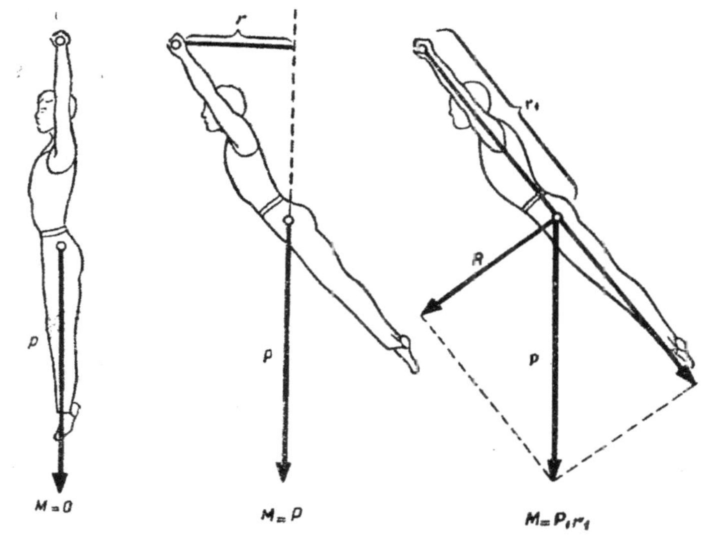

Fig. 102. Action of forces while hanging from the bar

For this reason, muscular groups and chains vary continuously, their formation often only involving a part of the muscular fibres, as in, only those which coincide the direction of traction of a motricity structure for a complex move. Passing from one movement to another requires permanent change in the composition of each muscular chain or group. For this reason, we can say that each movement, simple or complex, has its own group or particular chain and that the biomechanical analysis of the load reveals motricity components of movement or of position respectively. Knowing this, it is possible to imagine and create complexes of exercises, apparatus and methods of training, which can be superimposed one on top of the other if it's possible or to move away from the habitual basic movement. If this data is not considered then habitual, parasitic movements are formed which hinder the achievement of more advanced technique.

- The main muscular chains of the body

Posture and movement of the human body are carried out by musculature distributed around the articulations in muscular groups and chains; the latter vary depending on the movement which use different neuromuscular elements motricity units, in other words.

a. On the dorsal surface of the trunk there are the two strong muscular chains of the vertebral column extensors, which, through the multiple directions of the muscles of the vertebral grooves, participate in all the movements of the spine; so the interspinous system executes extension, the intertransverse system the lateral inclination, the transversospinous opposite direction rotation and the spinotransverse system rotation in the same direction. When working with gravity, the muscles of the vertebral grooves ensure flexion through the release contraction. In rotational movements of the spine, muscular chains of the transversospinous and spinotransvers systems are continuous with the oblique abdominal wall muscles on the ventral trunk.

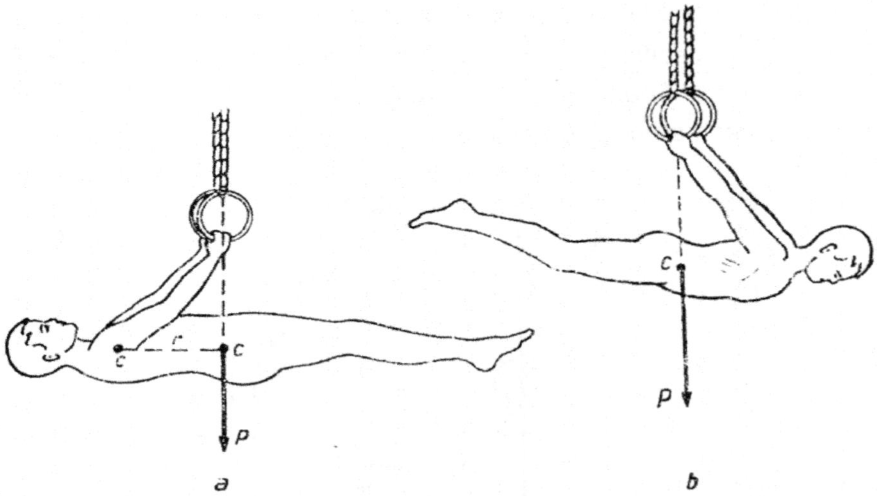

Fig. 103. a) forward horizontal hanging position; b) backwards horizontal hanging position– gravitational force; c – articular axis of the shoulder; r – arm of the force of weight; BCG. – body's centre of gravity.

b. On the ventral trunk, along with the two vertical muscular chains of the rectus abdominus, the antagonistic muscles of the spines extensors, there are two strong muscular chains which intersect, which, along with the dorsal obliques of the trunk form spiral chains. So, the external oblique muscular chain of the right side is continuous with the internal oblique of the opposite side, while in the dorsal part of the trunk it is continuous with the transversospinous system of the same side.

In general, to perform a twisting motion the trunks muscle groups form two spirals which encircle it from the mastoid process to the pelvis; all muscles with fibres parallel to the direction of the spiral with be synergic in the right-left twisting motion of the trunk.

The muscular chains of the trunk are continuous with those of the superior and inferior limbs, in this way unifying the whole body in movement and posture.

c. In humans, the muscular chains of the upper limb are capable of performing precise and complex movements which are perfected in the process of working.

Simple movements from each joint are bound in complex movements of the upper limb, of which the most important are:

1. Prehensile movement (grasping) and moving the upper limbs to the trunk
2. Pushing movement, which is carried out when lifting weights and in throwing; it is usually carried out with participation from the trunk, which amplifies it, and the inferior limbs, which fix the body to the ground. Execution of this move requires the participation of the muscular chain which raises the arms high (elevation), formed of the muscles which tilt the scapula (serratus and trapezius), scapulohumeral abductors (deltoid and supraspinatus) and the extensors of the elbow; at the wrist and hand they produce a block in flexion.
3. The Hitting movement has many varieties and is associated with a rotating movement of the trunk.
4. Throwing movement varies according to the object thrown. In any kind of throwing the muscular chains of the trunk and lower limb are involved.

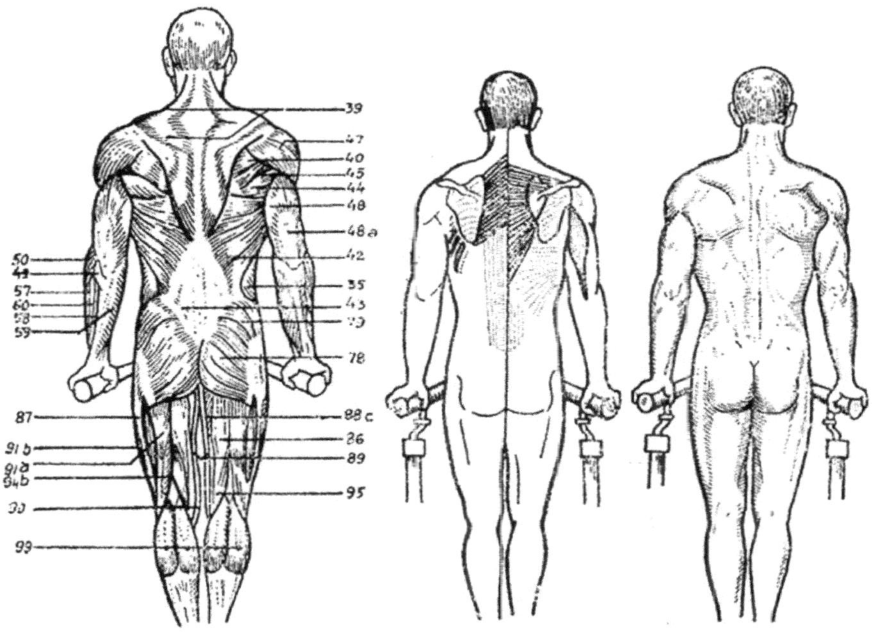

Fig. 104. Kinematic chains and distribution of the musculature while supported on parallel beams. (according to K. Tittel)
50 – biceps brahi.; 49 – anconeus.; 57 – second external radius.; 60 – extensor digitorum communis.; 58 – extensor carpi ulnaris.; 59 – flexor carpi ulnaris; 87 – Fascia lata; 91 b – vastus lateralis; 94 a – biceps femoris; 90 – sartorius; 99 – triceps sure; 39 – trapezius; 47 – deltoideus; 40 – infraspinatus; 45 – teres minor; 44 – teres major; 48, 48 a – triceps brahi; 42 – M. latissimus dorsi; 35 – oblicus externus; 43 – lumbosacral aponeurosis; 79 – gluteus medius; 78 – gluteus maximus; 88 c – adductor magnus; 96 – semitendinous; 89 – gracilis; 95 – semimembranosus.

Upper limbs can also fulfil a role of support but are rarely used during work but more frequently in sport. This is how we can have upper support (hanging positions) or inferior support (standing on the hands). D. Muscular chains of the lower limbs. In the past the distant past of phylogenesis, the lower limbs had the role of support, as is the case in all quadruped vertebrates. The architecture of the lower limb adjusted as bipedal stance and work developed, without affecting their role of support. Also, the development of the upright position required the development of a powerful musculature in the lower limb, which would correspond to the energy required, to which was added nervous coordination to ensure the balance of the upright position and movements. The development of work perfected the muscular chains and the nervous coordination, while physical exercise completed it through the complex requirements of effort and balance.

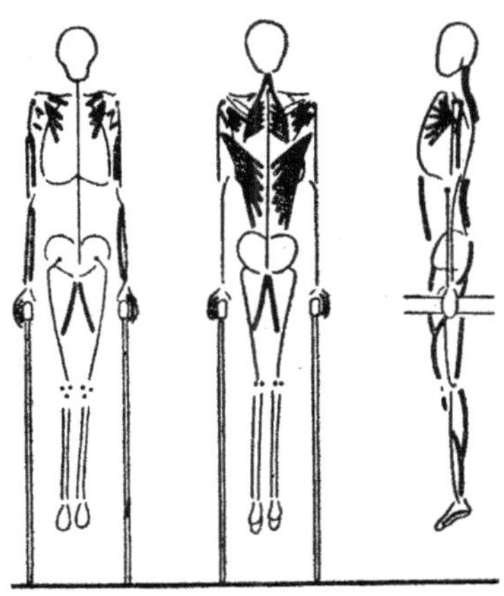

Fig. 105. Supported position on the parallel bars and the muscular chains which carry it out.

Bipedal walking produced a series of changes in the skeleton: accentuation of the curves of the spine, dorsoventral flattening of the chest, enlargement of the pelvic belt. The sacroiliac joints were strengthened with powerful ligaments (sacrospinos and sacrotuberos), likewise, the coxofemural joint (iliofemural, ischiofemural and pubofemural ligaments). In humans, the pelvis only moves concomitantly with the lumbar spine. While the lower limbs have mobile articulations, their range of movements is lower than the upper limb. The skeletal components of the foot underwent substantial changes in the form of the development of the two arches (sagittal and frontal). Ligaments and muscles of the sole maintain the normal curves of the arches of the sole. The greatest solicitation of the foot occurs when maintaining balance while standing still. The foot is very mobile and has a specific importance in the static and dynamic positions of the human body, particularly during sport.

What characterises the components of the muscular chains of the lower limb is the distribution of the flexor and extensor muscles in two antagonistic chains, in which there are three groups of muscles each, which is why they were named triple flexor and triple extensor chains.

Because of their major role in the support of the body, the lower limb is more important than the upper limb. The ratio between the weight of the skeleton and the musculature for the upper limb is 327.7:1000 while for the lower limb it is 519.8:1000.

The sole has a specific importance in the static and dynamic roles of the human body, especially during sport. Muscular chains of the lower limbs fulfil important static roles as well as different movements, some of the most characteristic of which are the following:

1. Impulsion, the primary movement of walking, running, jumping and numerous other actions executed by the body and its segments. It is carried out by the triple extension chain which ensures impulsion from the ground and concomitantly activates the musculature which stabilises the segments, which is necessary for maintaining balance but not so important in force.
2. Dampening (absorbing shock) which, after impulsion, is the most important activity contributed by the muscle chains of the lower limb. It is met in walking, running, jumping and numerous other types of movement. Through dampening the speed of the movement is reduced, in some types of movement, dampening must be removed (walking, running) while in other movements, it represents the final stage (jumping). The muscular chains which provide the dampening are the same as those used in impulsion, namely the triple extension chain, the difference being that impulsion is the activity dynamic overcoming while dampening is dynamic release, which slowly stops the reactive arrest force.
3. Kicking with the lower limb (football) has a great variability, due to the fact that it is not always executed on the normal axis of flexion and extension of the segments, but in numerous directions concomitant with medial or lateral rotation of the lower limb. The muscular chain which carries out the kick is made up of the flexors of the thigh on the hip, extensors of the lower leg and the dorsal flexors of the foot. The muscular activity has a ballistic characteristic through the powerful initial contraction, after which the movement continues from inertia.

Maintaining a stationary position is one of the main activities of the lower limb. It is carried out by the static contraction of the musculature, where the principal role is contributed by the triple extension chain. Fixation of the body on the ground is carries out by the muscular chain of the adductors of the thigh which act on the closed kinematic chain, which is represented by the two lower limbs and the pelvis. The actions of fixation on the ground and ensuring a vertical position have a greater importance in sporting activities.

- Methodology of biomechanical analysis.

Biomechanical analysis is, in essence, a complex study of the somatovisceral factors and the environmental factors which intervene in carrying out motricity activities, of the established relationships between them, of the way they participate and what effect they have on the human organism as a whole. The purpose of this analysis is to find ways to optimise movements in order to obtain a maximum sporting efficiency. Biomechanical analysis encompasses the following important sections: mechanical analysis, muscular analysis, functional analysis and pedagogic analysis. For teaching reasons, we will present these stages separately, despite being convinced that there are no clear boundaries between them, each having elements which must be interpreted as a unit with a view to establishing optimum results. Likewise, to systematise the material, we will refer initially to the biomechanical analysis of static labour (maintaining certain postures, superior or inferior support respectively), and then the biomechanical analysis of dynamic labour (analytical or synthetic exercises).

Stages of a biomechanical analysis

Mechanical analysis – constitutes, in turn, a descriptive analysis and a critical analysis.

I. Descriptive analysis
   1. Defining postures by establishing the base of support and the positions of the various segments in relation to one another.
   2. Determining the following elements
      a. External forces which need to be overcome, respectively exterior resistance and weight of the body segments conditioned by their position in space, specifying their direction, value and area of the body involved.
      b. Conditions for maintaining equilibrium,
      c. Distribution of pressures on points of support
      d. Direction and values of the unbalancing actions
      e. Levers involved

II. Critical analysis, of which the content is defined by the following element
   a. Defining frequent mistakes which break the rules of voluntary effort which maintains posture.
   b. Establishing the possible adaptations which could be made to the mode of execution of motricity actions according to the constitutional morphology of the athlete.

We exemplify the above points by mechanically analysing a standing position with a left leg outstretched.

1. A. the trunk is inclined in the prolonged lower leg; the hips slightly tilted, back is straight, the shoulders are down with the shoulder blades well fixed, the head, torso and right leg are in a straight line (all of these segments are in extension to the other)

B. external forces are executed vertically from top to bottom, with a high intensity due to the strong forward inclination of the head and consequently, the segments of the trunk which affect the left lower leg for all the body weight, pelvis for the segments of the trunk and back of the neck for the head. Balance is good, the base of support is long, the centre of gravity is slightly lowered, the triangle of support is tight, the unbalancing action is lateral, the greatest pressure is on the forward foot. Third degree levers are created at the ankle and calf.

2. A. the most frequent mistakes which can occur are: the base of support is too narrow or poorly placed, the shin is insufficiently extended, the head and trunk may be flexed or too extended.

B. Triangle of support for obtaining maximum metric efficiency will need to be adapted to the athlete's constitution. For example, at his waist or if is the case in the presence of a valgus or varus.

III. Muscular analysis indicates in detail, with certain anatomical precision, principal and secondary locomotricity factors of movement of the muscular groups which maintain or vary the bony levers.

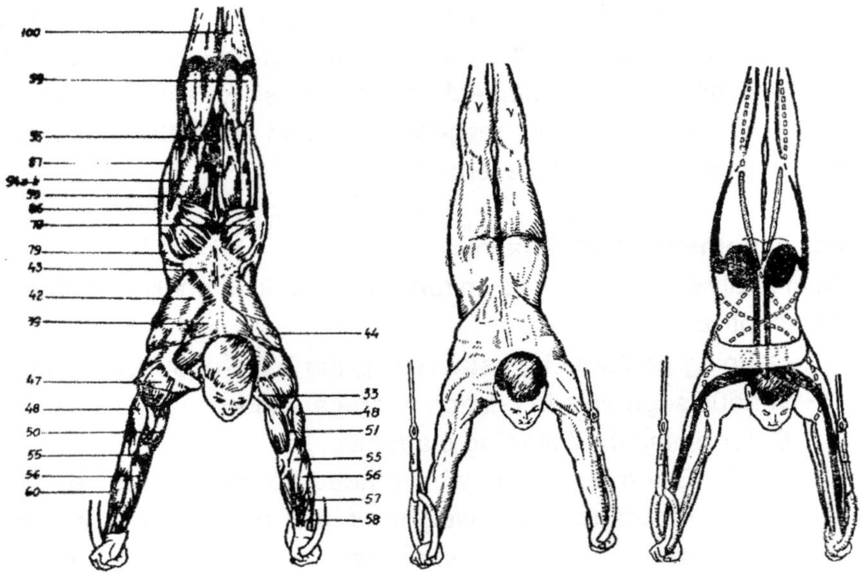

Fig. 106. Distribution of musculature and kinematic chains in the position of support on the rings. (according to K. Tittel):

100 -m. triceps sure; 99 – m. triceps sure; 95 – semimembranosus; 87 – Fascia lata; 94 a– b – biceps femoris; 90 – sartorius; 86 – M. tensoral fasciei lata; 78 – gluteus maximus; 79 – gluteus medius; 43 – lumbosacral aponeurosis; 42 – latissimus dorsi; 9 – m. trapezius; 47– deltoideus; 48 – triceps brahi; 50 – biceps brahi; 55 – brahioradialis; 56 – M. first external radial; 60 – extensor digitorum communis; 44 – terres major; 33 – pectoralis major; a) – pars descendens; b) – pars transversus; c) – pars ascendens; 48 – triceps brahi; 57 – brahialis; 55 – brahioradialis; 56 – M. first external radial; 57 – M. second external radial; 68 – abductor policis longus.

This analysis refers to, in part, the laws of muscular contractions, and also to the actions needed as a result of the external forces and to maintain balance. Muscular action can be static (for maintaining position) having as a direct substrate, the tonic contraction or dynamic, with its base in kinematic contraction. For static labour, the muscles can be classified according to their action, in fixators which stabilise the respective position and balancers, which oppose the unbalancing actions. For mechanic labour, the muscles are classified into: motricity, which determine movement, fixators, which ensure the base of support and the immobile segments, respectively fixed points of insertion for motricity muscles; balancers with a similar role to those in static labour, breakers, which regulate the grade of movement and oppose the motricity muscles. We specify that in dynamic labour, we recognise three types of action: concentric (leads to the segments being brought together in movement), eccentric (breaking) and ballistic (concentric action which is preceded by the eccentric movement, by nature conferring a greater amplitude than, for example, contraction of different portions of the pectorals in the javelin throwing exercise).

Exemplifying the muscular analysis of static labour while in the standing position, with left leg outstretched, we can specify the following muscular groups:

1. The fixators: for the left lower leg- extensors of the sole on the calf (triceps sural), the calf on the thigh (quadriceps), the thigh on the pelvis (gluteus maximus, which opposes flexion of the pelvis on the thigh), for the right lower leg- - extensors of the sole on the calf (triceps sural), the calf on the thigh and flexors of the thigh on the pelvis (psoas, iliac), for the trunk – extensors of the spine, and for the head – extensor muscles of the head (splenius capitis, trapezius).
2. Balancing muscles, which will oppose the unbalanced lateral actions, will be those of the plantar arches, abductors and adductors of the sole and abductors of the thigh, gluteus medius and minimus, tensor fasciae late.

For mechanical and muscular analysis of dynamic work we will concisely follow an analytical and synthetic exercise in order to establish methodology.

Analytical exercise, more simply, that which we will study constitutes in the movement of the straight arms away from the body using an extensor (rubber cord)

I. In the framework of the muscular analysis, testing the movements has a special importance. This is done by measuring the amplitude of the movement of the segment of the limb or body part, this is called testing (from the Latin testare: to witness), allowing the graphic inscription of the limitations of movement and establishing insufficient muscular objective.

A special goniometer is used for the analysis, made up of two mobile arms which have a protractor at the point where the arms articulate. The two arms are placed on the long segments of the body which will do the movement, following the mobile segments, showing the amplitude of the movements which is given as gradients by the protractor. The objectification of movement and the gradient of movement are measured through tests on each muscle, which are underlined and are edited concisely and illustratively for each case in turn.

Method of interpretation of the results is done on a conventional graded value scale between 0 and 5 in turn:

-0: Cannot perform any movement at all (total immobility)

-1: does not perform any movement but muscle can be seen to contract under the skin (clinical paralysis)

-2: movement can be performed only with the help of someone else (passive movement)

-3: completes the movements but only in as much as to overcome the effect of gravity (for example the forearm can be flexed against gravity)

-4: completes the movement, even if there are varied resistant forces to overcome, but remains under normal limits.

-5: The movement is carried out normally, overcoming all maximum resistance possible, considering that this force depends on gender, age, training etc.

We mention that in order to ascertain the force of the movement, testing must involve a manoeuvre which overcomes normal movements carried out by a muscle, composed of a muscle with fibres with different action or a group of synergic muscles. The procedure is also used for the demonstration of muscular definition. The manoeuvre of opposition is carried out with progressive force (which can be measured with the help of weights or a dynamometer). At the same time, with the help of the goniometer with protractor, the amplitude of the movements is also measured. In carrying out the test, it is important to establish:

-position given by the subject

-whether you are testing isolated or global movement

-Counter pressure which opposes the movements in order to ascertain the action and definition of the muscles

-trunk and radicular innervation of the tested muscles

-vascularisation of these muscles, with the origin of the vessel or vessels which irrigate them

In this way the two most important moments are

1. Lateral lift of the straight arm, creating a progressive traction on the cable of the apparatus, the arms move laterally until the extent of the articular movement of abduction of the scapula-humeral joint, when the hands pass the plane of the shoulders and the other segments of the body remain immobile.
2. Without marked breaks, returns to the normal, initial position, opposing the sharp retraction of the rubber cord.

II. Descriptive analysis develops according to the described methodology, with regard to the analysis of the levers of movement (third degree levers, in the shoulder, the movement of abduction, in extension of the forearm and third degree in the extension of the hand), we specify a principal motricity action, executed in the horizontal plane, consisting of overcoming the resistance of the rubber cord and a complimentary action generated by the elevation of the arm and the extension of the vertical segments of the body, respectively the lower limbs, trunk and head. Critical analysis reveals:

a. possibility of the following mistakes which reduce the exercise efficiency which, in mechanical labour, compared to static labour, is driven by the law of the smallest voluntary effort, so as to expend the least amount of energy to have the maximum efficiency of the movement

- too wide a base of support;

-trunk fixed in a position which accentuates slightly flexion or extension;

-traction saccades

-lack of amplitude at the end of the first time

b. The necessity of the following adaptations of the exercise for the constitutional type of the athlete

-regulation of the base of support according to the length and posture of the individual

-narrowing or widening of the walls according to the length of the arms

-regulation of the extensor resistance (the number of cables from his constitution) according to the strength of the gymnast.

Muscular analysis shows the following functional groups of muscles:

a. motricity muscles: in the initial time of the movement: the rhomboid and trapezius muscles act through concentric contractions- transverse portion (bring the shoulder back) the triceps, extensors of the hand and forearm, flexors of the fingers. Secondary action by the trapezius – the superior and inferior portion (opposes the drop of the upper limb), subspinous and deltoid (maintain the arm horizontally), in the second time all these muscles intervene through eccentric contraction (breaking)

b. fixator muscles (fix the point of insertion of the muscles): extensors of the spine (fix the trunk), rhomboid (fixes the shoulder blade), flexors of the sole (fix the solar arches) extensors of the sole on the lower leg, in the flexors and extensors of the thigh and pelvis (fixes the lower limb)
c. balance muscles: muscles of the arches of the sole, the abductor and adductor of the thigh on the pelvis
d. Breaking muscles: all the motricity muscles in function at the time of execution; the action is minimal, the exercise consists of overcoming the external forces.

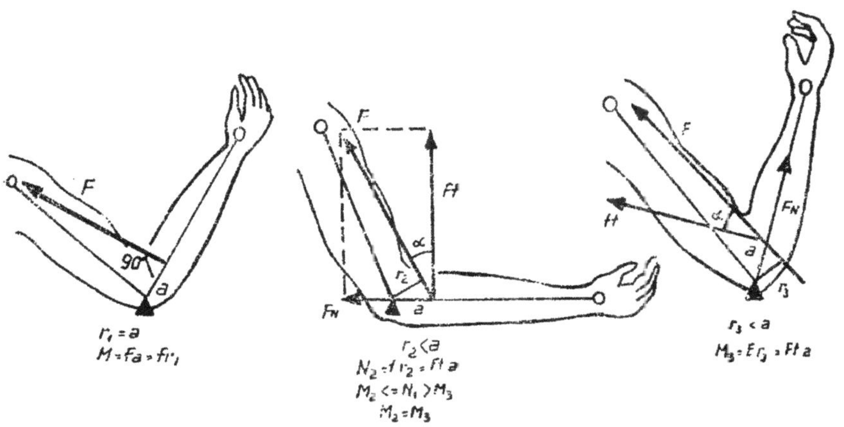

Fig. 107. Different ways to appreciate the force on a third degree lever. Action of force on the lever in a certain angle: left; medium-obtuse; right – acute

A. With regard to synthetic exercises we must emphasise that they are complex, that in their constitution are numerous analytical exercises, a fact which leaves its mark on the mode in which mechanical and muscular analyses are carried out. It is difficult in most cases to break down the exercises in order for each to be studied individually. For example, for sporting games or skiing it is difficult to analyse analytically each motricity action. For this reason the biomechanical investigation of synthetic exercise initially requires dividing it into principal phases which are then further deconstructed into homogenous groups of exercises (groups of fundamental motricity actions), in the framework of which are selected, for closer research, the most frequent and important movements and postures used in carrying out the sporting activity which we are referring to. Technological advances have put at our disposal the ability to record on film and later high speed cameras have facilitated an easier and more precise biomechanical analysis.

Mechanical analysis of a synthetic exercise follows the methodology which we have described, with the difference being that after the deconstruction of the exercise (in principal phases, fundamental homogenous groups and frequent more complex moves), for each division is specified, particularly, balance conditions, varieties of the position of the centre of gravity and the dynamics of the forces which need to be overcome, common exercise mistakes and adaptations in phases of the movement specific for the constitutional type of the athlete.

Similarly, for the conclusion of this analysis, it is utmost importance to establish the order in which this kind of movement requires certain motricity qualities (speed, tension release, skill, resistance, force). We exemplify some aspects of this complex analysis through the presentation of the start position for sprinting, which we will also come back to on the chapter regarding running. This position is characterised through a series of gestures which allow the runner, while in a position of complete immobility to obtain, instantaneously, a maximum speed. With regard to motricity qualities solicited, in order of their importance they are: speed, explosive force and skill.

The principal stages into which an exercise can be deconstructed are: (1) preparation and (2) impulsion. (1) Preparation can be further deconstructed into two fundamental groups of movement: a) waiting (the order 'on your marks') and b) swaying (the order 'get set').

1. a) waiting: forward foot is flexed and is supported on an inclined plane while the backwards foot, also bent, has the knee on the right of the calf of the forward foot; both upper limbs are in extension, slightly apart, having the thumbs directed interiorly, are on the ground, on the start line; the trunk is inclined forward, the head in slight extension.

b) swaying: pivoting forward on the fingers and the two ankles, backwards extension of the inferior limb, shoulders pushed anteriorly towards the start line, raising the pelvis and back horizontally, head raised.

2. Impulsion: quick removal of the base of support with a loss of balance, bringing the posterior calf forward, violent extension of the forward calf; correction of the trunks position and powerful launch of the flexed arms.

According to these analytical moments, the mechanical and muscular study of the complex exercise is continued. With regard to the critical analysis, frequent mistakes which need to be avoided:

-in the waiting phase: too long or too short a base of support, front foot too close to the starting line, hands in exaggerated abduction on the ground;

-in the swaying phase: imprecise and slow swaying, unsure support with flexed arms, pelvis higher than the back, head flexed, propulsion calf abducted or adducted to the trunk (poorly orientated)

-in the impulse phase: flexion of the head, angle of opening between the shin and the ground >45 degrees, premature correction of the trunk, slow sway of the arms due to keeping them straight. Likewise, the whole exercise needs to be minutely adapted to the constitutional type, the waist and the proportion of the segments of the athlete's body.

With regards to muscular analysis, it oversees the implication of muscles in fixation, balance and breaking, taking into account the complexity of the actions according to the principal phases analysed. It's very important to uncover the way in which the muscles are involved in executing concentric, eccentric and ballistic contraction. Knowing the phases of movement and the muscular anatomy, analysis is easily facilitated. So, in the waiting phase we discuss a static contraction of the following muscular groups: hand and finger flexors, extensors of the forearm, abductors of the arm and shoulder, plantar flexors of the toes, extensors of the sole, extensors of the thigh and extensors of the head. In the swaying phase a new posture is maintained with a slight loss of balance, the weight remaining on the upper limbs, to a lesser extent on the anterior lower limb while the back lower limb remains free to move forward in the impulse phase. The flexors of the fingers and hands, extensors of the forearm, abductors of the arm and shoulder are in static contraction. The anterior portion of the deltoid, executes an eccentric contraction, opposing the drop in front of the shoulder. Extensors of the sole, lower leg and thigh are responsible for the entire eccentric action, sixing the segments of the inferior limbs in an optimum position. The lumbar muscles fix the pelvis. In the impulse phase the motricity muscles will be

- For the anterior lower limb which carries out energetic concentric contraction: plantar digital flexors, favoured by the anterior eccentric action will thus, together, obtain a ballistic contraction.

- For the posterior inferior limb: flexors of the thigh on the pelvis, the calf on the thigh, the foot on the calf, all diminishing the length of the segment and favouring movement.

For the trunk: the extensors of the pelvis and spine; likewise the extensors of the head

- For the shoulders and arms there is a concentric energetic contraction by the lifting muscles of the shoulder and arm on the side of the oscillating leg and by the flexors of the forearm. Balancing muscles (muscles of the arches of the feet and the trunk) perform, on the one hand a sagittal balance (synchronism and opposition between the simultaneous movements of the arms and calves) and on the other hand a frontal balance (especially though the fixation of the arches of the feet). The breaking muscles represent in particular, a group of antagonists for the motricity muscles of the upper limb and intervene in the energetic balance of the arms. The fixating muscles act especially for the establishment of the anterior inferior limb after impulsion begins (extensors of the sole, extensors of the calf on the thigh and the thigh on the pelvis).

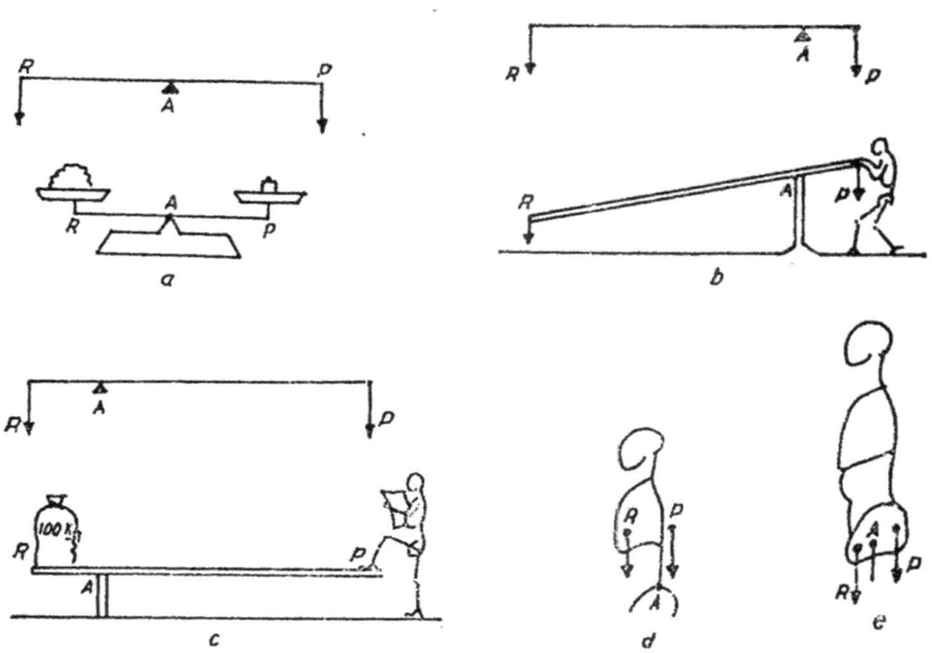

Fig. 108. Muscular levers

Another significant example of the synthetic exercise is represented by sporting games (tennis, volleyball, basketball, rugby etc). For example, analysing basketball mechanically and muscularly, results in the possibility of deconstructing the following fundamental exercises, throwing, running, and jumping. Throwing is done by one or two hands by lifting, lowering, directing and is preceded by a blockage of stepping in all directions. Running is speed and is combined with dribbling, faking or intercepting a pass. Jumps are vertical and lateral. Musculature is solicited as a whole (extensors, lumbar, obliques, abdominals, scapula-dorsi, scapula-pectoral, the arms, the forearms, hands and fingers, especially predominant in dynamic or Static effort made). Knowing all of these elements regarding the mechanics of exercise the action of each muscle in different phases of execution of movement motricity quality solicited we come scientific training exercises so that we can obtain maximum efficiency with minimum energy expenditure the. in this context analysis has ask as much in eliminating some vacations undermine the muscular mechanics as well as individualizing exercise according to the morphological mission of the individual.

Functional analysis consists of studying the specifics of the mode of participation the and apparatus during the execution of exercise. Death investigation has at its root the fact that the organism as a whole create a unified biomechanical system, while carrying out motricity activities presents adaptive modifications in all compartments. When solicited the motricity apparatus makes changes and all structures and functions of the human organism. Sway a muscle and you needs a richer irrigation which leads to acceleration the action of the respiratory, circulatory and metabolic processes (anabolism and catabolism). Likewise, physical exercise imposes nervous commands which ensure the regulation the multiple motricity actions. equilibrium, kinetic intensity, rhythm of exercise etc). The endocrine system is also highly in demand. In this way heiss, lendel blender and Zimmer demonstrate that athletes train a hyper functional hypothesis, thymus and thyroid, while milcu shows athletes have hypertrophy of the hypothesis, cortical suprarenal and thyroid gland as well as hypotonic gonads. Knowing the modifications which occur in the organism during activity permit optimization of execution permit the obtainment of maximum athletic efficiency.

In the framework of functional analysis, we first establish the motricity quality most solicited in that particular action and then predict the participation various systems and apparatus knowing the relationships established between morphofunctional modifications of the organism and motricity qualities involved.

A) In this way, speed trains the somato-physiological changes in the following systems and apparatus: in the CNS, considering the intensity and the rhythm of muscular concentration and in the cardio-respiratory, which accelerates significantly: the excretory system is minimally required.

B) expansion required primarily the CNS, which starts muscular contractions with amplitude and precision. Likewise, it produces functional disturbances in the respiratory system; the thorax being more often than not immobilised, (breathing is stopped), constituting a point of support for the musculature in action. these respiratory modifications attract important circulatory changes.

C) skill needed to coordinate finely is from the CNS

D) resistance requires the respiratory apparatus and somewhat the elimination systems of the body (sweating, excretion). The CNS is not at maximum capacity as the effort is stereotypical. Blood circulation is carried out in good condition.

E) Force established in a large and slow labour solicits especially local circulation while the respiratory system the system are only required in a reduced capacity.

Of course, in a dynamic labour more motricity qualities are required resulting complex participation from different systems and apparatus within the organism. As an example in order of the level of solicitation the motricity qualities involved some complex sporting activities

-Sprinting: Speed, skill, resistance, explosive force

-Running: resistance, speed

-Skiing: Resistance, skill, force

-Tennis: Skill speed explosive force resistance

From this comes also complex functionality and inter relationships which are established between different systems and apparatus in the organism knowing these aspects gives us the ability to scientifically direct effort, on the basis of individual morphofunctional criteria and particularities of the physical activities and the Constitutional type of the athlete.

Pedagogic analysis requires: 1. Distinguishing the dominant character of the exercise 2. Establishing the effects the activity 3. Explaining the grade in which an exercise corresponds age constitutional type of he who executes it.

1. In ratio to the dominant character of the activity, we specify the following exercises:

educative, use and reproduction and performance; from a somatic point of view we can achieve harmonious development or correction of physical deficits.

2. The effects on the organism from a particular activity can be a. morphophysiological b. regarding behaviour and aptitude

According to the type of sporting activity there are certain structural and functional modifications to the organism. This way, sporting games set off a mechanism of adaption to effort and modify as such the respiratory and cardiovascular (increasing the thoracic cage and as such the respiratory amplitude, increasing the volume of the heart in adaptive ranges and thus cardiac output). Exercises of force lead to a thickening and shortening of the muscles, which thins the body and the limb, elongates the body etc. likewise, physical activity perfects the nervous system (permeability of the sinapses, nervous connections, feedback mechanisms), developing thinking and intelligence. According to the complexity of the exercise, the central nervous system has a higher training. Numerous mental operations preceed the execution of an exercise. Receptors (seeing, hearing etc) are highly demanded, a fact which results in time to their development and acuity. Knowing the morphofunctional medications determined by the practice of exercise and the biological potential of the human being, solidified in his build, we can scientifically correlate these aspects in order to touch the maximum parameters of the organism and keep healthy.

3. The effects on aptitude and behaviour through sport are of mastering self-control, will, courage, tenacity, certainty, social skills and a team spirit.
4. The last aspect of the Pedagogic analysis refers to the measure in which a physical activity corresponds with the age and build of the individual.

The optimum age to begin certain sports varies largely. In this way, for volleyball, it is 8-9 years old, for basketball 11-12 years old, for rugby 18 years old and for swimming 3-4 years old. The age to which you can practice a sport also varies (e.g. Tennis until 80 years old, rugby 35-38 years old etc).

To draw conclusion regarding biomechanical analysis, we re-iterate that the interpretation and integrative correlation of obtained data from each stage (mechanical, muscular, functional and pedagogic) give us the ability to scientifically direct the sporting activity and obtain a maximum efficiency.

CHAPTER VIII.
THE ANTHROPOLOGICAL AND GENETIC DETERMINATION OF MAJOR CHARACTERS IN OBTAINING SPORTING PERFORMANCE.

Results obtained through the genetic determinations of some important character for sporting activities come from research obtained through various methods which I have presented previously. To continue we will make a synthesis of these aspects with special application in the selection and training of an athlete.

- Typological somatofuntional characteristics.

Regarding somatofunctional type and its hereditary determination, a new series of data has been obtained through various genetic methods (twin method, similarity between children and parents, family tree etc). We underline in this context, that the basis of motricity function is aquired somatically, physiologically and from the psyche.

Among principal somatic acquisitions are those which characterise the locomotricity apparatus, more powerfully conditioned genetically than adipose tissue. The correlation coefficient and sensitivity are higher, in this case for bone tissue than muscular but both tissues are more tightly correlated than adipose tissue.

Without doubt somatic acquisitions, as essential acquisitions, cannot be changed with the help of motricity exercises, other than to obtain transformation into a high-performance athlete. In this case it is necessary to select individuals with mass, height and body proportions which correspond to certain sports. A thesis was written stating that obtaining greater results in athletes is impossible when the somatic biological particularities were incompatible. Likewise, it was confirmed that changes to the bones under the influence of training were smaller with a higher hereditary Holzinger coefficient (*Dubinin* and *Kikijuk*, 1976).

As we know, the number of muscular cells increases rapidly in foetal development but is slower after birth, still, research is accurate in that muscular multiplication is possible even after the 5th decade of life (Adams and Ruecic, 1973), the discovery of which possibly explains remarkable results obtained in athletes even in their maturity.

Today it is considered a particularity of muscular structure determined genetically, especially the quantity of fibres and level of development of the system of distribution of nerves in muscle fibres, while the enzyme-metabolic particularities, to an extent, are influenced by training. During research, with the help of muscle biopsies, there was an absence of any difference in the muscle fibre density, the mitochondria and the cytoplasm between twins MZ and DZ in the same size sample from the same area. This is also valid for the proportional volume of mitochondria compared to the muscular fibres and mitochondrial and non-mitochondrial enzyme levels (SDH, MDH) (*Baeriswyl*, 1977).

The research discussed before, similarly to that of Gedda (1967), Komi et al, suggests that the interpersonal variety which appears in metabolic cellular particularities is especially conditioned by non-genetic influences (Klissouros, 1976). Still, on the other hand, research into musculo-skeletal structures, which constitutes the basis of motricity potential, shows that the structure of a person from a motricity point of view is powerfully controlled by genetics (Komi et al, 1976). From numerous studies it has been concluded that the maximum muscular force and percentage of muscular tissue is most evidently under genetic control. To begin with, considered to be short-term, anaerobic energy- during maximum effort for 2 minutes uses 50% anaerobic sources and 50% aerobic, during prolonged effort, covering the energy necessary is, especially, aerobic- from which it can be predicted which sports require individuals with well-defined muscular fibre system. The information above, which refers to the genetic conditioning of muscle fibre development and metabolism shows to what extent a process of selection is needed as how it is possible to stimulate development of the qualities through training. We must remember that while muscular force can be trained to an extent, it is not possible to change the number of muscular fibres, especially in those with a small number of muscles fibres.

An important acquisition for an organism in forming capacity for physical effort is a reduced sensitivity to hypoxia, as well as a capacity for thermoregulation. During large efforts, as a result of the transformation of energy, can result in heat which can raise the temperature of the body, even up to the temperature at which the water within would boil. It's still unknown to what extent thermoregulation is acquired, but one clue in this regard is the fact that there are significant differences between races, genetics and the location of sweat glands.

From research carried out on twins it is clear that other than the "construction" measurements of the body (65%) and the influence of genetic factors, one important genetic check proves neuromotricity function (muscular force, energetic effort, resistance to hypoxia, dynamic nervous processes) and vegetative function. Many authors have shown that at the base of superior physical capacity is the development of the acquired respiratory and circulatory systems of the organism. Also within this complex we mention the level of hereditary determination in the active body mass, which presents, according to various authors, a heritably coefficient between 0.70 and 0.85. To estimate it, determinations must be done on the parents before the age of 30-35.

In a wide range of indices studied in twins, the greatest genetic dependency manifests in the morphological components of the athlete. If express as a ration, in percentage, the number of indices which have reflected an hereditary influence compared to the number of indices from research, then you can see that for cardiorespiratory indices the value is equal to 34%, for neuromotricity – 58% while for morphological -65%.

With hereditary dependent: primarily, the length of the body and the extremities, body weight, diameter of the superior and inferior extremities, width of the pelvis and thighs, waist circumference, chest circumference, buttocks and shoulders and the various deposits of fat on different parts of the body.

The most important thing for selection and orientation of children in sport- in this compartment of research- we calculate to be data obtained from twins with regards to the structure of the body. It is (with the distinction of active body mass ABM), as established in the last years a new parameter of functional possibility of the human body. ABM correlated with CMO, with muscular force, resistance and other physical qualities. Distinction in body structure between individuals, nourishment, and, as research has demonstrated, genetics.

There have been a few methods of functional study used with twins, for which diameters and circumferences of the body and extremities were used as well as fat deposits. All methods of obtaining the components (with and without fat deposits), of the body have shown, statistically, certain distinctions between monozygous and dizygous twins. On the basis of results obtained, it was established that the structure of children's bodies from 6-16 is determined hereditarily.

The structure of the body is one of the criteria of selection necessary to establish the sport best suited for the individual. Already you can find much evidence that in the period of growth, some components of the body of children changes very little under the influence of physical activity.

A high grade of hereditary determination lies in the height of a child and the proportion of the body segments. The height of the body is one of the most representative anthropological characteristics and literature referring to its genetic determination is rich. Many studies were dedicated to estimating the coefficient of correlation between the height of the parent's bodies and their dependents, between descendants of different ages and from various socio-economic backgrounds (*Bailey,* 1954). From these studies its shown that these correlation coefficients between descendants and their parents are completely different depending on age and sex of the child as well as the socio-economic status of the population. Mueller gathered data (1976) from 24 studies conducted by different researchers in different parts of the world and discovered that these coefficients of correlation are in general greater in the European and American population than in others. The author mentioned that his conclusions were the incorrect matching of parents and the inadequate nourishment of children outside of Europe; Palmer (1934) showed that this correlation in the framework of families depends on the age, while Tanner (1962) suggested that intensity and duration of puberty was under independent genetic control.

Heritability of the height registers a pronounced growth according to the age of the child, indifferent of the method of interpretation. Coefficients of heritability reach their highest values in the adult group. That's why the role of environmental factors in determining the height decreases with age. Heritability coefficients, calculated for and older group, can be considered as the measure of heritability for height. Despite this, values differ significantly in accordance with the method of appreciation. Value of h2 calculated by the Penrose method and values obtained from the study of twins seem to be exaggerated due to the effect of assimilation of the surrounding environment and due to the existence of alelomophic dominance, factors which raise the correlation coefficient among descendants. H2 values calculated from the regression coefficient, in turn, do not consider the correct coupling of parents, raising the heritability by 0.04. As a result, the most objective value, charged with the least error, seems to be that calculated by Fishers method. This value raises by 0.66 in the largest age group and can be recognised as an additive value in the framework of the variability of height. The value is identical to Hb, calculated by Susanne (1976) on the basis of studies carried out on Belgian families.

Therefor there are several conclusions:

1. Correlation coefficient between the height of parents and their children, increase with age, reaching the highest values in the oldest age groups. Values in the younger groups are reduced and form on a similar level with the analogue values of the populations which don't belong to Europe.
2. Heritability indices of height increase with age, registering large differences depending on the estimation method used. The most probable appears to be the value Hb calculated from Fishers formula (1918) reaching 0.66
3. Height is polygenetically determined in the presence of a high number of dominant alelomorphs. Forming a phenotype of children's height in puberty is, likewise, influences by alelomophs which determine the duration and intensity of development. These Alelomorphs are tightly linked to the X chromosome and can influence the formation of anthropometric characteristics.

L. Sergienko affirms that the results of the numerous researches on the ratio of children and parents body height are almost the same. Coefficient of correlation which illustrates the analogies evident in the father son pairs are higher (0.450-0.461) Than father daughter pairs (0.200-0.382) while in mother son (0.310-0.480) they are smaller than in mother daughter (0.485-0.620).

The result is that height of the son can be estimated on the basis of height of the father, while the daughters can be estimated from the mothers. Still it should be taken into account that, at present, the new generation are overtaking their parent's physical development. Results obtained in research from over 100 sprinters, had a mathematical mean for time taken to run 100m of 11.03/s (interval between the best and the weakest being between 10.2 – 11.9) showed that the athletes running were taller (175.51) than their parents (172.40). The difference between the mean height of sprinters from the first half of the group (mean running time distance of 100m – 1072") and their fathers (177.9) raised to 3.7m and was higher than the mean height of the other 50 sprinters (175.4cm) and their fathers (172.9). the biggest differences between the height of the athletes and their fathers being in the first 20 sprinters.

In the first 10 sprinters (10.30s) the difference was higher compared to their fathers, a mean of 5.4cm while the next 10 with 4.2cm. the difference between the age of the sprinters and their fathers was maintained up to 30years.

Table 42

Correlation between the level of development of principal morphological features in different ages.

Age	Coefficient of correlation of values at 17 years old.		
	Height	Weight	Thoracic cage capacity
8	0.773	0.691	0.624
9	0.744	0.646	0.461
10	0.687	0.697	0.549
11	0.654	0.697	0.547
12	0.636	0.708	0.520
13	0.762	0.799	0.616
14	0.908	0.843	0.708
15	0.964	0.902	0.768

The results from here are that every 10 years the ascendance between children and their parents is 1 cm. Following the physical development in the last 10 years which has reached the greatest height of the body, we must remark that talented youth from a point of view of sports is well developed and surpasses their parents.

From here we conclude that while predicting height on the basis of information from the parents, we should take into account the rapid development of the youth who is active in sport.

There is a possibility to estimate the height of a sportsman on the basis of his parent's height and some formulas which have been presented above. Knowing the height allows for the other segments of the body to be estimates as shown in the chapter on anthropological morphology. Likewise, also for the establishment of somatic type, there have been studies which established a coefficient in the heritability of the skulls dimensions. It is a scientific fact that there are different types of skulls. This is important for sports, this way, a hit with the head, such as in football may be efficient in subjects with brahicrania.

Anthropological studies (*Szopa Jan*) carried out on the types of skill have proven the following: The greatest indicator of heritability, h2, was obtained through combined measurement of length and width of the head (h2~- 1.03), which upholds the theory referring to a greater genetic determination of the whole head rather than some of the measurements. This is in concordance with studies from other authors carried out on twins.

Indices of hereditability of the length and width of the head were, similar and large (0.85 and respectively 0.86), which indicates a role of genetic variety in the framework of characteristics.

The size of the h2 indicator modifies according to age of the child, reaching higher values in the children from the 11-14 age group or 15-18. This seems to be the accumulated effect of the actions of alelomorphs on age which determines certain measurements of the head and other, their level of growth.

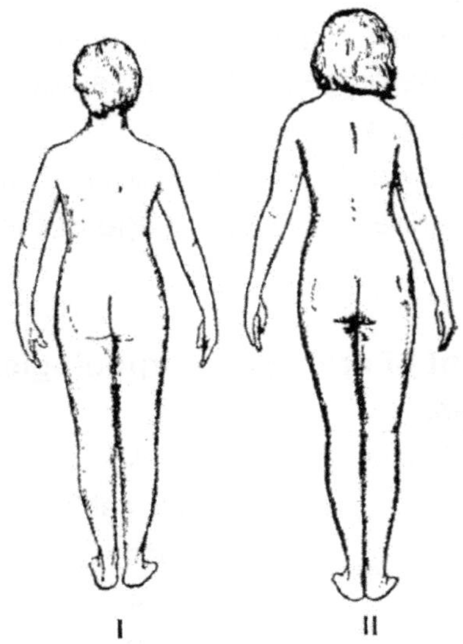

1. Type F (4) Supple, long, robust, round
2. Narrow shoulders, low
3. Well contoured waist long Short
4. wide hips
5. Buttocks with concavities, full and round
6. cone shaped femurs
7. Missing i.m.i. interval

Fig. 109. Female types F (4) (variant I and II).

Likewise, the determination of somato sexual type is also genetically conditioned and is essential in the selection of athletes. Genetically conditioned morphological parameters which define somatosexual type are essential to determine. This fact is necessary for different sports, as to obtain performance in certain sports a rate of masculinity or femininity is required. Thus, for example, in girls gymnastics, a hyperestrogenic subject with a high bicrestal-bitrochantarian diameter, large mammary glands etc will not obtain good performance. Or, in the framework of athleticism, performance on a superior level, female subjects with a more masculine body shape will succeed, as such a level of social determinism is also under genetic control.

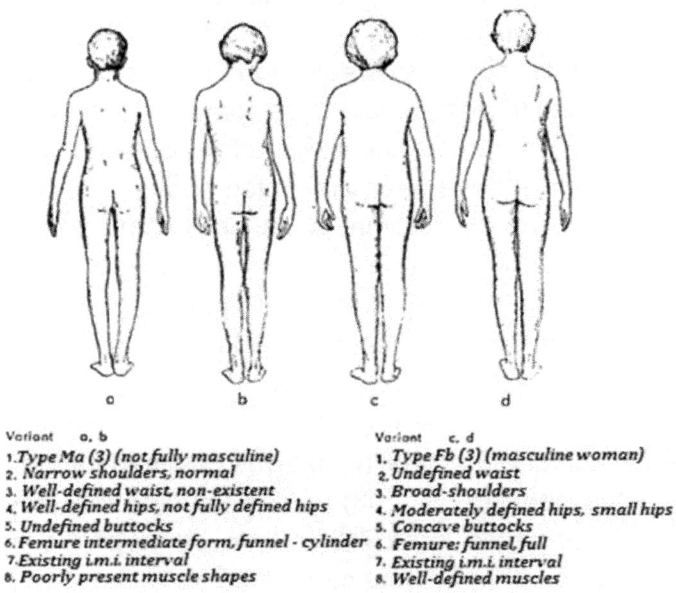

Fig. 110. a) Asexual masculine type M_a (3); b) Asexual feminine type F_a (3); c, d) Bisexual female type F_b (3).

From our research we have found that a grade of mother-daughter heritability of somatosexual type is between 0.85-0.90. We have established a simple method for determining the bicrestal angle (Elena Firea-Ifrim), which, when we make selections for girls' gymnastics, for example, it should not exceed, in the mother, a value of 60-65°. It is a method which permits a scientific selection, avoiding the surprise apparition of a hyperestrogen type at puberty, consequently, investing a moral and material capital in a subject who will not be capable of obtaining performance. Likewise, we recommend the Bayer-Bailey method of establishing somatosexual type. The applied method being before puberty permitting a prediction of this typology in the adult.

Bayer and *Baily* studied various aspects of the constitution lined to the differentiation and sexual maturity. They elaborated a procedure which permits the study of the androgynous variability and the typology of the individual on the base of a scale of androgenity. They had in mind, firstly, the proportion of the skeleton, while in the framework of differentiation they followed the rhythm of sexualisation, the sum total of the body's disharmonies.

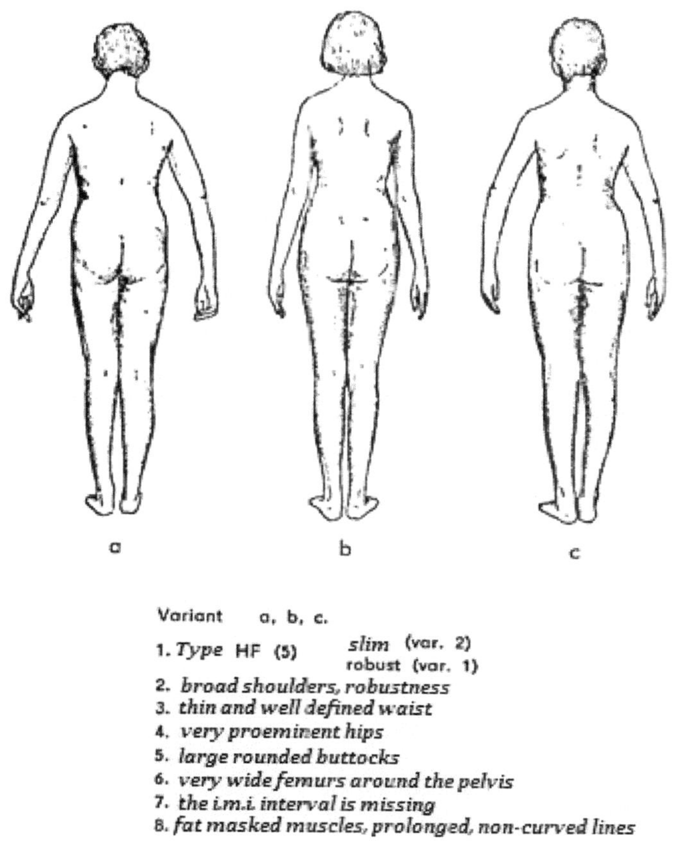

Fig. 111. Hyperfeminine type HF (4).

Starting from the concept of "mosaic androgyny" (*Dropert*,1941) which as at its basis the idea that every individual has both male and female characteristics regardless of the proportions, we have sought and outlined more concrete concepts of the constitution of sexuality, alongside those of somatic constitution (somatometric).

Eight items were studied, according to bayer-bailey method, in appreciation of which were considered the following elements: width, musculature, adipose layer. These eight items (among which we count the waist shape as seen from behind, form of the femurs, development of the muscular mass etc), evaluation according to the androgyny scale of the authors. The five types indicated by the authors which outlines a unique scale, continues for human androgenity having in its low values (1-2), a high grade of masculinity, defining, within the masculine sex, various grades of harmony between sex and sexualisation; while in the high numbers (4-5), a high, even exaggerated grade of femininity, presenting the same variability of grades of sexualisation. An intermediary number of 3 are attributed to cases of disharmony, where in the framework of sexes, evidences as a low grade of corresponding sexualisation of their own sex and more often than not with elements of sexualisation of the opposite sex. The advantage of this model is that having types with grades of sexualisation evidences elements of endocrine sexuality (allowing an abstraction of genetic sex), and offers numerous possibilities of correlation with aspects of psychological, behavioural and even psychological sex.

The authors have named these types in ascending order on the scale, hypermasculine, masculine, hypomasculine (undifferentiated), mixed (bisexed), hypofeminine (undifferentiated), feminine, hyperfeminine (see fig. 109-113).

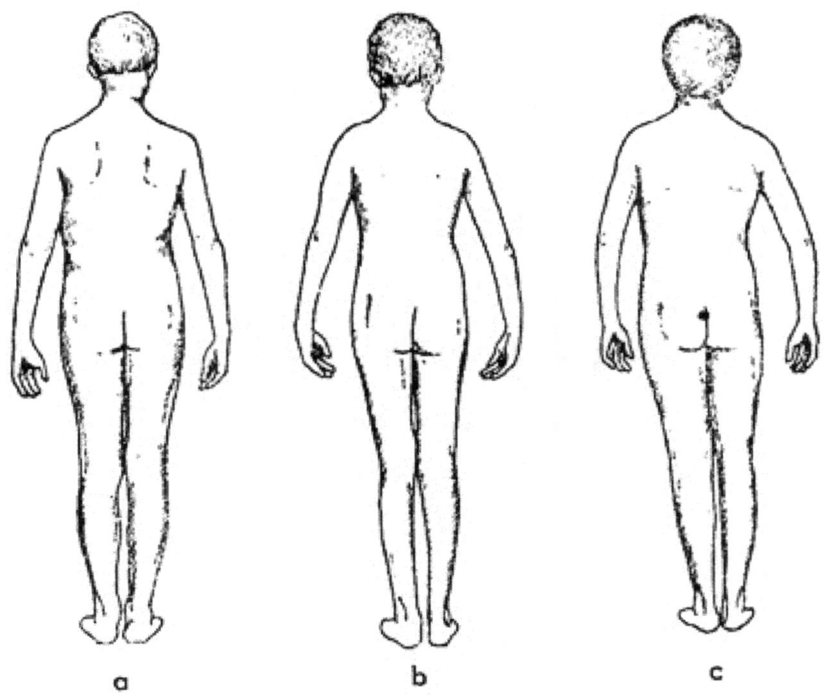

Variant a, b, c.
1. *Type* M_b (3) (*feminized - male and female characteristics*)
2. *broad shoulders*
3. *shaped waiste*
4. *feminine, wide hips*
5. *round buttocks*
6. *feminine femure*
7. Interval i.m.i. absent
8. *absent fat-covered muscle forms*

Fig. 112. Bisexed masculine type M_b(3).

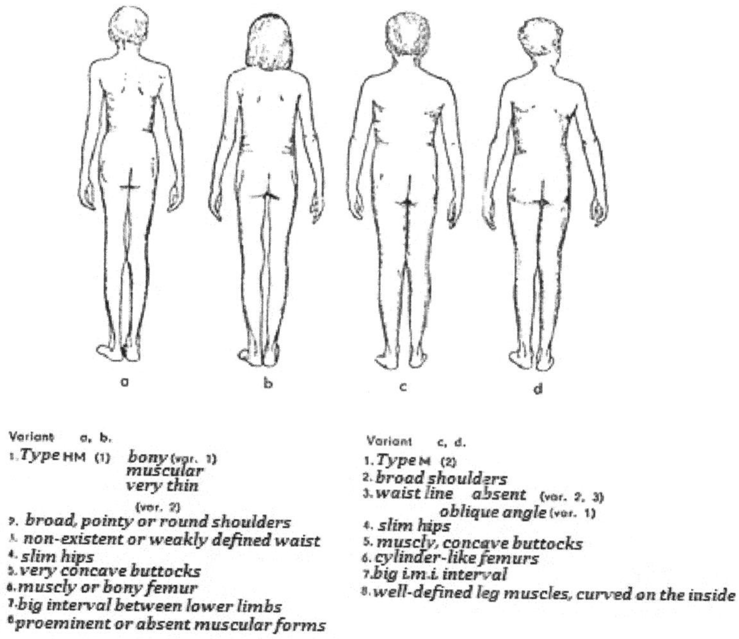

Fig. 113. a, b) hypermasculine type HM (1); c, d) masculine type M (2).

We give in table 43 the results of the evaluations indicated by the authors for ten types used as standards.

Representative types for different grades of androgenity
12–13 years old

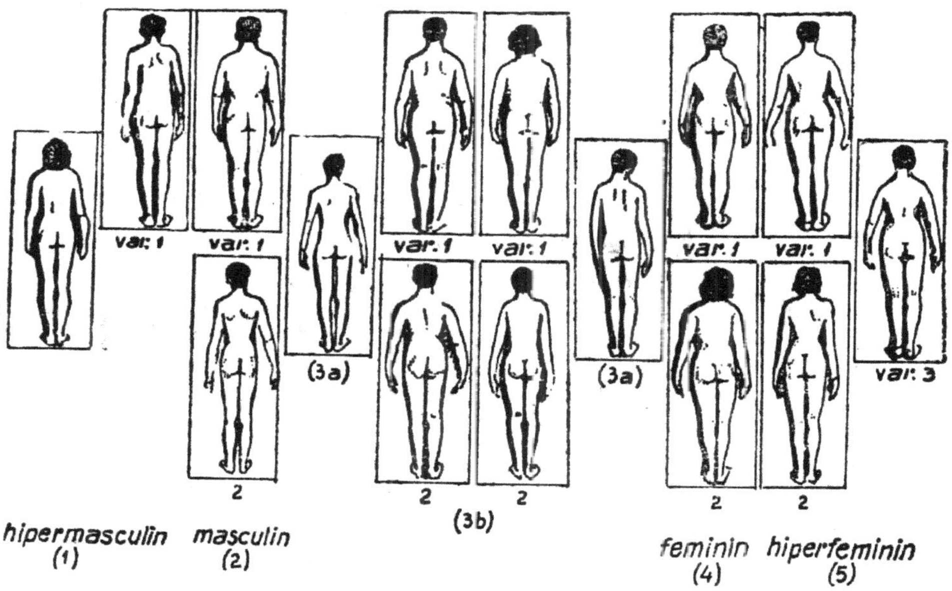

Fig. 114. Constitutional types of androgenity (according to Cornelia Guja).

a) boys at 11 years old, girls at 7 years old b) both sexes at the age of 18

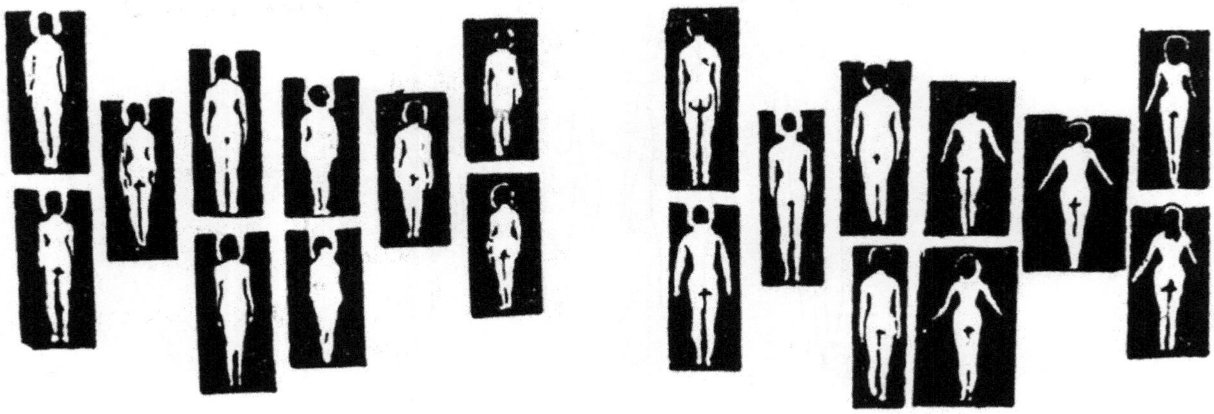

Fig. 115. Bayer-Bailey androgynous types.

Referring to the physiological parameters of the somatic type, which for teaching reasons we have addressed together with the morphological types, we comment below.

Table 43

	MH	MH'	M	MB	MA	FB	FA	F	FH	FH'
Habitus corporal back	1	1	2	3b	2, 5	4	4	4	5	5
Shoulder circumference	1.5	1	2	3b	3a	3b	3a	4	5	4.5
Line of the waist	2	1	2	3b	3a	3b	3	4	5	5-
Size of the hips	2	1	2	2	2-	3	3, 5	4	5-	5+
Shape of the buttocks	1	2	2	4	3	3	3	4		5-
Form of the femurs	1	2	2	3	2	3	3	4	4	5
Interval between members (m.i.) Unit m.	1	1.5	2	4	3	3	4	4	5	5
Bulging muscles (lower part i.m.i);	1	1	2	4	3a	3b	3a	4	5	4.5

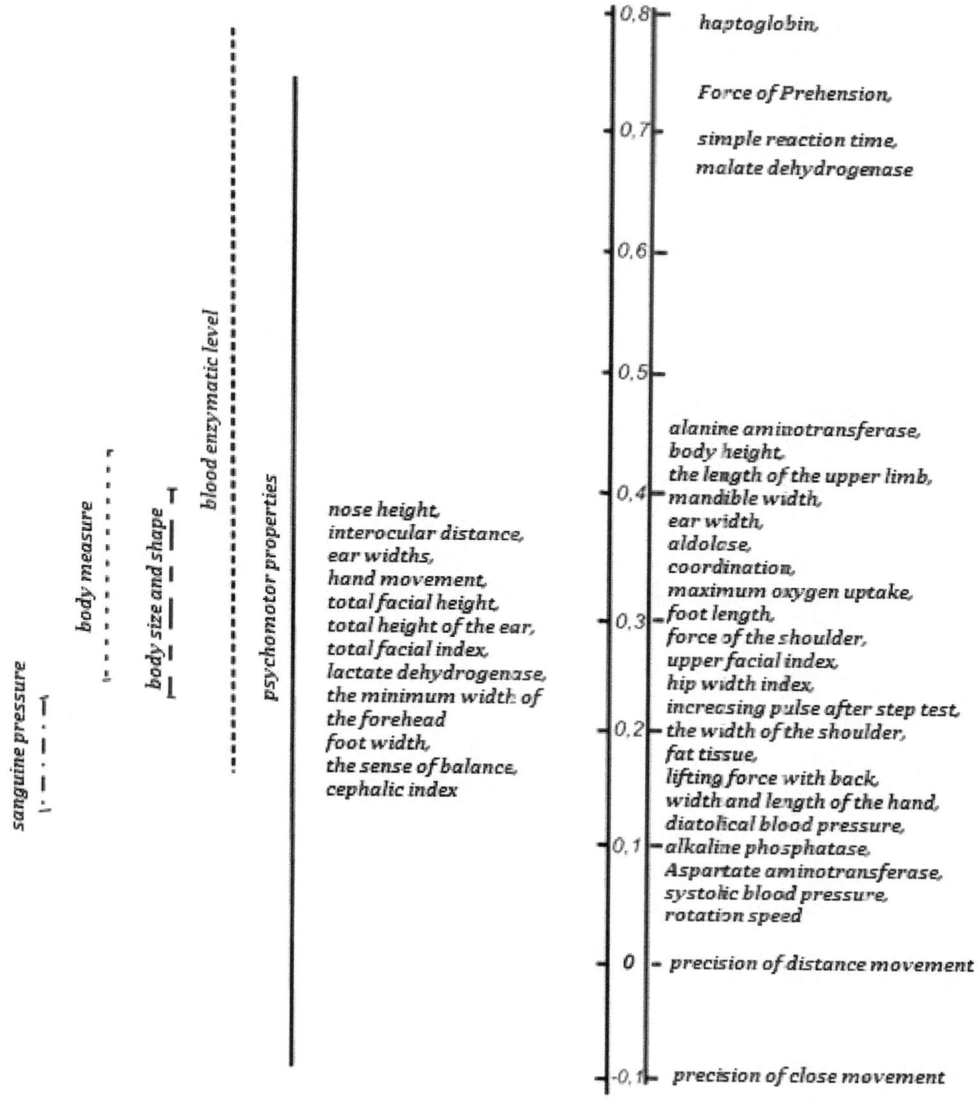

Fig. 116. Mean coefficient of correlation between parents and children for some characteristics (according to Wolanski).

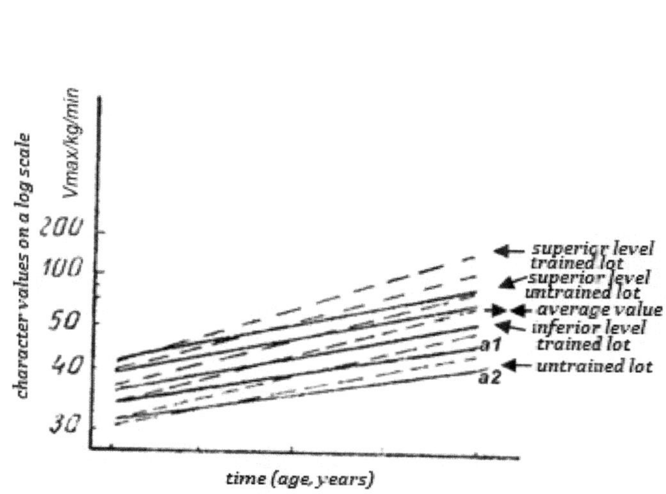

Fig. 117. Trained and untrained groups don't change their positions

It is difficult to make a net differentiation between studies which have as their objective motricity properties, on the one hand and studies of physiological-functional factors on the other hand. The majority of authors follow both somatofunctional and different final motricity acts, investigating diverse characters in their complexity at the level of organs or in their zones of histochemical structure (fig. 114-121).

The first study of this kind to date with regards to complexity and size, is without doubt that carried out by the authors Osato and Awono (1957). Their work encompasses detailed results of the different morphological and functional characteristics, the study group being comprised of approximately 100 pairs of twins. With regards to somatic characteristics, measurements taken referred to almost all principal body dimensions, such as length, width and circumference, radiological evaluation of the heart, dimensions of the lungs and stomach, studies of the skin folds, number and dimensions of erythrocytes, determination of haemoglobin levels etc. Functional research encompassed, among other things, motricity efficiency tests. As such, measurement of heart rate before effort, during effort and in recovery was also carried out; the same studies were performed on blood pressure and some respiratory tests. What is also interesting is the ECG and EEG, as well as the study of the reaction of the organism to various allergens. Some research also includes physiological studies and evaluation of fundamental characteristics of the personalities of twins. In many cases the authors also took into account sex, age and various types of environment of the subjects studied.

Results demonstrated that in almost all structural and functional properties investigated, hereditary factors have a significant role. Their contribution modifies according to diverse characteristics, an extremely important factor being the surrounding environment.

More recent research refers to a relatively limited number of functional factors related to the evaluation of the circulatory and respiratory apparatus or of some neuromuscular functions and their respective properties at a cellular level (electrical and enzymatic activity of the muscle tissue etc). In the majority of cases, these are factors related directly to a predisposition of an increased activity and motricity efficiency. Fundamental things in this direction are the two studies of Klissouras from 1971 and 1972, in which he addressed genetic conditioning of functional adaptability of the organism.

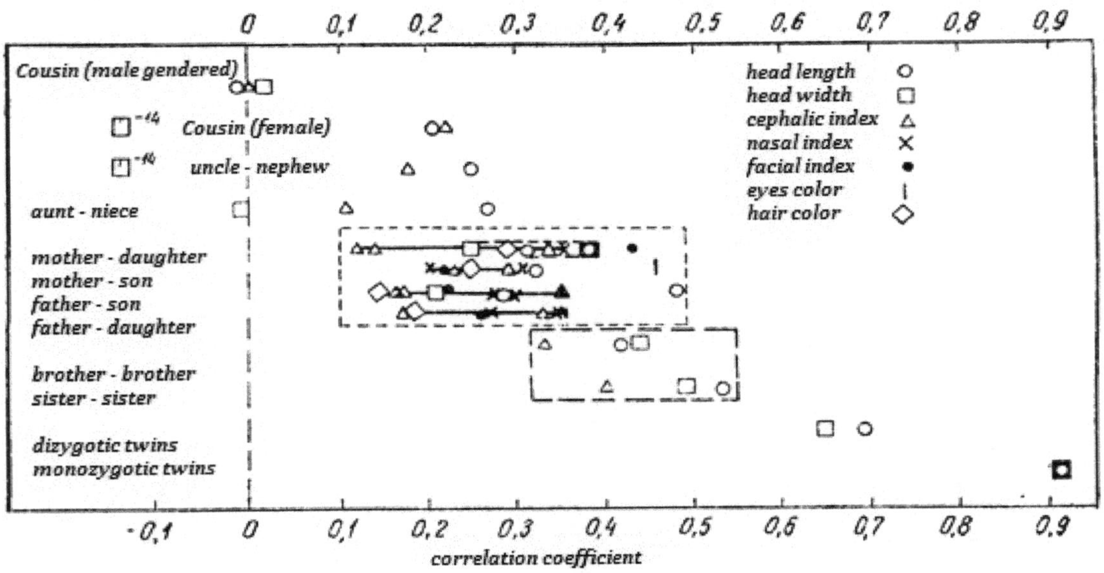

Fig. 118. Correlation between relatives regarding somatic characters (according to Wolanski).

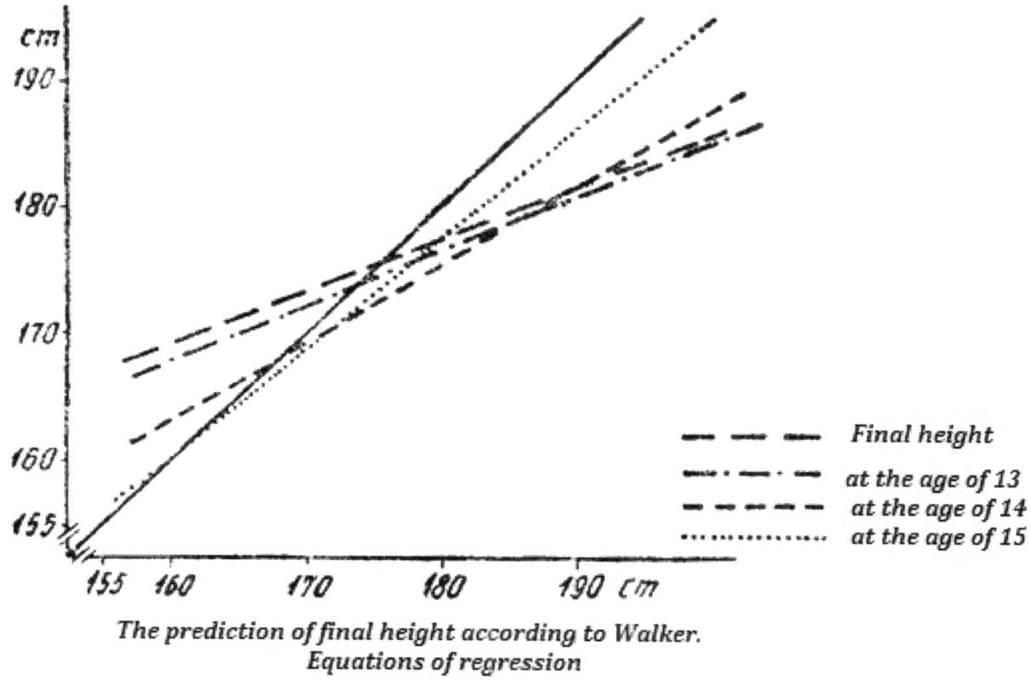

Fig. 119 The prediction of final height according to Walker. Equations of regression.

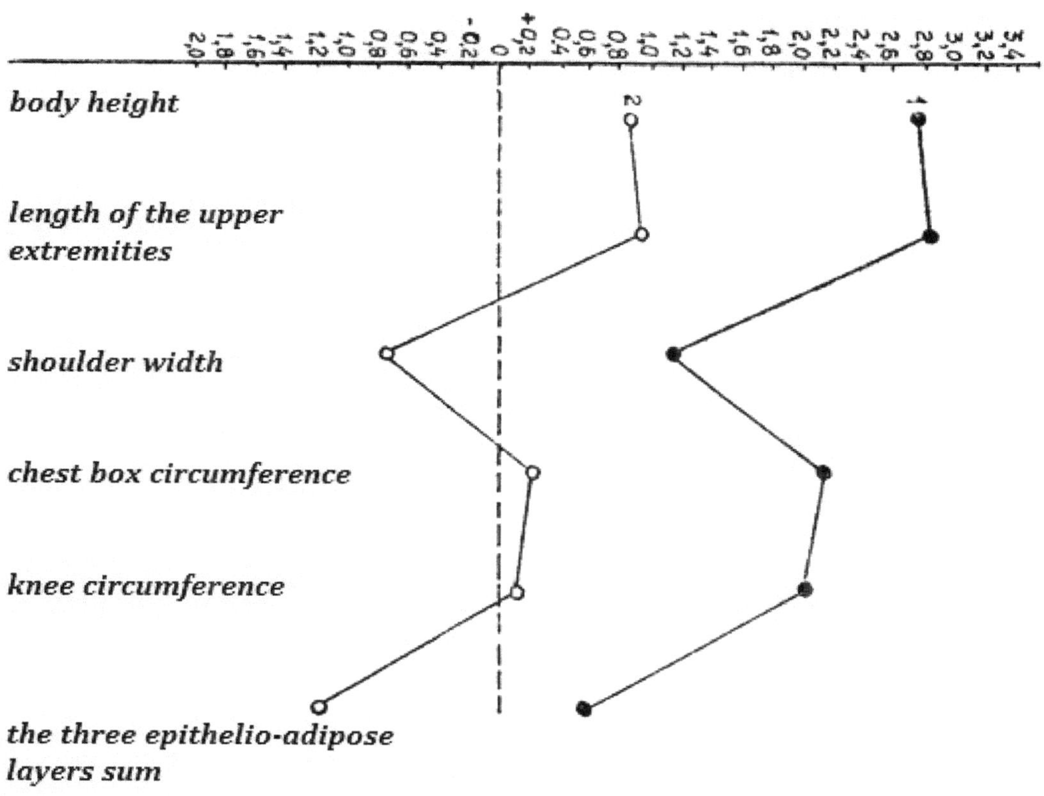

Fig. 120. Hereditary indices and determining existing values in a javelin thrower

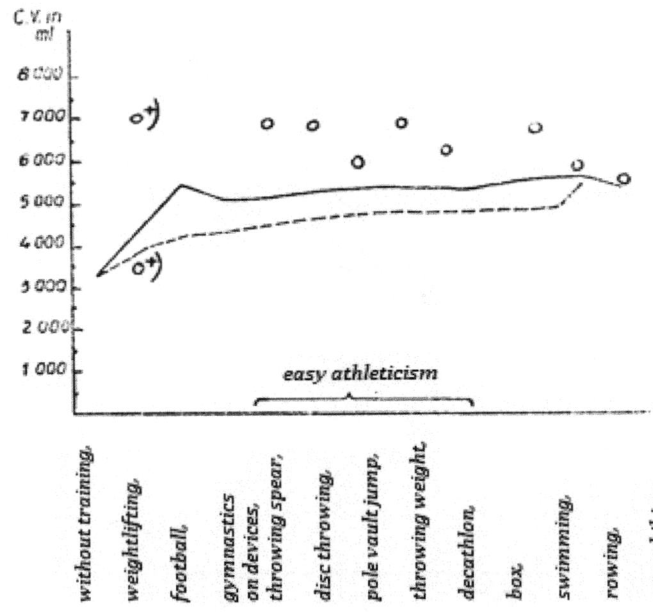

Fig. 121. Vital capacity of an athlete performance in various sports.

The first work of Klissouras (1971) encompassed 15 pairs of monozygous male twins and 10 pairs of dizygous male twins between the ages of 7-13. After a standard repetitive effort, they were evaluated under a ratio of parameters of circulation and respiration. Heritable coefficients established are the following: at a maximum heart rate -0.86, a maximum concentration of lactate in blood -0.81 and maximum oxygen consumption (radioed to 1 kilo body weight)- 0.93. These values are raised, permitting the establishment of the fact that genotypic predisposition of the individual, living in identical conditions have an important role on the individuality of the aerobic capacity of the organism.

In his second work (1972) Klissouras tried to study the situation in which the organism undergoes an intense effort in the conditions of training for sport and in particular is the functional level modifies significantly or if the modifications are limited to hereditary predisposition and initial stage. For the research, he used a pair of male monozygous twins, which, until the age of 15 were active in sport, practicing most together. After this period, their whole life was modified, one of them continued to practice sport while the other became inactive. Both were tested again at the age of 21, for a period of 17 months, and their circulatory and respiratory response was evaluated in standard resistance training. The results regarding the modification in the maximum consumption of oxygen were very interesting: in the untrained individual – 35.9 ml/minXkg- in the trained individual – 49ml/minXkg. The procentual difference is 37% - with regards to other factors, they registered oxygen-pulse 48.8%, an oxygen debt of 61% and a value of blood lactates of 67%. As you can see, in all cases, a great amelioration was created, but further detailed analysis of the absolute values showed that no intense training increases values much more than the general population. On basis of this, the author maintains that a given effort can considerably influence the functional adaptability of the organism, but that there are limits which cannot be overcome due to genetic determination. Due to this he considers that the old problem of measures in which an individual becomes an athlete, that the results of training should be viewed through the prism of contemporary genetic data which demonstrates that an individual with very reduced aptitude will not obtain, in the majority of cases, special results.

Environmental factors are essential fort the entire evolution and development of the human being, but they are not felt in the course of successive genetics, in as much that, for sport- which claims immediate obtainment of performance- the essential problem is the existence of a corresponding genetic basis and carrying out efficient training, according to genetic particularities which lead to obtaining maximum genetically determined potential (limited or reaction to genetic adaptability). Research of the maximum oxygen consumption in pairs of twins through the method “witness co-twin” with a different level of motricity activities and with different environmental conditions in the framework of the pairs was carried out along with other specialists.

Similar methods to Klissouras was used by *Sergienko* (1975). On a pair of female twins aged 16 he studied the influence of training on the development of muscular force and the maximum consumption of oxygen. As mentioned above, the aerobic capacity increases within the limits of the individual, compared to the increase of muscular force, it was considerably more reduced and unfolded in the course of a prolonged period.

A similar study is that of *Leight* (1977) In the framework of comparison of twins ages 16 from Scotland (monozygous twins, both junior Scottish running champions at 400 and 800 m), he established an astonishing similarity. Even though each was most efficient in a specific discipline and they carried out intense athletic training, the level of development of the maximum oxygen consumption and some respiratory tests was almost identical.

Mueller carried out an interesting experiment on two pairs of monozygous twins aged 20 and 23. He researched the influence of high resistance training for 4 weeks in various environmental conditions. One subject from each pair trained at an altitude of 2500, while the other at 20m. The individuals who were trained at high altitude demonstrated a high level of adaptability to demand. The maximum absorption of oxygen increased to 12% while the individual who trained at 20,m had an increase of only 2% and %. The research showed that in the framework of individual predisposition. Environmental factors still represent and important factor.

Howald (1976) studied the structural and functional properties of muscular tissue, among other factors they investigated some parameters of blood circulation and respiration. In the first research which the author carried out the studied 11 pairs of monozygous twins and six pairs of dizygous twins aged between 15-25, there were no statistical significances in the individual variations of the two types of twins (not even the ratio of maximum oxygen consumed nor in the oxygen-pulse). The second part of the research was the evaluation of seven pairs of monozygous twins through the “witness co-twin” method (one of the twins was subjected to 23 weeks of intense training while the other witnessed it). Observed modifications in the maximum oxygen consumed, oxygen-pulse etc, determined Howald to plead in favour of the influence of environmental conditions and athletic training.

There is a series of research which presents data regarding the coefficient of heritability of heart rate, pulse, ventilation, pulmonary maximums, maximum quantities of carbon dioxide expired. Important factors which determine variations are: age, sex, environment in which the twins live. Another cause can perhaps be represented by reduced relative accuracy of measurements related to certain aspects of the methodology around their obtainment. Referring to certain respiratory functions the results show, compared to circulatory functions, a lower grade of genetic conditioning (*Szwarz, Sergienko*).

Heywood and *Laurence* (1977) studied 52 pairs of monozygous twins and 68 pairs of dizygous twins of both sexes, their investigation being centred particularly on respiratory function of the organism (vital pulmonary capacity etc). They underlined the fact that these factors depend on the body dimensions, which we know are powerfully, genetically controlled. They expected the links between hereditary predispositions to be seen in ventilation function. This hypothesis was not verified and the conclusion of the research showed that hereditary factors did not exercise an important influence. A similar dissertation, having this time the objective to revaluate the organism's reaction to inspired carbon dioxide (together with a higher content of oxygen), is the study of *Akinstall* et al (1974). In a lot of 17 pairs of monozygous twins and 13 pairs of dizygous twins, they found no significant differences regarding the differences in pairs between the monozygous and dizygous twins. A remarkable hereditary factor was found in the expansion of the thoracic wall while the respiratory rate was influenced by environment.

Among these studies we can mention the research of *Engstrom* and *Fischben* (1977). Alongside the force of various muscle groups and the capacity of labour investigated via cicloergometer, they studied vital pulmonary capacity. The lot of twins was 39 pairs of monozygous twins and 55 pairs of dizygous twins, together with a witness lot of 508 boys aged between 18-19. Their comparison of the lot of twins during systematic training which the twins did in their free time was interesting. Conclusions showed that the differences in the maximums observed in the course of the study were in the capacity for labour and the muscular force, while the pulmonary vital capacity was not significantly modified. From this point of view there appears to be a marked hereditary value on the level of vital capacity.

An important factor which contributes to the influence of hereditary and environment on the circulating blood and respiratory factors is represented by the size and intensity of the effort in the course of which the subjects were tested. This fact is underlined by numerous specialists, particularly *Szwarz* (1972). This supported the fact that in the course of a low intensity effort, the hereditary factors are not really significant but in increases along with the intensity of the effort. At rest values of the heart rate, hereditary coefficients are reduced in all cases but at their maximum values, they increased considerably.

The author mentioned about also studied genetic conditioning on the regulation of circulation and breathing. In a lot of twins he studied the reaction of the circulatory and respiratory apparatus at a standard effort, registering modifications in the factors investigated in the course of the whole experience. He found a higher grade of genetic conditioning can be observed in the first stage after beginning effort and in a smaller measure after the termination of effort.

A factor which in general exercises an influence, if represented by age and step in ontogenesis, an influence which is seen in the majority of characters investigated. This aspect became an object of study for the authors *Klissouros, Pirnay* and *Petit* (1973). In the scope of their study they used twin candidate from Canada and Belgium of various ages between 9 and 52. Though their lot was not very numerous, encompassing only 39 pairs of mono and dizygous twins, the authors tried to establish to what extent age influenced the airs regarding factors studied (max. oxygen consumption, max. pulmonary ventilation, max. cardiac debit). With regards to the maximum consumption of oxygen, a significant difference was observed regardless of age, which means that the predisposing genotype influences individual variability throughout the entire course of life. Differenced regarding maximum pulmonary ventilation and maximum cardiac output were not significant, avoiding an visible influence of environmental factors.

Tightly linked to this study was another from the University of Montreal carried out by *Weber, Kartodihardjo* and *Kilssouros* (1976). The intention of the authors is very interesting and extremely interesting from the gnoseological point of view. They followed three lots of monozygous twin pairs aged 10,13 and 16 (each lot formed from four pairs of twins of that age).

Then one twin from each pair was subjected to conditioning for a period of 10 weeks. The objective of the research was establishing age at which the maximum increase to which the organism is receptive to environmental stimuli, as well as determining the measure in which age influence genotypic predisposition of an individual. Factors studied were: maximum oxygen consumption, heart rate, lactate concentration in blood and maximum pulmonary ventilation. They obtained the results from below. The trained subjects aged 10 presented an amelioration compared to the untrained in the maximum absorption of oxygen; subjects ages 16 presented amelioration in all factors compared to the untrained. The subjects aged 13, in puberty and undergoing important ontogenetic modifications, produced a corresponding increase in the factors mentioned, both in the trained and in the untrained. Comparison between these age categories showed that both the subject from the 10-year-old lot and those from the 16 year old lot had a higher amelioration in the maximum absorbed oxygen than those aged 13. On the basis of the results, the authors deduced that ontogenetic stage is an important factor in the development of important structural properties from a functional point of view of the organism.

What is still interesting is the second part of the study: they asked if the effect of the training was the same in the subjects with the same genotypic predispositions, in other words if there was an interaction between the genotypic predisposition and the influence of the environments? With this goal they used the data regarding the 4 pairs of twins who were 10 years old and the 4 pairs of twins who were 16 from previous studies. Through varied analysis, they calculated the total proportion of variability of the total consumption of oxygen linked to the component of the effect of training, the component of the environmental influence and the interaction of genotype-training. Data observed found the following: training 42%, heredity 51%, interaction 7%. It is clear that in extreme environmental conditions and intense training, the influence of genotypic predisposition in the variability of the maximum level of oxygen consumed is increased. On the other hand, the interaction of genotype-environment is not factor which significantly influents variability. So, we can suppose that in the conditions of different genotypes, modifications which result from the influence of environment and training are approximately the same.

As well as this, more research referring to the physiological-functional factors considered the elemental muscular function and the properties of the muscular tissue on a cellular level. The authors are *Komi et al and Howald*. The first investigation (*Karvinen*, 1973) was carried out on 15 sets of monzygous twins and 14 pairs of dizygous twins, boys and girls aged 10-14. The properties investigates the anaerobic maximum capacity determined by *Margario*, maximum force of flexion of the elbow and extension of the knee, integrated muscular electrical activity (biceps brahii) and the times of reflex and reaction. High coefficients of heritability were found for rotulian reflex -0.98, reaction time – 0.86 and maximum anaerobic capacity (evaluated by mechanical debit)-0.99. Authors also did a comparison of heritability ratio in the sexes. A genetic higher conditioning was found in the boys, which was explained through the fact that muscular function and manifestations of muscular force are tightly linked to the influence of sexual hormones and the particularities of the physical structure.

Another study (*Komi* et al, 1977) studied the results of muscular biopsies taken from a lot of 31 pairs of mono and dizygous twins of both sexes, aged between 15 and 24. They looked at, in particular, the percentage of types of muscle fibres and evaluated enzymatic muscle activity (vastus lateralis m.). Regarding muscular composition they discovered (% of fibres with slow contraction) that the hereditary coefficient was high, as much in boys as in girls: -0.99 in girls, -0.93 in boys, -0.97 indifferent of sex. No major hereditary influence was found in the level of muscular enzymatic activity. The work of *Komi* et al (1978) consecrated the research of the influence of isometric strength training on the different characteristics of muscular function and muscular tissue and was mentioned before. They applied the "witness co-twin" method; the influence of training was significant on all the investigated properties (muscular force, electromyographic activity and muscular enzymatic activity). Another research (*Karlsson, Komi, Viitasalo,* 1979) verified the fact that the results of the investigations on some phenomena at this level of differentiation differ, often considerably one from the other. The research is based on the reinvestigation of a lot of the twins who were used in prior a prior study (1977). Evaluated characteristics were the maximum anaerobic capacity after *Margario*, maximum extension of the knee, the time curve for isometric muscular contraction, integrated electrical muscular activity, cronaxia, percentage of fibres with slow contraction, levels of enzymatic activity (vastus lateralis m.). This research showed a significant influence of different genotypes regarding maximum anaerobic capacity, in which the heritability coefficient was increased to 0.98. There were no significant differences in the pairs of the types of twins regarding other investigated properties.

Montoye and *Gayle* followed parents and their descendants under the ratio of maximum oxygen consumption. The strongest relationship was found between sons and their fathers when they were under an age of 40 years old (r=0.066). The same factor constituted the objective of the research of *Wolanski* and *Kasparzak* (1976). Just as in other tests, in this test, the correlation is conditioned by the stage of ontogenesis, oscillating the correlation coefficient, as in from zero to almost one. There is a difference in the evidence regarding sex; it seems that until 18 years of age there is a large degree of similarity in the relationship between boy-parents, however after this period there the correlation daughter-parents increases, while in boys it is significantly reduced. Results overall appear equal when investigated afterwards, respectively regarding heart rate after a standard effort (step test). In this case, in the course of ontogenesis there is a higher degree of similarity in the son-parents relationship but correlation coefficient does not exceed 0.50. Regarding the daughters, a degree of similarity is observed but only around 15 years old.

The work of *Tanaka* et al (1976) dealt with some of the factors of circulation and systolic blood pressure. The correlation in a series of cases is statistically significant. On the other hand the heritability coefficient derived from the regression coefficient is fairly high (varies between 0.5 and 0.75), permitting the assumption of a high degree of heritability.

Among the functional properties at an organ level those which interest us are those linked to direct manifestations of motricity efficiency. In this regard, it seems that research on the basis on longitudinal stability is not paid enough attention. The evaluation of longitudinal stability together with the analysis of the correlation of data was carried out for the first time by *McCammon* and *Sexton* (1958, 1963). They established a high degree of stability of heart rate in standard effort conditions; their investigation encompasses high age limits from one year to adult.

Ulbrich (1967, 1971) studied these problems regarding the possibilities of students talented in sport. His work is interesting from a methodological point of view, presenting simultaneously factual results worthy of attention; working on a group of boys aged 11-18, the author arrived at the conclusion that circulatory and respiratory factors are very stable in the course of adolescence and that their development contributes in a special hereditary predisposition. Correlation coefficient found between the values of heart rate in different stages of development shows the stability mentioned above which is not disturbed even during puberty. On the basis of research into heart rate in standard effort conditions, the author elaborated a nomogram of development which can help in the prediction of development and the selection of subjects with a higher level of cardiopulmonary efficiency. The tendency in the development of 2 boys with different levels of heart rate is presented in the normogram mentioned above. They are similar to the tendencies of development in the case of running 1000m.

The research carried out by *Sprynarova* (1977) comes from the same research subject and the same place. In a lot of boys ages 11-18, subjected to different motricity regimes, this author studied a series of factors, among which were the maximum aerobic capacity (maximum oxygen consumption and oxygen-pulse maximum. As well as establishing that the stability of the characteristics mentioned above are relatively high (in general, it is still lower than the characteristics of physical constitution), the author also drew other interesting conclusions. They refer to the fact that a high degree of stability of individual development appears in the lot with medium motricity activity and from the point of view of age, during in puberty. Results of the investigation appreciated in the absolute values (not in kg body weight) and in the conditions of maximum effort showed a higher stability. Its true that the most adequate criteria for prediction of development of functional capacity, from the point of view of resistance capacity, from the authors point of view is considered to be the oxygen-pulse maximum.

Alongside the research mentioned above, other interesting investigations are those of *Sedov* (1976), having as the object some biochemical factors for the evaluation of the coefficient of longitudinal stability, in particular 17-ketosteroids (correlation coefficient reached a value of 0.55) as in the research by *Smirnova* (1976) when the development of the excitability of the locomotricity apparatus was studied. In both cases the authors established that the subject presents a tendency to maintain particularities of childhood until adulthood and that these factors are relatively "conservatory". Likewise, in the framework of the functional and typological parameters we mention the stability in hypoxic hypoxemia, which shows a level of development of the qualities of resistance. Hypoxemic resistance of tins was studied in the maximal apnoea tests (inspiratory and expiratory) and the expiratory resistance tests. In monozygous twins and dizygous twins there is no real difference., even though all tests on mono and dizygous twins suggest differences. Capacity to tolerate hypoxemic state is dependent on the grade of training, even though the individual with insufficient oxygen is very stable. Even though these results do not show with enough clarity (children, perhaps are unable to carry out the entire test due to not having being instructed prior to beginning) may allow for the prediction of the existence of an inborn capacity for hypoxemic resistance. Alpine residents who live their whole lives at high altitude create an adaption for the insufficient oxygen supply which those who live at low altitude do not. Yet still, children of high altitude areas show no difference to children from other regions with regards to haemoglobin and erythrocyte concentration. It is only after a prolonged stay in the mountains that they develop their adaptive mechanisms, indispensable for preventing hypoxia.

Adaptation reactions to hypoxia in athletes over the course of the years manifests as a specific constant. All of this allows the affirmation that individual differences regarding the level of resistance to the insufficient quantity of oxygen are, largely, hereditarily conditioned. Thus, they can be certain components of a selection process in children for certain sporting disciplines which require the development of high resistance. In ratio to physiological acquirements, on the basis of motricity premise, there have been a series of studies regarding the degree of hereditary conditioning of physiological phenomena at rest, during submaximal and maximal effort as well as rest after effort. All the results demonstrate that during times of great effort, genetic control and acquirements are manifest and not while at rest, the intensity of genetic conditioning having and intermediate place in rest after effort. Data obtained regarding the cardiac volume, debit, frequency and respiratory capacity were obtained by: parent-child correlation methods (*Kogan* and *Antipov*, 1974), through methods influencing genetic components in the change of phenotype of acquirements (*Wokanski*, 1978) and though the twin method (*Szwarz*, 1971, 1976; *Sergienko*, 1975). With the help of these latest methods it was established that the acquirements of the circulatory system are much more powerfully controlled genetically than those of the respiratory system (*Szwarz*, 1971).There are results which affirm that the process of beginning an effort is especially genetically controlled as is the process of regeneration (*Szwarz*, 1976). In this context we mention the research of *Szopa* regarding environmental genetic conditioning of aerobic capacity and some parameters of the circulatory system. This way, familial correlation coefficients for pulse before, during and after effort, for body weight, graphs of changes of the correlation coefficient in various periods of life, heritability coefficients of pulse before, during and after effort and capacity for aerobic activity and components of phenotypical variations. All information obtained has a special importance for the selection and training of athletes (table 44)

Table 44

Comparison of hereditary indices h^2
– results from data obtained from research carried out on twins

Author	Children's age	Pulse before effort	Pulse during effort	Characteristics
Szwarz, Kramov, 1970		-	-	0.79
Klissouras, 1917	7-13	-	-	0.93
Venarando, Milani-Comparetti, 1973	10-13 14-17	0.28 0.38	0.91 0.51	0.66 0.77
Sergienko, 1975	12-17	0.17	0.48	0.73
Kovar, 1984	7-10 11-14 15-19 7-19	0.05 0.00 0.10 0.06	0.30 0.27 0.65 0.37	0.20 0.24 0.47 0.28

Static equilibrium is another physiological parameter. It was determined through three tests:

1. Maintaining a position "standing on one leg"
2. The "swallow" test
3. In position 1 without stopping until balance is lost, the twins turned their heads side to side with a rate of one turn per second.

Dynamic equilibrium was studied through increasing the errors left and right while walking straight ahead on a straight line with eyes open for a distance of 15 m.

The results were the following: hereditary coefficient effect for static balance, determined through the three tests were: F-1,44, with p 0,05; F=1,70. With p 0,05; F=3,37 with p 0,01. From this data it is possible to presume that static equilibrium in it development, depends approximately with equal measure on hereditary and environmental factors. More significantly, environment influences the development of dynamic equilibrium (F=1,14, with p 0,05).

- Typological motricity characters

Genetic determination of the motricity development is conditioned by polygenic characters which depend on a group of many "weak" genes, which exercise an additive effect (cumulative). They are thus expressed in a medium ratio with the determinant genes, which are hereditarily transmitted to a person in a proportion of 50% from the father and 50% from the mother. This results in, theoretically, parent-child correlation coefficient of 0.5 while the mid-parent value (parent-child) should be 0.71. this last effect is likewise due to the fact that some of the genes inherited from mother and father can be identical (homologous). Thus some phenotypes sometimes present a discontinuity, which appear in the form of the presence of many peaks in the distribution curve of a particular characteristic. In this case characters are not submitted to Mendelian segregation (*Incuye*, 1973) (fig 122). Hereditary transmission of fundamental motricity characteristics hard to explain, due to the aspects of motricity activity they are not themselves separate. Usually the following characteristics of motricity activity are taken into account

1. Force: capacity to overcome great resistance
2. Speed: capacity of movement over a distance or a given angle, in a short interval of time.
3. Skill: capacity for voluntary coordinated, precise and elastic movements of the body, adaptive motricity actions in response to an adversary, anticipate motricity capacity, balance
4. Resistance: capacity to carry our long, often submaximal movements without signs of exhaustion.

Many authors consider still that only force and speed or force and resistance are the real characteristics of motricity activity, and consider the others to be mere derivations from those real characteristics. In the scope of genetic research, it is of essential importance to establish the elementary characters. This explains the tendency in research to consider some variable, such as biomechanical conditions: mass and body proportions, somatic type, development of muscular mass, coordination and precision of movements, reaction time and respective movements, sense of balance and rhythm, static, dynamic and explosive muscular force, maximum oxygen absorption etc. Hereditary transmissions of these 4 characteristics of motricity activity mentioned above are considered to be a combined manifestation of the number of elemental characters, each of them being polygenetically defined. For this reason, it can be compared more to genetic determination of intelligence. The hereditary transmission of intelligence was studied in more detail than that of the motricitys characters. The latter not only depends on the somatic and physiological traits of an individual but also on their psychic basis: imagination of movement, resistance and persistence (tenacity). Bearing this in mind the term usually used is "*hereditary transmission of psychomotricity traits*". Research carried out on the basis of the three principal methods: longitudinal studies with comparison of a group of identical subjects: familial and twin studies, all the three methods presents some advantages but sadly none are without deficits.

Results on the basis of research on twins. The apparition of twins in a population if very rare, still investigation of them is situated among one of the most frequently applied in the study of quantitative human characters. This fact is evidenced through the number of studies which had as a theme the study of motricity predispositions. In the last 50 years, a series of interesting, from a gnoseologic point of view, studies emerged, to which we should accord attention (fig 123-129).

Study of twins

Study of twins presents is with the best modality for verifying the hereditary importance and the importance of the environment around us, which determines, in some measure our athletic talent. Monozygous twins have the same genetic system. Big differences between them are determined by non-hereditary factors. On the other hand dizygous twins have diverse genotypes. On the basis for comparison of change observed in mono and dizygous twins, there has been a scale of indices of hereditability has been established. If the value is 1, cause of changes observed is hereditary, if it is 0 then the changes were produced under the influence of the environment. If the change is conditioned both environmentally and hereditarily then the heredity index is between 0 and 1: closer to 1 is considered an index relative to the force of genotype. Bearing this in mind, hereditary indices for the chain of physiological, biomechanical and morphological changes were calculated, which are linked on the highest level to physical skills.

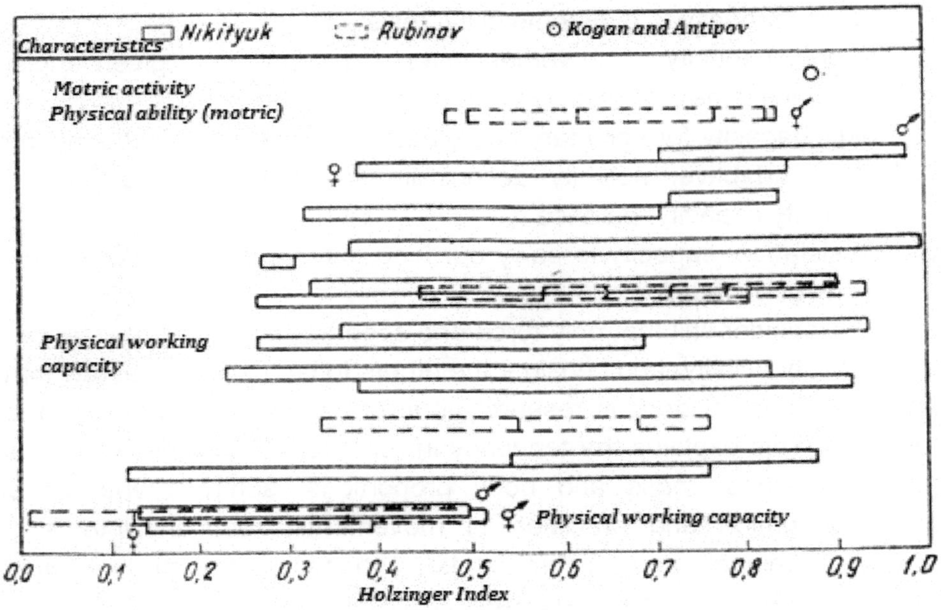

Fig. 122. Heritability coefficients with importance in sport (according to Wolanski).

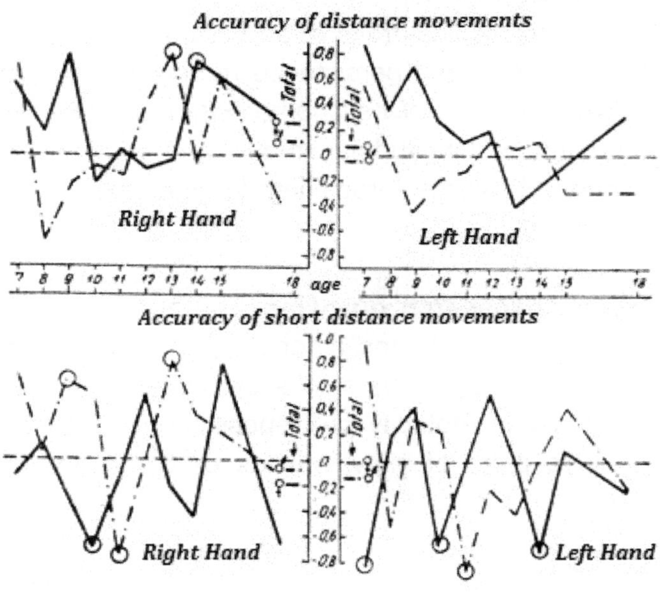

Fig. 123. Parent-child correlation regarding the precision near and distance movement of the right and left hand. (Wolanski, 1976, with modifications).

In two different series of research, Komi and collaborators obtained indices close to one (0.99 and 0.98) for maximal muscular force, measured through scale running tests. A value (0.97) was similarly obtained for the maximum force of the forearm muscles on the basis of speed-force tests (B. Joness – unpublished data obtained in the authors laboratory).

In their research, *Komi* and *Karlsson* took muscle biopsies from the vastus lateralis muscle from 20 pairs of twins (9 monozygous and 11 dizygous) and researched the types of fibres of the skeletal muscle. They confirmed almost identical percentage distribution of the skeletal muscle fibres in the cases of the monozygous brothers. The hereditary indices were raised to 99, 5% while indices for maximal force were almost a value of 97.8%.Bearing in mind that the muscular neuron uniformly innervates the type of muscle fibre, the authors suggested the component in the motricity unit in skeletal muscle is established genetically and that genetic factors have a decisive importance for the physical capacity of a man. Examination of other research carried out obtained high indices for morphological capacity and motricity agility.

The method of studying twins is based on the evaluation of the variants of correlations between the pairs of mono and dizygous twins. As a rule, the monozygous twins possessed 100% identical genes while the dizygous twins bore only 50% of these kind of genes (value similar to a brother-brother pair chosen at random); divergences in these two values can offer the key for drawing conclusions regarding the genetic determination of characters. Correlation coefficients between pairs of monozygous twins are usual underestimated while the correlation coefficient in dizygous twins are often overestimated, in relation to their real genetic similarity. For the evaluation of heritability the following formula is used in the study of twins:

$$H^2 = \frac{s_{DZ^2} - s_{MZ}}{s_{DZ^2}} \quad \text{or} \quad h^2 = \frac{v_{DZ} - v_{MZ}}{V_{DZ}}$$

or $$F = \frac{s_{DZ^2}}{s_{MZ^2}}$$

or $$H = \frac{r_{MZ} - r_{DZ}}{1 - r_{DE}}$$

where: s_{DZ} is the variation or standard error of difference between dizygous twins multiplied by; r_{DZ} is the correlation coefficient between twins *DZ* or between the two *MZ;*.

Sometimes in these formulae the correlation for errors was considered, a fact which did not bring significant modification in this approach. The value of methodology of the study of twins is incontestable, but the methods described above are etched with considerable errors for the reasons explained below. Existing differences are not in any way a measure of genetic differences. They express instead an unidentified proportion of genetic determination of environment which cannot serve as a measure of heritability even though they constitute in some measure in the case of family studies, as mentioned above. Another inconvenience of the fundamentals of the study of twins, as described above, is constituted by the fact that monozygous twins may have a common or separate amniotic sac, while in dizygous twins the sacs are always separate. In the case of a common amniotic sac, the twins are in competition for the same nutrients obtained from the maternal milk (*Price*, 1950, *Churchill*, 1965) and, as a result, one twin usually dominates the other. This diminished their similarity to varying degree, in an individual way, for each pair of monozygous twins with a shared amniotic sac. Mortality of monozygous twins is higher both while in foetal life as well as postnatal (*Nkikitjuk*, 1976), while the type of morbidity differs from that of dizygous twins. This shows that twins are not randomised groups from one "pool" of genes from the population into which they are born. The number of subjects with active X chromosomes is higher among twins (genosomal type of hereditary transmission – *Nikitjuk*, 1976). The comparison of mono and dizygous twins from the demonstration of differences is tied to considerable errors because they have shown that even in reaction of motricity stimuli (stimulation of bone development) there are differences between mono and dizygous twins (*Antipov* and *Kogan*) (cited from *Dubinin* and *Nikijut*, 1976); in the case of trained identical twins, there are many larger observed effects in monozygous twins than in dizygous. A fact which is very important for the study of motricity aptitude (*Kogan* and *Antipov*, 1974). Difficulties encountered in the study of twins from the genetic point of view are due to the fact that they are realised together and usually food and clothing are identical. For this reason, it's hard to outline the role of the genetic factor from the environmental one. The proportion of this factor is different in monozygous twins and dizygous twins and those raised in identical conditions. Mathematical methods used in this context have not as yet given results.

Among the first who studied the hereditary influence on the human motricity manifestations were Verschuer and Bossik. They studied the same problem, carrying out continuous research on pairs of mono and dizygous twins at a young age, observing their firs movements and evaluating the measure in which they correspond or differ. In the pairs of monozygous twins there was observes a much greater similarity in the pair with regards to the development of walking. According to Verschuer, in the pairs of monozygous twins here was a concordance of 67% in cases while in the dizygous pairs there was only 30%; according to Bossik the respective proportions were 69% and 35%. Both authors arrived at the same conclusion that hereditism exercises and important influence.

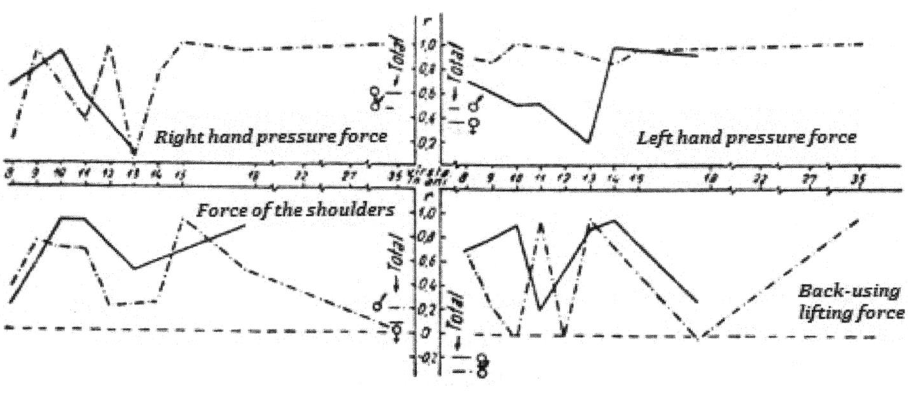

Fig. 124. Correlation of mid-parent-child regarding muscular force, static force and prehensilism, force of the back and shoulders. (Wolanski, 1976).

Frischeisen-Kahier studied the individual differences in speed and rhythm of simple movement of the hands. They established that considerably smaller differenced were obtained in monozygous twins while variable results were obtained from dizygous twins which corresponded to differentiation between brothers (sisters) normally. The similar results with regards to the evaluation of orientation in space of the movement (deviation of the hand from the direction followed) were obtained by *Molan*. Affinity within the pairs of monozygous twins was twice as comparable as compared to the dizygous twins.

A simple study is often cited, carried out by *McNemar* (1933). This author observed the influence of some effort continues towards the differences in the pairs between the mono and dizygous twins, in the framework of the 3 skill tests (activity of the hands and fingers. He examined the results obtained at the start and after the exercise. The data obtained shows the differences in the pairs of monozygous twins are relative and influenced very little by exercise, while those between the dizygous twins have tendency to diminish differentiation. This conclusion resulted from a similar study by *Brody*. The results showed that the possibility of acquiring certain motricity capacities probably lies under the influence of conditioned genetic and hereditary predisposition.

A similar problem refers to the genetic aspects of learning movements and the sensory-motricity predisposition was addressed by a German psychologist *Wilde*. He studied the time necessary for acquisition of simple motricity acts grouping similar pictures according to a pattern and evaluating progressive amelioration in repeated tries. It was noticed there was a considerably higher degree of concordance in monozygous twins than in dizygous twins.

Linked to this is a type of research and study of genetic conditioning of literalities (evaluated for example through hitting a punch ball). From the results obtained in his research it was established that the hereditary component is in general much stronger in general in the dominant hand. With regards to writing, fine coordination and demanding sensorial activities, there is big difference between the pairs of mono and dizygous twins. This proves the diverse influences of environment are significant in these cases. Other factors are the level of mastery of agility, differences in age, diverse conditions of acquisition of dexterity etc.

The study carried out by *Gedda* and *Neroni* (1955) on 56 pairs of mono and dizygous twins is centred on the unconscious involuntary movements. By recording on film, they were able to follow the reactions of the subjects while they would show them different kinds of pictures of twins and evaluated the grade of concordance On the basis of the of one pair from each type of twin. On the basis of the analysis of their results they reached the conclusion that genetic conditioning could be observed only in the manifestation of mimicry in the head and face.

Regarding human movement, *Spindler* (1955) occupied himself to a greater extent. Besides the observations of involuntary movements (mimicry, manifestation of emotion), his battery of tests included some ordinary skill tests (sewing, writing) and activities such as running, jumping, throwing. On the basis of the results of the study above, carried out on a relatively large group, the author considered that, in particular speed and rhythm of running are largely hereditarily conditioned (a similarity was found in 78% of the cases in the monozygous twins and only 12% of the dizygous twins). *Ledowskaja* (1972) studied the influence of the regime of speed and genetic predisposition of motricity activities. Motricity activity was evaluated by the number of steps taken and heart rate. The group included 10 pairs of monozygous twins and 10 pairs of dizygous twins of both sexes, ages between three and seven. The results showed that, even though individuals within the pairs differed one from the other, the difference is far smaller than those from different pairs (intra-pair differences were smaller than inter-pair differences). This can be seen by the data presented in table 45, as well as from correlation coefficients calculated (MZ=0.92, DZ=0.60). in conclusion the authors study showed that even though influence of genetic factors on the motricity activity is not, as seen from the investigations, especially pregnant, it must be considered (tab 45). The results are very interesting and useful from a gnoseological point of view, obtained through the study of twin, published in the last years by *Sklad*, from the academy of physical education in *Warsaw.* Alongside the constitutional body character and problems of physical development in the course of ontogenesis, he also studied motricity manifestations.

In his first work (1972) he bases himself in some older research, namely the studies of Frischeisen and Spindler. In a lot of 27 pairs of monozygous twins and 23 pairs of dizygous twins of both sexes with a mean age of 11, he studied the similarities in the ratios of movement in running. Through cinematographic methods and analysis of the results of running 60m (he evaluated the time, length and number of steps as well as the angles between the various segments of the body in certain phases of running). The results underwent statistic evaluation through the analysis of variants and the calculation or hereditability coefficient. From the results of the study it was observes that the individual running structures were only minimally modified. There is however a considerable different between diverse individuals. Kinematic structure of movement of the movement of running in the monozygous twin pairs presents a high grade of comparative similarities with the dizygous twins. With regards to sex, small differences within the pairs (intra-pair) were observes in the lot of boys. It can be deduced that speed, structure, rhythm or running are probably in some measure conditioned genetically.

Table 45

Comparative results of motricity activity in a lot of mono and dizygous (according to the results published by *Ledowskaja*, 1972)

Lot	Mean		Difference	
	Twin A	Twin B		(A-B)/(A+B)/100
Number of steps per hour				
MZ(18 pairs)	11 800	9 700	2 100	9%
DZ(10 pairs)	12 000	10 400	2 600	10%
Number of steps per day				
MZ (6 pairs)	2 600	2 200	400	8%
DZ (5 pairs)	2 400	1 800	600	12%
Number of pulsations per hour				
MZ(18 pairs)	6 900	6 400	500	3%
DZ(10 pairs)	7 200	6 200	1 000	7%

Note: Lot A encompasses twins from each pair who achieved higher values.

A second study by the same author addressed (*Sklad*, 1973) the problem of learned movement. The evolution of learning was studied daily for two weeks in 50 pairs of mono and dizygous twins of both sexes, aged between 9 and 13. Motricity tests included throwing a ball at a target, light tapping (tapping test) and an exercise of coordination with a thermometer. Repeated attempts were the basis for learning curves and for their statistical analysis. The results are very interesting, the differences in learning evolution between monozygotic and dizzy twin pairs are clearly observable; You can see the motion learning curves by the girls in monozygotic and dizzygotic twin pairs, the test being throwing at the target (evaluating multiple attempts to throw a small rubber ball into a basket placed a certain distance above the ground).

On the basis of its results, the author concludes that the skills to learn a new motricity act are under genetic control, but in terms of concrete task, they seem to be independent and quite specific. There is no general factor with universal influence on the learning of motricity acts, but a multitude of factors with a hereditary basis. The level of assimilation of a motricity act and learning speed seem to be more genetically conditioned in boys, and movements that require fine coordination and precision are more genetically conditioned on girls.

By the mid-1960s, interest began to focus on genetic conditioning issues of motricity efficiency, namely sports. Several papers dealing with this issue were published by *Grebe* (1955, 1956). In 1955 he published the results of a study of 34 pairs of monozygotic and dizigeneous twins of both sexes. He pursued the degree of concordance or difference between individuals within a pair in terms of their sporting activity. Subsequent research by *Gedda* (1960) is similar in terms of methodological approach. Using a questionnaire, he obtained information on 35 pairs of twins, reaching similar conclusions to *Grebe's* (the results of both authors are presented in Table

46). Both authors conclude that sports efficacy depends in particular on predispositions transmitted hereditary, which have the character of dominant hereditary predispositions. They influence an individual regardless of age or gender. Those respondents say that a sporting training process consists only in the development and development of these predispositions in optimal environment conditions (Table 46).

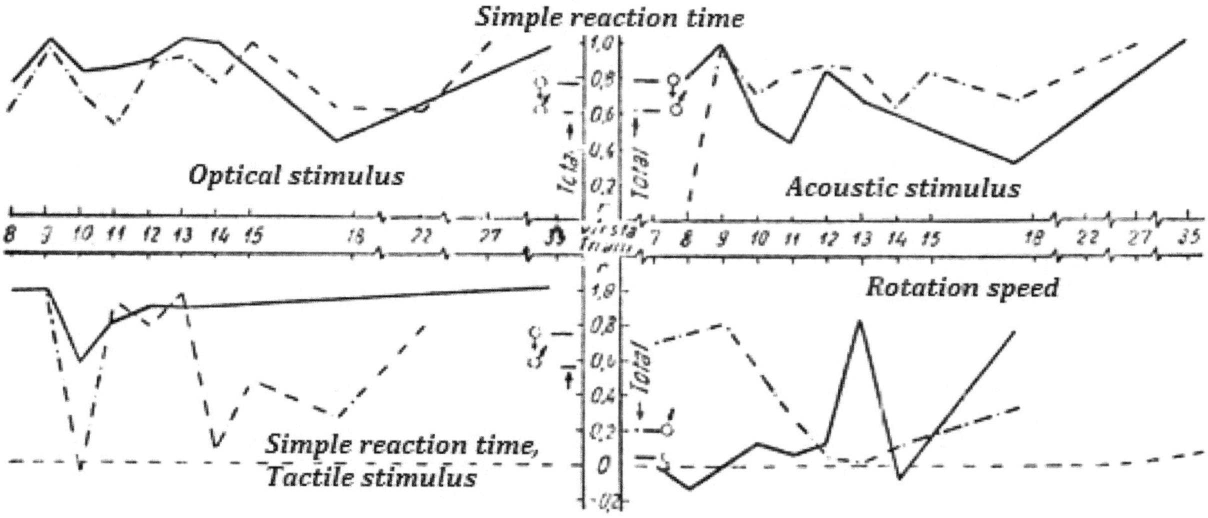

Fig. 125. The correlation of mid-parent children on the simple reaction time At different stimuli and spin speeds (Wolanski, 1976).

Table 46

Sports activities in monozygotic and dizygotic twins - percentage frequency in various categories (by the results of Grebe, 1955 Gedda, 1960)[3]

Author	Averages			Diferences		
	Total correspondence	Partial corres-pondence	Difference	Total corres-pondence	Partial corres-pondence	Difference
GREBE (34 pairs)	95	5	0	54%	30.8	15.4
GEDDA (319 pairs)	95	5	0	54%	30.8	15.4

A comprehensive and complete study of gemelarity, which pursued a number of structural and functional properties of the body, was carried out 30 years ago by a group of Japanese researchers led by Prof. Osato and Prof. Awano (1957). Their study also includes research into

[3] The author's results have been partly adapted so that they can be compared. Grabe evaluated the subjects as follows:

- total concordance - both twins practice the same type of sport at an approximately equal level of efficiency.
- partial concurrence - both twins practice the same sport, but at different levels of efficiency.
- Difference - either a twin or none does not practice a sport. Gedda also includes pairs in which none of the twins perform a sporting activity, and in the second category (partial concordance) it includes cases where a twin practicing a sports activity, and the other does not practice any sport.

50 m running results, various jumps and throws, performance in tests for local muscle strength, maximum strength of hand, torso extensions, and other factors. The results obtained in a batch of 121 pairs of monozygotic and dizygotic twins aged six 16 years (both sexes) were analyzed by Ishidoya (1957). The contribution of heredity was assessed by means of a mean percentage difference, expressed in pairs of monozygotic and dizzy twins. The author also studied the influence of different types of environment and age. Some of its results are shown in Table 47.

Table 47

Evaluation of heredity and the environment - influences on variability of results in selected motricity tests - study of twins (After the results of Ishidoya, 1957)[4]

Test	Heredity influence index	Proportion of environmental influence
Running 50 m	1.92	58.2
Long Jump	1.95	58.9
Throwing the ball	2.34	54.3
Pushing	1.82	59.3
One foot jump	2.13	56.1
Strength of torsoextensions	5.00	40.7
The force of prehension of the hand	3.53	52.9
Shoulder force	4.47	42.5
Trunk force kilocorp)	4.61	42.0
Shoulder Strength (per kilocorp)	3.66	42.2

From the analysis of the results it is deduced that heredity is undoubtedly a significant factor in most investigated motricity manifestations. On the other hand, the environment also has an important role in age dependency, with results varying according to the type of test. However, a lower degree of genetic control seems to manifest itself more during puberty, respectively at the age of 11-14 years. Compared with older studies, the authors of recent works try to raise new issues. While in the past the objective of the studies was to prove whether or not the influence of heredity is evident, contemporary research seeks to quantitatively assess the influence of heredity on the inter-individual variability of the results in certain tests and the corresponding properties or aptitudes. This allows assessing which one is more genetically conditioned and less influenced. This is also the possibility to influence by deliberate conditioning. In addition, the influence of gender, age, different environmental conditions and other factors is investigated. Depending on the Professional specialization of various researchers, the invested characters include various features of body composition, the results of motricity tests, or physiological and functional factors selected at a lower level of differentiation. In a number of cases, the characteristics of all the parameters mentioned above are established. Let us now quote the authors who have most influenced the state of knowledge of the current decade in assessing the motricity manifestations and the functional functional selections of the body. In addition to studying the influence of heredity on the variability of results in selected motricity tests, Kovar attempted to focus on some methodological issues concerning the study of heredity in relation to human motricity capabilities by comparing the different ways of calculating the heredity

[4] The author made a quantitative evaluation of the influence of heredity on the basis of Lenz's so-called Lenz's "force of heredity" ("Erbkraft" in original - Lenz, 1935). Percentage assessment of environmental impact is carried out after Verschuer (1927). Both methods are rarely used today.

coefficient by various methods. Relatively identical methods of mathematical statistical processing of data obtained through twin studies and the same research goal allow the comparison of results and the attempt to deduce some more general trends. To this end, we present the results obtained by various authors on the heritability coefficients obtained by various notations in Tables 48-51.

Table 48

Research on twins in a running engine test[5]

Test	Gender	Age	No. of pairs	Heretability coeficient	Author
20 m Run	F	10 (X)	49	0.83	SAVATEJEVA 1976
30 m Run	M+F	12-17	50	0.62	SERGIENKO 1975
60 m Run	M+F	12-17	50	0.45	WEISS 1977
60 m Run	M+F	10	3.000	0.85	SZWARZ 1972
60 m Run	M+F	5-17	61	0.91	KOVAR 1974
Alternative step running	M	11-25	30	0.89	KLISSOURAS 1973
1. 000 m Run	M+F	10-14	17	0.94	
7 min Run	M+F	10	3.000	0.93	WEISS 1977

Table 48 includes the data obtained from running tests. Most of these tests relate to shorter distances, serving to evaluate the speed of running ability; two of them are long run running tests, serving as indicators of total aerobic resistance capacity. However, it can be deduced from the data that the heredity factor plays an important role in the variability of the results in both the first and the second case. The heritability coefficients, except for two tests, are within the range of 0.83-0.91 for speed-type activities, and they are even higher and nearly equal (0, 93 and 0.94) in terms of resistance. In the above-mentioned analysis of the research results of the various functional factors related to the resistance capacities, we will arrive at an identical conclusion.

Table 49

Research on twins through tests to track the reaction and speed of simple movements

Test	Gender	Age	No. of pairs	Heritability coefficient	Author
The reaction of the superior member	M+F	8-16	194	0.70	SVANCARA 1966
	M+F	10-14	29	0.86	KOMI et. al. 1973
The reaction of the superior member	M+F	12-17	50	0.86	SERGIENKO 1975
	M+F	12-17	50	0.71	SERGIENKO 1975
The reaction of the lower limb	M+F	12-17	61	0.50-0.70	SERGIENKO 1975
The reaction of the lower limb	F	5-17	50	0.87	SZWARZ 1972
Speed of upper limb movement	M+F	12-17	30	near 0	SERGIENKO 1975
Easy knocking (by hand)	F	8-15	50	0.32	NOVOZILOVA 1975
Easy knocking (by hand)	M+F	12-17	50	near 0	SERGIENKO 1975
Easy knocking (by hand)	F	8-15	30	0.24	NOVOZILOVA 1976
Frequency of running on the spot					

[5] M - male, F - female. The number of pairs includes both monozygotic twins and dizigotic.

Table 50

Research on twins by dynamometric tests of muscle strength

Test	Gender	Age	No. of pairs	Heritability coefficient	Author
Prehension with your hand	M+F	6-16	194	0.24	SVANCARA 1966
Prehension with your hand	M+F	5-17	61	0.71	SZWARZ 1972
Prehension with your hand	M+F	10-13	23	0.43 }	VENERANDO.
Prehension with your hand	M+F	14-17	23	0.56	MILANICOMPARETI, 1973
Prehension with your hand	M+F	11-25	30	0.46	KOVAR 1974
Flexion of the elbow	M+F	10-13	23	0.42	VENERANDO.
Flexion of the elbow	M+F	14-17	23	0.80	MILANICOMPARETI, 1973
Flexion of the elbow	M+F	11-25	30	0.75	
Knee extension	M+F	10-13	23	0.67 }	KOVAR 1974
Knee extension	M+F	14-17	23	0.78	VENERANDO,
Trunk extension	M+F	10-13	23	0.44	MILANICOMPARETI,
Trunk extension	M	14-17	23	0.74	1973
Trunk extension	M	11-25	30	0.57	KOVAR 1974
Trunk extension	F	8-15	30	0.11	NOVOZILOVA 1976
Amount of main muscle groups	F	10 (X)	49	0.71	SAVATEJEVA 1976
	M+F	11-13	23	0.76	VENERANDO,
Amount of main muscle groups	M+F	14-17	23	0.87	MILANICOMPARETI 1973
	M+F	12-17	50	0.37 }	
The sum of 20 muscle groups (To one kilogram)	M+F	12-17	50	0.64	SERGIENKO 1975

Table 51

Research on twins by tests on joint flexibility and coordination of your hand and fingers

Test	Gender	Age	No. of pairs	Heritability coefficient	Author
Tacking the trunk forward	M	11-25	30	0.69	KOVAR 1974
Tacking the trunk forward					
Flexible hip joint	M+F	12-17	50	0.84 }	SERGIENKO 1975
Flexibility of the shoulder					
	M+F	12-17	50	0.70	SERGIENKO 1975
	M+F	12-17	50	0.91	SERGIENKO 1975
The task of the labyrinth	M	11-25	30	0.45	KOVAR 1974
The task of the labyrinth	M	11-25	30	0.64	KOVAR 1974

Other tests for speed skills are shown in Table 49. These are the results of the latent motricity reaction time measurement, which forms the basis for evaluating the reaction rate capability. In addition to the data obtained by Sergienko, all values of the heritability coefficient are between 0.70 and 0.86, which allows us to assume a significant genetic influence.

Completely different is the situation in tests that track the speed capabilities of frequency in simple movements of the extremities, in most cases the heritability is very low and, although it may have different causes, a more important contribution of heredity compared to other types of activity and other Skills can not be proven. Tests involving different types of jumps and throws serve as indicators for assessing the explosive forces of the lower limbs. In terms of jump-type activities, the heritability coefficients are again relatively elevated, oscillating on average around 0.75. This attests to the fact that a genotypic predisposition of a subject has an important role in the individual differences in the manifestation of the explosive forces of lower limbs. For the upper limbs, however, a similar conclusion can not be drawn. Because the author's data varies greatly, the above-mentioned fact may be due to some methodological deficiencies.

The data presented in Table 50 relate to tests that measure the ability of local muscular strength or other strength of dynamic strength. Except for two cases, the heredity coefficients are very high, showing a considerable contribution to genotype influence. An important aspect is the content of applied motricity tests, in which only a limited muscle group is active.

This supports the conclusion (Kovar, Sergienko) that there is a greater degree of genetic conditioning in elementary, simple activities than in complex and integrated activities. The largest data volume is undoubtedly provided by the dynamo-metric value of the maximum static force (Table 50). At the same time, the results are very contradictory. In some cases heritability is very low, suggesting a considerable environmental impact and intentional conditioning. On the other hand, other figures on the heritability coefficient are high, exceeding the value of 0.70. As such, here too, an important influence of heredity can not be disputed. It is assumed that the capacity of a single manifestation of a maximum static force with a prevalent isometric muscle contraction is under the influence of both genetic control and environmental conditions and factors, these two influences having an approximately equal participation. Finally, practical experience shows that this kind of force can be increased by training; At the same time, the upper level of such development has an individual limitation given by the norm of the genetic reaction. The above-mentioned findings are in an interesting way complemented by the works of Venerando and Milani Comparetti, according to which a higher heritability occurs in older twin pairs.

Regarding the flexibility of the joints there are relatively few data (Table 51). They come from the works of only two authors. However, heritability coefficients are high in all cases and, in particular, after Sergienko's conclusions, which addressed these issues in detail, articular flexibility appears to be among the most strongly predisposed genetic predispositions. This is probably related to the structural properties of the body, which are known to exhibit a greater proportion of genotypic differences in their interindividual variability compared to functional properties.

A prerequisite of the study of the genetic conditioning of properties included in the field of appraisals and coordination is, first of all, the explanation of the main theoretical and methodological aspects related to such a problem and the finding of appropriate motricity tests. From this point of view, it is necessary to evaluate the results of the tests in this field. There are only partial data obtained by two authors through different tests.

In addition to analyzing the results of heritability coefficients calculated in identical or similar type activities, other interesting data have also been obtained. Venerando and Milani Comparetti (1973), in works on the dynamometric evaluation of maximum muscular force, observed a higher degree of heritability in older twin pairs. An opposite trend was highlighted by the results of the tests of Sergienko et al. (1978) on joint flexibility. Also, Svancaro (1967) supports the hypothesis of reducing the influence of genotypic predispositions during ontogenesis. Kovar's work comes to similar conclusions.

Another issue concerns the influence of sex. By the fact that most authors conducted research on mixed twin groups of both sexes, the information was reduced. The comparison of the presented results does not allow for more general conclusions. In this case also an important factor seems to be the type of motricity sample and the corresponding motricity skills. This view is supported, for example, by data that found, in terms of articular flexibility, a higher degree of heritability in girls, while Cepulis and Kuklis (1976), when studying the maximum muscle strength, came to the opposite conclusion. In both the first and the second case, the explanation can be the sexual differences regarding the physical constitution, the structural properties, the functional properties of the body and the connection with the neuro-moral regulation.

Very interesting and valuable from the gnoseological point of view are the results of researches on twins by the method of different intrapereche environment conditions or the method of "co-pilot control". In a pair of monozygotic twins (16-year-old girls), under the same conditions and at the same level of observed factors, Sergienko introduced a different degree of motricity activity. After one year (when one of the twins was heavily trained while the other was physically inactive), he examined the level of maximum muscle strength and aerobic capacity (by measuring heart rate during a standard effort and after exercise, the maximum consumption of Oxygen, etc.). The results show that the increase in muscle strength was 17, 8%, thus three times lower than the increase in aerobic capacity. Based on this finding, the author concluded that the upper level of muscle growth is less determined by genotype than aerobic capacity.

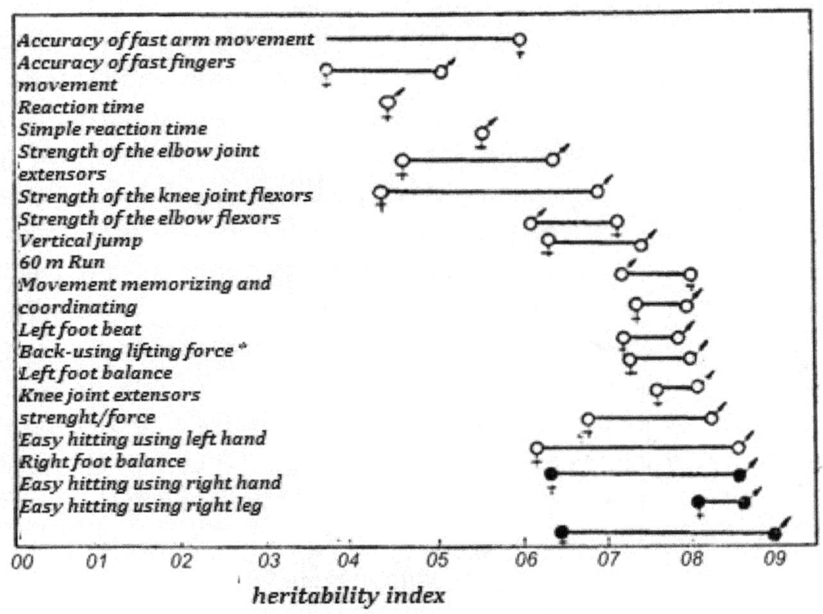

Fig. 126. Heritability of motricity properties (according to Stock data).

Klissouras has researched a pair of 21-year-old dizygotic twins who have been living separately since the age of 16. One of them did intensive performance training for medium-distance runs, while the latter never practiced any sporting discipline. It will be a puzzling fact that, for the brother who has never practiced sport, the respiratory capacity has reached 56.0 ml / kg.min and his trained brother 52.8. Two other cases are added to this finding. Two monozygotic brothers of 40 years have lived separately since the age of twelve and have led different ways of life. One of them has practiced intensive basketball training at the level of performance sports (from 12 to 30 years, from 18 to 30, being in the national basketball), while the second has a regime Balanced life. Over the past 10 years, none of them has ever used any form of physical activity. The test results indicate close maximum values of respiratory capacity (37, 8 and 41.7 ml / kg min - for the trained and the non-trained brother). Based on the findings of twin studies, we now know that such factors, including aerobic capacity, maximum muscle strength, and muscle fiber spread, are genetically determined. We also know that in the case of adaptation reactions, the training stimulus can only influence within the limits of heredity. From all these observations, it is clear that genetic factors play a decisive role in achieving sports performance. It is obvious that there must be fundamental biophysical provisions to become an outstanding athlete.

A similar research was carried out by *Browing* and *Whittle* (1972). Unlike the previous study, they followed the somatic characters and the results of motricity manifestations (hand pretension, knee extension, trunk muscle mass, speed of motricity reactions) to a pair of male twins. Comparison between the data on the subject of a sport and the non-sports subject showed that the structural properties related to the physical constituent characters are under genetic control more powerful than the functional manifestations of the body. *Komi* (1978) sought to study the influence of isometric training on the development of muscle strength. The subjects were two pairs of monozygotic twins and four pairs of monozygotic twins. The training consisted of the maximum isometric contraction of the knee flexors of the right lower limb (four times a week for three months). Only one pair of each pair was trained. The investigated factors were maximum muscle strength, electromyographic muscle activity and enzymatic muscle activity with respect to oxidative and non-oxidative metabolic processes. Isometric training has influenced the increase in the muscular force of the inferior trained limb by 20% and the other foot by 11%. At the same time, there has been an increase in electromyographic muscle activity (femoral law), as well as an increase in enzymatic activity in terms of oxidative muscle metabolism (established by biopsy in the large lateral muscle). Experience shows that the maximum static force level along with those processes at a lower level of differentiation can be relatively well influenced by training.

A similar research was carried out by *Stoboy* (1973). He studied multiple pairs of monozygotic twins how regular exercise is felt in the ratio of muscle strength to muscle contraction speed. From this study it follows that, in individuals with a higher effort (80% of the maximum effort), there is a positive correlation between force and the speed of contraction. The method of research on twins and the evaluation of results by mathematical and statistical methods involves a number of methodological problems. Some of them refer, for example, to calculation. We underline that the twin studies method undoubtedly provides valuable information, especially on the types of polygenic heredity, investigated on human beings, and is a classic method of analyzing genetic data. It allows the objective and conclusive research of the contribution of environmental influences and the heredity to the inter-individual variability of the various motricityic predispositions in humans and can not be replaced by any other method; In connection with a combination of identical and different environmental conditions within a pair, the longitudinal study and experimentally applied experimental conditions, e.g., a training effort, allow assessment of the possibilities of adapting an individual to the normal genetic response. The fact can not be altered by theoretical and methodological problems and assumptions, the realization of which is necessary for the correct interpretation of the results obtained by studies on twins.

The hereditary factor seems to act as a general factor that influences the variability of most of the investigated properties and capabilities. Therefore, individual genetic predispositions are the main cause of the motricity and functional level differences of individuals living in the same environmental conditions and possessing the same motricity experience. A deliberately applied physical effort and conditions can influence to a certain extent changes in the level of motricity predisposition, but it is obviously impossible to overcome the individual level of adaptation possibilities conferred by the genetic response norm. This does not mean the overestimation of the influence of heredity or the underestimation of the influence of environmental factors, since the realization of the genotypic predispositions of an individual is possible only in optimal environment conditions. As regards the contribution of heredity and the environment and the quantitative assessment of their influence, a multitude of factors interfere with this issue. In addition to some formal aspects related to the application of mathematical statistical methods and an appropriate additive model of the influence of heredity and the environment, as well as some minor problems, the main factor is the character and type of the investigated property.

Structural properties appear to have a higher degree of genetic conditioning than functional properties and functional manifestations. This is particularly evident in the characters of body composition, but not always in terms of cellular properties. Regarding the motricity manifestations, on the basis of which we assess the level of motricity skills, the factors that show a relatively large contribution of the genotypic predispositions to the inter-individual variability of the results are the speed and strength capacities tested in the course of a long run, the speed capacity The reaction, the explosive forces of the lower extremities and the flexibility of the joints. A relatively large contribution of heredity was also found with regard to the ability of local muscular resistance in simple and elementary activities.

With regard to dynamically assessed muscle strength, the results are not accurate. It can be assumed that this capacity is significantly influenced by both genotypic and environmental factors. A relatively large contribution of heredity has also been demonstrated for some of the skills of human natural movements, the speed, the rhythm and the structure of the movement, the speed and the pace of the limb movements, for some minimal predispositions And predispositions to learn about motricity activity. On the other hand, a more significant influence of the environment can be observed in complicated and integrated activities, which require a greater contribution of the various motricity predispositions than in the skills related to the speed of the extremity movement, the explosive force used In activities similar to throwing action and maximum static force, especially with respect to absolute values.

Regarding functional physiological characteristics, there was a higher degree of genetic conditioning for maximum oxygen consumption as a basic indicator of the body's aerobic capacity and general resistance capacity. The level of this factor can be influenced by training, but the heredity factor is still the main factor in terms of individual differences. Medium genotype interaction appears to be insignificant, but the influence of genotype can be observed throughout the course of life. Regarding the optimal period of development of aerobic possibilities, the assumption that it would be equal to the period of maximum changes of natural development can not be accepted.

An important influence of the genotypic predispositions was also found regarding other factors in the circulatory and respiratory system as well as in the anaerobic capacity of the body. As for respiratory functions, a reduced genetic condition was generally observed. An important factor seems to be the size and intensity of the effort applied. With its growth, the contribution of heredity is also increasing. S has also studied the genetic conditioning of blood circulation regulation and respiration.

Research on some structural and functional properties of muscle tissue, such as the number of muscle fiber types, electrical and enzymatic activity of muscles, has highlighted the prevalence of genetic factors. Characters at a lower differentiation level are more genetically determined and can be evaluated as such, compared to complex characters at higher differentiation levels, for example, at the apparatus or organ level

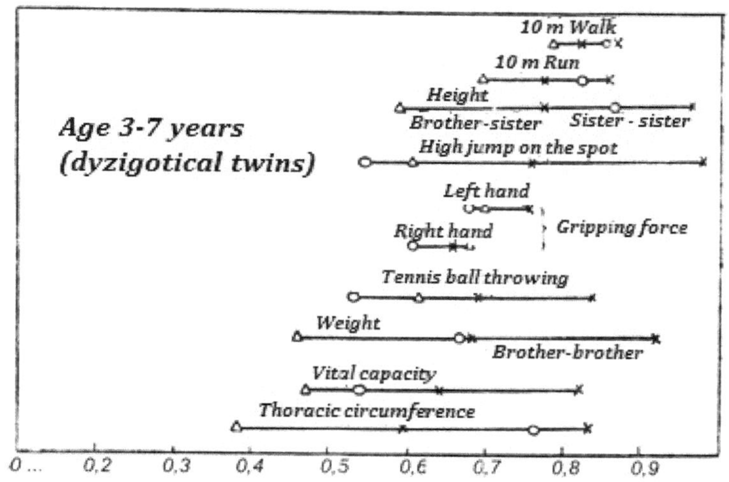

Fig. 127. Correlation of motricity and somatic characters between twin twins Aged three and seven years (according to Nikitjuk's data).

Concurrently with the influence of heredity, it has also confirmed, in a number of cases, a relatively large effect of training, especially in cases where the genotypic predispositions of individuals are similar or where the influence of heredity is not strong enough. It can also be assumed that the possibilities of genotypic adaptation are limited by the genetic norm of the reaction. The study of the influence of age, gender and other factors is just beginning; Drawing generally applicable conclusions in this regard still requires further research and a more unitary methodological approach.

As a conclusion of the evaluation of the results obtained by twin studies, one can say that some of the assertions made are questionable, especially as regards limiting the contribution of heredity. However, one conclusion that can be drawn from these researches is the following: reaching an extremely high level of development of a certain property or aptitude can only be achieved by an individual with appropriate genotypic predispositions and in optimal environmental conditions. From this point of view, the question of which factors is more important, the heredity or the environment makes no sense. Both of these factors are irreplaceable and act in a mutual unity.

Based on the research of similarity between parents and children, a series of data also emerged. The family study method is applied in two variants. One is based on researching entire families and correlating the characters of children from different groups with their parents or other relatives. It is believed that, proportionally, as the similarities of characters at the same level of kinship are higher and the more positive the dependence of the degree of kinship - the similarities of characters between relatives of different degrees - is more pronounced, the stronger their determination gene. According to the statistical model, the expected value of the coefficient of correlation between the characters of some related subjects is expressed by the general formula 0.5n for relatives of grade n. Thus, its value is 0.5 for the relation between siblings and for the relationship Parent children. For primary cousins and grand nephew's relationship, the value is 0.25, etc. The methodological difficulties of comparing children with their parents and siblings of different sex could be overcome by the use of relatively different scales, eg T-stairs. As the degrees of change through education, their parents and their children may be different, this factor can Generates non-genetic determinations. It was found that they are lower than expected (*Bielicki* and *Charzewski*, 1977). On the other hand, greater differences were observed in parent child values and brother brother correlation coefficients. This is due to the greater resemblance of environmental conditions and the way of life between brothers than between parents and children. Brethren grow at about the same time and in the same home, but the living conditions in this home change from one generation to the next. These changes in the economic system from one generation to the next are large enough, but differences in parenting correlation coefficients among children are not usually significant among families whose economic and social situation has improved, and families whose situation has remained the same (*Bielicki* and *Charzewski*, 1975). The correlation coefficients between randomly selected siblings are lower than the correlation coefficients between consecutive children in a particular family, which is further evidence of this problem.

Taking this into account, Wolanschi applied a new method of studying heritability. Until now, the correlation coefficients were used. Wolanschi shows that they should not be used as absolute values, but account must be taken of the influence of similar environmental factors and modes of life. On this basis it suggests the following formula:

$$Heritability = H_{p/o}\frac{1}{D_{p/o}}$$

where: $$D_{p/o} = \frac{\gamma_{ss} - \gamma_{po}}{\gamma_{po}}$$

γ_{ss} = Brother - brother correlation coefficient;
γ_{po} = Parent - child correlation coefficient.

According to genetic evaluations, the parent parent correlation should be identical to the brother brother correlation, because in the case of a sufficiently large number of observations, the same gene expression is the same (50%). However, the brother brother correlation is overstated because of the similarity of the way and living conditions, while parent parenting correlation is underestimated due to environmental conditions and particular lifestyles. The force of the genetic factor is highlighted by the value of this over and sub-evaluation, which must be small (insignificant). The higher the Dp/o or the higher the Hp / o value, the higher the heritability of the character. Another variation of the family study method is genealogy research (pedigree). To evaluate the characters of motricity activity, they have studied families of famous athletes. The athletes' relationship with non-contributors in these families is 1:1. Based on such studies, it has concluded that fitness for sport is hereditary as a dominant character, and motricity skills are determined by independent genes. It has also shown that in animals, motricity skills (research on the ability to jump dogs and horses) are hereditary as dominant characters (*Fedorov*, 1966). However, the results of studying the genealogy of athletes were frequently criticized. The argument against them was that they had not studied non-sportive families for comparison, so the results of studying the genealogy of athletes on motricity character and fitness were overestimated (Jorgensen, 1968). An intermediate method between genealogical research and twin research is that of observing the choice of a sports discipline or the interest in sports in twin pairs. It was found that 15% of dizygotic twins had a concerted interest in sports, while in monozygotic twins this concordance was found in 94% of the observed cases. In the research on the choice of sports discipline, monozygotic twins, the same discipline was chosen by 83% of them, while in the twin twins the same discipline was chosen by only 31% of the pairs pursued. The same specialty in a sports discipline was chosen by 87% of monozygotic twins and 66% of dizygotic twins. Similar results on sports achievements were obtained by 70% of monozygotic twins, but only by 22% of dizygotic twins (*Gedda*, 1960). The phenotypic external resemblance between parents and descendants is, in some cases, extremely striking, and has long been an object of research. The greatest attention was paid to the constitutional characters of the body, especially the height of the body; Among other properties, the most commonly investigated factors were some characteristics of personality, for example intelligence. A relatively large number of papers could be collected on this topic. Somewhat different is the study of different motricity manifestations or functional physiological characteristics related to motricity efficiency; In this regard, we have only partial results, which are generating further studies, but without allowing more conclusive results.

One of the first works worth mentioning is Cratty's research (1960). The author evaluated the effectiveness of male children and their fathers in four motricity tests (jumping in length, repetitive lifting, obstacle jumping, 100-yard run) and examined the results by correlation analysis. In jumping in length and running 100 yards, there was a relatively high degree of dependence (0.87 | 0.59); In the other two tests the correlation was reduced (0.38 and 0.04). Although the research's attention was different, given the relatively large size of the group (4,000 students and their fathers), the data obtained is interesting.

The study of *Jarosz* and *Wolanski* (1967) deals with elementary motricity manifestations. The aim of the research was to evaluate the influence of heredity and the environment on the ontogenetic changes of the proprioceptive perception quality in relation to the spatial characteristics of the movements (motricity precision). To this end, the authors surveyed 102 families with children aged over seven years. From the results and the correlation evaluated among all family members, some interesting conclusions were drawn. The conclusions show that there are considerable individual peculiarities between the properties characterizing the proprioceptive perception and the precision of the movement. They are especially genetically conditioned, while the influence of the environment and of the training is complementary. During ontogenesis these properties change to a certain extent; The greatest similarity between parents and children was found around the age of eight and after the age of 15.

Montoye, Mejznar and Keller (1975) carried out extensive research, consisting of the dynamometric assessment of the maximum static force level (flexion and flexion of the elbow) and physiological and functional factors of blood circulation and respiration. The number of subjects surveyed was quite high, namely, 2,500 boys and 2,000 girls and their parents. The analysis of the results was done in somewhat unusual way, without calculating the correlation or regression coefficients, however the conclusions were very objective. There was an obvious correlation between the level of parental and muscular strength of their parents, as well as between brothers and sisters. Compared to the height of the body, the correlation found is somewhat lower, but it does not differ from other features (fat, heart rate during exercise, etc.). A higher likelihood was generally seen in younger children.

From the point of view of enumeration of applied motricity tests and other evaluated characteristics (somatic characters, functional factors of circulation and breathing, etc.) as well as from the point of view of the current research scale (children and young people aged 18 years and parents Their results are very interesting, published by *Wolanski* and *Pizuk* (1973), *Wolanski* and *Kasprzak* (1976). These are data on the correlation between family members in muscular strength tests (hand force, shoulder force and back lifting force), tests aiming at the coordination and accuracy of hand movements, balance state of the body, flexibility of the joints, Motricity reaction velocity and several other factors. The authors attempted not only to assess the degree of similarity between related subjects but, in particular, to establish within the limits of ontogenesis the age periods in which the likeness is higher or lower. *Wolanski* believes that there is a so-called optimal (likely) period for developing various motricity skills. It follows from the above that the correlation between parents and their children changes to a certain extent, not only in terms of type of test, but also in terms of gender and age of children, and also depending on how the relationship with their parents is evaluated.

From these research results the considerable influence of heredity, which is manifested almost in all the motricityized predispositions investigated, as well as the importance of the influence of the environment. The greater or lesser influence of each of these factors depends, in particular, on the stage of ontogenesis.

The evaluation of the maximum static force (hand pretension, rear lift) and fine hand and fingering movements (paper pencil sensory tests, especially applied in psychological diagnosis) also constituted the object of the research *Kovar* (1980). The survey was conducted on 60 boys aged 16-17 and on both their parents.The results of the correlation and regression analysis are shown in Table 52.

Table 52

Coefficients of correlation and regression calculated on the basis of the relationship, Mother and son (Kovar 1980)

Test	r_{FS}	r_{MS}	r_{FM}	r_{PS}	$r_{FM, S}$	b_F	b_M
Hand dynamometry	0,309	0,067	0,264	0,326	0,285	0,313	0,015
Back dynamometry	0,071	0,164	0,261	0,180	0,164	0,031	0,156
Easy knock (number of strokes)	0,120		0,255	0,069	0,276	0,103	0,250
Load and maze (time)	0,241	0,216	0,442	0,342	0,268	0,181	0,136
Maze task (number of errors)	0,098	0,244	0,075	0,143	0,255	0,080	0,238

rFS, rMS, rFM - correlation coefficient between father and son, mother and son and father and mother;
rFS - correlation coefficient between mid parent and son;
rFM1S - multiple correlation coefficient between father, mother and son;
bF1bM - the child's regression coefficient relative to father and mother.
Statistical significance: x-p = 0.05, xx-p = 0.01.

The correlation found in the manifestation of the maximum static force (flexion of the elbow), evaluated in this case at a kilocorp, ie a relative value, showed an obvious resemblance between fathers and sons (r-0.682). This relationship is shown on a correlation diagram.

Drozdowski (1978), on 42 subjects, studies the relationship father, daughter, daughter, based on motricity tests. The tests used were the length jump - as an indicator of the lower limb's explosive force - and the bending forward of the trunk - as an indicator of the flexibility of the joints. The highest correlation appeared in the pre-torsional test in the relationship between daughter daughter (0.44) and daughter father (0.38).

Montoye and *Gayle* investigated the resemblance between parents and their descendants in terms of maximum oxygen consumption. The closest relationship was found between sons and fathers, when the latter were under the age of 40 (r-0.066). The same factor was the subject of the above-mentioned research by *Wolanski* and *Kasprzak* (1976). As in other tests, in this text the correlation is conditional on the ontogenesis stage, oscillating over the entire extent of the correlation coefficient, ie from 0 to values close to 1. There are obvious differences in sex: it seems that up to aprox About the age of 18 there is a higher degree of similarity in the relationship of parent boys, but after this period the correlation in the relationship of the parent daughter increases, while the likeness of the boys is very low. More equal results occur with respect to the factors investigated afterwards, respectively in terms of heart rate after a standard exercise (step test). In this case, in the course of ontogenesis there is a higher degree of similarity in the relationship of parents, but the correlation coefficients do not exceed the value of 0.50. With respect to daughters, a certain degree of similarity was found only around the age of 15 years.

If we make a general assessment of the contribution of works to research the similarity between parents and their descendants in terms of motricity test results, the following comments can be made. For most of the investigated skills, we have found statistically significant correlations that underlie our assessment of motricity skills and have demonstrated some degree of similarity between parents and their children. Regarding the contribution of environmental influence, the empirical correlation coefficients have approximated in a number of cases the theoretical values of the coefficient of affinity. This highlights the importance of hereditary predispositions and acquired from parents. On the other hand, in many cases there is no greater accentuation. Therefore, the important influence of the environment should not be overlooked either. It also results in a series of data based on longitudinal research. A group undergoing uniform training shows parallel changes of group members, although differences within the group become less obvious due to the faster development of subjects with a delay caused by environmental factors. The stability of the positions within the group is all the greater as the genetic determination of a given character is better (*Ulbrich*, 1972, *Swarz*, 1975). As such, in a group of identical individuals, those who have a reduced value of a certain character at the beginning of the observation period or experiment present this low value and at the end of the observations. The same applies to subjects with a high value of a character within the group (*Astrand*, 1963; *Volcov*, 1974, etc. - quoted by *Swarz*, 1976). However, the values of the characters in a group must not be distorted, in the case of different subjects before the beginning of the observation period, by a specific way of ife that differs from that of other members of the group. In other words, the group can not present internal differences caused by the effects of different living and living conditions before the start of the experiment or observation.

The degree of stability of group positions can be assessed by calculating correlation coefficients between character values at the beginning and at the end of the experience in the same individuals. For example, the stronger the correlation between the values of a character in the same individuals at the age of infancy or childhood and its value in adulthood, the greater the heritability of this character.

Genetic determination of the characters of motricity activity is also evidenced by the regression that occurs after the end of the training. It is well known that the results obtained in sports, youth practicing sports in clubs, are much less during the holidays, when the training is not supervised by an instructor (*Denisiuk*, 1961; *Raczek*, 1971; *Strzyzewski*, 1971). More evidence similar to the one above provides a short-term observation of trained characters. Under the same training, better-performing subjects perform smaller increases in character value than those with poor results. It is believed that the rate of improvement of the results is even slower as the degree of character development is higher in relation to the maximum possible degree in a given individual. This is a genetic mechanism for protecting the body against the undesirable effects of environmental or lifestyle factors. A disadvantage of the longitudinal study method is the difficulty of determining whether the way of life of all children in a lot was previously identical and whether they participated in the same exercise program. The result in sports is determined by many hard-to-measure health items. It can cause deviations in the development of a given character to be developed by training, and these deviations are not necessarily produced by genetic factors.

Data on individual peculiarities in the development of various motricity skills and their degree of stability during ontogenesis is based on the results obtained through longitudinal research. Studies of this type are much less numerous than research based on a cross-sectional investigation, but the major difficulty is that they generally pursue another purpose.

A number of authors have dealt with the question of the long-term stability of the results of different motricity tests and the possibility of indirectly assessing the degree of genetic conditioning based on human aptitude and motricity manifestation. Some authors have highlighted inter-individual differences in various motricity activities, finding that subjects maintain individual differences and peculiarities even in adulthood (*Gesell*, *Ames*). A research on a larger group of subjects, which has lasted several years, along with data correlation analysis, has provided extra and more objective data. The results show that individuals often tend to maintain their group position throughout ontogenesis and that a lot of motricityic predispositions are probably related to the genetic predispositions of the subjects. The starting point of the above mentioned conclusions is the relative stability of the results of some motricity tests, at the same time, it turned out that in other cases the stability of the results is diminished and therefore the possibility of influencing the given properties is relatively high. More in-depth analysis of accessible data is now required.

Based on published results, we can get detailed results of correlation analysis, along with other necessary information (gender, age, description of a test, research period, etc.). These data serve as a basis for a study of longitudinal stability coefficients for certain types of motricity activities and elementary motricity capacities. The values of these coefficients are shown in Tables 53 59.

As you can see, correlation coefficients differ between them. This has a number of causes, such as the duration of a research, different age groups, gender differences, differences in the selection of subjects, different levels of motricity efficiency, various motricity activities, tests and different ways of assessing Efficiency, etc. Differences between correlation coefficients result largely from differences that start from the theoretical characteristics of the correlation coefficient, such as the measurement of longitudinal stability. This is a selection feature with a certain error and confidence interval and its value depends, among other factors, on the correlated data variant. In view of these facts, the differences found are not as great as they seem at first glance (with a few exceptions). A very important finding is that, in almost all cases, the correlation coefficient exceeds 0.50, indicating at least an average degree of stability of the investigated factors.

In Table 53 are presented the results of the tests of short distance running tests (30,50, 60,100 m), which serve to evaluate the speed of running ability, as well as longer distance runs (100 m and 12 minutes run), as Indicators of total aerobic resistance capacity. In both cases, the stability of the results is relatively high, with the correlation coefficient ranging from 0.51 to 0.91. From the point of view of the investigated capacities (running speed, total aerobic resistance, running capacity) no obvious differences are observed, but on average, the girls' category appears to have higher stability values. The results of the jumping tests based on which the predispositions to the explosive strength of the lower limbs are evaluated (Table 54) correspond almost completely to the previous ones. And in this case there is a relatively high degree of stability in both boys and girls. A positive feature in the length jump test is a relatively high homogeneity of the calculated correlation coefficients (within the limits of 0.58 0.78). It argues in favor of the determined genetic nature.

Table 53

Longitudinal stability of the results in running tests

Test	Age limit	Gender	Corelation coefficients	Author
30 m run	7-12		0,55	RARIK, SMOLL 1967
30 m run	7-12		0,88	RARIK, SMOLL 1967
30 m run	12-17		0,52	RARIK, SMOLL 1967
30 m run	12-17	M F	0,69	RARIK, SMOLL 1967
30 m run	10-15	M F	0,70	RARIK, SMOLL 1967
50 m run	13-16	M	0,63	GLASOW, KRUSSE
60 m run	13-16	F F	0,71	1960
50 m run	11-14	M F	0,51	MATOUSKOVA,
50 m run	11-14	M	0,91	NEMCOVA 1973
100 m run	16-19	M F	0,82	MARTINEC, KOVAR
100 m run	16-22		0,74	1979
300 m run	13-16	M F	0,52	KOVAR, PODDANY 1977
		M F		MATOUSKOVA,
1 000 m run	16-18		0,75	NEMCOVA 1973
1 000 m run	16-22		0,74	KOVAR, PODDANY 1977
12 m run	11-14		0,64	MARTINEC, KOVAR
12 m run	11-14		0,67	1979

Table 54

Longitudinal stability of results in jumping tests

Test	Age limit	Gender	Corelation coefficients	Author
Standing long jump	7-12	M	0,66	RARICK, SMOLL 1967
Standing long jump	7-12	F	0,78	RARICK, SMOLL 1967
Standing long jump	12-17	M	0,73	RARICK, SMOLL 1967
Standing long jump	12-17	F	0,66	RARICK, SMOLL 1967
Standing long jump	10-15	M	0,74	GLASSOW, KRUSSE 1960
Standing long jump	13-16	F	0,61	MATOUSKOVA, NEMCOVA, 1973
Standing long jump	10-15	M	0,61	ELLIS, CARRON, BAILEY 1975
Standing long jump	16-18	M	0,63	KOVAR, PODDANY 1977
Standing long jump	16-22	M	0,59	KOVAR, PODDANY 1977
Standing long jump	11-14	M	0,58	MARTINEC, KOVAR 1979
Standing long jump	11-14	F	0,62	MARTINEC, KOVAR 1979
High jump	13-16	F	0,64	MATOUSKOVA,NEMCOVA 1973
Long jump	15-18	M	0,52	SIRIS 1973
Long jump	13-16	F	0,67	MATOUSKOVA, NEMCOVA 1973
Long jump	11-14	M	0,58	MARTINEC, KOVAR 1979
Long jump	11-14	F	0,84	MARTINEC, KOVAR 1979

The discarded tests, which serve to assess the explosive force of upper limbs, have a different characteristic (Table 55). Corresponding correlation coefficients are, on average, lower, but on the other hand some of them have a relatively high degree of accuracy (0.84, 0.78, 0.74). Taking this into account, it is difficult to draw a precise conclusion. Besides, there is less factual data on this type of test compared to the previous one.

Table 55

Longitudinal stability of results in discarded tests

Test	Age limit	Gen der	Corelation coefficients	Author
Throwing the cricket ball	7-12	M	0.47	RARICK, SMOLL 1967
Throwing the cricket ball	7-12	F	0.40	RARICK, SMOLL 1967
Throwing the cricket ball	12-17	M	0.40	RARICK, SMOLL 1967
Throwing the cricket ball	12-17	F	0.29	RARICK, SMOLL 1967
Throwing the cricket ball	13-16	F	0.84	ESPENSCHADE 1940
Throwing the cricket ball	11-14	M	0.78	MARTINEC, KOVAR
Throwing the cricket ball	11-14	F	0.74	1979
Throwing the grenade	16-18	M	0.50	KOVAR, PODDANY
Throwing the grenade	16-22	M	0.53	1977
Throwing the ball at the target	11-14	F	0.22	MATOUSKOVA, NEMCOVA 1973

Table 56

Longitudinal stability of results
In the test following the influence of a repeated or long effort

Test	Age limit	Gen der	Corelation coefficients	Author
Hanging the arm bent	10-15	M	0.65	ELLIS, CARRON, BAILEY, 1975
Hanging the arm bent	11-14	F	0.87	MARTINEC, KOVAR, 1979
Shoot up (hoops)	11-14	M	0.80	MARTINEC, KOVAR, 1979
Recovery (from sitting position)	10-15	M	0.63	ELLIS, CARRON, BAILEY, 1975

Test results that investigate the predispositions for local (static or dynamic) muscular resistivity or the dynamic strength of the resistance character are shown in Tables 56, 57. They show a high degree of stability.

The smallest amount of information refers to the longitudinal stability of joint flexibility: there are researches conducted by only two authors (Table 58). Determination of this type of motricity predisposition seems to be the highest compared to other evaluated properties. The cause is probably a close connection with the somatic character and the structural properties of the body constitution, which are generally known to be more conservative in their development compared to functional properties.

Table 57

Longitudinal stability of joint flexibility test results

Test	Age limit	Gender	Corelation coefficients	Author
Flexion of the elbow	8-12	M	0.75	RARICK, SMOLL 1967
	8-12	F	0.69	
	10-17	M	0.62	
	10-17	F	0.35	
Knee extension	8-12	M	0.54	
	8-12	F	0.69	
	10-17	M	0.74	
	10-17	F	0.64	
Flexion of the elbow	10-16	M	0.63	CARRON, BAILEY 1974
Extension of knee	10-16	M	0.51	BULGAKOVA,
Prehensiunea	11-14	M	0.74	VORONCOV 1976, 1978
	11-16	M	0.78	
Trunk extension	9-15	M	0.65	BALDWIN 1920
	9-15	F	0.45	
	11-14	M	0.77	BULGAKOVA,
	11-16	M	0.77	VORONCOV 1976, 1978
	11-14	M	0.62	
	11-14	F	0.69	MARTINEC, KOVAR 1979
gripping	9-18	M	0.63	
	9-18	F	0.57	
The sum of nine basic (main) muscle groups	12-15	M	0.85	TUDDENAM, SNYDER 1954
	12-15	F	0.79	JURINOVA 1977

Table 58

Longitudinal stability of joint flexibility test results

Test	Age limit	Gender	Corelation coefficients	Author
Flexibility of the shoulder	11-14	M	0.83	BULGAKOVA,
Flexibility of the shoulder	11-16	M	0.81	VORONCOV 1976,
Flexibility of the ankle joint	11-14	M	0.90	1978
Flexibility of the ankle joint	11-16	M	0.88	
Tacking the trunk forward	11-14	M	0.88	MARTINEC, KOVAR 1979
Tacking the trunk forward	11-14	F	0.78	MARTINEC, KOVAR 1979

The research carried out by Bulgakova and Voroncov (1976, 1978) offers a possibility to evaluate the longitudinal stability of the notation results, under the conditions of a systematic training and involving intensive solicitation, the group consisting of specially selected subjects within the population. Stability of results is high in all cases (only boys have been investigated).

Interestingly, in the case of longer swimming cycles, which for the most part require aerobic conditions, stability is higher than in the case of a route which is largely anaerobic (Table 59).

Table 59

Longitudinal stability of swimming performance results

Discipline	Age limit	Gender	Corelation coefficients	Author
100 m crawl	11-14	M	0.79	BULGAKOVA, VORONCOV 1976, 1978
100 m crawl	11-16	M	0.65	
200 m crawl	11-14	M	0.61	
200 m crawl	11-16	M	0.65	
800 m crawl	11-14	M	0.93	
800 m crawl	11-16	M	0.89	

There is another methodological approach, closely related to the results of the longitudinal stability assessment using the correlation coefficient. It consists in continuous research of subjects with varying levels of initial results in areas of the so-called nomogram of development. The interpretation of the results is the same as for the correlation coefficient; The only difference is "the level of differentiation of developmental changes". The measure is the number of individuals who have maintained their development trend and the number of those who have deviated to some extent. In the above-mentioned way, Jurinova (1977) investigated the longitudinal trends of developing the maximum static force of different muscle groups, assessed dynamo-metric. This author found that more than 70% of the boys and 60% of the girls maintained their limits in a battery of various motricity tests (running 50 m, running 12 minutes, jump in length, cricket, torso bending, lifting force with the dynamometrically assessed back), the proportion of subjects who stayed in those areas varied between 22 and 60% (various tests, both sexes) (Kovar). On the other hand, in some of the older researches (Kovar, Poddany, 1977), in relatively homogeneous conditions the following data were obtained: running 100 m - 89, 3%, running 1000 m - 82, 2%, jumping In length - 85, 7%, throwing the grenade - 82, 2%. These values are high, proving the considerable stability of the test results in that group (boys aged 15-19 years). An illustrative example is that of FIG. 129 showing the individual development of two subjects with different results at 1000 m (subject A - high value, subject B - low value). None of them has deviated from the area over the years.

Changes in motricity efficiency manifestations that accompany an individual during ontogenesis can also be evaluated from the point of view of their size and intensity. The question is to what extent the magnitude and intensity of the changes mentioned above are linked to a hypothesis on the relationship between genotype and environment and the conception that the possibilities of influencing a particular property are determined by its level of development.

A number of authors who have dealt with these problems, unfortunately, few, have concluded that the highest increases in the results of various motricity tests are usually found in subjects who are initially Weaker. In the course of subsequent development, however, they almost never exceed the subjects who were initially the best. It is assumed that one of the characteristics of a sports talent is also a higher level of adaptability and development of the respective predispositions, together with the predispositions for the acquisition of movements.

This is why this type of subjects has the highest increases. Siris (1973) pointed out the above phenomenon in terms of the possibilities of predicting motricity development and the need to select subjects with sporting talents. The pace of development is considered to be a very important selection criterion and usually insists more on it than on the initial level of a subject that is influenced by the previous motricity experience and the conditions in which the subject was raised. When we evaluate the results of the research on the stability of the different predispositions and manifestations of motricity efficiency, results obtained in order to study heredity, we can say that they are an important basis for further research. They support the findings of other methodological approaches and are also an impetus for further research, especially on the practical application possibilities (eg when selecting talented subjects for sports activities, etc.).

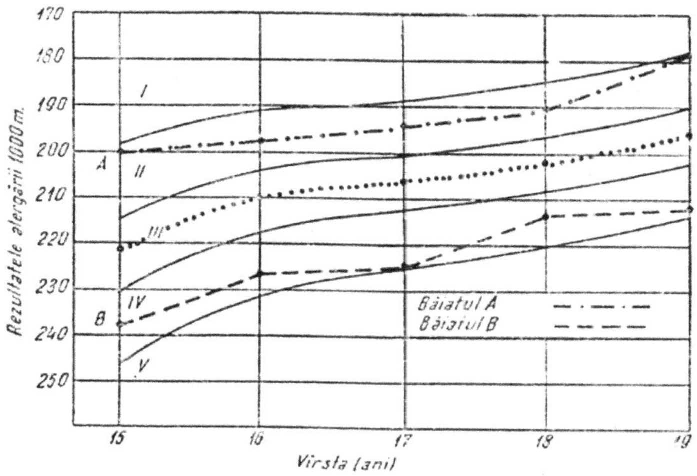

Fig. 128. Running results per 1000 m to two monozygotic twins (The rate of progression resulting in the degree of heritability).

The variability of the level of the various properties and motricity capacities during the overgrowth is shown to have considerable individual particularities in some cases. They are, on the one hand, generated by the genotypic predispositions of a subject (which is evidenced by the stability of the various properties) and, on the other hand, by the influence of the environment in the case of an imposed effort. Some of the motricity predispositions appear to be more stable ("conservative") and some less stable. Among the relatively more stable are the majority of structural properties (eg, somatic characters). This is the articular flexibility, the speed of running, some types of force velocity predispositions and functional predispositions of total aerobic capacity. As far as the abovementioned capacities are concerned, the level of final development depends to a large extent on the initial level, even in the case of optimal environmental conditions. From the point of view of individual development, it can be assumed that a subject has a certain tendency to be in a particular development area, the limits of which are determined by the genetic norm of reaction. The probability of deviation from this area increases with the diminution of the stability of the given character (property, ability) and extreme influence of environmental conditions.

The stability of various motricity predispositions is closely related to the possibility of intentional foresight and influence. The more conservative a property is, the better the prognosis, but at the same time the possibilities for influence and development are more limited. Thus, we come to the same conclusions as those based on the results of twin studies. The sporting performances of the best subjects in the population are, to a certain extent, the level of a person's motricity skills at a given time. The level proves to be relative, being time-bound, but there has always been a difference from the peak of the average population. A number of issues arise in connection with this, for example, what are the characteristics of these subjects, to what extent do they differ from the average population, on what their particular performance is based? These questions and others have played an important role in studying the selected characteristics of performance athletes and their families. Following the information on the issues mentioned above, we will turn our attention to facts about individual hereditary predispositions.

There are a number of examples of so-called "sports families" in sports practice. These examples often support arguments about the influence of hereditary predispositions and the genetic conditioning of man's sports skills. For the first time these facts were highlighted in the literature by Grebe (1956). After the previous study of the similarity of twins, he underwent a number of well-known athletes for genetic analysis using genealogical diagrams, explaining the dominant character of the transmission of sports predispositions. Sports talent appears in several forms, and therefore Grebe believes he is conditioned by several independent genes.

A complete and comprehensive study referred to the issue of "sports heredity" and was conducted by *Moser* (1960). In its introduction, it provides an overview of the historical development of breeding between races, and with this example it proves the hereditary basis and the dominant character of the transmission of motricity capacities. He then presents some genealogical diagrams of famous, randomly selected sports families, as well as examples of athletes from various sports disciplines. The total number is quite large - over 100 examples - but unfortunately the author did not attempt to analyze more objectively the data obtained. The conclusion of the research, based on the genealogy analysis and the results of Grebe, reveals the elements of efficacy of limiting sport efficiency.

A very concise and interesting paper dealing with the use of the findings made in the selection of sports talents was published by Line and Fleischman (1970). They relied on Grebe, Gedda and Moser's findings, adding personal examples. They predicted the use of family analysis to select talented young people for sporting activity and to study motricity skills in other similar Professions, for example artists.

An extensive and labor-intensive, organizationally, research into the genetic aspects of the limiting sports effectiveness of participants in the Olympic Games was carried out in 1968 in Mexico (*Garay, Levine, Carter*, 1974). In research, in addition to other factors, we evaluated the level of "sporting skills" of both parents with the help of a questionnaire and a three-point classification scale. The study included 1,221 athletes from different countries and a control group of 366 subjects. The results, together with the analysis of the statistical data, showed that there is some link between the sportive efficacy of parents and their children, but the data are not very conclusive. The authors explain the situation by the fact that performance athletes tended to underestimate the level of their parents, while the subjects in the witness group overstated it.

Some genealogical data on the hereditary predispositions of a sports talent are presented by *Kodym* (1975). It is based on a large-scale questionnaire survey of 200 former Czechoslovak performance athletes (155 men, 45 women). The data obtained relate, among other things, to the state of health, physical fitness and sports activities of parents and siblings. Regarding the health of parents, she was rated as very good at 74% of fathers and 70% of mothers; 65% of fathers and 55% of mothers were classified as very effective, and 12% of fathers and 8% of mothers were classified as poorly effective. Motricity activity was tracked at 40% of fathers, 26% of mothers and 33% of siblings. Approximately similar was the objective of a questionnaire survey conducted by Kovar in 1975. It included 128 performance athletes (83 men, 45 women); Data were processed on male and female categories and on individual and collective sports. To compare the batch with the average population, we used some previous data and additional information. The results of the research are as follows: In over 50% of cases, performance athletes' brothers (sisters) are also active athletes and their physical fitness is high (or at least average), based on questionnaire and qualitative assessment Within the selected categories. Athletes' performance sports performance is relatively high compared to the average population. The proportion is approximately 50% of fathers, 1/3 of mothers and 1/4 of both parents (mother and father), considering all cases. The frequency of a mum or father with reduced sport efficiency is very low and there is no case where parents are poorly effective. The number of subjects with sport activity in the entire genealogy investigated is on average higher than in the average population. At first generation (grandparents) is about 1/10, in the second generation (parents and their siblings) is about 1/3 of all cases. The research of performance athletes' genealogies is closely related to the study of other characteristics, which may relate, for example, to some biological aspects of individual development, to the particularities of body constitution, to the character and level of predispositions we consider to be the most important and decisive of limit sports performance. A series of information refers to the social, material and training conditions, to the environment in which a subject has grown, at the time he started sports training, to the training and training system.

One of the issues examined by Garay, Levine and Carter in the study of participants in Olympic Games was the influence of birth order on the level of sport efficiency. The problem is usually studied in terms of the psychic predispositions of an individual; In this case, however, it was applied to motricity skills. The results show that most athletes are children of the second birth; but if there are more children in the family then they are the firstborn. Based on their research and other studies, the authors conclude that the order of birth seems to be in some relation to efficiency, but the cause is unknown. It can be, for example, social influences (more care for firstborns, etc.).

The same problem was the subject of a research by *Billo* (1958) on over 1,000 performance twins. According to his data, 50% of performance athletes are the firstborn of the family. The factor was also investigated by *Kovar*, who found that 40.3% were the firstborn, and 37.3% came from the second birth. Relatively interesting results have been obtained through the research of body weight at birth and the evolution of birth. In most cases, the birth of athletes was normal without complications; In terms of weight, the average value exceeded the average (*Kovar*), especially female gender. More pronounced differences than among the mean values are observed in the weight distribution. A comparison of these data, obtained at performance athletes, with data on students at the Faculty of Physical Education and Sport in Prague, as well as with non-sophisticated girls of the same age in the average population is significant. It can be seen that the sport efficiency level route corresponds to that of the weight distribution. Regarding the fact that in most sports, subjects with a higher height, with a more developed muscular constitution and, implicitly, with a higher weight, achieve higher successes, an appropriate explanation can be found.

Other information is related to ontogenesis, illness, complications, health, etc. Some of these factors have been revealed in connection with *Kodym's* research, other data have been obtained by *Kovar*. In this respect, the athletes' statements about the character of their physical and motricityic predispositions in childhood are interesting. Most subjects claim that they were more agile and more "manual" and that they tended to acquire new motricity skills quickly (50.0%). This is especially evident in female sex, especially in individual sports (76.7%). In men's collective sports, basketball and volleyball, an important factor is the height of the body. There is also a link between polymorphic and quantitative characters. A relatively independent research group includes studies on the evaluation of the interdependence of polymorphic character manipulation, the so-called markers, with the level of development of selected characters having a type of polygenic heredity, ie quantitative characters. Thus, for example, mention is made of the relationship between certain types of dermatoglife or selected blood groups and the manifestations of sport efficiency. Greater attention has been given to these issues by the authors cited above, *Garay, Levine* and *Carter*, in their research into Olympic athletes. They took fingerprints at 1127 athletes in 92 countries, correlating the number of papillary lines found with certain sports predispositions. They classified sports as follows: explosive force sports, speed sports, strength and coordination.

Another object of their research was erythrocyte antigens (especially ABC, MN, Rh systems), erythrocyte enzymes and erythrocyte proteins (especially hemoglobin). As in the previous example, they also attempted to determine whether the empirical frequencies of the occurrence of the investigated characters differ for different types of sports and differ from the expected (theoretical) frequencies. Other results have also been obtained, which deserve attention. For example, *Kasierska* (1978) studied the most common type of dermatoglyphs in handball players. This researcher believes that some types may be characteristic of this activity.

The research of lip line types in a batch of sprinter women and handball players was conducted by *Drozdowski* and *Ziolkowska* (1978). Compared to the normal population, they noticed some tendencies that allow a link to be established between the character being investigated and the type of sport activity. The research was carried out on a lot of subjects.

A large-scale research, with the aim of studying the links between blood antigens and the results of various motricity tests, was conducted by *Silla* and *Teoste* (1976). They surveyed 1978 schoolchildren aged 17-17 under the blood groups 0, A, B, AB, and test results on dynamometric muscle strength test, speed and coordination of hand movements, various runs, Jumping, throws and several other parameters. Comparison of the mean values of the results of the various motricity and blood group tests mentioned above has shown that the level of motricity skills seems to depend very little on the frequency of occurrence of blood antigen variants. There is some connection to a young age in boys. Concerning the frequency of blood groups, in the case of speed and coordination activities, the most frequent group was group B, and in the case of force type activities, group AB.

Lukojanov, Sarec and *Kononova* (1976) correlated the research of markers with the investigation of the intracerebral differences of the twins. On a batch of 26 pairs of mono-zigzag twins of both sexes, they watched their motricity development, especially the beginnings of sitting, orthostatism and walking. At the same time, they studied the type of dermatoglobes; Based on their results, they claim that this factor can be correlated with the level of motricity development. However, the authors do not explain this in detail.

The method of genealogy analysis is used in the case of performance athletes, to which the notion of sports talent is usually associated. The results of the genealogical studies show that there are other subjects with motricity skills in the families of these athletes. Their number is considerably higher compared to the average, normal population, which is demonstrated by an illustrative example of the so-called sports families. The deficiency of the above mentioned studies is especially the fact that the method of genetic analysis is not appropriate for quantitative characters, because it does not allow the influence of genotype influence on the influence of the environment. The results obtained may be used to illustrate and support the concluding results obtained by the previous methods. From this point of view it can be deduced that the achievement of a higher level of sport efficiency is most often related to a certain number and a certain structure of the genotypic predispositions, which manifests as hereditary predispositions and which the descendants inherit from To their parents and ancestors.

The above statement is in line with the results of research into the characteristics selected at performance athletes. Achieving sport performance is proving to be conditioned by the fulfillment of vital biological, vital and ecological conditions. These factors are decisive for achieving and developing the genotypic predispositions of a subject, and for the most part they can not be replaced. Also, a high degree of heritability has both the concentration of cortisol in the blood (the main hormone involved in the effort) and the elevation of the level of this hormone during the effort. Thus, h2 is between 0.57 and 0.60 and the correlation coefficients mother / child, father / child and ranges between 0.54 and 0.84, which is essential for the selection in sport, where the level of the effort capacity Mainly by hormonal constellation (cortisol, catecholamines, thyroid hormones, androgens and estrogens) is essential (*B. Raczynski* et al.).

*

* *

Concluding on the heritability of the motricitying typology, we emphasize, even at the risk of repeating itself, the following elements that we consider important. Given the differences in the results obtained by the method of studying twins, by correlating parental children or by various psychomotricity tests, it is not possible to present a uniform synthesis of studies conducted so far. Most of the divergent results were recorded in twin studies, but this method has so far provided the most data on motricity skills. The question now arises whether such a divergence of results is evidence of failure or whether, as *Nikitjuk* (1976) stated, it is due to differences between different populations, which would mean that heritability will be different depending on the development of a Certain motricity character in the population concerned. The assertion is not unreasonable because the assessment of heritability in twin studies depends on the variant, and this may depend on the value and degree of differentiation of character in different populations. The context shows the need for a critical approach to attempts to assess the role of genetic and environmental factors without taking into account the living conditions of the studied populations. It would be completely useless to expect an identical heritability of a character under different conditions because the genetic factor usually acts with equal force (and in any case is structurally homogeneous), while the environmental factor Or the way of life is extremely labile. Therefore, their proportion in any condition and therefore in any population may be different.

In the results of *Wolanschi's* studies by child parent correlation method, the strongest genetic determination among all the psychomotricity characters studied was observed at the muscular force of the hand, measured with a dynamometer (the force of the flexor of the hand and forearm). Genetic determination of humeral muscle strength was lower, and that of lumbar muscles weaker. The greatest resemblance between parents and children was observed with regard to hand and shoulder strength, at about 10-11 years old, and in terms of lumbar muscle strength, at about 13-14 years of age.

A slightly weaker parent parenting correlation was conceived for the reaction time to acoustic and optical stimuli. The correlation of tactile response time was moderately intense. A particularly high similarity between parents and children is observed at the age of 11-14 years of children. There are correlation coefficients for children, raised, for the speed of hand movements, and the coefficients of rotation speed around the longitudinal axis of the body showed a significant correlation coefficient. Controversial views on genetic determinations of the force and speed of movements resulted from studies on twins. Some authors conclude that the genetic determination of the force and speed of movements is similar (*Eysenk* and *Prell*, 1951), while other authors have found that the speed of movement depends more on genetic factors than the force of movements (*Sklad*, 1973; *Savatiejeva* 1976; *Szwarz*, 1976). It has also expressed the view that power is more dependent on the speed of genetic factors, as demonstrated by twin studies (*Osato* and *Avano*, 1957) and studies on the likeness of the son father (*Cratty*, 1960). *Osato* and *Avano* considered that the highest differences between the pairs of monozygotic and dizigito twins were found to be discarding, followed by differences in shoulder and back strength, and the smallest differences were found at the speed of running. *Cratty* observed a greater correlation with dynamic strength than speed, and the correlation to force testing was the lowest in the test battery used by this author. The answer to this question lies in the type of tests used to evaluate these two characters. First of all, as we know today, the separate characters have correlation coefficients for parents older than the groups of characters. This has been demonstrated, among other things, for the size and shape of the head and face (*Siniarska*, 1977) - the diameters have shown higher correlation coefficients. It is also known that genetic determinations are greater in elementary motricity skills than in associated skills.

From twin studies it can be concluded that the above results could shed light on this controversy, as it was demonstrated that maximum heritability in all rapidity tests was recorded at 10 m (*Nikitjuk*, 1973), followed in Logical 20 m (*Savatiejeva*, 1976), 30 m (*Zaciorskj* and *Sergienko*, 1976) and 60 m. On the other hand, heritability is higher for the 60-100 m race than for skiing. The heritability of the force also depends on the type of test performed, being higher for the strength of the hand (its value is of the heritability for the 10 to 30 m run), less for the force of the knee and elbow flexors and extenders (heritability for Running 60 m) and even lower for the strength of the back muscles and the explosive force measured by throwing the ounce ball.

An interesting result was obtained by Sergienko for the total force of 20 muscle groups and for the force expressed in kilocorp. The heritability of the force of certain muscles and the relative force (per kilocorp) is much higher than the total muscle force. It can be said that the strength of the hands, the speed of a simple reaction and the speed of the short-distance running have the greatest genetic determination. uch genetic determination decreases when the treadmill increases and when "bigger muscles or whole muscle groups" are recruited or the total force of the various muscles. It thus offers the possibility not to engage in basic combinations of movements but to engage in complex combinations of forces that require force and speed. Explosive force measured by high jump or long jump shows a relatively strong genetic determination. On the other hand, the explosive force of the upper limbs, measured by the throwing distance of the ounce ball, has an exceptionally low heritability. These results were obtained in twin studies and require confirmation by other methods.

Interesting results have also been obtained by studies (on twins) that determine the speed of light impact (on both upper and lower limbs). Fast hand movements performed in thermometer tests as well as twin studies have shown a high heritability (*Wolanski*). Flexibility has a relatively high heritability index. The value of this index is much higher for the movements of the humeral joints than for the column. Visual motricity coordination has a moderately intense genetic determination (tests on a thermometer without a mirror), with particularly high correlation coefficients being observed between the ages of nine and 12 and in adults.

For the sense of balance measured by rotation tests and walking on a narrow beam, we found a high genetic determination (*Wolanschi*). A similar parenting of older children was observed at the age of 10 11 years. Testing of twins by orthostatism on one leg showed a strong genetic determination of the sense of balance. The sense of balance is an elemental element with strong genetic determination. The precision of the movement has a high heritability index. Heritability of skill is high. This skill is obviously complex because it is made up of many elementary characters. Wolanski presents contradictory data in this respect.

Analysis of the genetic determination of motricity skills in humans suggests that general motricity activity has the strongest genetic determinations (*Kogan* and *Antipov*, 1974), followed by the force and speed of movements. Some parameters of skill (co-ordination, balance) and resistance have a strong genetic determination. Resistance to obesity, as it demands a maximum and long effort, can be assumed to have its strong genetic determination. In the studies published so far, men have usually shown a higher genetic determination of psychomotricity development than female investigators, although some studies have obtained reverse results. It is usually considered that precision movements are more strongly genetically determined in girls, while movements that involve force and rapidity are more strongly determined in boys. There is no gender predominance with regard to coordination.

Due to the role of certain genes present in chromosome X, there is a greater similarity of characters to female twins than to males. There are similarities in the correlation between male and female pairs of monozygotic twins, while in disseminated twins the likeness is usually much higher between female twins than between males. The difference between VMZ - VDZ correlation coefficients among girls is lower than between boys and girls (*Nikitjuk*, 1976). At the age of three to five and six or seven, the correlation between pairs of twins decreases, which probably corresponds to "school effort" (*Wolanski* 1962, 1964, *Tanner* 1968). Differences between twins diminish (correlation increases) at the age of seven and eleven, and then grow again until the age of 16-18. Characteristically, the smallest resemblance of psychomotricity characters between parents and children is observed in the prepubertal period (*Wolanski*, 1976) and during puberty, a little earlier for psychomotricity coordination and later for reaction and efficiency time. Similar results have been obtained in studies on electrophysiological and psychophysiological characteristics.

Cyclical changes in heritability have been observed even with regard to bone dimensions (eg metacarpal bones). These changes vary for the different dimensions of the same bone (*Bulayeva, Antipov* and *Krasikova*, 1976). From birth to pre-puberty, the role of the genetic factor increases, while the age of puberty decreases. In Soviet research, this decrease was observed at the age of 10-15 years in boys and 12-13 years in girls (*Nikitjuk*, 1974, 1976). Thus, a reduced heritability is observed in prenatal life, early childhood and puberty, periods that are known to be related and increased susceptibility to environmental factors. This correlation does not seem to be accidental. There is considerable concordance between changes in child parenting correlation coefficients and the dynamics of developmental processes with the aging of offspring (*Wolanski*, 1976). Rapid growth periods, which are likely to be genetically determined (*Wolanski*, 1976), usually precede periods of diminished similarity of the psycho-motricity characteristics of children and parents. Changes in resemblance are probably a secondary, delayed consequence in particularly rapid development periods of a certain character. Since the rate of development is genetically controlled, it can be said that the leap within itself is a mechanism for increasing the organism's susceptibility to environmental factors and lifestyle, a mechanism for increasing the adaptability of the body. It is obvious that characters with stronger heritability and lifetimes in which the parent-child similarity is increased, create unfavorable situations for factors that stimulate character development. Rather, selection methods should be applied based on these external characters of the individual's life with favorable conditions for, for example, a certain type of sport.

- Correlation between asymmetry, lateralisation and motricity development

Functional ambivalence and somatic asymmetry are considered examples of genetic determinations of development. It is important that these phenomena and their anomalies, such as functional asymmetry and morphological asymmetry, be explained as a contribution to studies on the heritability of motricity characters. It was noticed that the correlation of parental children, in many of the motricity skills studied by us, is stronger for the right hand than for the left hand. This is true for motricityized visual coordination, for precision of movements and speed of movement. Higher heritability of straight-hand force than left-hand force was also deconstructed as well as a higher heritability of the rapid movements of the superior and inferior right and equilibrium (in the orthostatism test on a Foot - *Stock*, 1973 - it was shown that the right leg orthostatism is more hereditary transmissible than that on the left leg). In many twin studies, it has shown a higher heritability of the right hand characters compared to the left hand. Exceptions to these studies were found only for mild injuries.

The genetic determination of lateralisation is also evidenced by the presence of morphological and functional asymmetry in young children before the age of walking (asymmetry crossed - *Wolanski*, 1957) and the absence of an increase in the degree of asymmetry with aging, With the exception of athletes and workers who carry heavy manual labor with one hand. Morphological and functional asymmetry decreases with age in men in rural areas and increases in those in urban areas. This is closely related to the motricity function and the positions adopted during the work. The functional asymmetry of the extremities is intensified in the course of office activity and in urban life conditions to a greater extent than in manual labor on farms, where both ends are more uniformly engaged in work.

The similarity of parenting children also diminishes with aging in terms of the precision of left hand movements. This observation supports the hypothesis that lateralization (functional asymmetry and dynamic asymmetry) is mainly genetically determined because the right hand, which is used more frequently, has more similar functions in parenting than the left hand, which is less used. Potentially frequent use of the right extremity should be reflected in greater differences between results, with a consequent decrease in heritability. The result obtained in this regard is analogous to the results of tests on the rest and post-exercise values of the physiological characters discussed above. This is further evidence that not only functional and somatic characters are under genetic control, stronger than the least used in motricity activities. In connection with this, functional asymmetry may become more pronounced during fatigue.

Morphological asymmetry, which persists without modification or even diminishes with age, despite the increasing lateralisation with age (functional asymmetry) in the population (*Wolanski*, 1972) proves that there is a limit to the stimulation of somatic structures development. This again supports the need for high sporting performance, the first stage in training athletes. In a second stage, selected subjects should undergo selective training, depending on their somatic and physiological predispositions for a particular sport discipline.It is important to note that morphological asymmetry increases at the age of puberty, at that time of life when the similarity between parents and children diminishes (*Wolanski*, 1976). This shows that better results can be obtained through motricity exercises performed at the age of puberty or generally at the age of diminished heritability.

In the issue of asymmetry, there is considerable interest in observing (but requiring confirmation) that, in general, subjects with the dexterity of both extremities are less effective than subjects with a net dexterity prevailing at one end. Measurements suggest that lateralisation may be associated with some more general neuromuscular specialization for physical fitness, but it is not known whether it will include a general or special aptitude. However, on the left, the activity of the alpha waves on the electroencephalogram is lower and the reaction to the hyper ventilation is increased. On the right, the EEG activity is more intense in the left hemisphere, which is not observed in the left (*Subiranc* et al., 1952). This could suggest a difference between the right athletes' predispositions compared to the left-handed ones. Regarding the correlation between symmetry and skill, we note that the latter is also defined by some researchers with the term coordination or agility. To highlight the coordination or agility, we also used the following tests:

- Rotation during jump (also described for highlighting symmetry). This is done on a 1 m, 2 wooden platforms with an engraved circle having a diameter of 80cm and along its circumference a gradient from 0 to 360° separated for the two right and left directions. Each subject performs rotation as a jump in both directions.
- Zigzag running on a set track, timed with photoelectric cell up to hundredths of a second
- Running with rotation.

These last two tests also require changes in the position of the general center of gravity and thus the balancing of the vestibular device. The three samples were used to test the fighters by giving a global score on which selection is made (*W. Staroste*).

Table 60

Elements that condition the coordination of motricity act

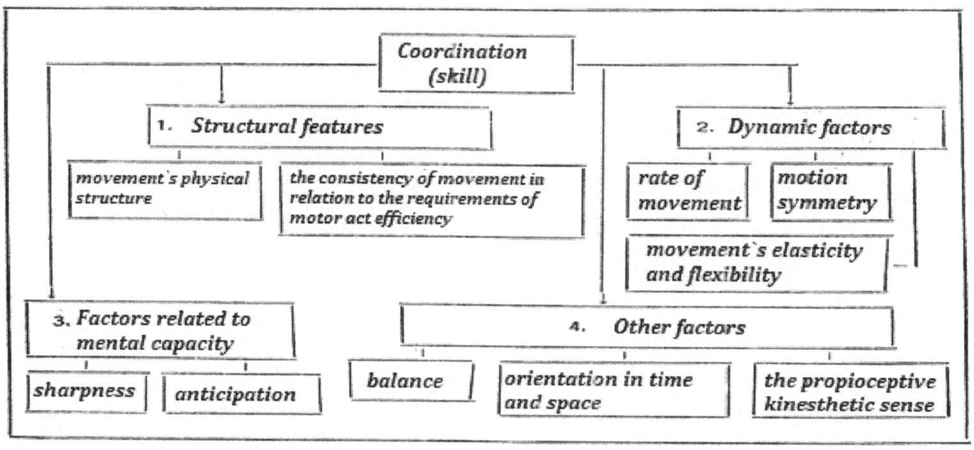

Table 61

Results of motricity movement indicating the degree of symmetry and coordination on top performances in various sports disciplines

Sports discipline	Rotation in degrees				Granting on a scale	Place
	right	left	difference	Right-Left		
Artistic skating (seniors)	695,5	767, 3	71,6	1463	96	1
Judo (seniors)	407	449	42	856	57	2
Classic fights (juniors)	396	483	16, 6	810	54	3
Free Fighting (seniors)	371	406	34, 9	778	52	4
Free Fights (juniors)	365	390	22	758	50	5
Judo (juniors)	362,3	387, 7	25, 4	750	50	6
Free Fighting (seniors)	366	380	13, 1	747	50	7
Ski (jumping from the senior trampoline)	372	369	3	741	50	8
Canoeing (juniors)	343, 6	358, 4	15	702, 2	47	9
Kayak canoe (seniors)	343, 6	339, 7	3, 9	683, 3	45	10
Ski (jump jump jumping)	339, 4	340,6	1,2	680	45	11
Canoeing (juniors)	324	348	24	672	45	12
Weightlifts (juniors)	334, 4	329, 6	4, 8	664	44	13
Weightlifting (seniors)	305	319	14	624	42	14
Rowing (seniors)	304, 8	316, 8	12	621,6	41	15

Typical psychological characters

We will not present this issue in its complexity because it belongs to psychology. We will only stop on the very close interrelationships between mental capacity and skill. As we have previously explained, skill is not so much a motricity quality, but rather an expression of complex functional results involving mainly superior nervous activity, balance, coordination, and extra-pyramidal leadership circuits. The muscular factor and the locomotricity system, as a whole, have a lower contribution, being just the effects of a complex command.

In this context, we emphasize that recent research shows the high degree of hereditary determination of superior nerve activity. We consider that, in assessing the level of brain function, one can really use the level of intelligence that is, in fact, a global parameter, by intelligence, understanding the individual's adaptability to different situations in the external environment (*M. Maliţa*). In sports activity and especially in certain branches, such as sports games, fencing, boxing, etc., the ability to make an adequate response to the adversary's actions is essential, in this context, motricity intelligence is only the stereotype of general intelligence, which explains Why this is essential for determining success in various sports disciplines. Of course, there are a number of difficulties related to the current state of knowledge, both in terms of defining and measuring intelligence. Undoubtedly, we must admit that the measured intelligence only partially covers all the cognitive skills and that the investigated individual's tests are not a strictly authentic expression of his intellectual possibilities.

The tests used are various, of which we quote *Binet - Simon, Terman - Merill, Wechsler*, all aiming through a set of varied tests to measure the global intellectual capacity of the subject, general intelligence. The results are currently expressed by the intelligence coefficient (CI) represented by the ratio (multiplied by 100) between the mental age and the actual age (Figure 129, 130). The distribution of the intelligence coefficients among a certain population is normal, ie it is expressed by a Gaussian curve whose average - m - which is confused with the median - is 100 for an unselected sample of an "accidental" population. Indeed, tests are built and staggered in such a way that the performance distribution is made according to this law, and more precisely that the type deviation is 15 or 16. In this normal distribution, nearly 70% of the flock has a C.I. Between m a and m + a (here, 85 and 115), about 95% between m 2a and m + 2a (70 and 130) (*Larmat*). Subjects with a C.I. Over 130 are indeed an intellectual elite. Under 70 or 80, C.I. Expresses a more or less pronounced debility.

Among the many factorial systems - none of which seem to be yet likely to express the true diversity of cognitive skills - those that have been most used in intellectual genetics work are PM A. (*Primary Mental Abilities*) Of Thurstone and the one working with *Differential Abilities Tests* (DAT). In the issue of asymmetry, there is considerable interest in observing (but requiring confirmation) that, in general, subjects with the dexterity of both extremities are less effective than subjects with a net dexterity prevailing at one end. Measurements suggest that lateralisation may be associated with some more general neuromuscular specialization for physical fitness, but it is not known whether it will include a general or special aptitude. However, on the left, the activity of the alpha waves on the electroencephalogram is lower and the reaction to the hyper ventilation is increased. On the right, the EEG activity is more intense in the left hemisphere, which is not observed in the left (Subiranc et al., 1952). This could suggest a difference between the right athletes' predispositions compared to the left-handed ones. Regarding the correlation between symmetry and skill, we note that the latter is also defined by some researchers with the term coordination or agility. To highlight the coordination or agility, we also used the following tests:

- Rotation during jump (also described for highlighting symmetry).

This is done on a 1 m2 wooden platform with an engraved circle having a diameter of 80 cm and along its circumference a gradient from 0 to 360 ° separated for the two right and left directions. Each subject performs rotation as a jump in both directions.

- Zigzag running on a set track, timed with photoelectric cell up to hundredths of a second
- Running with rotation.

These last two tests also require changes in the position of the general center of gravity and thus the balancing of the vestibular device. The three samples were used to test the fighters by giving a global score on which selection is made (*W. Starosie*).

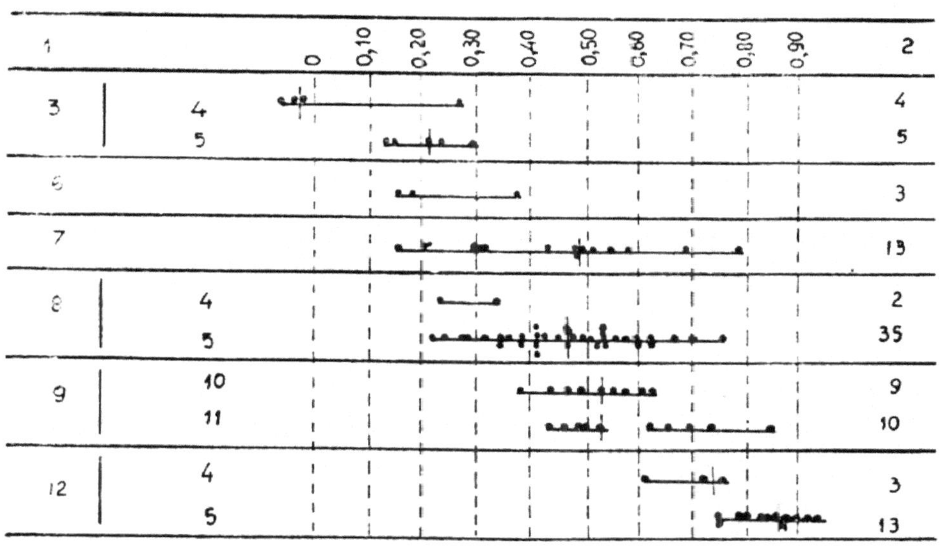

Fig. 129. Distribution of heritability coeficient on intelligence.

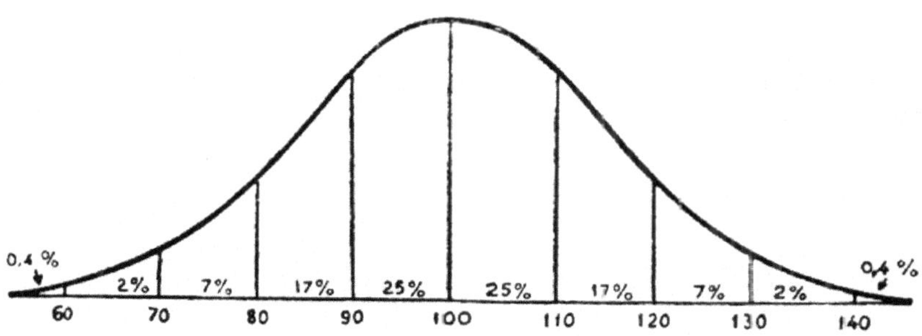

Fig. 130. The curve of intelligence coefficients in a population group.

In the issue of asymmetry, there is considerable interest in observing (but requiring confirmation) that, in general, subjects with the dexterity of both extremities are less effective than subjects with a net dexterity prevailing at one end. Measurements suggest that lateralisation may be associated with some more general neuromuscular specialization for physical fitness, but it is not known whether it will include a general or special aptitude. However, on the left, the activity of the alpha waves on the electroencephalogram is lower and the reaction to the hyper ventilation is increased. On the right, the EEG activity is more intense in the left hemisphere, which is not observed in the left (*Subiranc* et al., 1952). This could suggest a difference between the right athletes' predispositions compared to the left-handed ones. Regarding the correlation between symmetry and skill, we note that the latter is also defined by some researchers with the term coordination or agility. To highlight the coordination or agility, we also used the following tests:

- Rotation during jump (also described for highlighting symmetry).

This is done on a 1 m^2 wooden platform with an engraved circle having a diameter of 80 cm and along its circumference a gradient from 0 to 360 ° separated for the two right and left directions.

Each subject performs rotation as a jump in both directions.

- Zigzag running on a set track, timed with photoelectric cell up to hundredths of a second
- Running with rotation.

These last two tests also require changes in the position of the general center of gravity and thus the balancing of the vestibular device.

The three samples were used to test the fighters by giving a global score on which selection is made (*W. Staroste*). The method of family inquiries is undoubtedly the first whose principle comes to our mind, and it is known that *Galton* used a - but without too much rigor - to establish his hereditary thesis. It consists of comparing, among a large number of families, the intelligence of the children with that of their parents and that of their brothers and sisters. It is therefore based on C.I. To some and to others.

Here, as an example, the conclusions of one of the most carefully conducted investigations, that of *Conrad* and *Jones* (1940). They subjected to intelligence tests 977 people aged three to 60, belonging to 269 families in the rural districts of New England. The correlation coefficient between C.I. Of parents and children is 0.94 and the same value is found for the correlation between siblings (it is 0.45 between same-sex children and 0.54 among children of different gender).

In most of these surveys, close results have been obtained. In their journal Science (1963), *Erlenmeyer Kimling* and *Jarvik* retained 12 of them, in comparison to C.I. Of parents and children and 35 to that of C.I. Of children in the same family. For the correlation coefficient between parents and children, the values are elapsed between 0.25 and 0.80, the average being 0.50.

For the correlation coefficient between siblings and siblings, the results are between 0.30 and 0.78 averaged at 0.49. Thus, from the results of family inquiries a very clear conclusion emerges: statistically, children are intellectually resembling with their parents, as well as with their brothers and sisters, more than with aliens of the same age. More specifically, the correlation coefficient found between C.I. Of the compared categories is very close to the coefficient (0.50) that we could expect to find, starting from a certain genetic model, if the similarities between C.I. Would only hold the possession of common genes.

Several studies have been conducted on temperaments, alcoholism, mental illness, spatial perception, intellectual characteristics, etc. But the fundamental object of psychological genetics has been the issue of mental capacity, especially because of the widespread conviction that social success in society Industrial modernity is increasingly dependent on the ability to reason. According to this conception, cognitive ability determines the ranking at the finish line in the "race for life" Thorndike spoke about. From a technical point of view, intelligence could be taken as an objective due to the creation of tools that are said to measure differences in cognitive capacity; These tools have been called intelligence or intellectual quotient tests (Q.I.) (Quotient Intellectuel).

First Q.I. were developed in 1903 by *Alfred Binet* in France. Its purpose was to identify among those with unsatisfactory school results those who are likely to benefit from a recovery activity. The test highlighted memory, vocabulary, and the ability to distinguish associated elements. This test was then modified in the U.S. by *L.N. Termon*, to become Q.I. of *Stanford Binet*, which is still valid today. By adapting *Binet's* test, *Termon* (and, in general, those who have undergone mental testing) introduced a subtle but fundamental change of destination. From a test that initially aimed to find dyslexic children who could benefit from a recovery, it was turned into a method of classifying all children according to an intrinsic mental capacity scale, supposedly independent of education and experience. Convincing that Q.I. measure something intrinsic to the individual, regardless of any influence on living conditions, is not a random feature of Q. 1 tests but lies at their base. Intellectual coefficient expression derives from the operation consisting in dividing the gross result obtained by the test into a factor that is age dependent. Thus, the test is offset for each age group, depending on the major changes that occur during the development of intelligence. Those who developed these tests also canceled the influence of gender, eliminating the questions that boys and girls give statistically different results. It is also stated that these tests are neutral in culture, some are even considered independent of the linguistic baggage of the test person, which of course is wrong with verbal tests. A considerable effort, however, allowed for the development of nonverbal intelligence tests, so as to avoid the cultural differences.

An individual who repeats at short intervals Q.I. Obtains sixth results; But as more years pass through the evidence, the more the results will be different, especially if the second test is done in adulthood. The different parts of a Q.I. test, like vocabulary, analogies, structure recognition, etc., are in a relative correlation with each other, as they are in a relative correlation and different tests, whether verbal or not. This correlation between tests or parts of tests should be evidence that they measure all a general background intelligence (called "factor g") that manifests in different ways but which itself constitutes a characteristic of the organism that is not susceptible To develop with age or to be influenced by the environment. Thus, the ideology of the tests tends towards a biological explanation of the differences in the results. This makes it easy to "demonstrate" the hereditary character of intelligence.

- *Evaluation of heredity* Q.I. average Q.I. is 100, and the standard deviation is 15 points on either side of the average; Its shape in the bell is called normal distribution. These characteristics are not very conclusive, as the tests were designed and the notation system was adopted in such a way as to produce a normal distribution of the results with an average of 100 and a standard deviation of 15. It is to be remembered that when The Japanese version of *Wechsler's* intelligence scale for children was developed, it was conceived in such a way as to lead to this normal distribution to children from Japanese schools. Convinced that establishing heredity Q.I. Would have important consequences for social practice, some psychologists have made considerable efforts to divide Q.I. In a genetic fraction and a determined fraction of the environment, so as to establish the ratio between the genetic variant and the total variant, or the heritability (H2).

The higher the degree of affinity between individuals, the higher the correlation coefficient between Q.I. of those individuals is higher. Median correlations between parents and children or between bivitelini twins are approaching in all cases with a genetic predictability of 0.5. Unrelated individuals have a lesser correlation; Instead, the correlation is very high in the case of true twins. All Theories of Causality Q.I. but predicts an increase in correlation depending on the degree of kinship, so these data do not give us too many elements.

For QI heritability assessment, comparisons have been used very frequently on the one hand between people with the same degree of genetic affinity but different living conditions and on the other hand between people living in the same environment but not related. Test results

Q.I. To the latter does not of course have any correlation when they are grown separately but has a correlation of approx. 0.25, when the tested individuals were raised together.

Comparison of existing correlations between Q.I. Adoptive parents and children adopted on the one hand, and biological parents and their own children, on the other hand, also shows the effect of living conditions. At the other end of the stairs, Q.I. Of true twins have a correlation of 0.88 when they are raised together and 0.75 when raised separately. This again reveals the effect of a common family environment. If we look at the results, we can see that there are several ways to evaluate QI's heritability, which all agree to assign a fairly high value. The 0.25 correlation found between unrelated individuals raised together can be considered as a direct assessment of the influence of a common environment. Univitelin twins raised together share both genes and the environment; In this particular case, the correlation is approx. 0.87. Considering the effects of the same environment, we can estimate heritability as 0.87-0.25 = 0.62. Another method can also be used: the standard comparison between univitelini twins and bivitelini. The median correlations being 0.87 and 0.53, can thus be written as:

$$H^2 = \frac{rU - rB}{1 - rB} = \frac{0.87 - 0{,}53}{1 - 0{,}53} = 0{,}72$$

So it results for H2 of Q.I. A significant value.

Another way to address the issue of the hereditary environment is based on the study of capacities manifested by monozygotic twins separated from the early and raised in different families. The results obtained by Newman, Freemon and Holzinger are significant. The mean of differences within pairs between C.I. Of the 19 pairs of separated univitized twins (most before the age of one) was 8.2 points (or six after Woodworth's correction), while for unmarried children living in distinct families, she was in the order of 17 points.

The correlation coefficient within the pair expresses these findings more precisely. (Newman, Freedman and Holzinger, Burt, Shields) and the average value of Erlenmeyer Kimling and Jarvik (Table 62).

Table 62

	Newman and col. After correction		Burt		Shields	Erlenmeyer - Kimling and Jarvik
MZ twins raised separately	0,77	0,73	0,86	0,77	0,77	0,75
For comparison: Brothers and sisters raised separately			0,42	0,41		0,42
MZ twins raised together	0,88	0,92	0,92	0,94	0,76	0,87
DZ twins raised together	0,63	0,62	0,53	0,55	0,51	0,53

The conclusion appears clearly: the influence of heredity seems to be very strong, because among the separated twins raised in different families, monozygoties endowed with the same genotype have C.I. (R = 0.75 0.80 approximately) than non-twin siblings and sisters sharing only half of their genes (r = 0.42 approximately). Also, based on twin measurements, several authors have calculated the heritability value of C.I. Here are some results:

- *Newman, Freeman and Holzinger* (1937): from 65 to 80% (68% with Binet's test);
- *Woodworth* (1941), based on the "corrected" results of the previous: 60%;
- *Burt* and *Howard* (1957), with two different tests: from 77 to 88%. We note that, as far as the intellectual level is concerned, there is a tendency towards "marriage between those who resemble". The correlation between C.I. Of the spouses is, indeed, quite high: usually in the order of 0.40 to 0.50. This tendency towards "assorted marriages" alters some correlations, for example, covariance between brothers and sisters. For, to the extent that this phenotypical similarity corresponds to a similarity of the genotype - which is obviously lower, since the sought-after heritability is inferior to unity - to the same degree, the parents will share a proportion of genes (favorable or unfavorable) superior to those that result from Marriages "at random".

Children will therefore have more than half of their alleys. Also, heritability models built by geneticists should consider this trend towards homogamy. It follows that, due to the convergence of more research (population studies of the twinning method), we know that intelligence depends on hereditary factors and that - under equitable social conditions - it is distributed regularly (in Gaussian curve, according to the statisticians) from The lowest levels at the highest levels. At the same time, we must signal an essential factor, which strikes on the value of the intelligence coefficient results. The attempts to estimate heritability are based on the hypothesis that differences in performances of comparative subjects allow the evaluation of differences in intellectual skills. But this means forgetting the important role of motivation. As rightly pointed out, children do not solve any problem with intelligence alone. Not only knowledge acquired by them, largely dependent on the cultural environment, provides them with tools for this task, but also their curiosity, their willingness to understand, the habit of reflecting their success. Solving problems depends, in part, on the motivations they have developed in the course of their mental evolution. These motivations may at the same time have a hereditary basis and an ambiguous origin: they are, in any case, distinct from a cognitive aptitude that, of course, does not exist in pure state. They give us an additional reason not to accept the high values proposed by some authors for the heritability of intelligence too easily.

The elements presented above fully justify the need to test the intelligence coefficient in parents to estimate and predict what the child will become at peak performance. Certainly, there are a number of imprecisions, but doing this intelligence test, simple to execute, is likely to diminish the unknown. For sports, fencing, boxing and other sports, where skill-based skill-based intelligence is essential, this selection test is required.

Lately, in the definition of intelligence, an essential parameter is the ability to anticipate (*Mircea Maliţa*). In sports, and especially in some of the sports disciplines, such as games, scribbling, boxing, etc., anticipatory ability is essential to victory, as predicting the opponent's intention and anticipating it is often the decisive factor in achieving performance. Anticipation is the ability to cope with new situations, perhaps not met; Is the test stone for innovative learning processes. Anticipation is the ability to meet the future, to predict the chain of decisions and actions. It not only involves learning from experience, but also "experimenting" with substituted or imagined situations. A particularly important feature of anticipation is the ability to explain unforeseen side effects or "surprise effects" as some call them.

Moreover, anticipation is not limited to encouraging desirable directions and avoiding potentially catastrophic directions: it "invents" and creates new alternatives where they were not at all. In other words, anticipation saves the valuable process, but time consuming, lived experience, anticipation helps to avoid shocking, traumatic and costly lessons. In adaptive, unanticipative learning, all we do is "react" and seek answers when it's too late to apply solutions. We show great insensitivity to small but critical signals. Since innovative learning highlights the possibility of acting in new situations, investigating what is possible or feasible to happen becomes one of the main pillars of the learning process. At present, however, anticipation does not play a sufficiently important role. Some are tempted to reduce anticipation to the faculty that forms the foundation: the imagination. Anticipation, of course, requires imagination, but it must not be confused with it. Anticipation can be just as cold, prosaic, and full of data as accounting evidence. Many of the examples of anticipation are like archaeological excavations: both are based on the search for palpable facts, although one projects us back in time, while the other one is ahead. Anticipation in the form of projections, forecasts and scenarios is already fundamental to future studies, but is by no means limited to this area. In fact, there are anticipatory branches for all human activities.

Despite this thriving renaissance of anticipatory activities, our current learning concepts and processes do not seem to take too much advantage of them. Learning is not sufficiently anticipatory in the overall processes of the decision-making society, nor in education systems.

Anticipation is more than an act of mental simulation. It is an omnipresent attitude.

Anticipation is far more than the probability measure. It is, above all, the creation of possible and desirable future forms, as well as the choice of plans and actions designed to produce them.

The transition from simple design to more and more refined is seen in the field of modeling and simulation. Currently, modellers are faced with the most important prediction test: can models be developed to help formulate and create new events that are not yet on the list of desirable or unwanted events? Anticipation, as an important part of innovative learning, is inseparable from an increasing emphasis on conjectures, assumptions, scenarios, simulations, patterns, directions, plans, and forecasts. By emphasizing the importance of anticipatory capacity in defining as much as possible the reality of intelligence, which implies adaptation and anticipation, it is necessary to test the athletic potential of the anticipatory potential through the existing physiological and psychological methods.

Only such a vision allows us, both in the selection and the training, to find the optimal ways to develop and select subjects with a high level of biopsychometric skill of skill, especially in sports where they are pregnant. We mention that this quality recognizes a high degree of heritability, which requires a rigorous testing as complete as possible in the ascendants' genealogical tree.

CHAPTER IX.
SOME ANTHROPOLOGICAL AND GENETIC ASPECTS ON SPORTING SELECTION

Achieving performance in sport is conditioned by four important factors: the athlete's attitudes, the training developed, the athlete's attitude (interests, aspirations, motivation, the social situation of the subject concerned, the social environment of the subject), the social and material ambience Which is the sport activity (*Epuran Mihai*).

Of these four factors, an increasing role has recently been given to the aptitudes and the totality of genotypic and paratipical characters that provide the necessary potential to achieve performance in a sporting branch, characters to be potentially estimated on the occasion of the actions Selection. At a recent FIMS Congress held in Rome, it was concluded that in achieving performance, 70% of the selection and 30% of the training are available to allow the upper limit of genetic adaptability for the potentially hereditary characters possessed by a subject. Based on the anthropological genetics data presented above, it is clear that peak results in a field can only be obtained by a subject with exceptional genetic equipment. Hence the special importance of sports selection. We emphasize that, in anthropological view, selection is a process that must be carried out throughout sports training, in this sense it is necessary to have a thorough knowledge of the anthropological age-specific features of the body that I have presented in a previous chapter. Selection must be as effective as possible; If it is currently averaged over 1 out of 100 subjects, it should become 1/1000 1/10000 in the future to avoid as much as possible the investment of labor, moral and material capital in subjects who, at The age of maximum performance, do not become optimal anthropological guys on the sporting industry and are not competitive on the basis of somatic, motricity and psychic qualities, in great confrontations for the achievement of high performances. The selection also has a series of limits related to:

- late maturation of skills and personality dynamics;
- the analytical investigation of the somatic, motricity and psychic type, which is not entirely conclusive, since, in the body, as it is said, since the great Aristotle “the whole is not equal to the sum of the parts”;
- analytical parameters may not be appropriate, but overall the body responds to superior performance requirements and vice versa;
- the contradiction between the voluntary nature of sport and the great responsibility of the performer; Sometimes, the athlete, for lack of responsibility, does not engage in plenary so as to capitalize on his full biological potential to achieve performance.

The selection can be:

1. Spontaneous, which is done exclusively thanks to the subject's desire to practice a certain sporting branch.
2. Empirical, what is done by a coach with a great experience, who selects a subject that apparently does not have the somatic, motricity and psychic qualities necessary for the respective sporting branch.

We emphasize that neither spontaneous nor empirical selection should be ignored, because the human body is particularly complex and its knowledge is totally far from being realized; In the case of spontaneous selection it is an inner motivation which, with special volitional resources, can be decisive for the perforation, and in the empirical selection the “eye of the coach with great experience” acts, which, Through the synthesis it carries on the body, can conclude more than a sum of analytical tests that we perform at the scientific selection, whose role we do not minimize in any way by giving the importance to the coach's experience;

3. Scientific, aimed at establishing the somatic, the motricity and the psychic type, based on the tests that I have presented in the chapter of anthropological constitutional typology. We reiterate the idea that the three sections defining the constitutional type have a different weight in different sporting branches and, at the same time, there is the possibility of comparing these three parameters between them.

We emphasize that scientific selection is essential to achieve performance, as I pointed out initially. In our country, thanks to the researches of Prof. Dr. Nicu Alexe and Assoc. Prof. Ion Dragan, there is a national system of selection consisting of tests and methods of biological diagnosis and technical sports proofs for each branch of sport, which proved efficiency.

In the following, we present a series of data that complements this system on anthropological and genetic basis. As we know, as selection is a process, we still mark certain stages of selection depending on the age of the selected and the sporting branch concerned, materialized by what we define as initial, secondary and final selection, the final one having to achieve the optimal anthropological type On the sport branch.

The current trend is, for a number of sporting branches, to make the initial selection at a lower age, linked to the complexity of the technical tactical training in most sports and, on the other hand, Motricity drives and the development of physical qualities should be done gradually, well-dosed, in relation to the anthropological peculiarities of age, even from the pre-pubertal stage. In this context, it is questionable whether the topic selected for sports at a very early age will become or not an optimum anthropological type which, at the maximum perfection level, can be truly competitive at the highest level. The decline of the unknown in this field is due to a better knowledge of the hereditary background, which can be achieved through a selection based on anthropological and genetic bases. We present the main stages of genetic selection and the main morphological, physiological, motricity and psychological parameters, with high genetic and corollary value, and thus value in selection. We will seek as far as possible to point out only those biological parameters that have been extensively analyzed in previous chapters, detailing only what has not been presented. The methodology of anthropological and genetic selection is carried out over several stages:

1. The biochemical analysis of the constitutional type is able to provide us with corollary information on the genetic configuration of the individual. The importance of this investigation is special. We quote, for example, that the potential rate of insulin production, an important factor in sports performance, ranges from very broad ranges, from 10 to 40%, which are mainly related to hormonal interrelations with pituitary, thyroid, adrenal, and liver. In the same vein, we can quote the individual conditioned genetic variations, resonant in the efficiency of sports training, regarding iodine concentration (2.5 11.5%), plasma catalysis, serum lipase, beta6 - conjugase (carbonic anhydrase, Interstitial and so on). We also emphasize that each normal individual has a specific endocrine constitution based on anatomic, functional and biochemical peculiarities of each gland and complexities of complex endocrine factors within very wide limits (1-10). Knowing these individualities and, corollary, the genetic structure are of overwhelming importance for achieving the maximum performance of the sports training.

2. Cariogram, a genetic technique by which microscopy is detected, by current or marked thymidine, of the 46 chromosomes. Regarding the cariogram, it indicates, first of all, whether an individual is normal or non-genetically chromosomal, a fact that is particularly important for sports, where a perfect state of health is required. Also, the chirometric determinations (chromosome measurement) give valuable insights on the potential and dynamics of certain somatopathological features such as height, for example, correlated with the shape and dimensions of the U chromosome.

Also within this framework, a special consideration is the determination of genetic sex; It is known that in sports, many female performances (athletics - throws, jumping, kayaking, academic canoeing, swimming, etc.), exceptional performances are achieved by athletes with a high masculinity. The masculinity rate can be determined and predicted by Bayer Bailey's method of establishing the constitutional type presented by us. The high rate of masculinity translates into waist, proportions of body segments, superior motricitying qualities of highly restrained sportsmen (with very marked feminine characters) where the diameters of the pelvis are large, the volume of the mammary glands is considerable, the body mass is reduced in favor of the adipose tissue etc. The fact is also true of male sex, where high-feminine subjects are not competitive with lesser motricitying. We propose in this sense the generalization, as a prospective investigation, of the determination of androgen and estrogen by the Bayer Bailey method, which gives almost certain indications from the antepubert stage on the evolution of the constitutional type - in terms of the degree of proportionality of its somatic sexualization on the masculine or feminine line (It is known that both male and female body possesses both masculine and androgen hormones - and estrogen feminizers - only their proportion varies from sex to gender, there is also the possibility of intersexuality). It follows from the above the importance of determining the genetic sex on the path of the cariogram, both for the determination of masculinity and femininity as much as possible, especially for the detection of intersexual cases.

The problem has become reality since 1936 at J.O. In Berlin, when he began to suspect that a number of Olympic champions would have XY male sex. Subsequent research (*Jorgensen* and *Eberle*) attested that 2 3% of performance sports are intersexual. Normal genetic sex is characterized by the presence of XX chromosomes in female sex and XY in male. If genetic sex is normal, even if the masculinity rate for a sportsman is very high or for athletes, femininity is increased, there are no problems with the right to participate in competitions. These high rates of masculinity or femininity are explained by the high levels of androgen and estrogen hormone secretions. However, if the sex is disturbed, for example in an athlete we encounter male chromosomal confinement XY, it is eliminated from competitions, which is explained by the net morpho-physiological advantages it has in the competition, compared to normal-sex sports.

Diagnosis of genetic sex is done by both the cardiogram and, more easily, the Barr test. The Barr test, entered into the practice of investigating athletes at major competitions, is based on the finding that one of the two chromosomes X of the female organism is inactive (Mary Lyon) and condenses to form X chromosome which is a triangular formation glued to Internal face of the nuclear membrane. It is very noticeable at the level of the cells in the oral mucosa which, especially colored, have a hypercalcemic triangular area in the membrane of the female membrane, which is considered positive Barr. The male sex, which has only one X chromosome that is active, does not have that corpusculus and is therefore a negative Barr. Performing this test is of particular importance at the time of selection because it eliminates the possibility of investing moral and material capital in a sportsman who, due to such genetic disorders, can be eliminated from a large competition, thus constituting an important loss for those who have prepared a Great performance. Such cases were the first time in the world athletics championships in Budapest. Also in the determination of the genetic sex there is a method similar to the Barr test for highlighting the Y chromosome. The cells in the oral mucosa, especially colored and now viewed with fluorescent light, have a small fluorescent point due to fixation of the fluorochrome on the long arms of Chromosome Y. The number of points is equal to the number of Y chromosomes. Thus, there is one point in a man, and one normally does not. We mention that the XYY formula exists in man, which also translates into the existence of two fluorescent light points in the above test. Male subjects of formula XYY are normalized, but have been found to have a waist size above 1.90 and have motricityized strength and resistance to very elevated parameters. Research on athletes reveals the existence of a higher percentage of those with outstanding performance, especially in the samples where the strength and strength of this formula is required. Hence the importance of detecting by this method subjects having the XYY formula and directing them to the sporting branches where strength and strength are demanded, and they have superior possibilities to achieve it.

3. Family survey correlated with the somato-physiological characteristics of the individual; In this respect, the investigation of the genealogy tree, correlated with some anthropometric characteristics, provides significant relationships to the biological potential of the individual. Also within this framework is the constitutional type. In defining the constitutional type, investigation based on anthropological methods is essential. In this context, sports anthropology is becoming more and more pronounced. We quote some relatively recent research that highlights the extremely complicated relationships between anthropology and sport. Achieving performance can no longer be conceived without an in-depth anthropological knowledge of the human individual. The genetic determinism of anthropological parameters is becoming increasingly known, and the correlation between the constitutional anthropological type and the performance in various branches of sport is an element of the first order for achieving some sporting performances. Critical analysis, a mandatory component of biomechanical analysis, sets out the particularities of the execution of different physical exercises, in relation to the constitutional anthropological type, in order to achieve higher parameters in sport.

A method of great value is the study of twins (the performance of the 20-year-old Polish twin sisters, *Małgorzata and Dorota Tlałka*, the slalom world champions at the Sarajevo Olympics, the twin brothers Phil and Steve Mahre in the US who have won the medals Gold and silver at the special slalom in Sarajevo, etc.), namely, the evolution of the morphological and functional characters of the monozygotic twins compared to the dizzy ones. This method can appreciate the erection of some morpho-functional characters based on the differences between the twin partners. Numerous studies have been undertaken, including some of the biological parameters of physical value. Some conclusions could be drawn on the weight of the physical training influence on some of these components or, as Klissouras expresses, the "functional limitation genetic limit".

It has been shown that for each character there is a superior limit of genetic adaptability that can not be overcome. Attaining it undoubtedly competes with favorable environmental factors. Thus, the scientific explanation of the capping phenomenon in sport is to achieve this higher limit of genetic adaptability, which, regardless of the volume and intensity of the effort put into training or other paratipical factors that intervene, can not be overcome. We emphasize that environmental factors, including training, have a determining importance on evolution through the extremely complex phenomenon of mutations, but for sport and performance, it is of immense importance to select subjects with the highest possible genetic adaptability for anthropological characters Which condition performance. Without repeating the data presented in the previous chapter, we underline the fact that, at the stage of family inquiry of genetic selection, the somatic, motricity and psychic qualities of ascendants (parents, grandparents) and collateral relatives (brothers, sisters, etc.) With the correlation and heritability coefficients that allow us to make predictions about the somatic and psychosomatic potential of the selected subject. The foundation of this anthropological and genetic viewpoint is becoming more and more solid lately. It is appreciated that motricity activism, which ultimately is one of the basic parameters of biomotricityity that condition sports performance, recognizes an important genetic conditioning.

The anaerobic mechanism of muscular activity is also heavily dependent on heredity. As a result, aerobic and anaerobic processes are predominantly determined genetically, as demonstrated by the genetic determinism of the percentage of white fibers with a rich mitochondrial apparatus and red fibers loaded with an increased amount of myoglobin. We mention that lately, the stage of investigation of aerobic and anaerobic capacities has only begun to go beyond the determination of components of significant energy equipment in the effort. This highlights the role of the SH and S-S groups, which bring together a heritability coefficient of 85%, and it seems to balance the whole balance of essential amino acids and fatty acids.

It can be concluded, on the basis of these data, that in cyclic sports disciplines, the energy selection criteria (aerobic, for sporting disciplines requiring resistance and anaerobic for cyclic sports disciplines and short time) are quite safe. It is, of course, natural for man's old faculty to run, first, under the influence of genetic factors, while other more complicated ones, such as throwing, jumping, etc., which depend to a lesser extent Of energy processes, - under greater influence of environmental factors. Indeed, the analysis of world and Olympic records from the beginning of the century to the present day shows that the improvement of the results at the throwers has produced 55%, long distance runs only by 12% and sprint with and less - 7%.

It has long been known that in the training process, some qualities develop relatively easily, and others, on the contrary, are very inert and are subject to the influence of training. Thus, speed and skill are very stable, with a very high degree of genetic determination, which requires genetic selection to be performed. As a result of the studies on twins, it was revealed that the influence of genotype on the regulation of vegetative functions was reduced to low efforts than to great efforts. The aspect is very important in connection with the continuous increase of efforts in training in modern sport and the continuous increase of sports results. Only people with proper genetic baggage can remove those hardships they face towards sporting performance. Performance is not only the result of strenuous training, but also of discovering the athlete's determined genetic possibilities. Within this framework, a special mention must be made of the determined genetic reserves of the athlete and of the possibilities to be valued, knowing that even in the sport performance performance the body mobilizes on average about 80% of its metabolic capacity. Also, in this context, we must emphasize that adaptive reactions to athletes over the years show a specific constant. All of this allows us to affirm that individual differences in the level of resistance to insufficient oxygen are largely hereditary. Therefore, they can be safe components in the selection of children for sports disciplines that require a great development of resistance.

Genetic research also shows that compared to the speed, strength, energy (aerobic and anaerobic) energy indicators that are predominantly hereditary, the resistance test indicators are more under the control of external environmental factors. In terms of morphological biotipology, the degree of hereditary determination of the proportions of the body segments and of each segment is now proven. Thus, the height of boys at maturity is equal to:

$$\frac{\text{Father's height (cm)} + \text{Mother's height (cm)} \times 1{,}08}{2},$$

And the height of girls at maturity is equal to

$$\frac{\text{Father's height} \times 0{,}923 + \text{Mother's height}}{2}.$$

Such indices exist almost for all the proportions of the body segments, of which the cranial indexes are under the most stringent genetic control (Fellow Institute data from the U.S.).

There are, of course, variations depending on the determined genetic population. From the table presented, Jan Szopa (Table 63) concludes that the coefficients of correlation between body height in parents and offspring increase with age, reaching the highest values in the highest age groups.

The heritability index of body height also increases with age, with large differences according to the estimation method. Most likely, the Hb value, calculated according to Fischer's formula, amounts to 0.66.

Table 63

Components of phenotypic variation of body height and heritability indices calculated by various methods (after Jan Szopa)

Age grup	Method							From the regression coefficients h^2	From the studies on the pair of h2 data collected by Orczykowska Swiatkowska 1968
	Fischer (1918)			Penrose					
	G_T – Complete genetic variation	H – The heritability coefficient	Ho – The heritability coefficient encountered in an accidental mating	Vd – Variation due to dominance	h^2	$(dr)^2$	Xpe		
3-9	0.80	0.38	0.36	0.42	0.78	0.41	0.09	0.38	0.80
10-16	1.11	0.56	0.53	0.55	1.12	0.39	0.39	0.79	0.87
17-x	1.13	0.70	0.66	0.43	1.18	0.27	0.04	0.78	0.86

Also, in this context we mention the Briant method which showed that the volleyball morphology compared to the control group is megamorphic, harmonic and longiline orientation. The stature is very high (after the Martin scale), the trunk and the limbs are well proportioned (the index = 51.2) and the trophicity is poor (*Rohrer* = 1.18). The harmoniously configured constitutional type has predominant dimensions that express the development in a sagittal sense. The prevalence of thoracic width over its depth and abdomen width explains the trend towards the longline constitution of these athletes (*Martin*, 2007).

By doing standardized anthropograms on age groups, a more efficient selection process can be carried out on sporting branches. The yield increases with their correlation with the degree of hereditary determination of the proportions of the body segments and correlation with the genetic determinism of some physiometric parameters and motricityic qualities. The correlation of these data with the active body index, with a high degree of genetic determination, is of particular importance.

We also note the research that proves the existence of some homeopathic drug constitution, which opens, through their genetic determination and laboratory identification, immense possibilities of efficient and rational use of effort supporters; But if they do not know the genetic biochemical individuality of the body, they can lead to serious disorders.

Determining the degree of heritability of skill-related intelligence also has a special role to play in the selection of athletes, especially for sports requiring mainly skill (the Larmat method).

Dermatoglyphs, who are recognized for a very high heritability coefficient, have also entered the genetics acquisitions. In the last decade, researchers have been interested in the use of stable genotypic indicators, which do not change in the process of ontogenesis and accompany the high development of the motricitying qualities of sports selection and orientation. Studying the dermatological features, *E. Iukojanov, J.D. Sareţ, V. N. Kononova* (1976) revealed the accelerated development of motricityity in children with high frequency of ulnar networks. *B.*

A. Nikitjuk and *V.I. Filipov* (1982) highlighted the dependence between the number of skin ten of the ten fingers and the development of speed and force ratios. *Nikitjuk* studied 13-15 year old teenagers, Ukrainians from Verhnedneprovsk district, Dnepropetrovsk region. The driving qualities were appreciated by the following tests: running 60 m, jumping in pitch, throwing the tennis ball, running 500 m (boys) and 300 m (girls). A total of 256 adolescents of both genders were studied. According to the magnitude of the deviation of the motricity quality from its average arithmetic value, more or less according to the size of the average square deviation, groups of persons with high, medium and low values of these qualities were delimited. The fingerprints and fingers of the investigated persons were recorded according to the method of T. D. Gladcova (1966). The following dermatoglyphic indexes were analyzed: 1) fingers drawings; 2) the place of finish of the main palm lines; 3) the ten-finger comb indicator; 4) the size of the angle etc; 5) drawings on the palms of the palms. Observations have shown that in the 60 m running, indicating the speed level, better performances are achieved by high-frequency boys, such as the ulnar and radial networks. In jump-length jumps showing strength in speed and explosive force, the presence of the arc-type digital model is associated with a higher perfor- manance in both boys and girls. In boys, the model of the ulnar network type also accompanies the higher performance. When throwing a tennis ball that highlights the explosive force, the arc-shaped design can be correlated, both in boys and girls, with the level of performance. In running 500 m in boys and 300 m in girls, marking the resistence, it did not notice any dependence between the type of the drawing and the performance.

In the 60 m high-performance boys, it was often noted that line B was completed in field 7, line C in line 9, line D to 11 (for details on dermatoglyphs, we mention the *Papillary Fingerprint*, by *I. Ţurai*, Medical Ed. 1981). In jump-jumping, high-performance boys frequently encounter line B ending in field 511, line D in field 9. In throwing the tennis ball, high-performance boys often notice the completion of line B in field 7 and line D in 11, and in girls, line A in field 2. In running on 500 m boys and 300 m girls there is no correlation between dermatoglytic particle size and performance. These data show that there is dependence between the level of the development of the motricity qualities and the summation indicator of the palm circumvolutions - SCS. In 60 m running, SCS shrinking is associated with improved performance for both boys and girls. The long jumping with the elk shows the same correlation and the same way when throwing the tennis ball. *Atari* dependencies are not recorded when running on 500 m boys and 300 m girls.

There was no connection between the size of the palm angle and the development of the right hand qualities of boys and girls. Similarly, no diagnostic dependence has been identified in the assessment of the driving qualities related to the drawings of the hypotensive, tattoo, II, III and IV eyelids of the fingers. So, a good speed indicator (after the 60 m running performance is represented by: the frequency on the fingers of the ulnar and radial mesh designs, the end of the main palm line B in the field 7, the line D in the field 11, the decrease in the number Combing on the skin of the 10 fingers (boys), the girls reducing the number of combs on the skin of the 10 fingers. High performance jump in elongated length are accompanied by boys by increasing the intersections of the drawing on the fingers of the arc type and the nets, Line S in field 511 and line D in field 9, decrease the number of combs on the ten fingers, in girls - by increasing the frequency of design intersections on arc-type fingers, lowering the SGS summation indicator In throwing the tennis ball, the high performances are Accompanied by the frequency of the digital arc models and the reduction of the SCS indicator. In 500 m, boys, and 300 m. There have been no links between dermatological indicators and sports performance.

As is known, average sizes level individual peculiarities. In order to define the diagnostic significance of dermatoglyphic markers, the level of development of the motricityic qualities of individuals with the complex of dermatological symptoms presented individually evolved. S proved on the researched works that in boys having the net shape (ulnar and radial), in the 60 m running, the small performance occurs in 8.6%, the average 43.4%, the high 48, 0% of cases on the small SGS indicator (from 109.7 to 131.7 combs), the low performance is 7.4%, the average 59.2%, the high 33, 4%; In the case of line B termination in field 7, small, medium and large performances are respectively 13.1%, 57.8% and 29.1% of the cases; The termination of line C in field 9 is respectively: 6.3%, 49.7%, 44.0%; The completion of line D in field 11 corresponds to 12, 5%, 53.1%, 34.4%. In long jump jumps, individuals with ulnar and radial networks showed low performances in 11.7%, averages in 79.5%, tall in 8.8%; Boys with a digital arc design showed average performance in 85.7% and high at 11.3%; In the case of a low SGS (from 128.9 to 145.0 combs), the low performance was 11.3%, on average 77.4%, high in 11.3% of cases, with line B finished in the field 5, respectively 16.1%, 71.0%, 12.9%; In boys with line D completed in field 9, the three performance levels were respectively 20.8%, 70.9%, 8.3%. In the shooting of the tennis ball, the arc-shaped boys reached the average performance of 66.6% and the upper one in 33.4% of the cases: individuals with SGS lowered (between 99.4 and 129.4 combs), 63% achieved low performances, 75.00% average and 18.7% high; In boys with line B completed in field 7, the three levels were respectively 8.0%, 76.0% and 16%; In individuals with line D terminated in field 11, in 8.7%, 73.9% and 17.4%.

In girls, in the long jump, those with line A completed in the field 2: 66, 6% average performance, 33.4% high; At a low SGS (79.9 86.1 combs), mean performances were recorded in the tennis ball, individuals with reduced SGS (between 76, 5 and 100.7) had lower performances in 7.7 %, Averages 61.5% and higher in 30.8% of cases.

The complex of dermatoglific markers in high-performance individuals has also been studied. S proved that the 60m high-performance boys, with 31.3%, had all five highlights, 25.0% - three and 44.7% - two bullets. In jump-jumping, 25.0% of the boys had five scorers, 25.0% four, 50.0% three. In throwing the tennis ball, 75.0% of the high-performance boys had all the scorers, and 25.0% were two. It follows that the genetic markers of motricity quality can be digital drawings (ulnar and radial networks), SGS, line B in field 7, line C in field 9, and line D in field 11. For speed - (Arc and net), ending line B in field S11 and line D in field 9, SGS; M - digital arc designs, SGS. The indicators shown along with other genetic markers (serologic, odontoglific, etc.) can and should be used to maximally highlight people with potentially high motricity skills (Table 64).

Table 64

Chest indicator in teens with varying degrees of growth (V.I. Filipov et al.)

Indicator	The general indicator						Summative indicator		
The size of the growth	Left hand			Right hand			down	medium	high
	down	medium	high	down	medium	high			
	9.10	63.3	52.7	73.7	65.1	46.5	144.7	128.4	99.2
	68.6	64.0	57.0	66.0	69.9	57.4	134.6	133.9	114.3
Chest circumference	68.3	60.3	71.7	68.8	61.7	73.0	137.1	122.0	144.7
Head circumference	74.4	61.0	58.5	73.9	64.9	58.1	148.3	129.9	116.6
Pelvis width	69.2	60.9	62.6	72.7	61.9	62.4	141.4	122.8	125.0

Growth rate prognosis in children and adolescents has a theoretical and practical value for medicine, physical education and anthropology, for which attempts have been made to establish the interpolation between some dermatological indicators (score of the comb) and the increase of the somatic indicators. In the high, middle and low growth groups, the overall left and right hand comb score was determined as well as the summative score for both hands. The significance of the differences between the indicator and the selected groups was determined by the Student formula. Existing data show a marked decrease in the comb index as measured by body length increases. Thus, in adolescents with low and high growth levels, the differences in the overall score of the comb were 18.3 combs (p 0.01) and 33.2 (p 0.001) for the left hand; Between medium and low levels, respectively, of 10.6 and 18.6 with p 0.001 in both cases. Concerning the summative score, the differences were: 16.3 (- medium, with p 0.05), 45.5 (lower - upper, p 0.001); 29.2 (medium - high, p 0.001).

As far as the width of the basin is concerned, there is a significant decrease in the number of combs from the lower to the middle level in the right hand. For the summative indicator we can see the decrease from the low growth rate to the average and high by 19,1 (p 0,05) and 16,9 (p 0,05). So the reduction of the overall and summative index of the comb can be taken as a genetic marker, which accompanies the increase in length of the body, the circumference of the head and the width of the basin.

When genetically correlating in a selection action the morphophiological data of the parents with those of the children, it is necessary to consider the acceleration phenomenon in whose genes the melatonin discovered by Swirtze plays a very important role and the phenomenon of non-fetal, Which constitute morphogenetic realities of the contemporary period. Also, considering population genetic determinations, it is necessary to establish the anthropological typology specific to the regions in our homeland. and we can not extrapolate identical data from other countries. For example, Wolker's regression curves that allow the pre-height growth at certain ages based on the knowledge of height at a particular moment of childhood, studied and researched by Tittel on the German population, have proven not to be fully consistent, being Necessary adaptations which have found a wide applicability in physical education and sports.

These genetic determinations and estimates of constitutional typology are strictly valid on population groups. Knowing the genetic background of the individual and of the populations, we can make more rigorous sports selections and then act with the help of the environmental factors in the most efficient conditions, reaching the higher limits of genetic adaptability, the role of the environment being especially important under the conditions of action on a hereditary background favorable. It has been shown that the existence of a certain configuration of dermatoglobes with over 10 vortices, easily evidenced by existing methods, prefigures a very high waistline. Thus, dermatoglyphs decipherment can be a very important selection criterion at a young age for sports where performance is conditioned by the existence of the longilin anthropological type. Also, the genetic determination of the plant vault type is of great importance for the selection in sports because there is a correlation between the plant vault configuration and performance. (Fig. 131-133) We also mention, in this context, the genetic determination of biorhythm and the special importance of its knowledge for the efficient conduct of sports activity.

It follows from the above the importance of the family survey (establishment of the genealogy tree) in the sports selection. I have just pointed out in this chapter some meto-logical aspects, since the elements of detail in their entirety are found in the previous chapters of the book, the reader will also use them for the orientation and development of the sports selection (the somatic, functional and psychic parameters with a high index of hereditary determination).

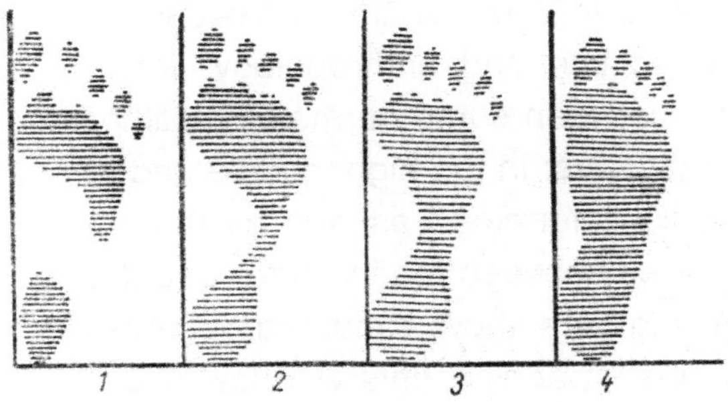

Fig. 131. Next plantar (after St Milcu and E. Walter).

4. Human anthropological and genetic investigations constitute the fourth stage of genetic anthropological selection in sport. They reveal important peculiarities of the human body according to pedoclimatic conditions that have acted within generations. Population represents the ensemble of the genes of individuals that enter into its constitution. It develops through panmyxia (heterosexual marriages), consanguinity (marriages between close relatives leading to degeneration) and homogamy (homozygous marriages). In the populations, directional selections (given by spontaneous abortions), normative selections (favoring the occurrence of intermediate phenotypes), differentiated selections (favoring the appearance of extreme phenotypes) and heterosis, all leading to the existence of some Specific biological characters of that population, which are likely to differentiate it from other populations. We note that Fr. I. Rainer made some references to characters of importance in physical education and sports. Thus, he points out that in Oltenia we encounter with high frequency persons who possess the quality of coordination (the so-called skill) with higher parameters, and in Banat we encounter more often the type of longilin somatic type with the qualities of detent (explosive force) Higher level. We emphasize that isolates [isolated geographic areas where relatives are married, ie the phenomenon of consanguinity with a very high Molecot coefficient] is characterized by the presence of human subjects with degenerative aspects, hereditary diseases and lower psychomotricity potential.

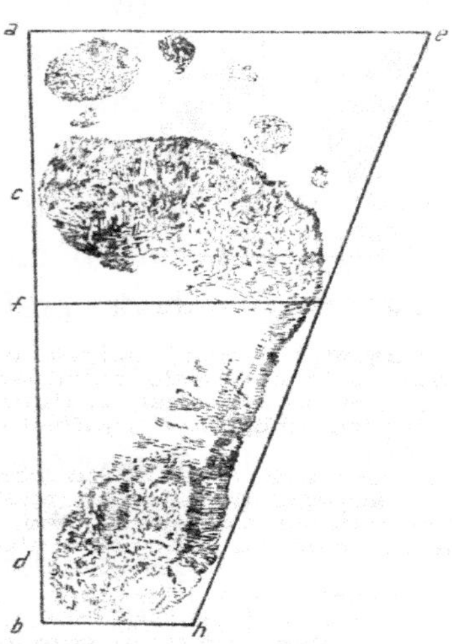

Fig. 132. Plantar footprint

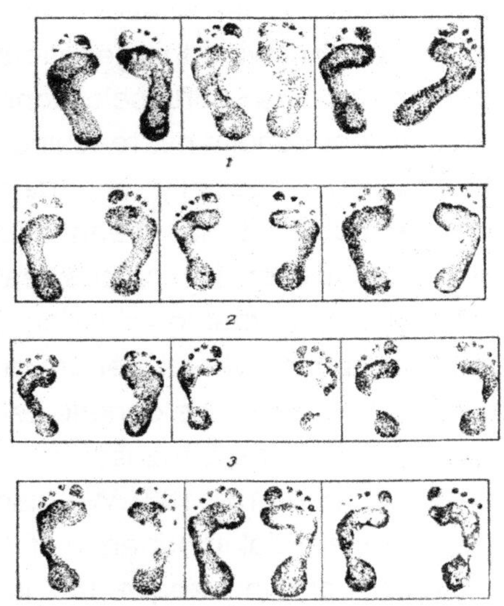

Fig. 133. Planetary trails to the top three (After St Milcu and Walter) 1 - Disc Throwing; 2 - Speed alerts;3 - Jumping in height; 4 - Jumping in length

The phenomenon of heterosis, or fecundation produced between an egg and a sperm-maze, from individuals as distant as geographically and even racially different, leads to the birth of descendants with a superior psycho-mental and motricity capacity. It is also noted that certain somatic, functional, motricity or psychic qualities have a higher level in certain breeds. Thus, the black race has a higher percentage of white fibers in the muscles and has a particular configuration of the Achilles tendon, which gives it superior speeds, having an upward net in sprint athletics.

In this context of genetic investigation, we highlight genetotrophic explorations whose scientific substantiation was made by Williams' recent research. Genetotrophic theory is of particular importance for the scientific direction of sports training, knowing that a primary environmental factor is nutrition. In order to achieve a harmonious body development and cultivation of particular physical qualities, Williams proposes optimizing the action of the food factor according to the following methodology:

A) selecting individuals with special skills;

B) biochemical exploration of genetic and metabolic particularities;

C) Establishing a differentiated diet according to the individual's genetic meta-bolstic peculiarities, so as to enhance the somatic qualities that we want to develop.

It results from these research that it is necessary for the athlete's diet to be in accordance with its somato-physiological and genetic particularities.

In conclusion, it results that anthropology and genetics open very high perspectives to raise a higher ranking of sports performance, respectively, to achieve great performances. At the same time, through their methodology, these disciplines objectively highlight selection methods, increasing, in terms of economic efficiency, the investment of moral and material capital in subjects that will not be in a state of failure during the preparation for big results. We must point out that, although very modern and developing, domains have an old tradition in our country. Professor Francis Rainer, the first rector of the National Academy of Physical Education - one of the oldest institutions with this Profile in Europe - has undertaken the first research of sports anthropology and genetics. His anthropology course, held in the third year of that time, synthesizes current trends in sports anthropology and presents some notions of genetic selection in sport.

- Individualization of training in order to develop the motricity skills, in relation to the anthropological and genetic determinism of motricityity

Speed. Regarding the ways of developing the speed, we mention the following: speed exercises, to constitute an appropriate stimulus in the development of this quality, must be of maximum intensity, not exceeding 10-15 seconds; The repeat method is basic. Rest periods should take into account the fact that in order to achieve training results, a high level of cortical excitability should be maintained at all times and the oxygen requirement should be restored. Pauses reduce cortical excitability and restore oxygen debt - so the effects are both positive and negative. S has shown that if the entire oxygen debt is restored in a given time, the value of this recovery is 65% in the first third of the time, 30% in the second third and 5% in the last third.

Starting from this, it is recommended that breaks do not exceed two-thirds of the full recovery time of O2 debt in order not to decrease cortical excitability and also to make an active rest by walking, running smoothly, by even engaging Of other vascular groups. However, when the fatigue by accumulating this 5% of O2 equipment is felt, the coach has to interrupt the training because otherwise it will develop the resistance in speed mode and will not develop the speed. The training also has to be done in terms of optimal functionality and management of the nervous system, given the importance of the nerve structure in the improvement of the speed. Given that speed is strictly genetically determined, there is a danger, especially in the early years of age, that high intensity, often repeated and exclusive exercise exercises lead to the formation of a steady dynamic stereotype, namely to the "barrier" Speed " which is below its genetic adaptability limit, thus below the maximum potential of the athlete. Thus, the very large volume, focused exclusively on speed exercises, can have this consequence which, at first glance, seems favorable, by holding fast results, but leading to a subsequent capping.

To prevent this, in the pre-pubertal and pubertal stage it is necessary to achieve good general physical training and multilateral training; Speed performance must be achieved mainly through this type of training and less through strict physical training based on speed as athletes reaching the age of performance; The speed barrier is prevented by performing a speed training in the power regime and less by using in training the exciting exciting specialty for the competition. Thus, Demeter shows that runners have to rarely use full-stroke speeds, but put emphasis on speed-jumping training by jumping with the ball, work with hardships, specific preparatory exercises. We conclude that the speed barrier is a consequence of high genetic speed determination and occurs as a result of the large number of repetitions of the specific speed exercises with maximum quantum scales. Its extinction is achieved by temporarily interrupting the training between three 12 months in the ante and pubertal stage and exercises that ensure that the adult's maximum speed is exceeded (volleyball, traction, etc.).

It should also be borne in mind that the execution of a maximum speed movement is conditioned by the overcoming of resistances such as body weight and inertia, external environmental factors, etc., which requires force, so that the development of speed can not be abstracted The force of that subject. Hence the need to develop the force as the speed develops, all the more so as the force is clearly superior to the speed. Undoubtedly, this extra force must be achieved on the same motion structure that aims to improve speed. This requires at the same time a profound knowledge of the succession of the muscular groups in action, so that the force of each of them develops, and in the order of action of the muscles, the effects of the speed increase similar to those of the rockets. At the same time, optimal neuromuscular coordination is essential because it ensures relaxation of successive muscle muscles, which allows a ballistic contraction (example: maximal extension flexion) with maximum efficiency in terms of both speed and force.

Regarding the aspects of the particularities of the stages of growth and development, we note that in the pre-postwar period the speed effort is at the forefront. The works of *Nicu Alexe* (2008) show that in this period the speed of movement is constantly increasing, the 40-60 m distances are well tolerated by the body and have favorable effects on the growth process. In this regard, a special emphasis will be placed on speed development, avoiding long-lasting and long-lasting efforts that would overwhelm the insufficiently developed cardio-respiratory system at this age. The fact that both the development of strength and resistance at this age, due to the anthropological features of different systems and devices, occupies a smaller place justifies fully placing the center of gravity in speed training.

In the pubertal stage, the anatomical function of the body still allows the development of velocity, dynamics and mobility of the cerebral cortex being at a very high level at this stage. All forms of speed (reaction, execution, displacement, repetition) can be developed so that the reaction time reaches the values found in the adult (*Farfel*). It is noted that the speed efforts, with short durations with sufficient breaks, with the alternation of different types of motricity activity, ensure the rapid development of the speed, morpho-functional modifications in the body being favorable to the development processes from this age. Optimal speed assistance is between 60 and 80 m. The development of velocity and speed in force rapidly increase the anaerobic capacity during this period. *Arinkin N.I.* (1969) found a better adaptation to a standard effort (7,500 kgm in 15 minutes on a cyclogergometer) in puberty pupils (13-14 years) after having been trained by speed and speed efforts Force, towards the group that was coerced with resistance efforts. Cardiac frequency has reached higher limits, pulse and blood pressure recovery has lasted longer, and voluntary apnea has been substantially shortened in students trained by speed and force. Instead, other parameters that mirror the stimulation of large vegetative functions, such as systolic volume, venous and capillary pressure, "the circulation speed and circulatory flow of the forearm have proven to be more favorable for students undergoing repeated resistance efforts" (*Demeter A.*).

In the post-graduate stage, a very small progression in speed development can also be achieved. The rate, being mainly genetically determined, is maximally obtained as a progression rate in the antepubert and pubertal stages. The emphasis in this period is not so much on the speed of reaction, but rather on the repetition, execution and displacement, as these forms of speed depend to a greater extent on the neuromotricity coordination and the force that is developing during this period. Also, the resistance velocity develops as the anaerobic resistance increases at this age. Running distance can be increased up to 200 m at that stage, since the anaerobic alactacid neuromuscular effort is well tolerated, with the nervous and muscular system being well-consolidated morpho-functional.

Of course, significant advances in speed performance can be achieved by subjects who are just starting sports training during this time. Force. The methods of force development are:

Static methods. Isometric contractions lead to local circulation difficulties, oxygen intake is low, and metabolism takes place under anaerobic conditions with accumulation of lactic acid and pyruvic acid. Oxygen deficiency and catabolite accumulation are thought to constitute muscle fiber functional exciters, which, in the overcompensation phase, lead to capillary vasodilatation and hypertrophy of muscle fibers by increasing saroplasm and uroglobulin, conferring fibrous red blood cell histology with efficiency Increased in the realization of force.

However, isometric contractions lead to increased intrathoracic and intracranial pressure, striking the venous return movement. It is disturbed by the cortical and subcortical activity, which can also be emphasized on the EEG, hence the need to customize the isometric effort according to age (it is contraindicated in the antepartmental stage), gender and individual typological characteristics (it is indicated for the trained athletes). Lack of movement during this effort is not an element favorable to the development of motricity skills. In view of these considerations, both positive and negative, it is good for the static effort to succumb to the dynamic effort, to be customized and preceded by adequate heating.

Dynamic methods. I'm using isotonic contractions. The methods are also based on the mentioned biochemical and physiological aspects. In beginners, the method of repetitive average effort to fatigue is indicated, using 35 40% load of the beginner's force. The method has the advantage that the large workload engages in extensive metabolic changes, the last elevations being of maximum efficiency because of the high excitability of the nervous system, which synchronously engages a large number of motricity units. Of course, the drawbacks are related to long training time, increased fatigue, and high recovery time.

In performance athletes, the method of maximum effort is at the forefront. The maximum load is considered to be the one that the athlete can lift two times in a favorable mental state. Particular attention should be paid to biomechanical aspects, for a more efficient technical execution, by making levers suitable for the prevention of musculoskeletal injuries and the eardrum, respectively the breaks between the lifting series; The maximum load, as I said, represents the ideal biological excitator for both the nervous system and the vascular effector. It is possible to use the lifting of the maximum speed using a dynamic effort of speed. Exercise structures close to the specific movement must be used. This increases the force in the specific motricity skills. It is very good to increase the speed at the end of the motricity act. It is used together with methods of increasing maximum force and maximum speed. Regarding the development of force in the antepubert stage, there are a number of controversies. Some authors, especially the classics, consider that the efforts of force carried out before the complete ossification processes endanger the process of growth and development, slowing down or even stopping it.

Recently, however, research shows that a force effort duly matched with anthropological peculiarities is even a favorable functional stimulus of growth processes at this age. What is contraindicated is the use of heavy weights, which can lead to musculoskeletal and bone trauma in this antepubertary stage. Force force begins at a load of over 33% of the maximum force of a muscle group; Some misunderstandings can only be misunderstood by the notion of effort, but only the efforts made at over 66% or very high, over 90% of the maximum capacity of the muscular groups involved (the overload principle). However, in antepubert age students, the use of 35% 40% of the maximum potential load is tolerated, having a beneficial influence on somatic growth and functional development of the organism (*Demeter A.*).

In the pubertal stage, the development of force is imperative. We mention that during the puberty the motricity activity suffers a reduction due to somatofunctional changes, such as in girls, the development of the pelvis and mammary glands, the acceleration of the growth process and the occurrence of disproportions between the body segments, etc. The relative strength (relative to body weight), especially of the extensors, decreases. Because of this, moderate force exercises, performed with light weight dumbbells, are welcome. Of course, it is contraindicated to work with great strains, overloading the muscles and tendons. In the post-graduate phase, observing the principle of gradual increase of effort, force can be developed under its many aspects, both by increasing volume and intensity. The development of the force is due to muscle hypertrophy, which has as its substrate the intake of proteins and anabolic hormones, associated with the exercises of force as an exciting factor of the environment. However, heavy weight (impulse, toothed, thrown) weightlifting may be avoided, which may have negative effects on the spine, keeping the principle of successive and alternate development of segmental muscle groups, while taking care symmetrical. At the same time, isometric contractions leading to intrathoracic and intracranial hypertension, creating difficulties in venous return, and therefore throughout the circulation (Valsalva effect) and oxygenation of tissues, will be avoided in 16-18-year olds, Saw that the respiratory system is, in particular, insufficiently developed.

Resistance. Starting from the elements described above, training for resistance development should consider increasing aerobic capacity, biochemical structural recovery after exercise, and lifting the will threshold. In this sense, it is necessary to carry out a large amount of work, the passage of high speed portions, fractional training with varying intensity repetitions.

Among the methods used, we mention a few:

The long run method that runs in the aerobic area up to an intensity of 70 75% of the maximum oxygen consumption and which only causes the increase of the number of oxidative enzymes without acting on glycolithic ones. In order to educate the will, training of this type is useful even for performance athletes, but in order to be a biological stimulant for the strength of effort intensity, 85 90% of VO2 mcm must be carried out in the endurance area. The variable effort method requires rapid adaptations to increased oxygen consumption (varied ranging), but maximum demands are low and variable intensity, the method can be used only for beginners or for educating the will. The interval training method consists in varying the intensity of the effort by varying the duration, resting interval, repetition tempo, pause content (active or passive) so as to achieve both an aerobic and, alternatively, anaerobic mechanism Moderate and submaximal lactic acidosis and pyruvium, which also positively influence the resistance capacity, potentiating aerobic mechanisms - leading to the biochemical transformations of the intermediate fibers into red fibers.

They will be used, along with the four-minute aerobic time, for a few seconds to two three-minute anaerobic periods; Short rest periods after four six minutes that will accentuate aerobic and short breaks after up to two-three minutes that will increase anaerobiosis; Variations in speed over time, which will be subcritical, resulting in pure aerobic activity; Critical, located in the endurance and supracritic area causing anaerobiosis; Repetitions varied in number, based on the same principles (dosed so as to maintain the body in the endurance area); Attention must be paid to the accumulation of lactic acid in the anaerobic area, which is not a perfect match between the pulse and the lactate concentration which, in the absence of biochemical dosages, raises particular difficulties in conducting the training; Breaks also in content, can be achieved by passive rest or active rest, by running at slow pace, with the pulse reaching 110 120 pulses / minute.

We recall a physical effort of more than five years, with the demand of at least 1/7 of the muscular mass, in which the cardio-respiratory intake is required in a proportion of 50% of the total exercise capacity, is stress resistance (*Demeter A. - Hallman W.*). And with regard to the development of resistance, the opinions of the authors are controversial. Some fundamentally contraindicate the resistance effort in the antepubert and puberty period, based on the anthropological features described and on the possibility of disturbing the growth and development process, while, lately, it is increasingly accredited the idea that, under appropriate dosing, Resistance is favorable at this age.

Demeter has synthesized the views of the authors lately. *Mellerowicz* (Germany) points out: “There is no phase in the period of human growth that, for medical reasons, prohibits long distance journeys.” *Nocker* specified, as early as 1957, that resistance training at antepubert age is not detrimental in itself, damaging only the intensive form of the resistance effort. American specialist Jokl, as well as Swedish Astrand, recommends the start of resistance training for girls prior to the setting up of puberty, due to the existing favorable predispositions. Applying a resistance effort (4,720 m running) daily to a group of girls aged 12-14, *Valik* achieved very good results without signs of physical overload.

Maiorov, experimenting with groups of pre-puberty and puberty (11-14 year old) schoolchildren who were instructed to work hard in the form of special training, has found remarkable progress after a period of six years. Thus, in the 11-12 year group, at the distance of 5 km, with which the effort started, at the end of the year it was reached without difficulty the distance of 14 km per week, and for the 13-14 year group, At 7.5 km, 18 km per week was reached, without any evidence of intolerance or impairment of pupils' health. Reiss, from RDG, launched the formula “Run as hard as you can”, with the following figures characterizing the normal possibilities of child resistance in the growing period:

boys:

- 6 - 7 years: 7 min of free running - 7 min;
- 8 - 9 years: 10 min of free running - 10 min;
- 10-11 years: 15 min of free running - 12 min;
- 12-13 years: 15 minutes of free running - 18 minutes;
- 14-15 years: 18 min of free running - 20 min;

- 16-17 years: 20 min of free running - 25 min.

Hollmann (2004) considers that the resistance effort, which lasts at least three minutes, has no negative effect on somatofunctional growth and differentiation if it does not take the form of a competition. The "non-physiological" distances - after this specialist - are between 200 and 600 m, where the highest oxygen debts and the most pronounced pH changes are found, which can be premise unfavorable to the development of children and juniors. The results of tests carried out by *Nicu A.* et al. (1970), on samples of children across the country, has led to growing concerns about the national organization of physical education and sports for the development of resistance to pre-primary students. In the pubertal stage, the development of resistance recognizes the same principles of proper dosing as in the pre-puberty period, the effort of this type constituting a precious biologic stimulus.

It is appreciated that a 6 - 30 minute effort at a moderate intensity that does not increase the pulse over 120 -130 pulses per minute is favorable to the growth and development process. Records by *Nicu A.* et al. (1970) on more than 37,000 pupils from all regions of the country have demonstrated that 20 minutes for boys and 10 minutes for puberty girls are accessible to the real possibilities of their body to respond. The authors found a surprising fact at first glance, namely that 2% of those tested had successfully run on very long distances (12-36 km) at a rate of 12 km/h without training without any cardio-respiratory disturbance.

It is contraindicated at this stage to perform a very high time (200-600 m), which requires intense cardiac arrest. If the running is of a long duration but in absolute steady state, it is not harmful. Allowing the athlete to adjust the tempo, we realize that the subject in question can also determine the tissue metabolic level in accordance with its aerobic effort, so that the resistance effort is not harmful but stimulating the body. In the postpuberal stage, given the anthropological peculiarities, the resistance effort - which requires a trofotrop metabolism (high energy economy), a inotropic circulatory network (capillary wealth) and morpho-functional, especially raised cardio-respiratory parameters - has no negative effects on functionality and Body morphology, but positive, on the contrary. We note that the resistance effort is indicated at this stage, especially since it has a positive inotropic effect (it leads to the increase of the capillary network at the level of different tissues and especially of the muscle tissue). To this is added that the recovery processes are carried out in much better conditions at postpuberting.

Skills. Regarding the methods of development of skill we notice that repetition is the basic element in the formation of the dynamic stereotype. Note that the number of repetitions of the motricity act is not exaggerated in order not to produce inhibition of protection at the S.N.C. level, and thus the training will remain without results.

For motricity skills with a high degree of difficulty and complexity it is necessary to complex the exercises made. Also, a particular emphasis should be placed on the athlete's understanding of technical tactical schemes so that the theoretical learning of these elements is required with training to train motricity skills and motricity stereotypes. The development of the athlete's intellect, due to the correlation between intelligence and skill, as well as prefectability marked by the environmental factors of superior nerve activity must be a priority. Educational and psychological factors play a major role in this. At the same time it is necessary to develop the equilibrium by means of appropriate exercises; The biomotricity quality, strength, and strength of fitness will be developed by training according to their importance for the sports sector in question, as, as we have explained earlier, they often condition the skill of the motricity act.

In the antepubert stage, skill can develop but encounters some difficulties related to the predominance of excitation on inhibition, concentration irradiation, low threshold of differentiation inhibition, having as substrate the morphological characteristics of the nervous system during this period. In this stage, for the development of skill, it is necessary to repeat the various exercises in order to train and fix the motricity skills.

Driving skills have a different degree of complexity. Some are simpler and may be considered as motricityic conditioning reflexes, others more complex, constituting activity, motricityic acts. The mechanism of their formation and fixation is that of conditional reflexes and the realization of dynamic stereotypes (*I.P. Pavlov*); It assumes the existence of a dominant nervous system (*Uhiomschi A. A.*), of excitatory and inhibition areas to which the function of certain muscle motricity units corresponds. Under all conditions, plasticity and receptivity of the bark in the pre-puberty period provides a rapid increase in motricity skills, but fixation is more difficult through the lower threshold of internal (conditioned) inhibition, which explains the need for repetition and learning of a greater number of motricity skills In order not to overload the cortical inhibition capacity, and so deficient. We also need to avoid the formation of incorrect dynamic driving stereotypes, achieved through superficial growth, because their cancellation and then the right learning requires a marked plus of energy and effort.

In the pubertal stage, the same anthropological and corollary features are maintained, the same ways of developing skill, but at a higher level, because the nervous system and the analyzers are net at a higher morpho-functional level. The plasticity of the bark and the predominance of the excitation favor the achievement of fine and precise movements. We will avoid the long-term demand for attention and concentration that is lower at this age, and it is necessary to increase the attractiveness and variety of exercises.

In the post-graduate stage, skill can develop in better conditions as the level of inhibition of differentiation and internal inhibition increases. The risk of overloading the nervous system decreases, the fixation of the reflexes is better, being able to form complex motricityic acts with differentiated stresses of different muscle groups. The fact is also favored by the great cortical plasticity existing at this age.

Increased neuromotricity coordination, linked both to the structurisation and functionality of the bark and to the analyzers, has a special role in the possibility of a supportive development of skill at this age (*Dill D.).* We also need to emphasize that in the effective management of sports training it is very important to achieve a concordance between the sporting effort effort structure and the training structure that needs to be individualized in relation to the sporting performance performance and the trained subject.

A valuable experience is that of coach emeritus *Mociani* in the field of canoeing. Analyzing the structure of the sample, it was concluded that 3.3% alactacid effort, 6.7% anaerobic lactate effort, 30% aerobic effort, 30% aerobic anaerobic effort and 30% effort in the endurance area Aerobiosis with anaerobiosis). As a consequence, annual pre-competitive training plans, etc., follow this structure, with the results being the best.

To this, the levels are added at the time of the secondary selection that takes into account the heritability coefficients; For example, if for the anaerobic capacity this coefficient is, according to our data, at 0.85 0.90, the subject in the secondary selection phase must have an anaerobiotic level of at least 85 90% of that required for the moment of reaching the value The world performer. Also, through this prism, it is estimated the possibilities of increasing the level of global information in the future, it is calculated mathematically, percentage of the training structure and selection requirements, in relation to what is predicted for the performance.

In conclusion, we need to make a few anthropological emphasis on the standardization and rationalization of training. Standardization involves the establishment, in quantitative terms, of effort structures, exercises necessary for the development of biomotricityical qualities, the formation of motricity skills and ultimately the acquisition of athletic disciplines and achievement at the highest level. Rationalization refers to the qualitative aspects of how to structure the training to maximize its effectiveness. The standardization and rationalization specific to the different branches of sport under conceptual design (developed by the Research Center of C.N.E.F.S under the leadership of *Dr. Nicu Alexe*) are ways of optimizing the training that proved their usefulness in various sports disciplines. There is a valuable experience in athletics (*Tatu Titus, Ardelean Tiberiu, Dumitru Alexandrescu*), canoeing (coach emeritus *Mociani Alexandru*) and other sports. Also, the introduction of algorithms in standardization and rationalization (Assoc.Prof. *Ferenc Elena*) represents a remarkable progress on the road to high performance. We emphasize, however, that both standardization and rationalization must be individualized to the biopsychomotricity particularities of the athlete, since the human organism, as it derives from its entire anthropological and genetic determinism, is a unique one. Because a load of effort or exercise training structure is indeed a functional exciton capable of raising the threshold of biopsychotricity, a strict individualization is required. The whole genetic anthropological biochemical individuality (*Williams*) bases this concept. Standardization and rationalization is an indicative framework of great value that needs to be customized in training for the sporting subject. At the same time, the volume and intensity of effort, the basic components of the training, must be adapted to the biological functional structure of each athlete. We do not discuss standards that evaluate certain motricity and psychological somato-physiological anthropological qualities that set the value limits of the optimal anthropological type on the sport branch (national selection system - *Nicu Alexe* et al.) And the performance or those that target the training, the degree Such as Lefunov samples, aerobic and anaerobic capacities in relation to performance requirements, etc., which, based on the knowledge of the biological complexity of the human body, are benchmarks throughout the selection and training system. The whole training process needs to be adapted to the potential biotric potential of sports subjects, which is an optimal way to achieve high performance.

Alongside the principle of individualization on anthropological and genetic basis of training, another essential element to be considered is the interrelation of mutual conditioning in the building and perfection of the human being of the three parameters defining the constitutional type, respectively, the somato-physiological qualities, Motricity and psychic. The development of biomotricity qualities through training determines the development of somato-physiological and psychological ones. Raising the level of psychic qualities - intelligence, anticipatory capacity, temperament, character, etc., through mental training and other methods positively influences the motricityity (*Mălina, Eiben, Siarosta*, etc.). It therefore results in the need to diversify training methods and tools in relation to the objectives pursued, with attention being paid to the full development of the organism on all three of these coordinates which are in close interdependence.

We emphasize the fact that, in the development of skill, a special role - given the determinant mechanisms of this psychobiomotricityity - is mentally trained. Concentration training in this context is of paramount importance because the degree of inhibition of differentiation depends to a large extent on the efficiency of the cortical command that is conditioned by the motricity act in terms of skill. Of course, selection is essential, emphasizing on this occasion, there being a strong interdependence between the training and the qualities of the subject. This is all the more evident as the development of psychotronics has recently led to electroencephalographic evidence, outside the alpha, beta, delta, and wave waves, which makes it possible to predict what another is thinking Person and fita, through which one can influence the action of another subject, thus substantiating on scientific materialistic basis telepathy and hypnosis.

In the anthropological direction of training and selection an important role is played by the homeopathic biochemical constitutional typology. Homeopathy is a science that starts from the fact that balancing the body, in a state of illness or physiological imbalances, is accomplished by administering substances similar to those that cause it (homos = similar, pathos = suffering). This rebalancing of the criteria: anthropometric, physiological (after the predominance of a function), anatomophisiological (endocrine, neurovegetative, etc.) of heat, considering the homeopathic constitutional type.

- **Homeopathic types are the following (Chirilă, 2005)**:

1) Carbon type, with the predominance of calcium carbonate in the bones. It is a brevilin, with short and thick limbs, with the lower half developed, with large teeth, a large abdomen, the arm with an obtuse angle in a forced extension, the temperament is balanced, and in the females the menstrual cycle appears late; Is consistent with the endoblastic.

2) Phosphoric type, with the predominance of calcium phosphate in the bones. It is a longilin, narrow-chested, with a rapid growth process, with long, fine hands, elongated phalanxes, oval teeth, rectilinear joints, straight forearm and arm. Corresponds to the ectoblastic type.

3) Fluoride type, with the predominance of calcium fluorate in the bones. It is longilin or brevilin, with a soft hand, with nails and teeth of irregular shape, with articular joints and the protrusion of the lower jaw. Corresponds to the ectoblastic type.

4) Sulfur type corresponding to mesoblastic.

Under the correlation between temperament and the biochemical homeopathic type it is highlighted:

A) Hydrogenenoid type - characterized by excess H ion (excess water and temperament characterized by hyporesponsiveness.

B) Oxigenoid type - characterized by the excess of oxidoreduction and over-reactivity.

C) Carbonitrogenide type - with excess carbon and nitrogen, with a balanced temperament.

Knowing this typology is important in sports and other activities under two aspects:

A - in the selection, because on the basis of these biochemical homeopathic criteria we can pretend on some morfofunctional and temperamental qualities;

B - in making the optimal recovery after the sports effort, by administering in low doses substances based on the above-mentioned homeopathic type defining elements.

In the same context, we mention the existence of constitutional typologies based on the knowledge of the topography of acupuncture points, which have now been demonstrated histologically; Have been shown to contain endorphin-like substances; Can be easily highlighted by recording their bioelectric potential and are arranged according to trajectories (meridians) showing individual variations.

In recovery processes after excitement, the excitement of points, by toning or dispersion, has been proven to produce very good results. In fact, the individual anthropological typology of each subject has to be taken into account in the whole recovery process after the effort, and biochemical research has recently defined specific constitutional typologies and correlations between them and the optimal scheme for restoring the biological structures under stress.

It will be remembered to use the most suitable means for the individual structural structure of the body, such as hydroelectrolytic rebalancing with preparations containing mainly K, Mg, Ca ions, metabolic substrates such as essential fatty acids, glucose, etc.; Vitamin complexes; Biological stimulators of the type of apitherapeutic preparations; Adenosine triphosphates, etc., all of which are based on knowledge of anthropological biochemical individuality of the organism and specific pharmacotolerance (Williams). Avoid preparations with immediate or delayed imbalance effects on the body's homeostasis such as anabolic hormones or excitatory hormones (amphetamines, etc.) that can only be used on the basis of precise medical information when dealing with pathological conditions Are out of the scope of physiological effort (they are, in fact, doping, which is sanctioned in sports if this practice is detected).

We conclude on the necessity of biochemical anthropological individualization (Wiliams), the means of rehabilitation that must be in a perfect agreement with the somato-physiological, motricity and psychological typology of the organism. To this is added food, in which the observance of Wiliams' genetotrophic principle, stated in terms of biochemical individuality, is essential for the optimal functioning of the human organism. We also emphasize the necessity of making determinations, especially of aerobic and anaerobic capacity, during the training and in the competition, because the values highlighted in the laboratory, which constitute selection standards, have limits related to the degree of effort utilization. For example, a footballer may have an anaerobic capacity of 45 kgm/kg body, but in training or competition he/she does not develop more than 35 kgm/kg of body, thus not being competitive. This lower use is related both to its mental capacity to mobilize and to the existence of genetically determined reserves. Hence, the need to correlate laboratory determinations with those conducted directly in competition or training and genetic anthropological routing of effort to maximize mobilization of the genetic reserves determined, knowing that, in general, even in a peak sports effort there are 15-20% of the The capacity of the body to remain unused (in the normal activity of the body this metabolic genetic reserve reaches 35-40%).

The broader view of this issue explains, on a scientific basis, emphasized in this paper that the development of biomotricityological qualities condition and influence the increase in the level of psychological and somato-physiological qualities, which justifies the special care that needs to be given to the biodiversity potential of the population and especially Of the younger one, in order to ensure a good demographic fund, a decisive factor for the prosperity of a nation. In this context, physical education and sport are essential factors in achieving this goal, as it acts directly, under the conditions of a dosing of the individualized effort efficiently, on the biomotricityical potential and, implicitly, on the somato-physiological and motricityic qualities, completing in its entirety The human organism. In essence, this is essentially the justification of the importance of motricity anthropology, the movement being the very nature of the human being alongside spirituality, a fact reflected in the Greek antiquity, which emphasized the “mens sana in the corpore sano”.

CHAPTER X.
ANTHROPOLOGY - FIELD OF INTERFERENCE BETWEEN BIOLOGY AND PHILOSOPHY

Dialectics of the relationship between determination and structure in anthropology

If we look for two concepts of intense theoretical solicitation in the field of modern science, we should stop in particular at the determination and the dialectically correlated concept of structure. They prove to be dialectically opposed by some defining features. First, determination is a process, so it is carried out diachronically, while the structure is a mode of compilation, the emphasis being on the synchronous aspects of the systems. However, the synchronic diachronic relationship (analogous to the logical historical relationship) is evident in some features.

Secondly, the determination aims to subordinate the notions, ranging from those with wide sphere and poor content to those with a smaller sphere and richer content. In contrast, the structure co-ordinates if, in determining relations, the relationships are caused by cause (without thereby accepting an equivalence of subordination causation) in the structure are interactive (which does not exclude the interaction cause effect of the relationship of determination).

Thirdly, while the tendency of determination is to emphasize the contents, by their successive enrichment, the tendency of structuring is to emphasize the forms, the configurations, through more mathematical abstract analyzes (mathematical logic). We can also note that the determination follows the dynamic, uninterrupted aspects of transformation of objects, phenomena, notions, while the structure stops at the invariants - relative to certain operations - of the transformation processes. Then determination determines, first of all, the continuous aspect of phenomena, and the structure, the discontinuous, etc. Being part of the themes that urge the scientist to philosophical reflection, and the philosopher firmly on the preoccupations specific to natural sciences, the quoted concepts are likely to suggest the convergence of philosophy and science in the synthesizing effort of modern thinking.

The question that arises from the beginning is whether biology or other science provides the most sustainable basis for such a synthesizing enterprise, and if it would not be more natural to expect the unification of knowledge through philosophical approaches. This is all the more so since, in the literature, there are no-one opinions (*K.F. Schaffner*, 1969), according to which biology is still chemistry and physics, thus a kind of chemistry or physics in which the systematization of elements plays the decisive role. Organization or structure is defining for biological organisms, but they remain, in the sense of reductions, some chemical and physical systems. Here the behavior is determined by the isolated physico-chemical constituents, adding their topological causal structure. Although the answer to the question of whether biology provides sufficient groundwork for the synthesis of knowledge must first of all take into account the fact that such unity or synthesis can not be based only on the universal matrix of the creative spirit, but must start from the diversity of the objects under investigation. It is necessary, then, to take into account the somewhat central position of biology in the hierarchy of sciences, and not least the fact that its "fundamental" question is precisely the relation between the organic structures with the status of synchronous models and the philogenetic evolution, Determined diachronically.

Other specialists (*L.V. Bertalanffy*, 1952) begin to appreciate the central position of biology from the fact that it first relies on mathematics, physics and chemistry, whose laws are indispensable to the research of life, and then fuel the foundations of psychology, Anthropology and even sociology, not to mention philosophy: "The phenomenon of life is a meeting place for those conceptions that, according to the usual distinction, lie in the exact sciences with one leg and one with the other." If the last century had a conception of a world contaminated by physics theories - in which the game of mechanically controlled atoms seemed to point to the last reality, and its data - an ideal model for extraphysical domains, sciences today are confronted with notions such as Organization or gestalt, of certain biological origin. So, if the past is known with biology of tribute to physics (mechanistic vision), psychology (vitalism), or sociology (selection and struggle for existence), today is itself called to contribute substantially to the improvement of a "world concept" About the world. The ultimate goal of biological research is to contribute to the elucidation of higher aspects of knowledge, such as the place of man in nature, symbolism as a fundamental feature of human evolution and mind, and the relationship between evolution and civilization, Biology and history, natural and social sciences; Biology is thus one of the sciences capable of contributing fully to the foundation of a general theory of systems, meant to inter alia transcend the classic Cartesian dualism spirit body.

Biology reveals the tendency towards a unitary conception of the world by promoting the same general principles that manifest itself in all the realms of science, as the general theory of systems. It should be of logical mathematical nature, and then formulate and derive generally valid principles within a complex of elements in interaction. The general principles themselves, although related to the system, prove independent of the nature of the constituent elements and the relations or forces between them, from where the structural confortability or the "logical homology" of the laws of different scientific domains. Some of the concepts underlying the general definition of the system and attesting to the homology of structure of scientific principles and laws are: totality, sum, progressive mechanization, centralization, ruling parties, hierarchical order, individuality, finality, equivalence. So the systems are complex of interactive elements, benefiting of a non-random nature; they are divided into two broad categories: closed and open. Live organisms are open systems capable of subsisting by assimilating and disassociating material components from the environment, unlike the closed systems of traditional physics that do not engage in environmental exchanges: according to principle II of thermodynamics, they will attain the state of equilibrium remaining Constant in time, ie stagnant macroscopically, depending on the initial conditions. Open systems can achieve a constant stable state, but will never enter rest, developing into states of maximum entropy, likelihood, and increased clutter. However, in the sphere of life there is an apparent deviation from principle II of thermodynamics: open systems present anti-entropic processes, developing into orderly states, differentiation and organization. The appearance of contradiction is blurred, however, by the application of so-called irreversible thermodynamics, in which the balance of production and transport of entropy is negative. Given that the specificity of the viva consists in a continuous organization, ordering of the disparate elements in relation to the self of the environment and that the measure of the disorder or the probability of a state in which the elements of the system are found is given by entropy, evolution can be considered as an increase of Negentropy. From this point of view, the whole organized world is a fluctuation in the general course of the Universe.

Life can increase negative entropy (order) as a result of the irreversible process of restitution in the form of irradiation of solar energy. But as we all know, in nature, all processes, except for some insignificant, prove that entropy can not be diminished. In the environment, positive entropy, ie disorder, increases. Therefore, the change of entropy in the open system as a whole is zero. Hence the establishment in such systems of a hierarchical order, that is, stratification by the overprinting of the higher layers, which take the role of leading parts. A certain way of unifying sciences, under the sign of philosophy, is to interfere with science;

Because there are many points of contact between philosophy and science, resulting from the fact that philosophy is not limited to the general human valorisation of knowledge, but a practice itself.Having a clear synthetic coordinating character, it will be in the realm of science through the research of scientific data in order to establish meaning, and will go beyond adopting a "speculative" vision with the search for the human relations of knowledge. It is a thesis consistent with the modern finding of the removal of concrete knowledge, with the continuous abstraction of the object of science and the appearance of the so-called operative structures (logical mathematics), isomorphic with the perceptual data. For what ultimately means the abstraction, if not an abandonment of the empiric by conceptualization, through the transcendence of the phenomena into an implacable speculative impulse, by what can be called the deeper, more accurate, more complete nature, being necessary For the living intuition. This is a process that facilitates the unification by mutual deduction of the laws and scientific concepts that are in continuity, that is, the correspondence of the cognitive substance.

Taking on such a current theme as Abstraction and the Unification of Modern Science of Nature, Werner Heisenberg notices the process of abstraction of the contemporaneous science of nature and - related to it - the proper abstraction of art, which is related to them from the point of view of the content. As far as biology is concerned, although it should be the least abstract science, it contains the very relationships that express itself in the abstract language of atomic physics: the only reason is that a unitary explanation of fundamental biological phenomena can be obtained; From which it follows that the actual unification of knowledge - whose broad range covers sciences, philosophy and not less art - is accomplished by absolutism. But its character proves to be entirely objective, as the character of mathematics, which together with philosophy, guides the process from complementary sides.

The fecundity of biology for discussing essential issues of philosophy and the theoretical complexity of its integration in the unification process are illustrated by the well-known work of Jaques Monod, Hazard and necessity; The central category of this study of biological "philosophy" is determinism, analyzed from the point of view of underlying categories such as absolute hazard and absolute necessity. The work cultivates both existentialist and structuralist philosophical suggestions; The proposed determinism is not seen, therefore, in terms of causality, though not only through structural interactions. As far as its attitude to the main issues of the philosophy of science is concerned, it is characterized by the emphasis on the duty today, more than ever, for the scientists to think their own discipline in the whole of modern culture, to enrich it not only with important knowledge under Technical point of view, but also ideas from own science, ideas that can be considered as meaningful from a human point of view.

Thus, the author considers, as the most concluding conclusion of contemporary biology, the assertion that the starting point, the basis of evolution in the biosphere is pure hazard, singularity, absolute but blind liberty, the essential unpredictability. Here is the only possible source of changing the genetic text, of any novelty in the living world: one example would be that between the determinism of a mutation in DNA and that of its functional effects at the level of protein interaction we can only identify an absolute coincidence Meaning that the two series of events are totally independent. The determinism of evolutionary series in nature - the extension of the statement and society makes it even more vulnerable - it would only support single, totally singular facts, which can only be supported by total ignorance of necessity and progress, and not least of statistical law. Such a position obviously suffers from determinism, one of the most serious consequences being the promotion of the thesis of total unpredictability, the absolute impossibility of scientific prediction; which, in passing, is also turning against the practical work of the brilliant Nobel Prize laureate, which is *Jacques Monod*. Expanded to social phenomena, to human issues, the author's position reveals an eclecticism that makes it oscillate between existentialist individualism and anti-structuralist anthropocentrism. The patos of militancy for objective, anti-animist knowledge, in which man renounces the claim to be the ultimate cause, the exceptional purpose of any knowing act, does not justify scientific conclusions such as: It is true that science attacks values. Not directly, for science is not a judge and must ignore them; But it ruins all the mythical or philosophical categories, which the animist tradition, from the Australian aborigines to the materialist dialecticians, placed moral values, debts, rights, prohibitions.

Another hypostasis of the biosphere, complementary to it, is, in *Monod's* view, the one defined by invariant properties that is absolute necessity. It means that, for example, the genetic code is forcibly constituted, but later it will be recovered by virtue of absolute necessity; Apart from this, a second may be mentioned, namely that, although subjected to mechanical reproduction, the code still suffers a quantum alteration. This means that in the "compensation" of the imperfection of the mechanism for preserving the correction of the code, any alteration will be taken over by DNA by the proteins: Out of the pure hazard field, the single accident enters the necessity field, the most implacable certitudes.

What is to be emphasized - and the scientific reality is illustrated by the current - is that, although new species appear after committing translations of the genetic message, these mistakes are to be captured, preserved and converted hereditary over a long period of speciation. Also, we can not lose sight of the fact that, at any level, the world asserts itself as the dialectical unity of order and disorder, necessity and fulfillment; That is why it is wrong to claim that the basis of the chemical organization of living structures is exclusively hazard, while their biological composition would be strictly necessary; Or that at the level of the genetic code, any novelty occurs only by virtue of the hazard, while at the level of hazard selection it would be completely absent. In the same vein, it seems to me to be very vulnerable to the maximum biosphere customization, which does not contain any foreseeable class of objects and phenomena, but would be just a particular event and as such a contingent. Researchers believe that the abolition of general connections in nature eliminates not only the basis of predictability, but also inductive practice, the use of empirical data as the basis for inductive generalization. Since admitting only "regularities" as forming what he has established in things not only does not fully justify inductive reasoning but undermines their own legitimacy.

The irreversible and absolute opposition between hazard and necessity is also non-dialectic, because the distinction between subjectivism and all its nuances and dialectics lies "inter alia in the fact that in dialectics (the objective) and the difference between relative and absolute is relative." Equally relative is the distinction between the particular and the universal, the connection of the individual and the individual with the necessity: "Every individual is bound by thousands of particular passages of another kind (with things, phenomena, processes), etc. In all of this there are already elements, embryos, notions of necessity, objective connection of nature, etc. The random and necessary element, phenomenon and essence already exist here, because, saying: (...) this is a tree leaf, etc., we remove a series of random clues, separating the essence from the phenomenon and opposing each other". Therefore, it seems to me the position that the mutation would be unlimited, while at the level of selection any novelty in the form of altering the structure of a protein would be tested for compatibility with the system. To claim that between the determinism of a mutation in DNA and that of functional effects is only an absolute coincidence, it means ignoring, among other things, that the theory of structures, as indestructible units of morphology and physiology, alters traditional optics on their opposition or inadequacy. To these we can add the finding that what is happening at a level of life may prove necessary at the lower level, as the need at a level is haphazard at higher levels. Molecular genetics uses information theory to elucidate some of these theoretical aspects with certain philosophical implications. The indeterminism stimulated by the net disjunction between absolute hazard and absolute necessity receives, in this way, serious refusals. As is known, in higher organisms genetic information is encoded as a code in the bases of chromosomal nucleic acids. DNA, as a direct molecule, transmits the information on two channels: one along the germ line, from DNA to DNA, ensuring continuity of cell generations and transmitting hereditary information from children to parents; on the other channel, the metabolic activity of the cell, in fact the synthesis of proteins through RNA and DNA in somatic cells, is carried out.

The scheme shows that the environment can not usually interfere with gene action, which is easier to support in the case of the transmission of hereditary characters from one generation to the next. Only incidentally, undiagnosed, mutations may interfere with environmental factors in the modification of genetic patrimony and, exceptionally, they can be conducted according to deliberate intentions. Without exhausting the problem of necessity-dialectic, such examples suggest a heuristic approach to it.

There is, however, another important aspect of heredity, which gives the possibility to determine hereditary phenomena through the extragenerational information factors: it is the differentiation of various cell lines specific to specialized tissues, coming from the same zygote, from the same genes content and chromosomes. On which channel the influences that decide the activation of some or the other in the genes of the complete set, it does not follow either the schematic or *Weissmann's* theory, to be sought on a third way of the hereditary information, namely, the interaction between the pericelous environment And constituents of the cell. Only by admitting the transformation effect of local environmental factors is explained, for example, the following experience: we take a fragment of ectodermic tissue to be transformed into skin and transplant it to an area where the embryo Nervous if the surgery was done on time. As far as the differentiation of the transplant is concerned, it will be diverted according to the new environment, becoming nervous tissue not only in that generation, but in the very heredity of the cell. In such cases, the specialists speak of "connecting" and "disconnecting" the genes through metabolic processes in the cytoplasm; Although it is not about structural changes but only about changes in gene functions, we can not ignore the determinism of environmental factors, able to convert the incident into elements of the hereditary necessity: "We must assume that these factors, although incapable of influencing Transmission across the DNA-DNA channel may, however, exert a selective influence on the leakage rate of information on the second channel, from DNA to protein. The detailed structure of each protein that the body is able to synthesize is specified by a corresponding segment of DNA, but a number of nuclear, cytoplasmic and environmental factors all have a say in deciding which proteins in the whole range Possible, will be synthesized in a given cell and will be the dynamics of this synthesis."

That such issues, which may be added to others, must be questioned when it comes to the philosophical integration of biology, it emerges from the needs of any science to reflect upon its epistemological condition, to begin and to state a conceptual regime More lucid. But we do not ignore the fact that, by working with logical and philosophical categories, general theories do not yet affect the much-desired philosophical integration.

As we can see, the resizing of the principles of evolutionism in recent decades has led to a much more elastic conception of its mechanism, to the unification, in the name of common epistemological criteria, of points of view that seemed otherwise irreconcilable. Weismann, Bateson, de Vries and many other geneticists reduce the evolution of combining the constituent elements of the genetic code, ultimately the deoxyribonucleic acid; It follows that any adaptive and progressive step of the organism would preexist from the beginning of any living form, not a gain but a mere revelation of original latencies. From which he concluded that the new constructive or "creative" evolution would be excluded. The logical analysis of the hereditary information structure reveals data that seem to confirm such a thesis. Indeed, the discreet structure of genetic information, expressed in the form of the postulated postulate of genetics, indicates that "any hereditary character is a certain logical combination of a set of these characters, genetically indivisible." But although the structure of the chromosomes perfectly matches the structure of hereditary information, it is not possible to exclude the possibility of plasmagene, which makes an irreversible breach in the main postulate of genetics. This is because it allows the "continuous" non-mathematical heredity, which explains the violation of the first postulate of genetics that reduces the evolution to a question of probability theory: "The current state of the researchers in the field of the implications of evolutionary necromosomal heredity indicates certainly its role..."

As early as 1939, *Darlington* had delivered the idea of an evolution of the genetic system itself, including the genome, and the latest conquests of molecular genetics, biophysics, its cutting-edge branch, quantum biophysics, biochemistry bring to light the existence of intermediate states From the unorganized field to that of life; It turns out that the genetic system has its own evolution, being not only a source, but also a product of evolution. (Cf. *Jean Piaget*, op., P." Genetics and the theory of experimental evolution," says *L. von Bertalanffy*, is exclusively interested in the mutational changes in the existing genes. But, unquestionably, evolution looks at not only the changes in existing genes, but also the creation of new genes."

In the process of emergence of genetic material, stages similar to those of the emergence of terrestrial life can be identified. Thus, the origin and evolution of the genetic code can not be detached from the natural history of organisms: "The vicious bodies do not depend on time. Living bodies are indissolubly linked to time. None of their structures can be detached from history, "says *Fr. Jacob*, one of the scholars who contributed to the elucidation of "mysteries" related to the structure of the genetic code.

Three stages of the appearance of genetic material can generally be distinguished. The first, started about four billion years ago, would be an earthly atmosphere almost free of carbon dioxide and free oxygen, but rich in hydrogen, methane, ammonia and water. With the help of solar radiation, ultraviolet radiation, electrical discharges and temperature variations, such an atmosphere is likely to favor the synthesis of organic substances such as amino acids, nitrogen bases, organic acids, fatty acids, sugars, forming a kind of "Organic soup"; Monod calls it a "probiotic soup". In the second stage, we are witnessing the synthesis of elemental and then some more complex protein substances, such as nucleotides, polyphosphates and others, while enriching the atmosphere in oxygen then in ozone (this forms a high layer of ultraviolet radiation filtration). In the last step, the synthesis of the proteins themselves and of the polynucleotides, initially without enzymes, then under their catalytic influence. From the interaction of nucleic acids with proteins, more stable complexes have been formed than each component. In fact, genetic material is still closely linked to proteins that catalyze its synthesis, and as far as genetic information is concerned, it is completely transferred to protein.

Within this nucleoprotein complex, nucleic acids take on the role of matrix due to their relatively strong chemical stability, and the proteins have assumed structural and enzymatic properties due to chemical lability and superior reactivity. All this leads to the continuous evolution of the complexity of organic molecules, reaching the first living organism that was nothing but a protein system; Its maintenance and continuity will depend on genetic information from nucleic acids. In a tendency so justified to avoid "inelastic" excesses, some current philosophical orientations, such as that of genetic epistemology, reject Orthodox neo-orwinism, consciously breaking modernized neolamarcism. The concrete scientific basis is provided by the positions of some prestigious biologists such as *Waddington, IL Whyte, Mair* and others about the existence of an epigenetic system or the epigenetism resulting from the interaction of heredity with the environment, and moreover from the manifestation of a cellular regulation capacity of mutations, whose mechanism remains unknown, an immanent force. This vision, before highlighting the recrudescence of Neo-Marxism, is an overstepping of what *Jean Piaget* calls the simplistic methods of "neo-wavinism " The evolutionist hypothesis, based on hazards and selections, will be substantially improved by the circular patterns of self-regulation, which attest to the existence of a specific developmental circuit established between the inborn and the acquired. The "circularity" of such explanations will be even more evident if one takes into account the fact that the phenotype appears as a replica of the genome to the influences of the environment, and on the other hand, the selection refers only to phenotypes and emanates from An environment chosen and partially modified by them. It results that between mutations as internal variations and ambiance, a complex of circuits, expressed in particular by recombinations, is established; Hence the thesis of a genetic assimilation of the external influences and, inevitably, that of the heredity of the acquired characters. The epistemological conclusions we may draw from these references are as follows:

A) evolutionism still preserves the wealth of theoretical implications, which is why no investigation of the philosophy of science can reveal either its dialectical materialism or its materialistic spontaneity, its methodological significance, but it is only valid from one Point, as Aristotle synthesizes: "above the matter is the spirit"

B) by the synthesis that he makes between continual and discontinuous - in fact between historical and non-historical, function and structure, such as the relation between adaptation and hereditary heritage, goes beyond the diachronous synchronous dilemma (which is hindered by some current philosophical currents);

C) The main concepts and categories that define the contents of evolutionism, including it in the very core of materialist dialectics, seem to me the following: causality, structure, determination and determinism, interaction, continuously discontinuous (in an indestructible unit), contradiction, Quantity, quality, leap, legitimacy, necessity-happening, synchronic diacronic, etc., on another plane, they operate naturally and dialectically;

D) the concepts of determination and determinism are central to evolution for the following reasons:

1) determinism includes in its sphere both the cause and the conditions, the causality, together with the interaction is the central category of the evolution, as well as the internal or external conditions of the development, from where the conclusion that the determination, manifested through the cause, of the interaction, Conditions, information, law, etc., is a key concept for understanding evolution, which however can not explain everything and is based on parapsychological creation.

2) determinism includes within its sphere the notion of structure, as it indicates the modalities of constructing the dynamic systems taken as a whole. But structuring a system involves knowing the relationship between pattern and genesis, between code and meaning, between structure and function or essence: established against the variation of elements, the structures also imply immanent transformations, while being finalized in the process. As a whole, evolution proves determined and determinant, that is, it manifests itself both as a structured activity and as a structural activity, in the sense that it contains the model of any transformations of its components as a process; Therefore, in the evolution of the world, it is important not to

organize but to transform.

3) determinism includes within its sphere and the quality, in the Hegelian sense, that determination is nothing more than the successive attribution of qualities to "indeterminate being", meaning becoming. Indeed, differentiation, diversification of the world means the transition from one determination to another, but also their unity, the synthesis of the different determinations between them, as well as the qualitative diversity of determinations, with quantitative amorphous, not "nothingness". All the dynamics of the evolution, of the spectacular becoming of the qualitative diversification of the world, in the process of its uninterrupted determinations, can be expressed by some Hegelian ideas, such as "becoming is a silence without stopping... the passage that takes place within the unity of being and nothingness", Appearing as the very being determined. Between becoming and determination is a relationship of interconditioning, that is to say, from becoming acquainted is determined by qualitative diversification; In the same process, however, determination determines becoming or evolving by the fact that the products of becoming, that is, the objects of the real world, are only moments of the whole, of the evolution taken as a unitary process; Because evolution is not only birth, but also the disappearance of species; That is why evolution is not only the uninterrupted assertion of novelty, it is not just a specialty, a suite of mutations that will become implacable in all other forms of life, so organic belong to evolution and the opposite phenomena: spectacular, fatal errors, falsities of Life in uncertain directions: reality, says Hegel, is considered to be only something positive, something that would exclude negation, limitation, lack. The negation, taken as a simple lack, would be what is nil. But it is a determined being, a quality determined only by a non-existence. Such aspects of the becoming of the violin are under the concrete sign of a determination that Spinoza has formulated as "omnis determinatio est negatio", and in modern terms are definitive as magnifications of negative entropy. In fact, it is an increase in information (negentropia) as the power of organizing the living, on the account of energy consumption, ie the increase of entropy (disorder) in the environment;

E) There are great similarities between evolution and progress, which can go as far as identifying the two phenomena; But it must be borne in mind that it is not a continuous series of quantitative changes that will lead to the continuous improvement of the organisms (which, as we have seen, would be a false, irrational infinite progression, in the sense of its inexistence in nature), But by a limited sequence of time and space of organizational levels, evolving not as a scale from and to infinity, but as an asymptomatic curve, tending towards the balance between entropy and adaptation, between information and finality. Finally, there is a steady increase in the negentropy (the order of order) corresponding to the anthropic gap between man and the coacervate, which justifies the metaphysical parapsychology and Socrates' axiom, which states, "I know that I know nothing."

Ontogenesis - complementarity or opposition between materialism and idealism, between science and religion

Ontogenesis is a process that takes place at the level of every living being - be it animal or vegetal - from the time of gamete formation to its death. It goes through two stages: progenogenesis, namely the formation of gametes and proper ontogenesis, from joining the gametes to the exiting of the individual. It is worth noting the existence of the common side between the animal and the vegetal world in the context of the above-mentioned process - called the genetic structure. The genetic code is found in various forms in all living matter. Interestingly, the basic chemical elements, carbon, hydrogen, oxygen, nitrogen, as well as a multitude of mineral substances are found in both the living matter and the inert, inert. The difference between the two categories of matter is that the living essence of life occurs through the combination of chemical elements, amino acids and proteins, whereas in the inert, these organic compounds do not exist.

The evolutionary theory, founded by Darwin, Lamarck, Cuvier, Linné, etc., describes the evolution of species, from the lower to the most complex, in the following sequence: C, H, O, N, coacervates, fish, batracians, reptiles, birds, mammals, anthropoid monkeys, hominids, neanderthals, humans of Cro Magnon, Homo sapiens.

This exclusive materialistic theory considers that all animal and vegetic species are the result of a long evolution. Despite the above, cladistic theory emphasizes that there is an absolute correlation between everything that exists - animal and plant species - on Earth, and that correlation is that which ensures the ecological balance and adaptation of all species to their living environment. Growth and development process are strictly established:

1. The same structure and the same number of chromosomes: man has 46, of which 44 are autosomes and 2 ganosomes.
2. Genes have a different sequence ordering, but a structure such as strong or pyrimidine base, deoxyribose and adenosine triphosphoric acid.
3. Embryonic development is also strictly structured and ordered: mourn, blastul, gastrula, neurula, necrosis process (septum primum, secundum, spurium), induction process (not statement □ nervous system).
4. Postnatal development also adheres to several rules: a superior limit of adaptability for each character; A limited influence on the environment and only on a generation scale; Correlation between genotype and paratip (phenotype).
5. Structure of the nervous system: rhinencephalus and hippocampus, considered as archaeocortical formations (old, primitive) that have a role of great complexity, even greater than that of neocortex.

If a comparison is made between the human being, considered by the mystical evolution to reach the highest level of development, and the rest of the living world (animal and vegetal) it is found that man is not the exclusive possessor of the capacities to think and, implicitly, Is not totally superior:

1. S have experiments that have proven that the plants emit actionable currents, that these currents prove a way of communication between man and plant, demonstrating the establishment of certain bilateral relations, such as the sensitivity of plants to human suffering And their response to inappropriate human behaviors.

2. The animal world has a system of thought and communication. It is enough to quote Fabre's research on the bee's life, and one can demonstrate the way the hive in the hive thinks and communicates: the division of labor, the work-bees' dance that shows the place where food is rich, the division of the work into a hive, etc.

The materialists believe that all these types of behaviors are instinctive, but they ignore the fact that instincts also have their own substrate of creativity, and that, in addition, even in humans, the instinctual area of the hippocampus or instinctual subconscious determines essentially cortical activity, even spontaneous creativity, often called intuition.

3. It is straightforward to think that there is a language of communication between plants and animals. Recent research clearly demonstrates the existence of this language, which we are still far from understanding. In terms of thinking, the intelligence whose definition is the ability to adapt to different situations, we can assume that as with the human world, where there is great variability, the vegetative and the animal one offers a great diversity depending on the species

that make up them. In the preface to the "Human Comedy," Honoré de Balzac compares the human individual and the animal communities. And he takes as a starting point in this analysis that, just like the animal world, where there are species so distinct in each other, in our world, every individual in a group of individuals can be compared to an entity of the animal world.

The differences between the two worlds consist of:

1) - In the animal world, the mouse combines with mice and binds mice

- In the human one a mouse can combine with a lioness and give birth to chickens.

2) - In the animal world the lion is the king of animals

- In the human world, a mouse can become a lion

3) - the world of animals and plants ensures the ecological balance of the planet

- man is the only being who destroys this balance

Numerous researches have also been carried out in the field of parapsychology, science which addresses phenomena that can not be explained by the knowledge system that we currently have; Parapsychology states:

A. There are many papers, including those of J. Fowels, describing phenomena. We quote a few of them.

B. Telepathy, telechance, hypnosis are far from being explained by material realities. For example, remote transmission and interception of thoughts is a reality, but their material explanation is not possible, because the phenomena we can call "where", "biological currents" pass through solid bodies that, Are opaque for all kinds of irradiation.

C. Intuition, in turn, is an inexplicable "given" or "fact" if we remember that the discovery of insulin by Sir Frederick Banting, a Canadian orthopedic physiologist, was made as a result of a dream in which he "sees "That he can obtain the active principle of hypoglycemia in the pancreas extract by ligating the Wirsung and Santorini channels. When Banting told the above-mentioned scientist JJR Macleod, director of the Toronto Institute of Biochemistry, he did not ignore such antimaterial vision and gave his best student CH Best a chance to study in detail with Sir Frederick Grant Banting, "dream"; They have experimentally, through the detailed method above, managed to extract... insulin! At the same time, the great Romanian scholar Paulescu discovers insulin through the alcohol fractionation method, this simultaneity being the starting point of a big dispute around that epochal discovery, which was the subject of the 1923 Nobel Prize for Medicine, which was awarded to Banting and Best.

If we add to these phenomena the direct communications that some individuals have in special circumstances with God, things become even more complicated. In this context, I will quote the experiences of Donald Walsh, an American billionaire who has experienced the beggar's life to later return to the status of a billionaire, at a time, considering that God was unfair to him, addressed, directly The loud voice and, miracle, heard the Voice of the Lord, who answered all questions. The discussion of the Supreme Being was eventually published by Welsh in his famous book Conversation with God. My opinion, after reading this book, I recommend, is that all human thinking, all the philosophy of work, the vision of humanity and morality, are of a divine nature.

E. Without going into detail, I must point out that the prophets are real people. Moses existed, he heard the Voice of God in the desert and received the Ten Laws on Mount Sinai; Jesus is also a real, concrete prophet, whose existence can not be explained by materiality but only by his divine nature; In turn, Mahomet, Buddha, are all real characters, just as it is, coming closer to our times, St. Anthony of Padua; And the examples are numbered.

F. Returning even today, the existence of Sai Baba, who has three residences in India, is a reality. I personally saw this character, whose appearance is announced in the Old Testament, and the history of his miraculous actions was published by an American scientist, doctor and psychologist, who had frequent meetings with Sai Baba.

If we consider all of these elements in their entirety, we will have to ask which one is more true, which is more valid: materialism or idealism, who considers our material world as "a divine fire shade that Is the spiritual world of God "a magnificent comparison made by the father of idealism, Plato; In the same vein, the question is whether the truth belongs to science or religion.

The answers to all these questions were given by the great philosopher Aristotle, considered founder of materialism, but who said that the spiritual is above matter. If we assess the phenomenon of ontogenesis, in this context, it will be clear that there are certain material regulations that are explicable, but it is also a hazard to admit exclusively evolutionary theory. If we look at the ecological balance in the same context, if we admit the parapsychological realities and the religious beliefs, it follows that the world was created by God, but that, undeniably, over the millennia, adaptations have been made. The genome, the essence of creation, can be influenced by the environment, and paratipic factors, respectively.

The Vatican now operates an institute that uses today's knowledge of science, seeking to penetrate into the essence of the Divinity and confronting the limits existing in our possibilities of knowledge. Eisenberger's research on the steps, the levels of matter, in fact, leads us to the demonstration of God.

We conclude that there is a complementarity between materialism and idealism, between science and religion. Material laws exist, but above them, they observe the spiritual laws of the Divinity, which guide the earth globally in its entirety, after me, the entire Universe. In this vision I will quote the words of great philosopher Andre Malraux as saying: "The 21st century will be religious or not at all." It is only through faith and religiosity that we can convey to human beings the wisdom of not considering our alpha and omega of the universe, and of understanding that we must fulfill the missions of the Divinity, which in essence signify: agreement among nations, Respecting the rights of the universe, understanding through the Universe all living matter and do not know, and promoting a culture of peace and tolerance in accordance with the principles of all religions. We consider the comparison of the Swiss writer Dŕrrenmatt, after which God is an elephant, and we humans, blind beings, who worship him according to the rituals of different religions, because we have managed to know Him to some extent through our own experiences, or, metaphorically, Put his hand "on one of the forelegs, or the hind legs, or on the trumpet, or even on his ivory teeth.

CHAPTER XI.
ANTHROPOLOGICAL INTERPRETATION OF DENTAL MEDICINE FROM PALEOLITIC TO MODERN PROTECTION

1. Introduction

The first dental pain occurs with the first cavities observed on the skulls of fossil humans, who lived 100,000 BC years ago in the Middle Paleolithic; The Broken Hill skull (Figure 137, 138) from Oriental Africa (Rhodesia), a Neanderthal with progressive cranial elements, had two approximate cavities in the premolar II and the upper molar I.

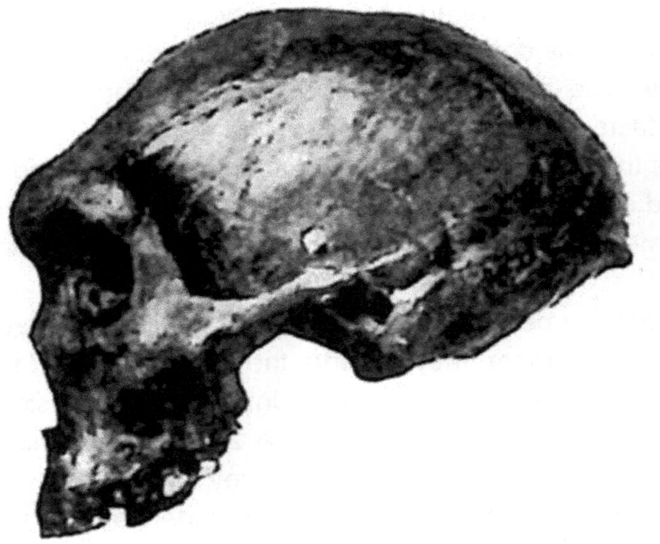

Fig. 137. The skull of an individual in Broken Hill in Oriental Africa (Rhodesia), Neanderthal, which lived 100,000 years ago and has many progressive elements present at Homo Sapiens Fossilis; This cranium revealed the first dental caries.

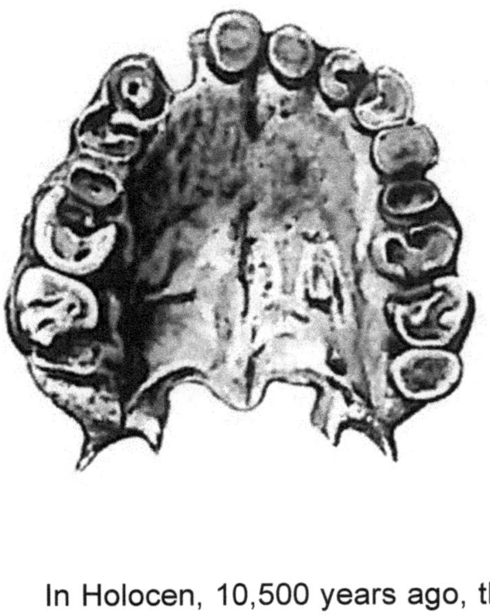

Fig. 138. Upper Maxillary of Broken Hill (Rhodesia) with cavity cavities in the upper premolar and upper molar; Associated with well-shaped dental areas of wear, forms that we often encounter at Homo Sapiens Fossilis.

In Holocen, 10,500 years ago, the dental decay rate reached 5%, so that in the Neolithic (5,000-2,000 BC) this percentage would increase to 10%; In the Bronze and Iron Age (2,000 BC), the frequency of caries reaches 20%, and in the prefeudal age (700-900 BC) we witness the doubling of the caries frequency index to 50% -55%; After the Napoleonic wars, when the use of potato and sugar from sugar beet was generalized, the dental caries reached 80% -90%, a frequency which is maintained in Romania and today (Fig.139) (Firu-14-1983).

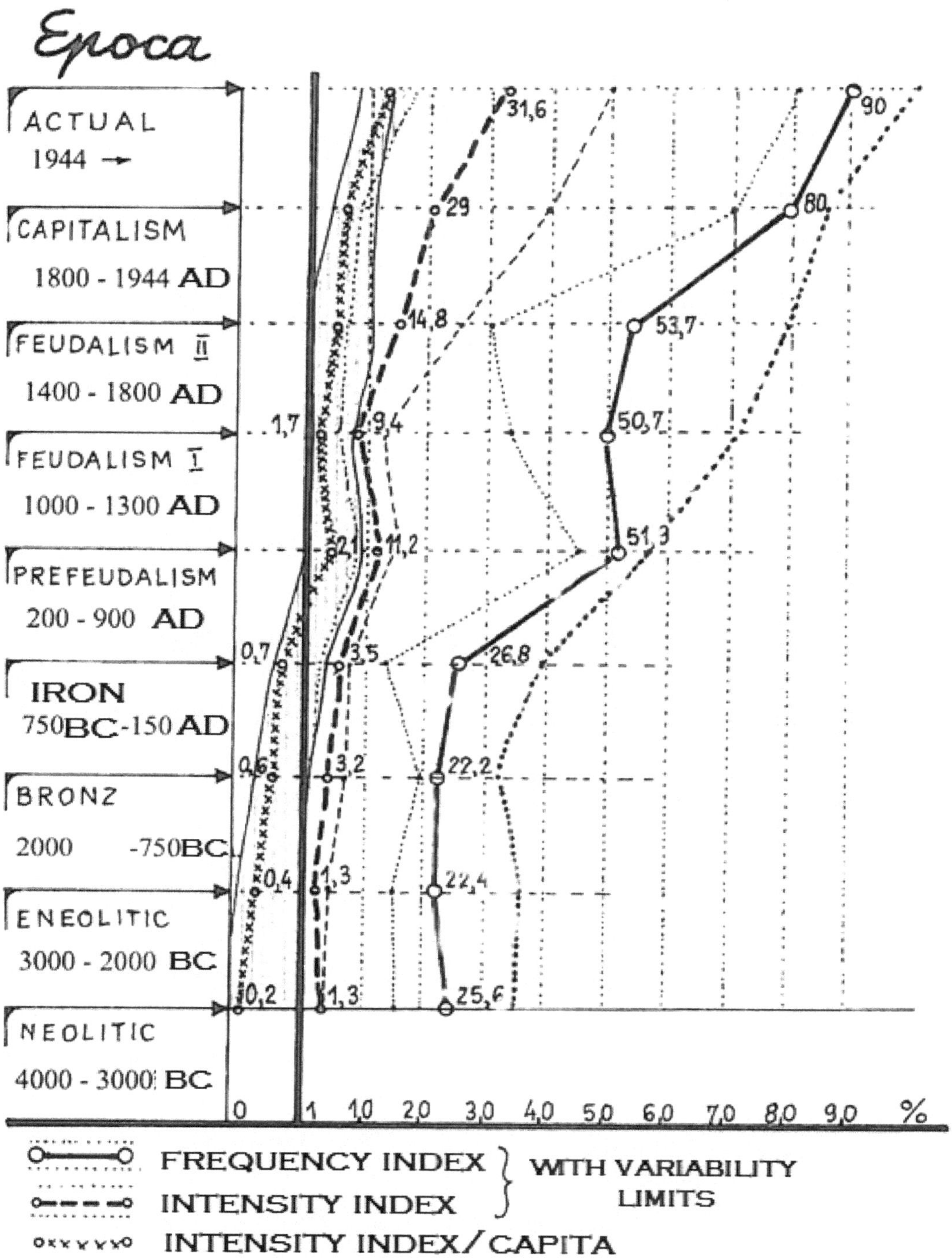

Fig. 139. Chart representing the evolution of dental caries from the Neolithic age to the present age in Romania; The introduction of hydrocarbons more frequently in the diet of the Neolithic populations to date, has led to the increasing evolution of this disease, causing very high pain (Firu-14-1983).

The progressive progression of this disease is probably due to the increasing consumption of hydrocarbons, which remain on dental surfaces for a long time. Dental caries may be considered to be the oldest disease tested on teeth, from fossil to current man; the tooth being the most representative human organ that resisted all weather, including fire. The dental caries also produce the most intense permanent pain known to humans, and it can be said that the need to cure dental caries has become imperious since the first human communities. Interestingly, in the early ancient civilizations, in Mesopotamia, China or America, the Aztecs, the

Incas or the Maya, the idea of caries prevention was linked to food debris on the teeth; removing these remains would prevent dental caries, an effective method today, based on in-depth studies (Rauscher - 29-2002).

2) First dentists

The first dentists thus appear in the imperial courts with metal, wood or goose feather toothpicks; These dentists were included, along with the harem of women, as men to serve the major state of the army leaders; They were recognized after the toothbrush, as a pendant; The Assyrian Emperor of Nineveh, Assurbanibal (669-627 BC), who had such "dentists" in his suite; The toothpicks have remained until today, all official tables having hygienically packed toothpicks (Figures 140, 141).

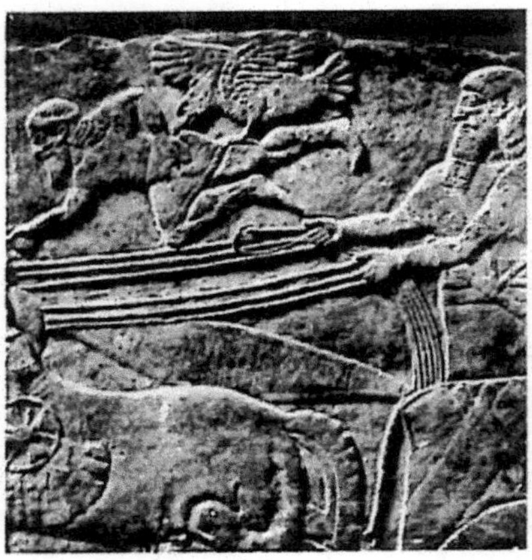

Fig. 140. Asurbanibal, king of Assyria, leading his own battle car while an eagle is flying over the battlefield to show him the most favorable way. Basorelief of the century. VII BC (After W. Krauss, 2001).

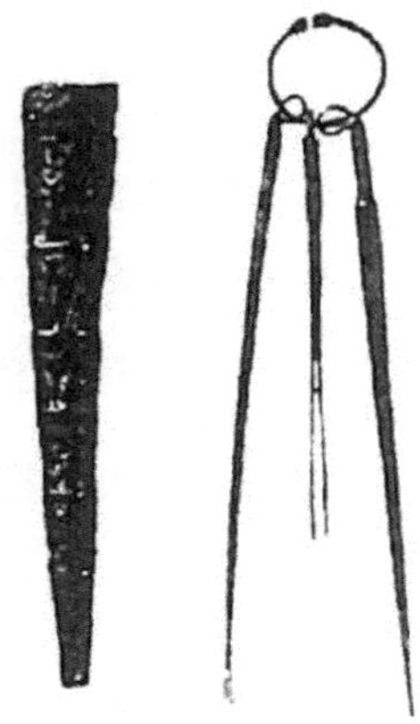

Fig. 141. The oldest toothpicks (about 3000 BC), discovered in 1888 in the temple of Ningual in Ur (Babylonia). These toothpicks were worn on the throat by the first "military" dentists being included in the king's suite in Ur (after Coredero).

Antiquity necktie carriers may be considered the first "military" dentists included in the suite of chiefs of armies.

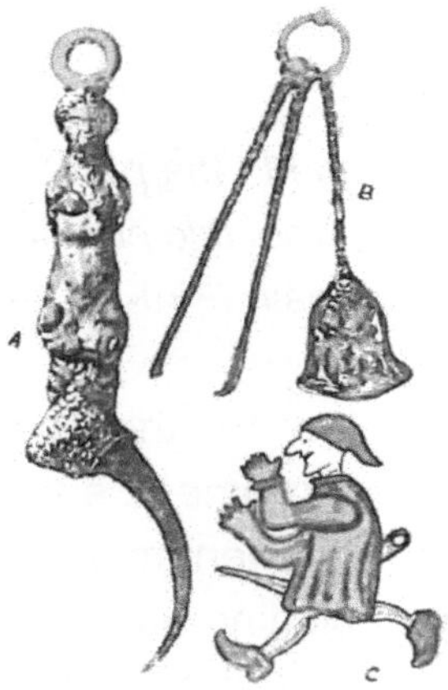

Fig.142. A. Golden Toadstools in Inca (Peru) in sec. VI d.H., worn on the neck as a pendant; B. Scarves, ear cleaners and tongue rack, gold, worn on the throat in the Renaissance (15th century); C. Scorching metal, nail and ear cleaner, used in sec. 18 in Germany.

In the 2nd millennium BC, Hammurabi, the king of Babylon (1792-1750 BC), dug a cuneiform inscription in stone with a text of 80 articles in which he published his famous law "eye for eye, tooth for tooth"; Are texts of this age where a doctor recommends soldiers, even civilians, to use beer and wine to revive their activity (Grivu, 16 - 1996). Dental extraction was performed by hand; In this era, these "dentists" were a so part of the royal suite, since a Syrian doctor advised the child of an Assyrian king, VIII BC, to take out the diseased tooth, which is the cause of the inflammation of the hands and feet; Dental focal infection was so known 2500 years ago. At the same time, the Scythians, installed 2000 years ago in Crimea, had warriors who drew their teeth by hand; Proof is painting on a Greek vessel discovered in Kul-Oba-Crimea (fig.143).

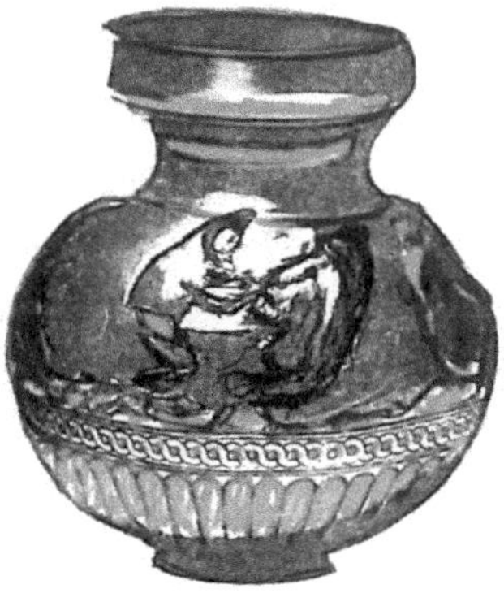

Fig. 143. The Greek vault found in a tomb in the great Kul-Oba (Crimea) mound. The bas-relief is the scene of the dental extraction of a fighter.

In Egypt, dentistry took a special moment with Imhotep, the surgeon's surgeon, who laid the foundation for wounds, fractures, including those on the face and neck; He was also the architect who made the plan of Egypt's oldest pyramid, Sakkarah, of the pharaoh Zoser (3,000 BC). However, the chief of dentists and physicians of the royal palace of Zoser was Hesi-Re, who also had a suitable instrumental for dental extractions and treatments, with mummification of dental pulp; These treatments were made by a "layman", not by a priest, without "reading" the prayers to the gods to forgive the sins punished by them for their sins; Moreover, during this period, golden ligatures of the molars or incisors were discovered in *Gizeh* (2720-2560), in cases of dento-alveolar fractures or paradontoze (Fig. 144, 145, 146), Described in the papers Ebers and Schmidth, presented in the Berlin Museum.

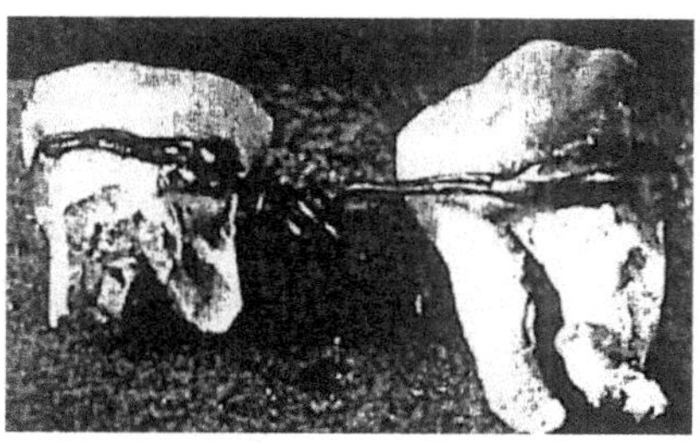

Fig. 144. Gold wire ligatures (circa 2720-2560 BC), discovered at Gizeh - Egypt in the Ebers and Schmidth papyrus, presented in the Berlin museum (after Cordero).

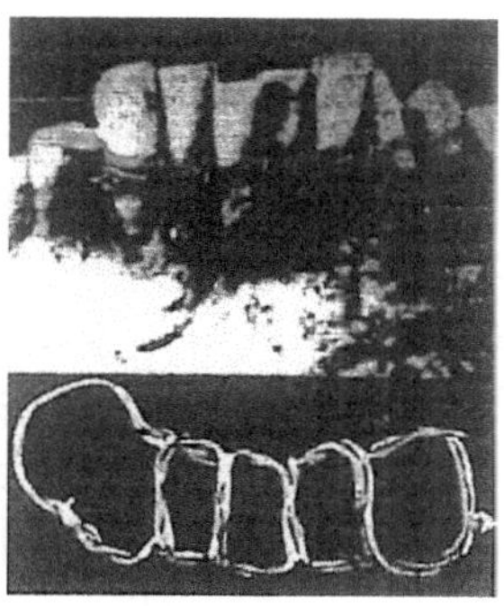

Fig.145. The oldest dental work discovered in Egypt at Gizeh (2700 BC) in the papers Ebers and Schmidth, presented in the Berlin Museum (after Cordero).

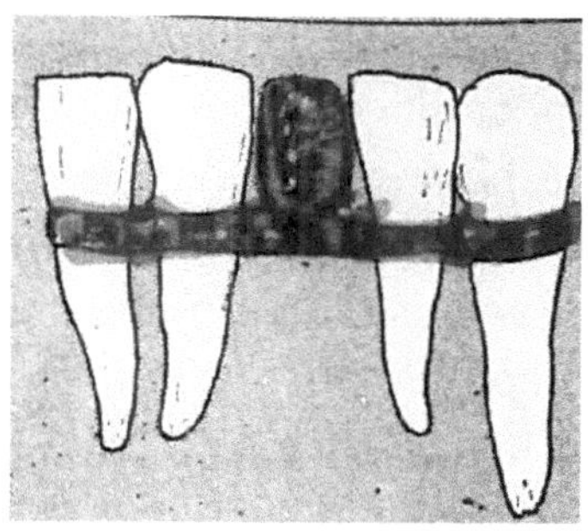

Fig. 146. In Italy, during the first millennium BC, the descendants of the Sumerians, with their herds of cattle, emigrated to Tarquinia, near Rome, where they developed a yafelite culture; In one of their graves were found dental prostheses attached to natural teeth with gold strips.

3) Greco-Roman dental medicine

1. Dental medicine in ancient Greece.

In the Mediterranean islands of Crete and Cyprus, the Greeks commerce with the ships, using the bow with bronze arrows and daggers, for their defense; The traumas were frequent, so that warriors used the calcareous rock powder as a hemostatic wound; After removing the darts, the dirty wounds were washed with old black wine, which had tannin, astringent as a haemostatic and even antiseptic; They applied leaves of aromatic plants on the wound, which had trophic and antiseptic action at the same time; In addition, these leaves, covering the plague, prevented local dehydration and the formation of a bleeding crust. All these empirical therapeutic methods are also used today by those who go on a mountain in trips and do not have the appropriate medical kit with them today.

In Homer's Iliad, the wound-healing treatments are described, and on some Greek vessels, Achilles is presented by the arm of his friend, Patrocle, with canvas feathers. During this period, Greek medicine was based on beliefs and customs where the gods played an essential role in the production of diseases and their healing. In Greece, the healer was Apollo, the god of the sun; In this era, the saying goes, "where the sun does not enter the disease." Apolo was considered to be the savior of health (Apolo prophylax). The Greeks worshiped Asclepius the son of Apollo with the Coronis, a mortal nymph; He taught medical art from the centurion Kiron; Asclepios is carved on the metropolis in the temple of Epidaur, sitting on a chair (4th century BC).

Being half-dead, Asclepius married a mortal, having two boys and three girls; Of them, Machaon was ready to heal war wounds from arrows, spears, or flares. His name disappeared, evidence that he did not bring important services to the treatments known in antiquity; Hygea remained because he had patronized general and oral hygiene; She had a pupil, Telesphores, represented on the gates of the Greek and Roman cities as a hooded child of the Dacians. Panacea deals with herbal medicinal herbs; Her name remains as something that has no healing pleasure; The other two children, Padaliros and Epione, were completely forgotten, not being representative of the healing of the sick (*Sandulescu*, 32-1940).

The cultural and philosophical movement developed in the Pericles century (6th-5th centuries BC) gave freedom to people to heal and bring the "man" to the center of activity: "man is the measure of all things." Under this account, in the island of Cos, Hippocrates (fig.147), the son of a physician who heals people with "thermal baths", he initiated and developed a rational medicine, which until today remains a reference science (*Sandulescu* - 1960).

Hippocratic medicine includes 67 books, which set the basis for disease prevention through the balance between diet and physical activity, in a fresh air area with forests, with springs of flowing water; Not by chance the competitions on Mount Olympus, where Fidias carved the famous statue of Zeus, took place in such a clean air; The sporting competitions are, in fact, a preparation for the battles that will follow, for the defense of their homeland. Fractures of the jaw were resolved by immobilizing the teeth with gold or linen; Reducing the temporomandibular dilation was done as we do today. Hippocrates makes the first observations of orthodontics, establishing the ratio between the dental eruption and the child's age.

Hippocrates describes the dento-alveolar incongruences, associating them with the narrowing of the upper jaw, with a deep vault and often with "otoree"; Also believes that dental plaque can produce periodontitis, recommending the necessity of dentition (*Sandulescu* - 32-1940). Aristotle, (322-284 BC), the perceptor of Alexandru Macedon, brings a series of new data on dento-maxillary anatomy and proposes the extraction of teeth with "pliers", pliers to be introduced by the Romans in the legions theirs, with the name "denticeps".

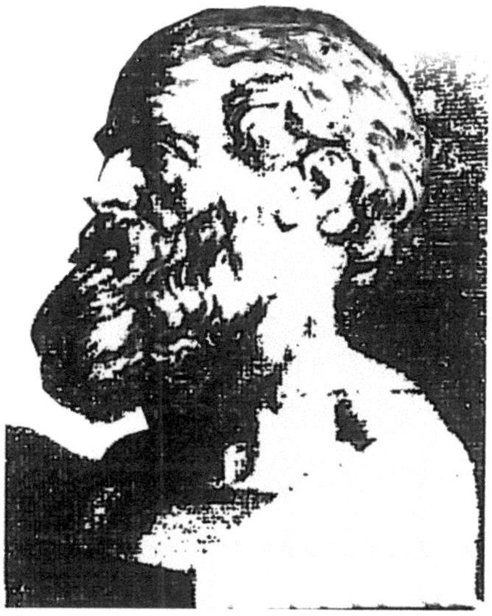

Fig. 147. Hippocrates, the creator of medicine based on clinical signs and a rational diagnosis; He develops a "secular" medicine laying the foundations of modern medicine.

Aristoteles skillfully described the late eruption of the molars of minds with their accidents observed in the young fighters, prepared by Philip II, fighters with whom Alexander Macedon conquered the Oriental Ancient World, defeating the Persian armies and replacing their empire with the Greek Empire, From India to Macedonia.

In 333 BC Alexandru Macedon establishes the city of Alexandria, which will become the largest port and cultural and commercial city in the world; This city became famous through the built lighthouse and the famous library of this city, made by Ptolemy, one of the generals of Alexandru Macedon, remaining to rule Egypt; This general became a pharaoh, and his descendants founded the Greek dynasty Ptolemy, the last pharaoh being Cleopatra, after which Egypt became a Roman colony. Under the leadership of the Ptolemy, for three centuries, Alexandria became the most important medical center, gathering in the library of this great city all the manuscripts existing in this field; Hippocrates' 67 volumes, under the name of "Corpus Hipocraticum", are housed here, where epidemics, diseases of the eye, fractures, joints, including dento-maxillary are mentioned; Here are also included the first laws of Professional ethics, also known as the "Hippocratic Oath", which he "swears" today about all promotions of doctors, including dentists.

2. Dental medicine in ancient Rome.

The great Greek doctors are brought to Rome as slaves, yet they become doctors of imperial families; Celsius becomes the doctor of Emperor Octavian Augustus; In the sec. II dH, the Emperor Marc Aureliu brings to Rome the famous physician Claudius Galenus Nicon (131-200 dH), who collected in all 67 volumes all ancient medicine, volumes which were consulted by medical students in Europe XVIII d.H.

Roman medicine during periods of civil-military ascension in the 5th century BC - II d.H., focuses on beliefs and habits based on empirical observations. The first written documents on Roman medicine appear in the sec. II BC after the Battle of Leucopetra (146 BC), when the Greek cities, including Athens, were occupied by the Roman troops, and when the Romans began to import the culture and therapeutic methods of medicine in Greece; Horatiu said "Greece capta ferro, we win the cap" "Greece was conquered by iron, but (Greece) conquers the victors." After this conquest, the Romans introduced into their legions the "dentists", who pulled their teeth with iron pincers, introduced by Aristotle to Philip II's court, pliers they would call "denticeps"; Will of course also take some antiepidemic measures, engaging Greek doctors to treat their wounded in the struggles that will continue for five centuries. In the sec. In Rome (91 BC), the Romans set up in Rome the first military medical school, in particular, by employing the doctor, Asclepiade of Bitinia, formed at the Alexandria school; At that time atomistic theory was in vogue, inspired by Thales' philosophy in Miletus, a theory known as the "soldier"; They argued that all organs are made up of moving atoms, atoms that come from the cosmos through the pores of the skin, and through these pores also leave the human body in the cosmos (I. Charchet -21-1997).

When the pores of the skin diminish, the atoms no longer circulate and the disease occurs; When pores remain open, at the entrance and exit of atoms, man is healthy; This theory was most probably inspired by Yang Yen's Chinese theory, where "energy" (Yang) penetrates into the living, receptive (Yen) human body and exits the body in the cosmos, after the physical and mental "energy" Produced in the human body; When these "partially consumed energies" are blocked, the "painful" places in the body appear sick; The Chinese bring, as a therapeutic method, "acupuncture" in the current; The Greeks do not propose any effective method in their solistic theory. Also in the sec. IHH, and I dH, Pliny the Elder (23 BC-79 dH), the Mesina fleet admiral, dead at the eruption of the Vesuvius volcano (79 dH), philosopher and naturalist, speaks in the seventh book Of the 37) about milk teeth and the treatment of wounds, actually copying the known methods from other books.

Aulus Cornelius Celsus (25 BC-50 AD) was the doctor of Emperor Octavian Augustus; Formed at the Alexandria school; Celsus brought to Rome the latest medical techniques and theories of his time. In the eight volumes written, Celsus reserves, in two of them, volumes six and seven, the dento-maxilo-facial problems, which are still valid today. Celsus makes incision of dental abscesses, including fistulas, after which performs dental extraction and curettage of the alveolus; In periodontitis he causes cauterization, and in the dento-alveolar fractures he makes connections with golden wire; He questions the cause of a disease, leaving the dictum "sublata causa tolitur effectus" - "suppressing the cause suppresses the effect"; That is why he does the extraction of the teeth that produced the dental abscess. Celsus first describes the carotid arteries that "carry the blood up" and the jugular veins that "carry the blood down". He makes the differential diagnosis in blood leak in the mouth; In headaches or abdominal pains, in coughing; In vomiting or "ulcerations" in the neck or nose, blood may appear in the mouth.

In articular dislocations, including temporomandibular ones, Celsus says that these dislocations occur "violently" either by tearing their ligaments or by "loosening" them. During the emperor Augustus Octavian, stationary nurses with military doctors were established, where soldiers who became nurses in legions were trained to treat their wounds and to extract their teeth with denticeps (figure 148).

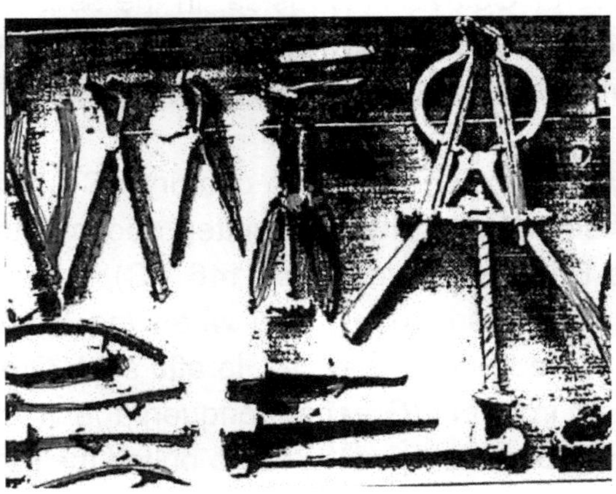

Fig. 148. Surgical instruments used by Romanians, each legion being endowed with such dental instruments.

Also in these stationary infirmary in Rome and other cities of the empire, dental homotransplants were routinely made, extracting healthy teeth from slaves to be implanted in the edited spaces of rich people; To maintain these homotransplants, ligatures with hair of horse, silk or gold were used; Such ligatures were also routed to patients with paradontosis, on their natural teeth; We do not have material evidence of these methods, because the Romans were incinerated; In the martial epigrams, or in the satires of Horatiu, Juvenal and Persuis, these methods are mentioned. Fragrances were used by Romanians, especially after Cosmus markets these products, later called "cosmetics". So use mouthwash with saffron, red roses or extracts of pistachios, myrtle, mastic, anise, etc.; The parsley leaves were chewed to relieve the smell of the mouth (hay fetish).

Caring for her mouth, her perfume was common in the good world of Augustus Octavian's era, while Ovidiu wrote in "The Ars Amandi" "the care you give to this agreeable person can be guessed by observing the pink incarnation of the lips, the gums as blue glow Of the two rows of pearls that illuminate their little face" (free translation from Latin).

In ancient Rome during Augustus Octavian, there was also a dental office on Mount Aventin, served by dentist Cascellius, who practiced dental fillings with lead, hence the use of the word "plumbare" to define the dental filling. In this cabinet were used various "dust" tooth cleansing and even tree stems, probably "sweetwood" to "rub" the teeth.

Claudius Galenus Nicon (131-201 AD), a famous physician of Roman antiquity born in Pergamos in the Middle East, makes medical studies in Alexandria and Smirna (Izmir) to be called by Emperor Marc Aureliu as a personal physician, still serving on His son, Commodus. Galenus did a medical school in Rome; For studying the anatomy, Galenus dissects with his pupils a pig. Galenus adopted "Hypocratic medicine based on clinical signs and symptoms and a rational diagnosis; Presented the two theories in the production of diseases, solidism and humoralism, without supporting them; Galenus is the creator of medicine, mostly medicinal herbs, creating the discipline known today as Galenics; His volumes (manuscripts) reached 67, contain the therapeutical theories and medical methods of his age, having the merit of reminding all the doctors who preceded him from antiquity; For 1500 years, his work was the "book of all" of all the students and doctors who trained in this noble Profession; Arabs and Christians accepted the medical work of Galenus, which was also known in India and China in translation (Bratescu - 6 - 1981). Until 1700 there were "Galenists" who did not accept other therapies except those written by Galenus; In Europe, medical school students were trained in the manuscripts of Hipocrates, Galenus and Avicena; The basis of Galenus' therapeutic principles was:

- "Contraria contrariis curandum est", the law of the contrary; The fever should be treated with cold compresses, high blood pressure should be treated with phlebotomy, etc.
- Disease is an imbalance of humor in the body, treatment is the balancing of humor, a method that is currently used in endocrinology.
- Knowing the diseases, the efficiency of the treatment methods, should be done only on the basis of the experiment; The clinical experience of a physician is fundamental.
- Galenus made a distinction between disease and lesion, hence later, Virchow established the classification of diseases after tissue lesions (*Bratescu* - 5, 1987).

4) Person-Arab dental medicine

After the collapse of the Roman Empire, the Arabs, under the banner of Islam, occupied the former Roman colonies, forming two great kingdoms in Cordoba (Spain) and Baghdad (Syria), where they developed hospitals and dispensaries for the sick, considering medicine science science; In this respect, translated almost all the medical manuscripts of time into Arabic, while at the same time committing to their court the best known Persians, Greeks, Syrians or Jews; Of these are Rhazes (850-923 AD) who wrote "Al Havi," the comprehensive book for his students in Baghdad. Avicena (Ibn Siva), a Persian of origin (Buhara), lived in the 9th-10th centuries AD, introducing pulse and urine research into the patient's clinical analysis, continuing to analyze the patient's Hippocrates temperature (*Abu AH Avicena* - 1962).

Avicena wrote "The Canon of Medicine" in five volumes, the third book being reserved for head and neck diseases; The "canon of medicine" was also written in poems of medicine (1326 poems), which were taught as poetry. This "canon" has become the basis of medical education in Europe for 700 years, being translated into French and English; Avicena's manuscript reached the first stage in Montpellier, where Arab merchants sold epic spices on the mountain of the Mediterranean bay, then called Mont des Epices, from which the name Montpellier was derived. In the sec. 12 dH, the first medical school in Montpellier was established, where Avicena's canon became the book of "captain" and from where the canon circulated in all European countries, in England, Germany, etc. (*Duţescu* - 12 - 1979)

In Europe, during this period there were many wars between the feudal states, so that the fractures, shakes and wounds caused by arrows, swords, spears were frequent; Avicena's books establish the therapeutic principles of these diseases; In verse 1312, Avicena says: to repair a fracture, you must first succeed in reducing it. In verse 1313, Avicena says: continuing to place bone fragments so that they can resume their place; Cut the bones that hurt the saw. In verse 1321: the dislocation is reduced by pulling until the scraped bone resumes its place, after which it must be maintained for a certain time.

5) Dental Medicine in the European Middle Ages

After the collapse of the Roman Empire, cultural life is being degraded and hunger, epidemic diseases, tuberculosis (tongue), plague (1347-1352), smallpox (black plague), typhoid fever, leprosy and all known debilitating diseases; Blinds, scolios, cockroaches, paralysts are appalling appearances in the paintings of Breughel; It is shown here that these sick people became beggars because their families were banishing them, believing that they had become ill because of the sins they had done, and did not want this sin to be transferred to the members of the family; "There is no doubt that sin is the primary cause of disease of time," said John Chrysostom.

In this period of "underdeveloped country" feudal "oases" appear, where the normal life of people continues with the medical therapeutical methods continued from Hipocrate, Celsus, Galenus or Avicena; However, most poor people resume popular beliefs and habits, resume charms and witchcraft, reintroduce supernatural forces in the form of magnetism; A group of Italians are coming out to tease their teeth and stones under their tongue with their hands and offer the sick to various multipurpose plants; These were the charlatans, who made aberrant treatments without therapeutic value.

In the 10th-15th centuries, medical schools were developed in Salerno, Bologna, Padova, Montpellier, Paris, where "red-hot" wounds or hemorrhoids were started; Lead-based purgatives were recommended in all existing diseases to "cleanse the intestines" and apply bleeding (phlebotomy) to the plethora (hypertension)

In dental pain, Rugerro of Salerno (12th century) used fumigants with noxious substances to kill the "worm" that produced the pain in the tooth (Fig.149, 150). Also in Italy the teeth were pulled out by hand (figure 150).

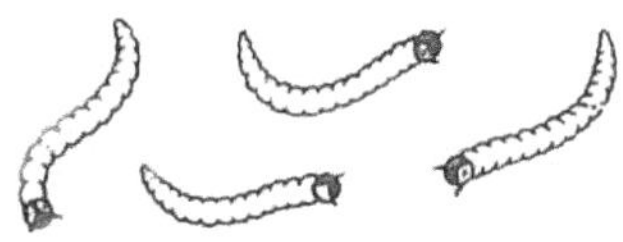

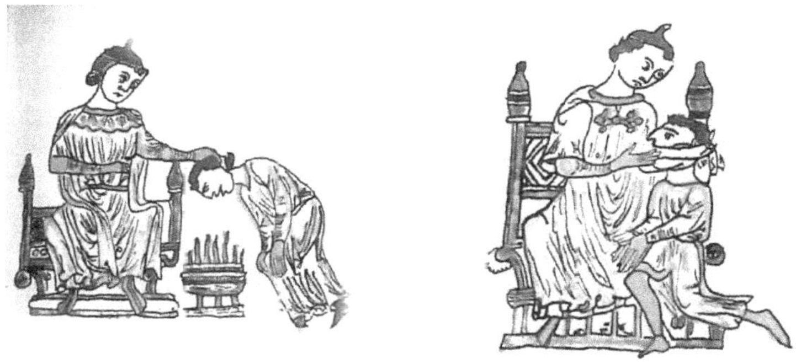

Fig. 149. The dental worm, after Cordero.

Fig. 150. Incision of a dental abscess with nail (From the surgery treaty of Rugero de Frugardo, 1100-1200).

It is no wonder that in the sec. XVII King Louis II of Louis VI (picture 151) addressed to the charlatans in the Paris parish to take out his carious and painful teeth before re-marrying Mme de Maintenon; Although he had an internist physician and surgeon (Dr. Marechal) in the palace, the king called a queen to pull his teeth out with his hand and instruments, and finally managed to make a buccal-sinusoid communication Has suffered the rest of his life; After the extractions he had suffered, he gave an edict that forbade the charlatans to make extractions; He gave an order to become a surgeon at a school attached to the Paris School of Medicine (Sorbonne). These schools were in fact surgeons who held the "short robe" final exam, unlike physicians who had a lot of anatomy and little surgery, and supported the "doctoral thesis" in a "long robe" (Ferenbach - 13-1986).

Fig. 151. Louis XIV King Sun, sec 16-17 Called a "charlatan" from Paris to take out all her mobile teeth before marrying M-me of Maintenon; The charlatan made a buccal-sinus communication of which he has suffered all his life.

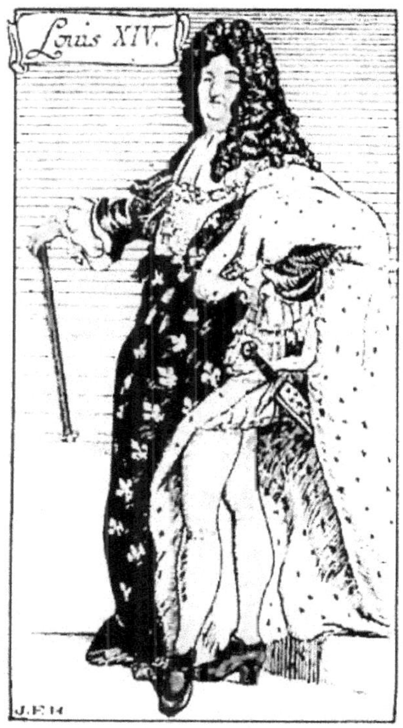

It is no coincidence that during this period, Stephen the Great of Moldova called a Jewish doctor from Italy, from Padua, to treat his wound with the red iron, according to the time method; Petru the Great, the Tsar of Russia, was also treated with red iron for hemorrhoids, and because of pain he pushed foreign doctors with the stick, making him "ungainly".

6) Dental medicine during the European Renaissance

The emergence of Christianity in the first millennium of this age brings a superior morality, based on love between people and good understanding; Man must reduce or completely inhibit the aggressive motions and animal instincts with which we are born; "I am the way, the truth and the life," says Jesus Christ to the true Christians; The "key" moment of the success of Christianity is the judgment of St. Paul of Rome on the leadership of Emperor Nero; Here the Roman judges asked St. Apostle Paul: "Do you want to sacrifice to our gods to escape with life?" St. Paul replied, "I have another God who preaches love among men, what It starts from our soul; You are dealing with the body of man, who brings sacrifices to the temple of Mars, the god of war and the temple of Venus, which glorifies the bodily love; My God promotes the love of the soul that remains forever". After Nero begins the degradation of the Roman Empire, barbarian peoples attack and occupy the territories of the old empire; The Goths and France will establish a Christian country in France, the Vandals occupy part of the North African territories, becoming Christian (the Aryan sect as the Goths); The Roman Empire of the East consolidated in Constantinople, managing to maintain it until 1453, when occupied by the Turks.

Christianity, with its humanitarian conception, is developing, and all time artists, from Giotto to Rafael and Michelangelo, portray Christos and his apostles in the paintings of the cathedrals, creating an atmosphere of total triumph of humanism. Renaissance discovers a new world, finds man, who may be non-aggressive (Jules Michelet); Moral principles are included in the nation's governing system; Executives who have agreed to specifically observe these principles have progressed today and are examples to follow (Switzerland and the US).

In 1462, the three great new roadmakers have died: Michelangelo, Calvin and Andre Vésale, roads based on freedom, equality and solidarity. Michelangelo, in Italy, led architecture, painting and sculpture on the verge of perfection, after studying art, the cult of antiquity and the anatomy of the human body. Calvin in Switzerland brought moral principles as the ultimate goal in conducting a social human community.

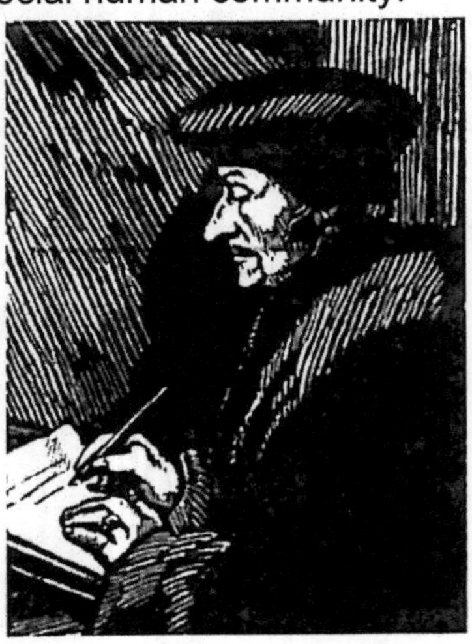

Fig. 152. Erasmus de Rotterdam (1460-1536), the famous reformer of theological education, criticizing scholasticism; He proposes to study matter through observation, developing the "humanistic" concept in social life.

Andre Vésale of Padua reformed descriptive human anatomy, laying the foundations of medicine, surgery and dentistry, whose progress is being seen today. During these reformers in art, morals and medicine, Erasmus of Roterdam (1460-1536), the reformer of education,

education and science, distinguishes the methodology of research on humanist principles. Erasmus of Roterdam introduces reason and observation, judgment and analysis into truth, being the declared enemy of "scholastics," used by the church clergy, on the principle of "believe and not search." In his work Elloge de la foie, reprinted in 1950-1962 in 52 editions, Erasmus proposes:

1. Respect and preserve works of literature and art, to be known, assimilated and developed by young people who follow us.

2. Knowledge of classical languages and language learning to know and interpret the works of our great forefathers and contemporaries.

3. Discarding the scholastic system, which teaches young people to recite everything they read as poetry without understanding the meaning of the words.

Passive reading should be replaced by rational assimilation of knowledge and confirmation of ideas through "reflection" and meditation, with direct observation of people, through discussions to better know them. Every researcher must study with "piety" and respect for those who say "truth" by repudiating any genius "scholar" who does not use reason (Gysel - 17 - 1980). In medicine:

- students must know the problems written by their predecessors, so their observations do not seem to be "rediscovered" by the new authors;
- any research should have the bibliography as accurate as possible, with appropriate comments and relevant discussions;
- any research must end with conclusions based on reason and truth, whether the result is positive or negative;
- Your colleagues (doctors or theologians) have to be respected for their ideas, thus addressing the first deontological attitudes in medical or pastoral life.

The beginning of the religious reforms with Luther, Huss, or Calvin deceived Erasmus, becoming sad and solitary (Figures 153, 154, 155). In this atmosphere of piety and respect for truth, "reborn" and medicine, starting with the fundamental foundations namely: anatomy, general pathology and surgery, making the first steps towards technical progress, which continues today at a dizzying pace.

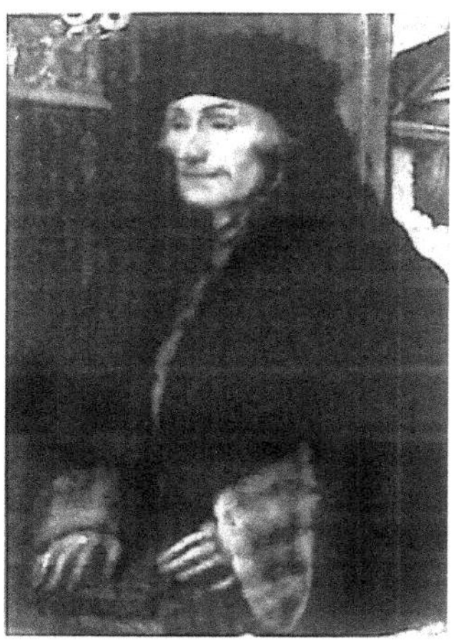

Fig. 153. After Hans Holbein's painting at Basel in 1525, Erasmus de Rotterdam is at the age he considered betrayed by his students who reformed, which is why he isolated himself in a continuous meditation.

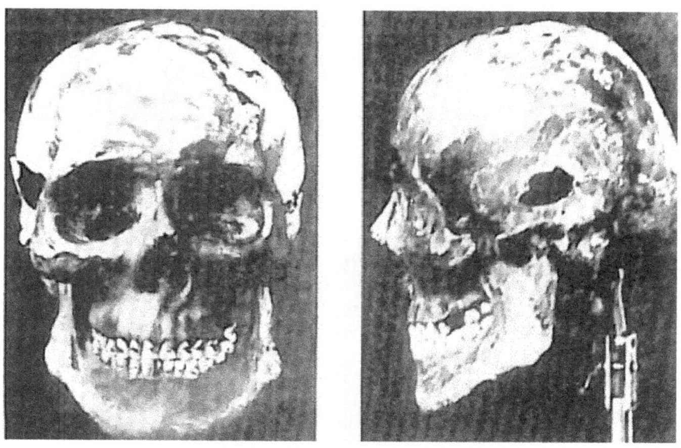

Fig. 154. In 1929 his skull was discovered. Erasmus de Rotterdam in the Basel cathedral curve, confirming the Nordic typology, eyed nails, thin lips, hyperleptoproscopy, elongated nose (N4D4M2)

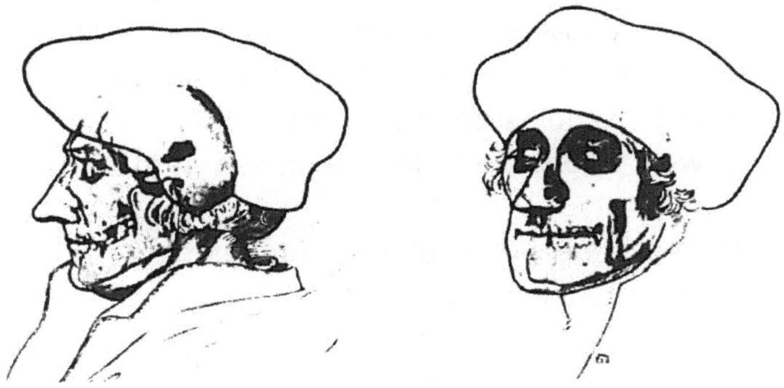

Fig. 155. Overlapping painting on Erasmus's cranial Profile in Rotterdam
Verify the identity of the skull.

7) From philosophical anatomy to artistic and medico-dental anatomy

In the group of representative anatomists of the sec. XVI-XVII we can remember Leonardo da Vinci (1452-1519) (figure 156), who "overcame the science and art of his time with centuries" (Ghiţescu), dissected 30 corpses, made molds by injecting hot wax into Lungs, blood vessels, and other cavity organs, for then to represent them through drawings and drawings that remained to this day very valuable by their accuracy; The mimics muscles are meticulously examined to know the facial mimics, the common language of all people of all time. Leonardo da Vinci's anatomy notebooks were only known in the sec. XVI, when they arrived at the Windsor (England) collection and when they were published, after the study, XIX.

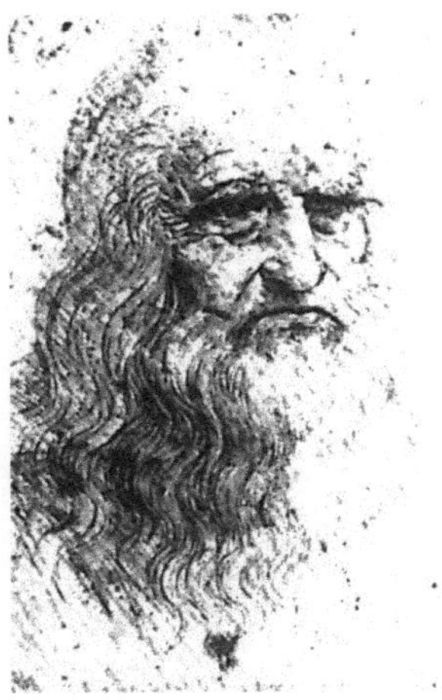

Fig. 156. Leonardo da Vinci, self-portrait, drawing made in 1512, kept at the Turin library.

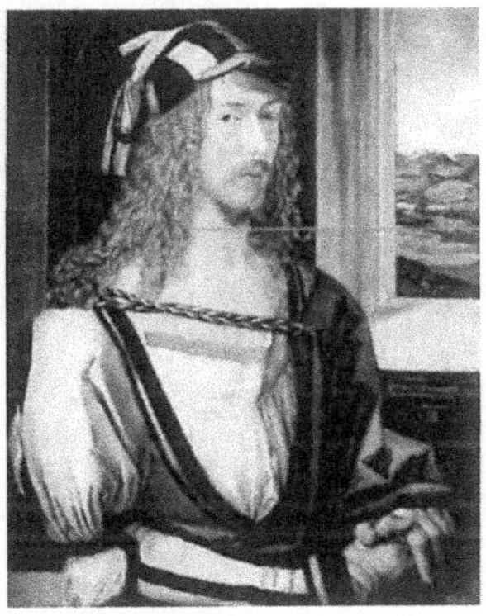

Fig. 157. Albrecht Dürer, self-portrait from 1498, exhibited at the Prado Museum in Madrid.

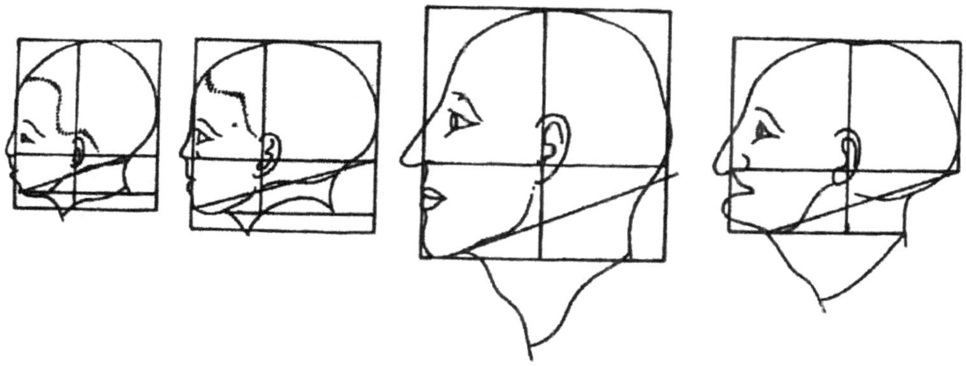

Fig. 158. The facial Profile changes from childhood to old age, from three, five to 25 And over 70 years, according to the loss of teeth after Albrecht Dürer.

Albrecht Dürer, (1471-1528) (fig.157), made a treaty in which it determines the proportions of the body, including those of the head (figure 158). *André Vésale* (1514-1564) was born in Brussels, continuing his studies in Paris and Montpellier; As a Professor at Padua, he corrected the anatomy of the teeth and jaws exposed in the volume "Humani corporis factory libri septem"; Here is the anatomy of all teeth (fig.159), although he considers that the tooth is a "denuded" bone, sensitive, with its own nerves; It excludes the existence of the incisor bone in the upper jaw (Figure 160), and the mandible is a single bone through ossification of the mentoniene symphysis (Figure 161) (*Gysel*-17-1980).

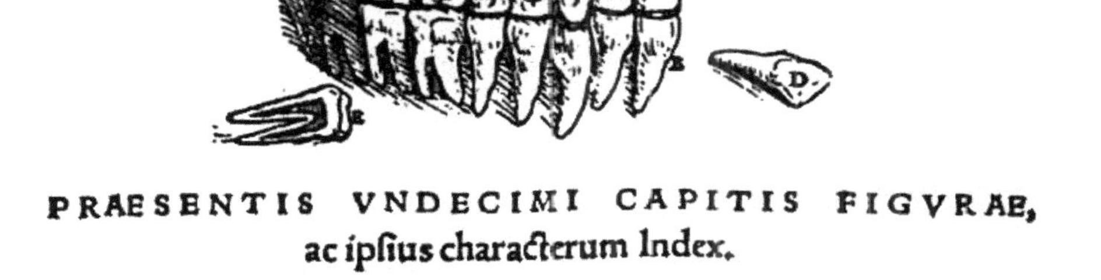

DE HVMANI CORPORIS FABRICA LIBER I.
DE DENTIBVS, QVI ETIAM ossium numero ascribuntur. Caput XI.

PRAESENTIS VNDECIMI CAPITIS FIGVRAE, ac ipsius characterum Index.

Fig. 159. Wood grading representing the superior and inferior teeth of man, Vésale describes for the first time the pulp chamber, after Gysel, 1980.

Vésale makes the first observations of the pathological skulls in the "Factory", showing that there are four pathological skulls, after the antero-posterior diameter (dolicocephal-brahicefalus) or their size (microcephaly or macrocephaly, hydrocephalus). Studying the skulls, Vésale presents the "thinker" in a wood engraving in the form of a standing skeleton, with a right hand on a skull and his left hand shattering his chin and face. Vésale's first successor is *Réaldo Colombo* (1515-1558), who is dedicated to anatomy, dissecting corpses with students from all over Europe to Italy.

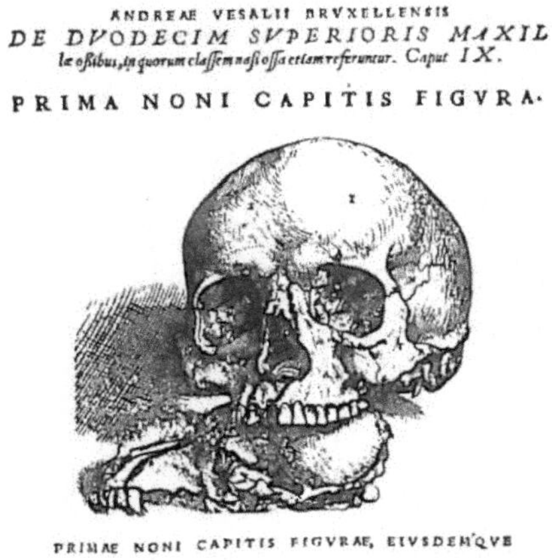

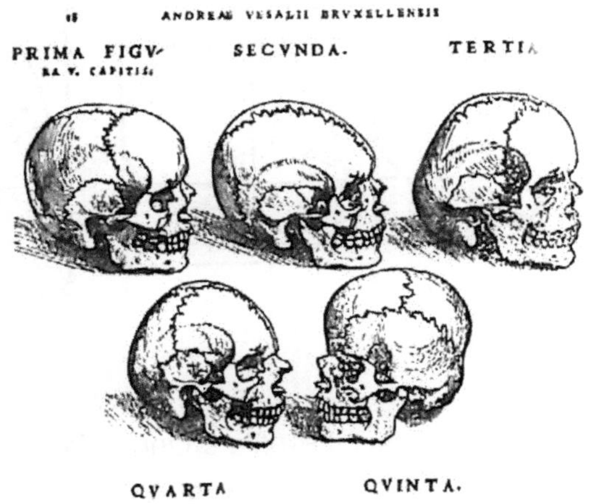

Fig. 160. Wood engraving in the volume of Vésale "The human corporis factory," where he claims for the first time that man does not have intermaxilar bone, as it does in the dog, according to Gysel, 1980.

Fig. 161. Wood engraving in its volume Vésale "The humani corporis factory", where Are presented a normal and other skull Four pathological, with longer cap or wider, smaller or larger, After Gysel, 1980.

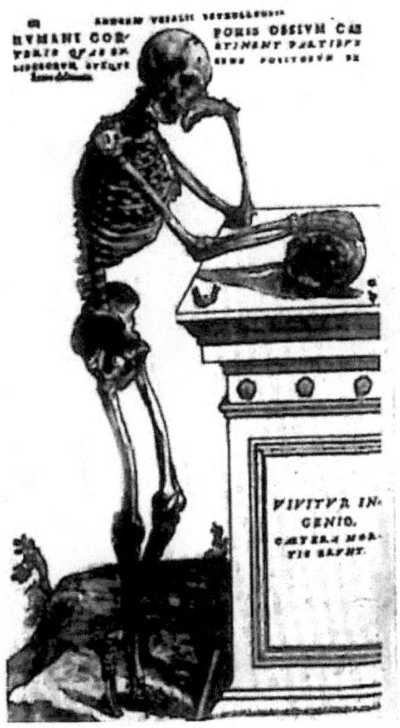

Fig. 162. The "thinker" skeleton represented by Vésale, in a wood engraving in his volume "The humani corporis factory after Gysel, 1980.

Bartolomeo Eustachio (1524-1574) writes "Libelus de dentibus" with a 42-page bibliography quoting Hippocrates, Aristotle, Galen, Avicena; Here he establishes for the first time that the tooth is an organ made of enamel and a tough, white tissue, like marble, which covers the dentin as a shell of the tree.

He also presents exactly the dental eruption with the follicular bag and gubernaculum dentis; A complete study is reserved for the mind's minds, distinguishing their inclusion in agenesis; He remains in anatomy with the description of Eustachio's trumpet, which makes the connection between the middle ear and the pharynx.

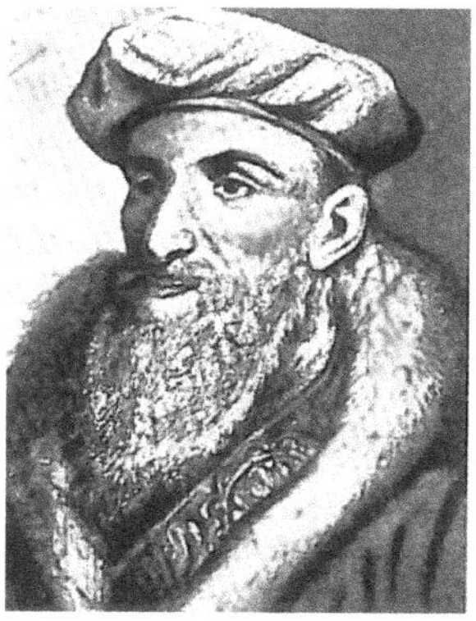

Fig. 163. Bartolomeo Eustachio (1524-1574), Wood engraving by Frederico Baroccio. He wrote the first full volume of dental biology "Libellus de Dentibus", after Gysel, 1980.

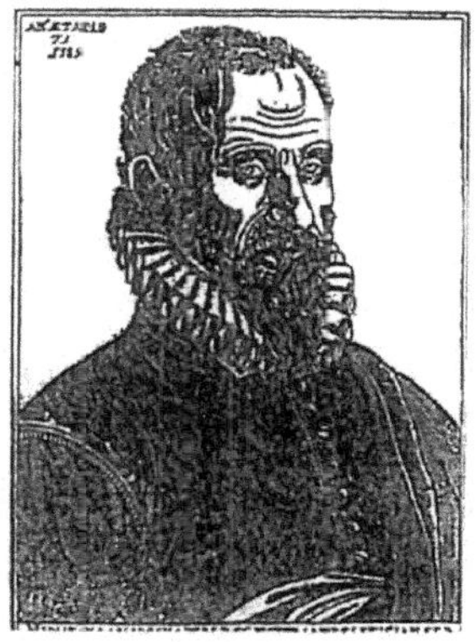

Fig. 164. Ambroise Paré (1517-1590), Renowned surgeon of Renaissance, After Zimmer.

*Ambroise Paré (*1517-1590) (figure 164) was a military-bearded surgeon, participating in various battles during the reign of Henry III; He treated the facial wounds, the alveolo-dental fractures and took out his teeth with the "pliers", being considered the founder of militant surgery in Europe; Ambroise Paré introduces dental prosthesis to patients with labio-maxilo-palatine clefts to help them speak; He studies the bones of the skull, completing Vesale, Colombo and Faloppia, establishing 15 bones, approaching reality.

Francesco Martinez (1518-1588) was the dentist of Philip II; He publishes a volume about "dental art" in 152 pages dedicated to Prince Don Carlos, the son of Philip II; He describes, in the form of dialogue, the evolution of temporary and definitive teeth with their pathological complications, giving indications for the prevention of dental caries; He recommends rubbing the "black stain" (carya) with boiled wine mixed with alum and cooking salt.

It performs the teeth extraction using special elevators (Fig.165 A, B); Also removes the debris from the dental caries with a special instrument (fig.166). In the wounds of the face, Martinez used Roman methods, washing the bloody wound with boiled wine, adding incense of incense, myrrh, rosemary, and especially copper sulphate, known as the "Roman vitriol".

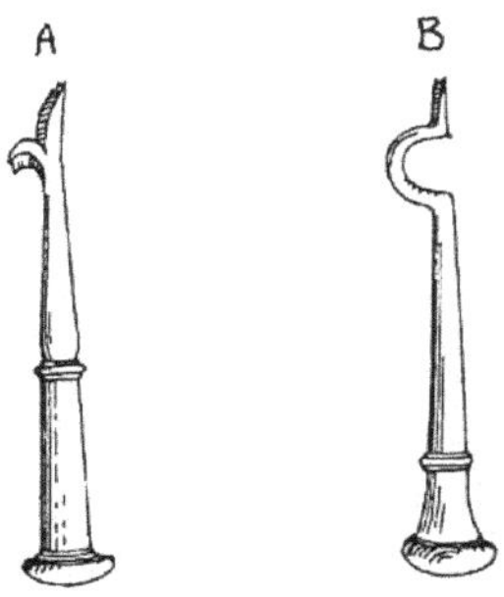

Fig. 165. Tools used by Martinez for dental extraction. A- for previous teeth; B- for posterior teeth (after Zimmer).

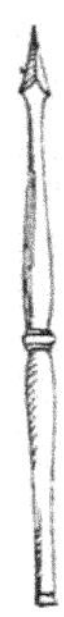

Fig. 166. Instrument used by Martinez to remove debris from a carious cavity (after Zimmer).

Gerolamo Cardano (1501-1576) wrote five volumes about teeth; 'De dentibus" and the joints "De morbis articularibus", considered a genuine encyclopedia of teeth at this time. He states that the tooth is an independent organ, like Faloppio; It is not "os denud", as Vésale said; He insists on the preservation of teeth through buccal dentistry and a healthy diet; In dental pain it recommends the recipe “aurea Nicolai” prepared by Nicolo Mirepsis from Nicaea in sec. XIII; It uses 68 ingredients by boiling plants and mineral or animal products, of which opioids are not available; The effectiveness of this “syrup” is unknown.

Gabriel Falloppius (1523-1562) is Vésale's successor, studying medicine after a monk training in Modena, where he was born, and in Padova, where he had Colombo, Montanus and Herophile as Professors; He was the physician of Pope Julius III and of the Este family, whom he “served” in her pilgrimages to Greece, where he was called the “Esculap of the Century”; As a Professor of anatomy at Padua (1514-1564), Falopius studies the four pathological forms of skulls described by Vésale and notes the cranial sutures, the filling of which determines the “flattening of the skull”; He describes and completes the bones of the skull with the sutures and muscles of the face. *Fabricio* (1531-1619), renowned surgeon and anatomist in Venice, was invited to treat Sigismund III from Poland, where he came to celebrate; He dissected over 300 bodies, showing more interest in the head and neck region; His studies relate to the functions of masticatory muscles and swallowing, illustrating these with hundreds of colorful pillars, appreciated today (figure 167). *Petrus Pavius* (1576-1617) (figure 168) is a Dutch student who studies at Leyda, having as a Professor Fabricio; He continues to dissect the corpses in a specially constructed amphitheater, dealing in particular with dental and skull abnormalities presented in a famous museum open to the public; The description of the maxillary sinuses remains its most important work, illustrated on hundreds of planes (215) and engravings in wood or metal.

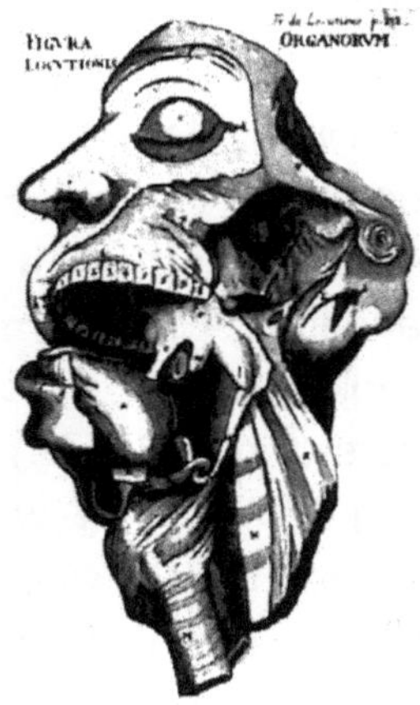

Fig. 167. Fabricio, surgeon and anatomist of Venice has conducted studies on the functions of masticatory muscles and swallowing (Gysel, 1980).

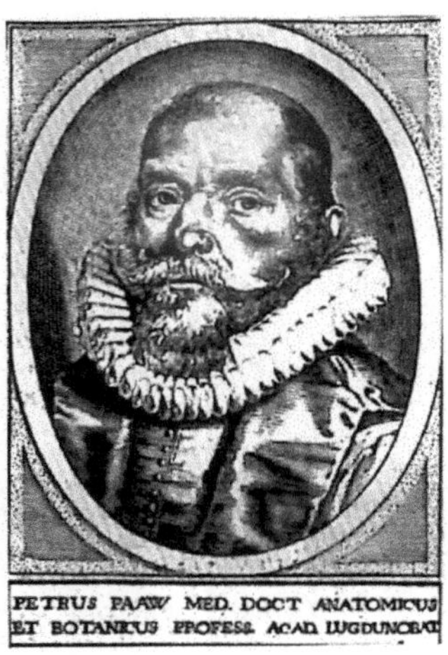
PETRUS PAAW MED. DOCT ANATOMICUS
ET BOTANICUS PROFESS. ACAD. LUGDUNOBAT

Fig. 168. Petrus Pavius, Professor of anatomy and botany at Leyda (after Gysel, 1980).

Johanes Scultetus (1595-1654) is one of the most renowned renascentist surgeons who invented an important set of instruments used in buccal-dental surgery (extraction pliers, elevators, upper or lower teeth spatulas in the area front or side (Figure 169).

Spigelius (Adrien van den Spiegel) (1578-1625) studies medicine at Leyda, Padova and

Bologna where he takes his doctorate; He will work as a botanical and anatomical Professor in Moravia, where he distinguishes himself by observations on tissues and organs and especially by the practical observations on the anatomy of the head and neck published by Casserius with colorful floorplanes where exact details; For the first time, Spigelius observes anatomical and physiological differences in man in terms of age, climate and temperament. Spigelius performs the first cranial measurements using four diameters that are "normally" equal.

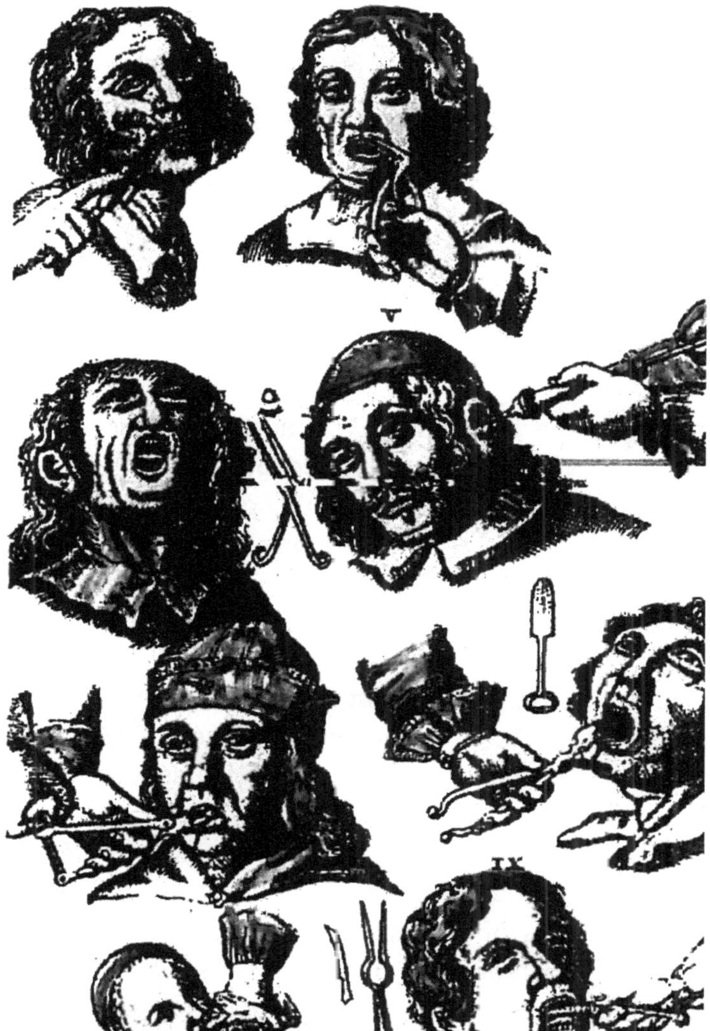

Fig. 169. Different instruments invented and used by J. Scultetus in buccal-dental surgery.

Facial diameter (forehead-chin), transversal (eurion-eurion probable), vertical cranial diameter, occipital hole vertex and oblique diameter, mastoid vertex-apophysis are, inherently, proportional and equal; Are variants of these diameters (elongated skull, shortened, broad or narrow face, etc.), variants found in populations in different countries; Crawny deformities such as flattening or elongation of the skull in children are due to the different habits of sitting down during sleeping and the use of different "bones" in children to avoid "cooling". Spigelius is among the first anatomists to notice the resorption of alveolar processes after the teeth fall. Spigelius announces the decline of the medical school in Padua, the hegemony passing to Bologna with Malpighi. The university of Padua opens with Vésale, a Belgian home, and closes with a Belgian, Spigelius.

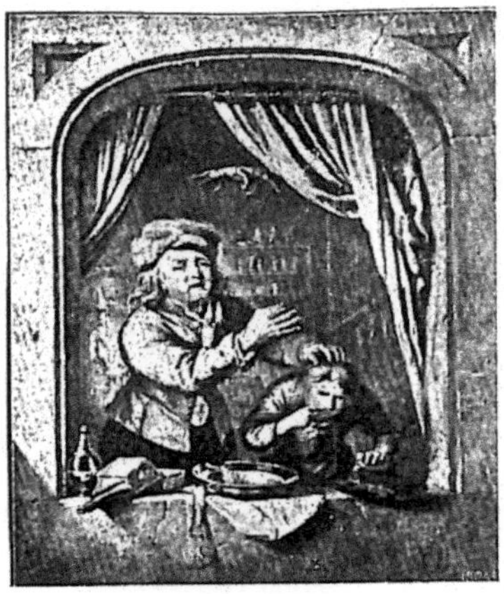

Fig. 170. Dentist and Child, Picture by Gerard Dou-Leyda (1613-1673), Rembrandt's pupil, who excels in patience and sensitivity to represent children; Here is the "dentist," a happy barber extracted a "toddler" a tooth; On his work table is a plate and a rudimentary instrument; On the wall behind the "barber" is painted a crocodile, the usual guest in a dental office.

8) Conclusions, renaissance dentistry

In the 15th-17th centuries the culture and art of Renaissance shine, beginning with Leonardo da Vinci and ending with Spigelius; During this period philosophical, artistic medicine with the anatomical description of the head and neck is also developed as a representative area of man, seen realistically.

Anatomy, physiology, general pathology and surgery are developing in new ways, based on the research of realities and truth, accompanied by beauty (aesthetics); Reality, truth and aesthetics form the triad of exact sciences, including the medical sciences guided by the humanistic concept initiated by Erasmus in Roterdam; Italy and the Netherlands (Belgium, the Netherlands, Denmark) are the promoters of this renaissance humanist movement, which has prepared the era of the development of science technology, which includes medicine (Janus - 21 - 1995). The anatomists of this period, starting with Vésale and continuing with Eustachio, Falopio, Fabricio and Spigelius, lay the foundations of head and neck surgery, which will also develop in this era with Ambroise Paré, Francesco Martiènez, Gerolamo Cardano and Fabricio, Surgeons who will tackle most of the surgical technologies used today in oro-maxillofacial surgery.

The early surgeons approached the dental extraction Professionally, introducing an appropriate instrument, such as Iohanes Scultetus, leaving the "charlatans" of the surgeons to continue to extract the populations of the fairs and cities; Towards the end of the seventeenth century, the doctor's Profession is regulated, by granting the doctor's title of "long robes" and the surgeon's Profession (beard-surgeon) obtained through special courses in dental schools, concluded with "short robes" surgical shavers. Dentistry thus makes a first step towards Professionalism with an average surgeon frame that will evolve from the title of barber-surgeon to the "dental surgeon" used until the last twentieth century.

In the Renaissance age the comparative anatomy of man and animals develops with Vésale and Fallopio; With Spigelius, human anatomy becomes the fundamental basis of medicine and especially of surgery, which develops in the coming centuries (Irsa - 20 - 1986). Physicians and surgeons with "long robes" provided medical or surgical care, including buccal-maxillo-facial surgery; The royal homes were frequently accompanied, on battlefields, by military surgeons; Even Leonardo da Vinci participated in the fighting in Anghiari, scenes of these battles were immortalized by pencils in the pencil; Ambroise Paré also accompanied Henry III of France and Philip II of Spain in the wars, treating facial wounds and jaw fractures, performing dental extractions as needed. Qualified dental care was done by local doctors in the royal homes in Italy and the Netherlands; In France, Germany and Russia, royal homes were assisted by interned physicians or foreign surgeons employing unique therapeutic methods, namely: purgatives in general diseases and red-iron cauterization in the treatment of wounds or hemorrhoids; Dental extractions were made by the queens called by the cracks. An example is the medical assistance at the court of King Soare, Louis XIV, where art and literature reached its peak, and where medical care remained at feudal level; Thus, Louis XVI was treated like all his children and grandchildren with purgatives, in the illnesses they had; The surgeon of the palace, Dr. Maréchal, treated Louis XVI hemorrhoids, making cauterizations with red iron, and for the extraction of teeth with severe paradonto, he was called a "charlatan" from the parlance in Paris that drew all his teeth Making it also a buccal-sinus communication.

In our country, in Moldova, Stephen the Great called a surgeon from Italy to cauterize his wound with red iron. At the court of Peter the Great in Russia he was also called a doctor from Italy to treat the sovereign from a urinary disease and the Tsar banished them with the "stick", making him "foolish" that he did not know how to Treat a sovereign.

Towards the end of the Renaissance, in Basel, Gaspard Bauhin (1560-1624) and Belgium in Antwerp, the great painter and anatomist, philosopher and artist Pierre Paul Rubens (1577-1640). Gaspard Bauhin (1560-1624) (figure 171) is part of a six-generation dynasty of physicians in Switzerland (Basel); Gaspard Bauhin, the brightest physician of this dynasty, begins Basel's botanical and medical studies, continuing in Padova, Bologna, returning to Basel where he teaches the anatomy of the man with the opening lesson "Oratio de Homine"; Is more concerned with the anatomy of the head and face, studying the skulls and muscles of the face a lot; Bauhin's merit is to present the anatomy of teeth, jaws and jaws with their sinuses much more extensively, using an immense bibliography from Aristotle to Spigelius, without introducing new notions, repeating even the mistakes of his predecessors.

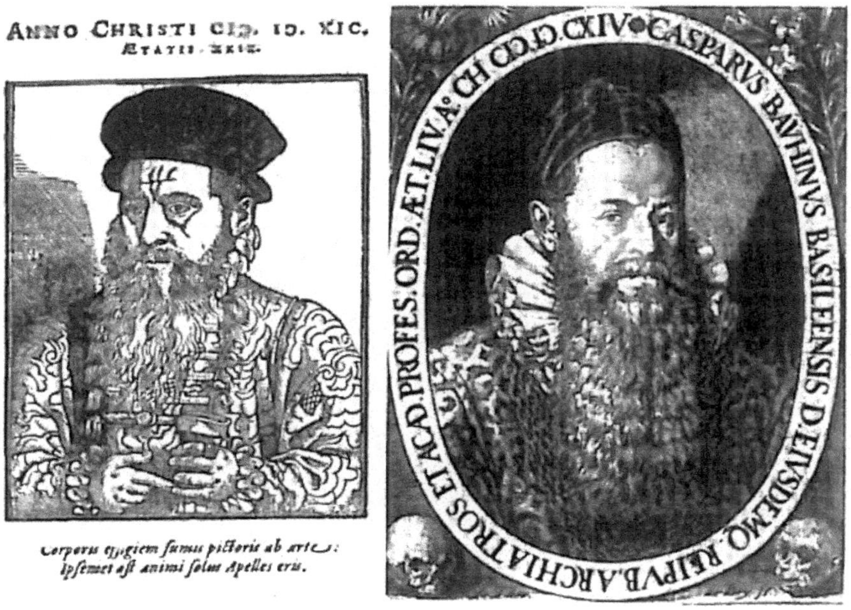
ANNO CHRISTI CIↃ. IↃ. XIC.
CASPARVS BAVHINVS BASILEENSIS D. EIVSDEMQ. REIPVB. ARCHIATROS ET ACAD. PROFES. ORD. ÆT. LIV. A° CH CIↃ.IↃ.CXIV

Fig. 171.
Gaspard Bauhin, 29-year-old portrait and 54-year-old portrait Engraving by De Bry (Switzerland).

Pierre Paul Rubens (1577-1640) is considered one of the five great artistic geniuses in Europe who studied artistic anatomy to use in their famous paintings; All these great Renaissance painters considered the face "the eye of the health and the character of man", that is why they made hundreds of pencils in pencil to put in their paintings people fit with their characters. Rubens has made hundreds of crooks with boys or women with a cross-border Profile, characteristic of the flames of his homeland (Figures 172, 173, 174 and b).

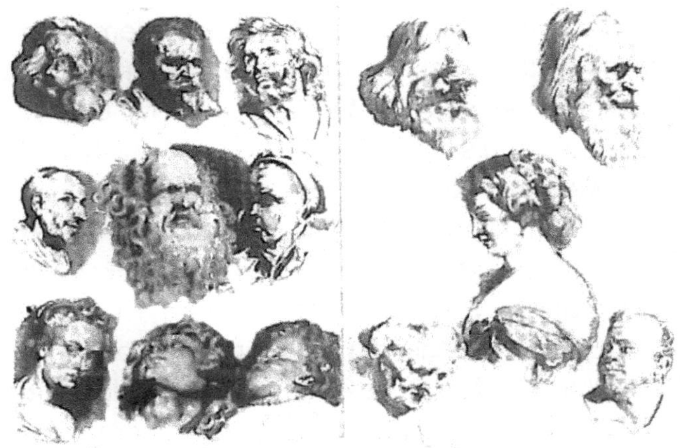

Fig. 172. The drawings in Rubens' book "Human Figure Theory" which draws men and women from Belgium.

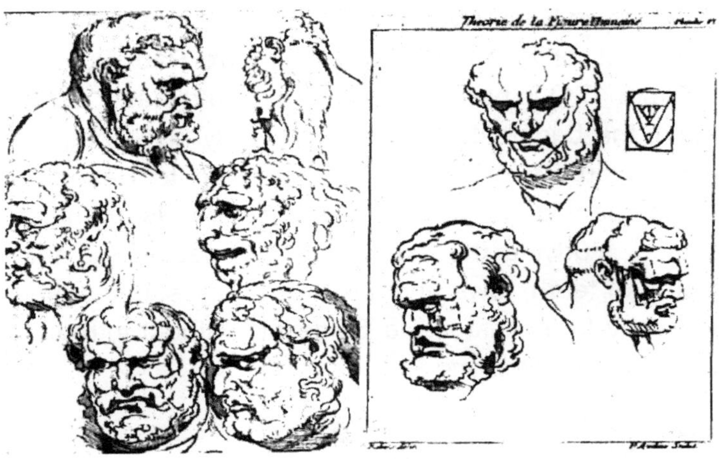

Fig. 173. Cover of Rubens Volume "The Human Figure Theory" with drawings, some etched, bearded, front and cross-border and semi-Profile, where "mimics" express different feelings.

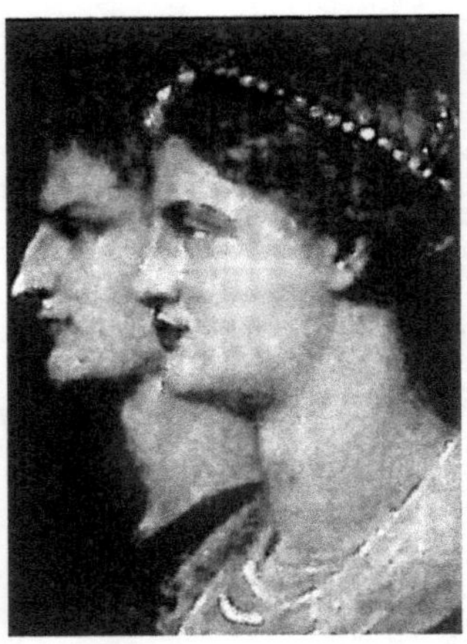

Fig. 174 a. Its Profile figures Tiberiu and Agripina, in drawing, Before being painted in the picture.

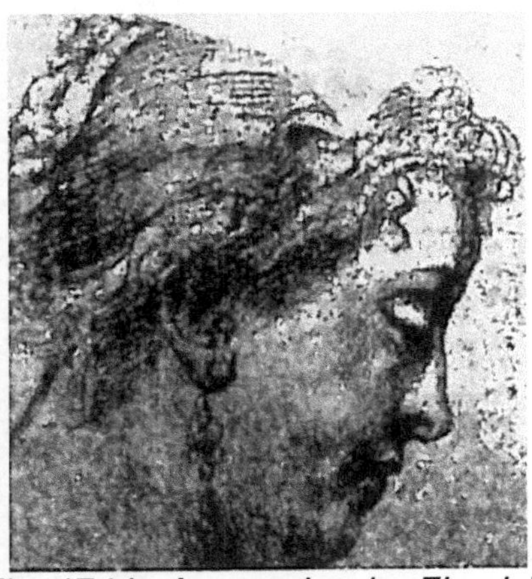

Fig. 174 b. A cross-border Flemish Profile, study for one of 1,600 paintings.

Born in Antwerp (Belgium), Rubens studies painting in Venice, Naples, where he is also employed in the Spanish embassy; Returning to Antwerp in 1608, at the death of his mother, Rubens remains here, where he marries Isabelle de Brandt (1610), the daughter of a great city clerk, making a portrait where his talent immediately stands; During this period he enters diplomacy and visits Paris, Madrid, London, where he is asked to paint portraits or different secular compositions; Henry IV and his wife, Maria de Medici, command the 14 paintings as a wall to decorate the rooms of the palace of Luxembourg; These paintings were then transferred to the Louvre, where four were displayed periodically in a large room on four walls; After the death of his wife in 1626 the plague, he remarried after four years with the beautiful lady of Fourment for 17 years at his 53 years.

In the next 10 years, Rubens has a feverish activity, painting 13,500 m2 of cloths, where he can immortalize real life with the joy of living; Unlike Rembrandt's countryman, who illustrated the tragedy of human existence; Being a happy man with a balanced family, Rubens painted sociable, balanced, educated, receptive characters with a desire to succeed in their lives; Painted admirable mothers and husbands who passionately love their husband; Though the themes were varied, historical, mythological, religious and even philosophical; The expressivity of the face was admirably illustrated in all 1,600 sails; His studies of artistic face anatomy were essential in rendering mimics with the expression of the most varied feelings or characters. Rubens painted realistically the representatives of the Habsburg royal house in Spain, having all the mandibular prognosis. The children appear in the lively, playful Rubens' canvas in the fruit garland of the Düsseldorf museum. Rubens met the good world in Europe, portraying the humanism of the represented person; He also suffered from human suffering, with gout, "broken" teeth drawn from "charlatans" and heart failure, of which he died in 1640, leaving a work in glamorous and good-looking pictures.

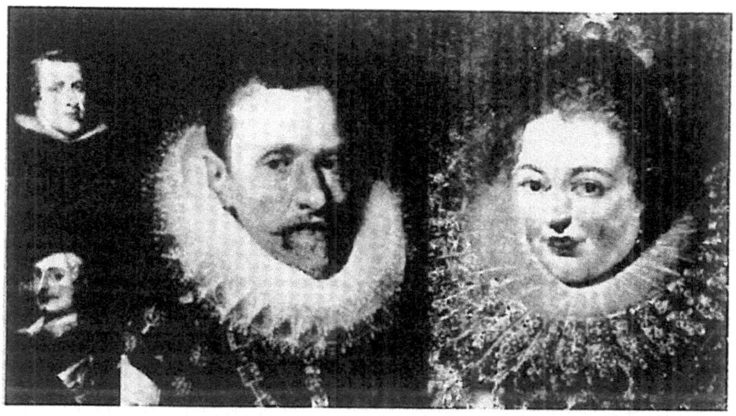

Fig. 175. Portraits of the Habsburg family in Spain; Albert and Isabella (archduke); Philip IV, top left in medallion and baby cardinal Ferdinand (left down medallion).

9) Dental medicine in sec. XVII-XVIII. Beginning of technology

The 17th-18th centuries began with the 30-year war in Western Europe (1618-1648), continued with the wars between Poland, Sweden and Russia in eastern Europe and complemented by plague epidemics in Spain, which will spread All over Europe, including Moldova and Muntenia in the following centuries.

These wars and epidemics have led to the impoverishment and decimation of populations in Western and Eastern Europe; However, commercial and industrial (manufacturing) cities are developing, mostly in England, where the population has doubled (from 5.5 to 10 million); In northern France the population increases from 20 to 25 million inhabitants; The population increases by several million and in the Netherlands; In the sec. 18 population in Russia increases to 36 million inhabitants with all epidemics; The increased mortality in these centuries was due to poverty, total lack of hygiene; The dirt in Paris even terrified the palatine princess, who said that "Paris is a horrible city; The streets have a pestilential smell that is breathtaking; The extraordinary heat causes the rubbish to rot in the streets with debris of meat and fish "; However, in these cities decimated by epidemics, the scientific medical life is awakened to find solutions for the development of a healthy life. In the past centuries philosophical anatomy developed first, then artistic with six main artists, to render human figures in motion and expressiveness; Then a descriptive anatomy developed, which corrected the mistakes of the predecessors of antiquity, Aristotle, Celsus, Galenus.

In the seventeenth and eighteenth centuries general and specialized medicine and histology are approached and developed, from the need to know the structures of the tissues in the organs; Blood circulation is described by Harvey; Explains the functioning of the muscles and joints, by Bonelli; In Bologna, Malpighi develops histology by writing "De viscerum structure".

The emergence of print allows rapid dissemination of discoveries, stimulates the development of fundamental medical sciences, biology, physics, chemistry, anatomy, philosophy and histology, creating a good collaboration between scientists who unite in a freely agreed consensus. New cities in northern Europe become medical research centers and scientists feel the need to organize themselves in societies or academies, of which the most important ones were founded in Rome, under the name of Academia dei Lincei, of the Clairvoyant (1603); Paris, Académie Française (1635), Oxford, Royal English Society (1662). They began publishing in printed journals, the first being in London in 1665, "Philosophical transaction", which appears today; The first medical journal "Journal des nouvelles decouvertes sur toutes les parties de la medicine" appears in Paris, the editor being Nicolas de Blegny; In the sec. The seventeenth new medical universities in Leyden (the Netherlands) in London, Edinburgh, Gottingen, Paris and Montpellier, universities organizing congresses, conferences, where biology and medicine issues are being discussed, "preformists" criticizing "epighenists" Fixists "defend against" Revolutionists".

In this atmosphere of scientific research, dentistry develops as a medical and technical branch at the same time; Is the merit of the graduates of the Faculty of Medicine in Europe, who will also deal with the anatomy, physiology and pathology of the dento-maxillary apparatus (Bologa - 4-1970). Knowledge of anatomy and physiology gave courage to surgeons to operate at royal homes; Felix de Tassy (1669-1703) operated Louis XVI for an anal fistula, which healed after many cauterizations carried out by the surgeon in Ver-sailles, Maréchal; King Solar approves the establishment of a Paris college (college) of surgery (college of St. Cosma), plus a "surgiens dentistes" school, which will form dentists to replace the queens in the fairy; In 1730 the first medical science societies were founded; In Berlin, Leibnitz, followed by the Paris Academy of Surgery (1731). In this period of scientific effervescence, the Edict of Nantes by Ludovic al IV-th is revoked; Following the emigration of the Huguenots from France to the Netherlands and to America; These being entrepreneurs and wealthy merchants, have developed the cities of the countries where they have settled; There is an economic and political decline in France after the death of Louis IV, with the onset of epidemics of plague, flu, typhus and dysentery, which decimated thousands of citizens; A smallpox epidemic is triggered in Britain, and in the European armies there is a scorbut, where military doctors can not cope, transmitting and recommending recipes to troops in the form of infusions or decoctions of roots or leaves of plants, plus milk and Honey without too much therapeutic effect.

During this period of economic, technical, social and religious reforms, the creator of modern technology-based dentistry appears; It is Pierre Fauchard (figure 176); Born in 1678, he studied at Paris College of Dental Surgery and, after a long practical experience, published in 1728 the first specialized work "Le chirurgien Dentiste ou traité des dents", which will become the basis of dental education (dentistry) in Europe in the next centuries

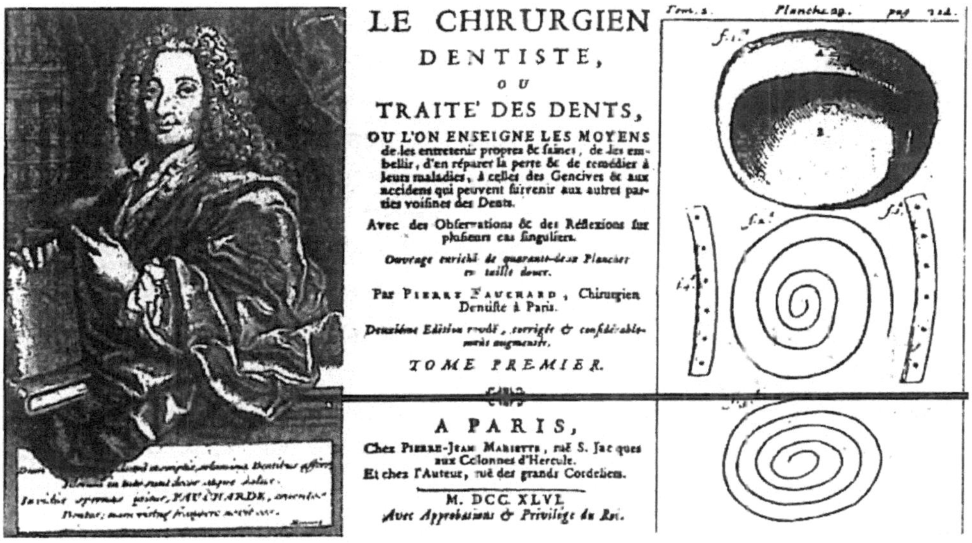

Fig. 176. Pierre Fauchard and title of his work (after Gysel, 1980).

Here Fauchard introduces for the first time in 1720 a hand-held milling cutter, which he uses to remove dental caries before filling; With other milling cutters he grinds too high teeth or approximate surfaces of the molars that have caries in this area (fig.177).

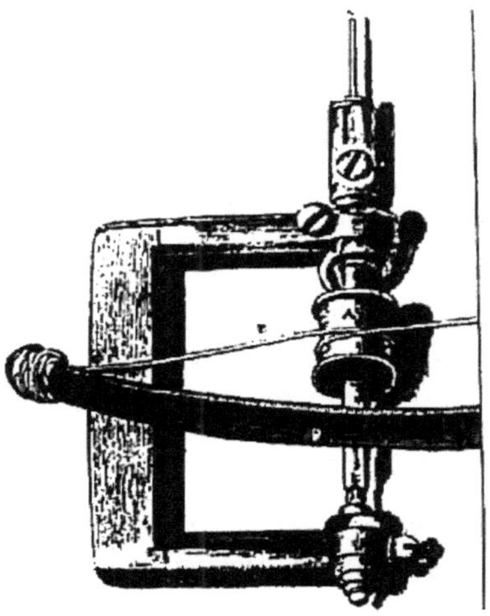

Fig. 177. Handwheel, which produces the rotation of a milling cutter that removes the debris into a carousel cavity built by Fauchard in 1720; After a few decades a leg tour will be built that will move the milling cutter and in 1877 there will be a tour with a mechanical device made by Morisson.

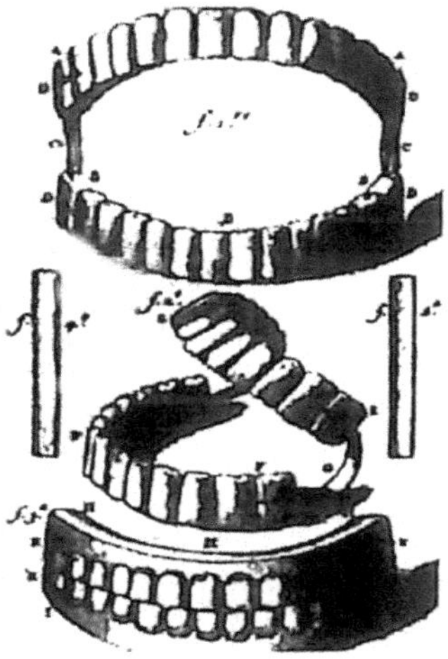

Fig. 178. Mobile prostheses made by Fauchard using pink porcelain and various springs (after Gysel, 1980).

In his volume, Fauchard describes precisely the temporary teeth, dental eruption and dental anomalies; Dental extractions with different pliers and elevators occupy an important place. In the prevention of dental caries, the author of the book proposes to wash teeth with a sponge dipped in water and "teaspoon" (distilled grape alcohol). Fauchard opens and was prosthetic, realizing the first full or partial porcelain porcelain prostheses in France (Fig. 178) (Firu, Bercus - 15 - 1970).

Robert Bunon, (1702-1748), is the initiator of pedodontics, establishing scientific bases in the prevention of dental caries and in the preservation of teeth affected in children. Born in 1702 at Chalons sur Marne, Bunon studied at the St. Cosma College of Dentistry in Paris, obtaining the diploma of a "dentist surgeon" with a "little robe", which distinguished him from the graduates of the Faculty of Medicine who wore the diploma Doctor a "long slave". In the "Tooth Disease Test" paper, Bunon makes a study of 5000 patients of all ages, reaching the following conclusions: Prevention of dental diseases starts from the pregnant woman, because the dental buds form in the intrauterine life; in the infant, breast sucking is necessary to prevent dental caries and dental abnormalities. In 1746 he publishes "Experiences and Demonstrations," where he correctly describes dento-alveolar incongruances, recommending for the first time the extraction of temporary or permanent teeth to allow for their alignment by gaining space.

Antoine Ferein, (1693-1769), studies medicine in Montpellier, where he obtains a diploma in medicine (with a long robe); He then sets up in Paris as a doctor and Professor of anatomy, dealing with the liver, arteries and large veins, and especially the lymphatic vessels. He was concerned about the movements of the "diagonal-transversal" mandible, describing rightly in the work "On the movements of the two jaws to open the mouth" the antagonist muscles of the dento-maxillary apparatus.

Dental art, as dentistry (stomato- logy) had begun to be called, was represented by "surgiens dentistes" in Western Europe, of which we mention: John Hunter (1728-1793), who made important contributions to the orthodontic-surgical treatment of dento-alveolar incongruences, frequent abnormalities in European populations at that time, due to exogencies favored by population migration from the village to the city where they were working as tradesmen Or merchants. The lack of space in the alveolar processes for the eruption of permanent teeth is due, due to Hunter, to the insufficient growth of alveolar bases (Figure 179).

Based on this theory, he recommends extracting the teeth from the outbreak of incongruity, namely the tooth distal to the ectopic canine; In higher proalveolodention, he recommends the extraction of the first premolars.

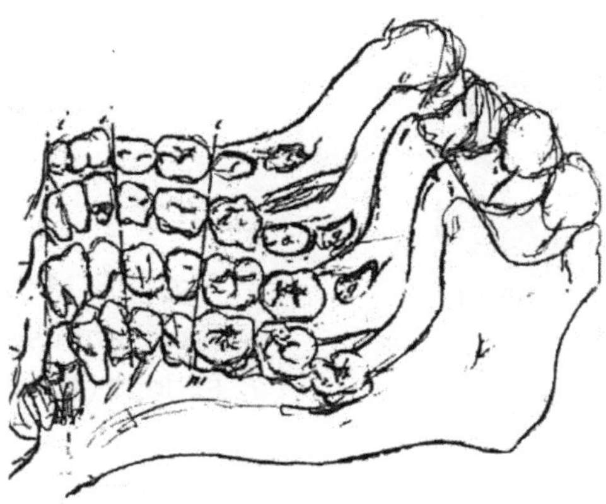

Fig. 179. Different overlapped mandibles (show that alveolar processes increase, As well as the "Condylian process of the mandible"), Hunter did not know at this time The resorption-opposition process of the upward branch of the mandible.

Robert Blake is studying medicine at Edinburgh College (Scotland), where he holds a PhD thesis titled "Inaugural Dentistry Dissertation," studying the growth of jaws, arguing that alveolar processes are growing in every way as permanent teeth erupt; The role of the sutures in the upper jaw and the mandibular growth cartilage, which provides the development of the bone bases of the alveolar processes, is not known.

Towards the end of the eighteenth century, dentists, trained at the European faculties of medicine, devoted themselves to the study of teeth, addressing in particular problems of disease prevention, of which caries, periodontitis and dento-maxillary abnormalities were subjects of scientific debate. Of these, one can quote: Tissot de Grancy, a Professor at the University of Padua, where in 1791 he published the "People's Opinion on Health" paper, drawing attention to the catastrophic state of the "dirty" teeth. Bartolomeo Ruspini, of Italian origin, trained in London in 1768 to publish the work "Treating teeth, structure and their various diseases"; He invented the oral mirror to examine the teeth. Philip Pfaff (1713-1766), was the dentist of King Frederic II, practicing stomatology in Berlin. He made dental re-implantations and the first movable prostheses of silver or gold as a base, and human teeth, extracts or teeth sculpted from the bovine or ivory femur. Louis Fleuri Lecluse (1712-1792) invented the lift, which bears his name. Bourdet (1722-1789) was the dental surgeon of Louis XV and XVI, much concerned with "mouth cleanliness." Thomas Berdmore (1740-1785) is attached to the court of King George III in England, attributing high sugar consumption to tooth decay. They also practiced dentist dentists in Sweden, Juel Assur, (1753-1837), at the court of King Gustav IV. In Hungary he practiced medical dentistry Matyus Istvan, more concerned with "mouth cleanliness".

In North America, a dentist school is developing this century, which will evolve much better due to the economic and technical progress in this area; Of these can be reminded:

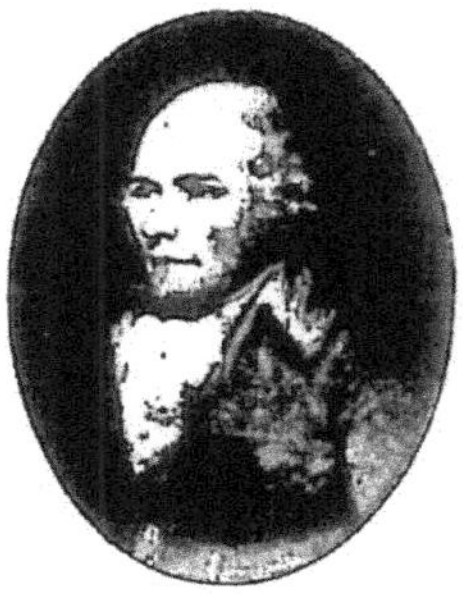

Fig. 180. John Greenwoods

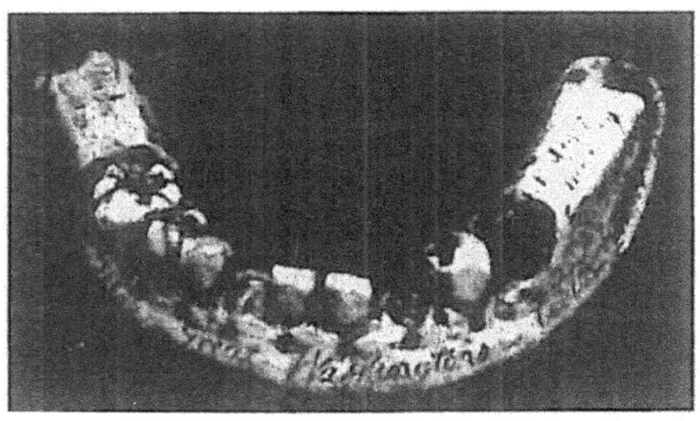

Fig. 181. G. Washington's dentures Made by John Greenwoods.

John Greenwoods (1760-1819) (figure 180), who performed the prosthesis of G. Washington, a prosthesis now kept at the New York Medical Academy Museum (figure 181); The body of this prosthesis was made of a hippo tooth, in which gold teeth were embedded; The only remaining tooth of Washington was integrated into the prosthesis. In Europe, Japan and America, partial mobile prostheses with a hardwood base, ivory or cremation (in Japan) were begun; In Europe were made partial porcelain pink ceramic prostheses and artificial teeth from bones of bovine animals, which were easily altered as the ivory was porous; Hippo teeth were more resistant and used in America.

10) Conclusions

In the seventeenth and eighteenth centuries, wars for hegemony take place between the feudal states that have been deprived of the populations where these struggles took place;

Population migration was caused by epidemics of plague, dysentery, smallpox (England), and scurvy in soldiers engaged in battles; All this has decimated the populations of the rich countries that waged the wars and reduced the financial resources; Towards the end of his life, Louis XVI revoked the edict of Nantes under the influence of his catholic catholic, and so the Huguenots had to emigrate to the countries that tolerated them; Christian reformers emigrated to the Netherlands, where they were well received; America was also a welcoming host. Reforms were capable people, laborers, good entrepreneurs and wealthy merchants, so they revived welcoming countries, where economic and social progress was immediately highlighted; Economic and social progress has favored the development of technical sciences that also benefited from dental medicine. For the first time now, the graduates of the European faculties of medicine (Padova, Bologna, Montpellier, Edinburgh, etc.) are concerned with the anatomy, physiology and pathology of the dento-maxillary apparatus; During this period the paths of evolution of dental surgery, pedodontics, orthodontics are opened, showing many dento-alveolar incongruences as a consequence of exogamy.

At this stage, there is the first dental treaty, published by Fauchard, which has remained current until today; He also introduces for the first time a hand tour which turns a milling cutter for the treatment of dental caries and for abrasion of teeth with abnormalities.

Now he is attached to the Faculty of Medicine in Paris and a "College" for dental surgeons, at Louis Ludwig's disposition, to replace the queens who did dental extraction without any technical training. Also in these centuries are the first medical associations under the name of Societies or Academies and the first medical and dental congresses with the first specialized magazines. These can be considered centuries of "awakening" scientists to develop medical research, bringing the first technical inventions in the field of dentistry.

CHAPTER XII.
ELEMENTS OF CULTURAL ANTHROPOLOGY

Anthropology, being founded as part of anatomy (Canon) and addressing the human phenomenon (Fr. Rainer, I.th. Riga), has crossed the borders of morphological, physiological, psychological, intellectual and genetic areas – in both the individual and entire populations (I. Drăghicescu). The definition of constitutional and structural typology entered the psycho-spiritual and social spheres, which are part of the purpose of the anthropological entirety (I. Th. Riga), thus representing the cultural anthropology of great complexity, interfering with philosophy, religion, literature and many other products of immaterial spirituality, that we wanted to present during the trial of defining the meta-psychological type.

In this context, the main elements of cultural anthropology refer to features of the social, spiritual, in conjunction with the definition of physical anthropology- rooted in physics. In fact, by making a digression from the anthropomorphic scope to the entire world (both living and nonliving) that is defined by mater, energy, information and time. Milcu and Neacşu replaced the factors that can explain the phenomena from a metaphysical realm, designing a system for teaching the objectives of cultural anthropology.

1. Manifestation of human social life

The events of social life include, on one hand, the social unity that formed the family, and on the other hand, social units larger than the family unit. The family is not permanent and unchanging, but is subject to social conditions, which are of concern to its variability. It is linked to religious, legal, moral and economic facets that characterize each ethnic group, this institution being viewed differently within various ethnic groups. During its evolution, the family concept has been narrowed down to other framework and duties. Members which formed the very numerous primitive clans were significantly reduced in modern conjugal family.

From totemic clan, mixtures of domestic functions - both economic and religious, have reached modern conjugal family, which lost its religious and legal function and has a reduced economic and educational role. However, until today, a family bond kept a strong moral influence over its members, which was due to the mutual affection of its members. It thus remains the most qualified institution for raising children. Although industrial progress has produced a weakening of family discipline, family remains, in essence, a moral group.

In many primitive societies, relations between the sexes are free, as long as the marriage was not celebrated. The loss of virginity isn`t considered important. In some primitive populations artificial deflorations occurred before marriage took place; in others, women earn their dowry by prostituting themselves. Marriage was designed by the family and for the family only; today it is made possible, in most cases, by mutual consent. By Westermarck, marriage is extending beyond the act of reproduction and birth of offspring. It is a universal phenomenon of the human species, a necessity for existential purposes. The phenomenon has its origins in the sexual instinct developed by the strong influence of sexual selection. The man shares with other animals the sexual instinct but differs from the latter in those distinguishing forbidden sexual relations. Human society sees relations between the sexes not as a matter of individual and biological choice, but as a product of social norms and ethics. Marriage includes, besides intercourse, the solicitude parents have towards their offspring. Parents caring for children are necessary for the survival and perpetuation of the human species through reproduction. In fact, we can say that reproduction has as an objective basis for survival of the species, and as a subjective basis the satisfaction of the sexual instinct. On the care that parents have towards their offspring, we see that marriage and family are closely linked, finding marriage rooted in the family unit. There are, in fact, nations in which the married status is achieved only by the birth of the first child.

By Westermarck, there was likely a moment when humanity knew a human mating season. Therefore, continually exercising the sexual instinct cannot play a significant part in the emergence of marriage. In fact, there are primitive populations where the sexual instinct was increased periodically. The fact is connected with the end of Spring, when we share an abundance of food, which makes all children born in this period more able to survive.

Primitive people from Greenland reached the maximum abundance in winter, so the children being born in September are actually linked to the abundance of food that exists in this region during autumn. However, apart from these populations, the rest of humanity shows no increased sex drive. With the progress of civilization, man is forced to withstand external influences and is not compelled to conceive children in a certain period. The origin of marriage must therefore not be sought in the continuous pursuit of the sexual instinct, but perhaps in the fact that the human species is characterized by a reduced descent and by a long childhood.

Promiscuity plays no role in social evolution. Belief in primitive communal marriage is based only on certain events in tribal societies where sexes freely cohabit before marriage. By most primitive people, maiden sex trade is completely banned or is very rare. On the other hand, taking into account the sense of universal jealousy, promiscuity appears unlikely.

Celibacy is also rare in primitive to civilized people when it occurs much more often due to economic and psychological reasons where celibacy causes boil down to lack of money needed to buy a woman. Marriage was designed by older members of the family and for the family only; today it is made, in most cases, by mutual consent. Choosing a husband acknowledges the existence of a common ideal of beauty within the human race, the ideal is to develop fully visible characteristic features of the body and sex. The differences in taste are closely linked with each group separately and human appreciation of harmony that exists between the physical type and living conditions. Most healthy type, one that best matches the external requirements, is the one who has the strongest power in action and natural selection. This selection is determined, however, by other factors as well: emotions, intellectual qualities, moral sympathy and age.

The shared horror for incest finds its origin in cohabitation. By Westermarck, people living together during childhood share an aversion to the sex trade. The monopoly of the prohibition is largely due to local kinship. In the latter case, the prohibition of marriage between relatives- by marriage or by adoption is due to an association of ideas that inhibits sex drive. Westermarck concludes that the prohibition of marriage between relatives is not a phenomenon based on experience, but on instinct. This law has almost universal value, but there are also exceptions. Thus, the primitive people who practice exogamy, incest is favored taking a camouflaged form.

For the appearance of incest, there are other hypotheses. Spencer believes that women who were captured in wars as proof of victory, each individual will seek to possess a strange woman of his tribe. This hypothesis is improbable, for women of a tribe would always remain unmarried, and the vanquished cannot get married again. Kohler sees incest prohibition policy as a method of preserving, which would tighten relations between tribes. But this hypothesis does not explain the moral attitude regarding inbreeding. Morgan believes negative results that occur sometimes in marriage inbreeding to explain the horror of incest. Finally, Huth sees the prohibition of incest, a law that prevents the same blood from marrying too soon. Incest only appears in human groups in which individuals pose a huge pride (as happened in the Egyptian unions of the royal family), thus isolating from people with excessive and flawed instincts. In primitive societies, man as a subordinate social structure is not treated as endowed with certain natural qualities, but is treated as a member of a class or family. Concept determined the choice of a husband until recent times, when civilization has insisted on individual rights. Husband may be chosen within the social group (inbreeding) or outside the group (exogamy). This latter form is, as Durkheim features it, the totemic clan. Certain human groups find preferential unions, as levirate (widow marriage brother) or surrogacy (marriage of a widowed sister of his former wives). Almost all women rely on primitive method of coercion, when it comes to purchasing of the future wife. However, there are many primitive societies, where we find a marriage based on the principle of choice. Marriages of capture, purchase or services are only the last forms that remain while more modernized marriage takes place. A method of time constraint, however, was replaced by a contractual method by moving from constraint to the contract that was passed in marital relations, from selfishness to altruism. However, even the last form, marriage alienates partly free woman. Resident spouses may choose to leave their home and go live with the wife's family; also it may go to the home and family of her husband. Most often, however, a fact especially common among civilized nations, the young couple will form an independent home.

A high number of spouses are due to a series of economic and social causes. The proportions of men and women are about equal in every human group, monogamy will appear as a natural fact. But the proportions can be modified, when many men are killed in wars or for reasons of superstition or difficulties of existence, primitives kill new born. In these cases, there can appear marriages between a woman and several men or vice versa. Polygamy (marriage of one man and several women) and polyandry (marriage of a woman with several men), appears besides the above cases and other cases of religious or economic stress.

Polyandry is a rare form of marriage (found only in Tibet); for we cannot believe that such lending of wives is widespread in primitive populations, which appears at times only as an act of generous hospitality. Polygyny is and was, on the contrary, quite widespread, especially in rich layers of certain human groups. Polygyny causes are man's taste for variety, unbalanced numerical proportion of the sexes, separation of the sexes during pregnancy, a woman's sterility, the advantage that it presents many working hands, the desire to have as many children and social differences. Such instances have found it difficult to maintain the relationship with more women, while needing assistance to pay a sum or provide a service to get a woman, violation of women rights and the natural passion of a man for a single person. In fact, many polygamous couples tend toward monogamy.

Monogamy is the most perfect form of marriage, since through it one can reach that goal that it pursues as a family group, namely, the continuation of the genetic line and individual happiness. Marriages groups have not been found in any primitive people.We cannot say that the man began to live in promiscuity, because there has been a process from polygamy that reached to monogamy. Monogamy is the natural form of marriage and polygamy is just an accident occurred as a result of economic or social causes. Because of the weight, gaining food aid is necessary for any kind of survival. Therefore, the family consists of parents and children, terms that shall be interpreted in a sociological sense, not biological. Therefore, a man who marries his brother's widow when the legitimate father of her children died becomes the father.

The parentage varies within the different ethnic groups. In most human groups the present system is patriarchy, the male lineage system. The patriarchate has its origin in property status and subordination of woman to man's natural impulses. In it we find the father's authority; his last name to his wife and children, he is the administrator of family assets and possesses the means for desired correction. Patriarchy is par excellence the lineage system of civilized nations. But within some nations we might find matriarch primitive systems of lineage, through the mother. This is characterized by a family authority that the mother possesses, who has a family fortune, providing governance of children with civil and political rights. Blood ties are not sufficient to form a family; they disappear in the face of economic and religious considerations, as maintenance of the properties change familiar heritage and ancestor worship. Based on these principles, the adoption of children is regulated in different primitive population, its purpose being to insure the cult of ancestors in families without offspring. The family, founded on common names includes, on the one hand, the descendants of a common ancestor, and on the other hand, foreigners who have entered the group by adoption. Kinship involves a community of goods, mutual assistance, the obligation to revenge insults to the group, community worship and duty to ensure the perpetuation of the family. The family ties the totemic community, which is based on social conventions. Totemic clan is a group of individuals who recognize kinship as a particular sign called totem, which is a sign or object that has been animated. Most often, the totem is an animal or plant of any group supposedly descended, and it serves as the emblem off the collective forms (Durkheim).

The ties that bind two consorts differ from those of lovers, in that they act out on sexually mutual obligations. The intimacy of conjugal relations is determined by social prejudices and the character or temperament. In all human societies, the existence of common interests, a strong bond is based on mutual affection. Such conjugal relations include a number of economic activities, moral, intellectual and aesthetic, recognizing marriage as a basic instinct less than all of these. Love for children as a general human trait is derived from the offspring preservation instinct. In fact, it is more likely that this is a selfish instinct, the individual loving, within his children, his own person. He sees in this manner of offspring conservation and transmission of individuality over time. However, there are some altruistic considerations in this sense, given that the individual is more often not confined to love their children, but it extends to the other consort taken or contemplated, in a previous marriage. The child receives education from his parents, but most often, external factors like school and church, supplement or even replaces altogether parental education. Education contributes strongly to the survival of the species in the preparation of the child in the struggle for existence. As humanity has evolved, education has increasingly foraged protection. Great inventions and industrial progress have resulted in significant changes in education. Depending on environmental education and a perfect adaptation to it as derived from differentiation and specialization and division of labor ideas. However, the conditioning process, which is performed during childhood, absolutely does not determine human behavior, which is to some extent conditioned by the circumstances of adolescent and adult life.

Ideal education involves education of the emotions and discipline over the critical phenomena. Besides the mind, we must consider the body as it affects us. This principle is based on samples of individuals who underwent pubertal initiation in primitive peoples. Initiation consists of an educated period, followed by a series of tests to which the child it is subjected. Following these tests is a ceremony during which the individual is declared adult. Many religions of civilized nations have kept this ceremony, of course, under different aspects. From all that was said above, it appears that all sentimental ties, economic and legal problems between parents, consorts and children, brothers and sisters make the family a strong social unit.

The main social functions of the family are the perpetuation of human lineage; obtaining the means to support family members, social and economic education of the young generation. What is the evolution that has followed the family unit? After Durkheim, totemic clan, domestic confusion of functions, religious and economical aspects, such as primitive family. Following the patriarchal family, the father is the head of domestic religion, sole owner and representative of the family. The patriarchal family would result in a paternal family, where we find greater independence of women and children. It follows modern conjugal family, based on mutual consent, the mutual debts, raising the dignity of women and the emotional ties between its members. The family unit is determined by different causes. Once religion ceases to be purely domestic, the dismemberment of the family begins to occur. Political causes determine family unit. Cases involving economic family unit determine the image of a primitive family activity. This unit is itself a primitive appearance who got destroyed by big industry.

After Durkheim, relations between members of the same family are regulated by ethical principles. Effectiveness of the moral life consists in forming the only familiar social transitions, freeing us from pure personality, giving rise to true sociability (Comte). Besides family life, social life also includes larger units, units with an economic organization, management and policy, making a different family. The company one find within society is a body outside which individuals can only have a purely biological existence. Social consciousness determines the structure of individual conscience and supplies the content. For these reasons, social life involves, primarily, an economic organization. In primitive societies throughout human group the common activity is to look for food. In civilized society, characterized by an extreme differentiation of functions, there are some social units serving exclusively the economy, and other units that play only a secondary economic role, such as the family and the state. In primitive societies, in the countryside, the family has - among other functions - to satisfy the material needs of its members. Big industry and the Professions or public workshop helped dissolve the family, making the family a social unit with a secondary economic role. The state's role in contemporary economic life remains quite high. By general work that cannot be executed by private initiative, the state protects agriculture, trade and industry, intervening directly in production. Actual economic organizations are: corporations, unions and cooperatives. These organizations are calling on moral forces: individual energy and spirit of solidarity which reconciles them by virtue of their educational (Gide).

Property regime takes all the economical, given that depends on the production, distribution and consumption of wealth. What often determined by the nature of the property is then output. The property is under political dependence causes more social or moral. Thus, legal or moral rights are collective property regime, met in primitive peoples to recognize addition to this property and individual. Assets can be tangible or intangible. Material goods are mobile and land. Movable property includes garments, utensils, weapons, domestic animals and slaves. Land assets are determined by economic structure of each nation individually. Thus, the primitive land is inalienable, the fields are jointly owned. Alienable land is not the primitive, under certain conditions. Thus, only when the meadows are becoming rare or when there is a decrease in domestic animals.

As the work arises from the game of needs and desires of satisfaction, it only appears as a necessity in terms of economic necessity which man sacrifices his minimum effort possible, however looking through this minimal effort to achieve maximum pleasure. The needs, desires and human effort will be by mutual determination, human economic nature. The basis of this nature is causes psychological as: finding personal economic benefits, searching rewards, praise and honor search, search and search activity to satisfy their conscience. We can say with Wagner that going from selfish reason for moral, economic values form a ladder of decreasing sizes. Economic values remain so largely related to our opinion religious, aesthetic or moral.

Trade has evolved and with it, the social evolution. The Stroller is related to domestic social structure; Fair trade is linked to the urban economy and trade is linked to sedentary economy. The first way of appropriating foreign goods was by theft. The exchange appeared only later. He appears not as an act instinctively as he was stealing, but as a rational act, as is done by the User voluntary, which is due to the desire to possess a new object, to get rid of an object or redundant to get rid of an object without immediate use. In primitive forms of trade, exchanges were made through barter. Feeling, in civilized societies, lack of exchange values was chosen for this operation first items desired by many people and later objects which by their rarity, presented greater value. From bartering was passed so the coin, standard value serving as a medium of exchange. Economists are four phases in the evolution of trade: the first phase is the domestic economy, which corresponds to production and rural family. In this case it satisfies one human group from economically; it produces for itself and its production consumes place. The second phase is the urban economy, growing with separation of different trades and the emergence of urban centers. The third phase is the national economy, which corresponds to state formation. Finally, the last phase is the global economy, which is based on the economic division of labor between countries. In its first phase, the trade does not have a commercial character itself, but rather a moral or religious one. He does not appear as such only once the third phase, when the man managed to use natural means of transport and created artificial means of transport. Trade appears in the history of human civilization as a factor of great progress and civilization. This quality establishes relationships between people whose degree of culture is often different. Thus trade promotes dissemination of ideas and customs and on the other hand facilitates peaceful relations much needed social stability, which constitutes the paramount of moral and intellectual progress.

Once the data above, we must see that social transformations suffered throughout history and who is due to other systems of social organization. Family unit has been changed through the life of the hunter to farmer, by establishing parentage blood and setting up family property -a clan regime. A patrilineal clan is a social unit consisting of a common ancestor, his children's children and descendant's males. Transmission symbol of membership of the clan is the preservation of the name of the father. But there are many clans in respecting native descent. The clans are extinguished once in a generation time, all children do not transmit the clan name. The links between clan members are the same as between family members, i.e. blood relation and adoption. But the clan unity is stronger than family, although this unit is bigger than family. Not to suppress the family unit, but is only a social unit superior to the latter, due to complication of social relations.

Clan functions are those of industrial and economic aid, political and legal between members that constitute it. Other functions of the clan are sending goods, vendetta and totemic. Clans rarely provide magical-religious functions. Primitive social institutions have a number of regular characters. Social groups are built on small and are based on kinship and race. They have classes or castes. Finally, in these groups, political power is mixed with the Economic and both are centralized. National unity achieved by the fact that they form independent political units. Clans can join to form a tribe whose purpose is to cultivate land. Even in this case, however, the clan prevents assertion of tribal sentiment. Another important reason that prevents merging clans is their mobility. The constitution of states and nations has always been preceded by some changes in habits, changes that led to the adoption of sedentary lifestyle.

The unit immediately above the tribe clan is founded on common totem. Most advanced stage of social organization is formed nations diffuse intermediate stage between tribal and national organization. The nation is a social group, composed of differentiated organs, but interdependent. After Hariou nation group is fixed to the ground, having spiritual kinship between its members, links which develops the idea of a national unit. Renan sees a nation as large sample of moral solidarity. But linking the German concept of a nation absolute determinism namely soil, language, race and history. Human individuals and groups would play by adopting this view, only a minimal role. French conception of the nation seeks social solidarity support in the individual subordinate to the free group, an agreement of wills of all individuals who constitute the group. Artistic instinct is a need therefore appears as indispensable to the human soul: we find artistic events in extremely remote epochs (Paleolithic). Although the artistic need is universal, each nation manifests in a different manner, according to the nature of the materials you have on hand, after the nature of the instrument, and after the group mentality. Due to artistic technique, the art has been linked to the evolution of craft. Since the artisan has mastered the technique, he was able to free trade and give free rein to his imagination. He could accomplish the birth of art. Thus, basket weaving decorations gave has given birth through the interpretation of the artist. Also decorating clay vessels with ornamental designs was one of the first forms of art and perhaps even writing. The artist introduces such values in his work, which nature does not know and which are strictly personal. All the above but do not entitle us to believe that we must assign, excessively artistic merit results of an activity whose value is more social and economic. On the other hand, freedom, which the artisan obtains when it reaches perfect knowledge of his Profession, does not always lead to the creation of an artwork. As of now, his imagination is free; it may be that instead of a work of art, the craftsman to create an opera or a vulgar image of its taste.

Each of artistic events thus has its origin, the aforementioned principles. Thus, dance acknowledges, on the one hand, magical-religious causes, the primitive part of the religious ritual and war preparations and, on the other hand, is evidence of social solidarity. Alternating dances of primitive men and women form a powerful auxiliary of sexual selection, as an expression of erotic arousal collective action. Finally, the dance has arisen during work jointly when one of the workers for rhythm work of others, mime works in their sight. Music found in ancient times is most often reduced to a single element, namely rhythm, given that serves more to accompany dance. This primitive music, using sounds simple, but can reach a highly complicated rate. In civilized people, the use of sound is wider, leading to marks and arrangement within the game. Harmony and counterpoint are emerging not only in civilized societies and represents the maximum complication in the musical structure.

Music has its roots in events both magical-religious, and labor and dance. It recognizes the often association with other social manifestations as war, transmission of sounds, dances, ceremonies and recitation flooring. Painting and sculpture recognize the main causes are magical-religious, they found their origin in primitive totem. Other causes which are at the origin of arts and crafts are ornamentation. The first poems were repeated rhythmic phrases, expressing sensations usually most vulgar and by referring especially to digestive functions. The songs are not unknown to primitive warriors; topics inspired by the beauty of nature or feelings of love not only exceptionally primitive meet. Literature was born from songs warrior or magical incantations of primitive peoples is represented by proverbs, riddles, lyric, mourning, satire, religious hymn and folk tales. Epic poetry, essay and novel are characteristic of a more advanced civilization. Of course, at first, literature is represented only by a handful of practical knowledge, which was transmitted by writing. It has become a source of pleasant emotions and aesthetics.

Religion is one of the most complex manifestations of the human spirit. After Feuerbach, the origin of any religion must be sought in the feeling of dependence that man is in the face of nature. Religious mentality is indebted to affective impulses that are directly related to preservation instinct. Belief in imaginary beings rooted in fear of any event of the unusual, disease or death. Man wants to preserve its existence by any means and religion appears as a product of human selfishness. Belief in the supernatural can be impersonal, as if magic, the act of faith is not indicative of an imaginary being. All processes used in magic namely imitation of desired event, charms, taboos, keep this supernatural impersonal seal. The transition zone between the personal and impersonal supernatural fetishism and is the personification of nature. Fetishism is only one aspect of animism, the first step towards idolatry. But he differs essentially from the latter two, by the fact that all idols are only the image of certain supernatural beings and even fetishes are these beings. After Comte, fetishism contributed to human evolution, the end state of nomadism and ensuring regime sedentary. Personal supernatural religion appears. This means all beliefs and rules that characterize human relations viewed from the standpoint of ethics; religion appears as a conduct penalty, sanction of supernatural origin. Essential and constant characters that we find in all religions are not based on any notion of divinity, or that of the supernatural, but the distinction between sacred and profane. Phenomena- such as religious beliefs relative to sacred things (prohibited) and practices which relate to items that faith.

To explain the distinction between sacred and profane, several theories have been issued. First we have the animist theories, then the notion of soul imagined by the idea of the sacred people. This theory is insufficient to explain the distinction between sacred and Profane, given that to many people there is the idea that the soul is destroyed with the body, a concept that is not in agreement with the idea of a soul separate from the body. Natural theories admit that people worshiped natural phenomena with which they had a feeling of fear or awe. And these theories are insufficient to explain the origin of the religious phenomenon, because once people would have noticed that sacrifices to the gods that inhabit nature without any result, religions ought to disappear. Finally, the theory of totemism and social origin of religion by Durkheim explained the concept of the sacred, relying in explaining them as the existence of a principle, mystical, general source of life, a principle that would result from the opposition, of the individual soul, Profanity and the forbidden. Thus, religions will be generated, religious ceremonies became part of man`s social life and soul of mysticism.

The source of religion becomes the system itself, with merely symbols of the religious character of society. In fact, the social function of religion is to maintain and strengthen social solidarity. The most primitive form of religion is the animism, which is the belief that there is a double soul, able to break away temporarily from his fleshly envelope. Animism acknowledges that all material objects are also equipped with a double soul. As society develops, the notion of soul is reported from the nearest human objects, objects increasingly farther and then the phenomena of nature. The latter are thus superior deities, who are due a cult. In addition to these superior deities, we have a number of family deities, which are nothing but myth ancestors in the past. In this way polytheistic religions arose.

Finally, the most perfect form of religion is the monotheism, the notion of divinity is not reported to natural phenomena, but the one unknown leading universal phenomenon. In social evolution there is therefore a gradual transition through the stages of animism, polytheism and monotheism. There are so primitive populations, such as certain tribes that are defending monotheism. On the other hand, the belief in one supreme being or multiple gods is determined by the spirituality of believers. Those whose predominant trend towards unification, there is the belief in one god; those who believe in diversity of nature and soul, adores many gods (Huxley). The supernatural appears as a primitive form of religion and the interior due to the nature of revelation. The supernatural is full of inconsistency and selfishness amazes us by its goals. Animism is devoid of any element of moral education, ethics is only by public opinion and social conventions. The moral right arises only in higher forms of religion polytheistic and monotheistic. These religions match their goals by altruism and involve a coordinated effort mystical phenomenon.

The social role of religions is not, however, to ensure respect for morality, for religions have not been intended as disciplining companies. They are only the moral image of society itself, funding her own primitive nature, religion is moral indifference. The height of the spiritualized ethics of religions indicates only appropriate moral progress of societies. Moral power of religion always expresses a social reality; religions evolve with the evolution of societies. On the basis of totemism we find feelings of trust rather than feelings of terror. How a believer seeks the existence of a moral power, due to pressure from the collective consciousness of the individual, all spiritual life is dominated by a mystical mentality, known for Lévy Bruhl. Because universal religions can arise, as different peoples had to meet, relationships and exchanges are formed among them. These religions grow because as the tribes reached a certain degree of culture, the individual ceases to be a social group; it is increasingly more a distinctive value, and it appears the idea of a special destiny, not be confused with the perpetuation of the group to which it belongs.

In most religions we can distinguish four main elements: conception of divinity, dogmas, rites and myths. These four elements are not always together. Such mythical elements we find in natural religion, but not the mission, being linked to the presence of a certain territory, of any particular geographic location, any monument whose meaning has been forgotten by some rhythm for local custom or a historic event. The universal religions, myths are only linked to the person of the founder. Religion has survived being extremely useful human utility is that it makes one apt to a full life and it allows him to -and to achieve maximum human condition. Through its practical maxims and precepts of religion also favors the activity of nutrition and human reproduction.

The religious feeling of the individual would have only a vague aspiration, if he had not built a system of practices and dogmas, that of a church. Only religious practice brings us to the inner belief and continuously feed this belief. The idea that the church becomes inseparable from religion. Church is a society whose members are united in identical representation of the sacred world and its relations with the secular world. Members of the same church translate this common representation through the same practices. The ritual is the appearance of religion. Along with the ceremony, they appear where people gather to participate in an activity that interests them emotionally. Where there is emotional interest, this will strengthen the ritual, the ritual is unable to produce an emotion in itself. When the ritual becomes absurd, the intensity of faith is most often low. Ceremony supernatural prints its mark on very many aspects of social life. Such military events, poetic, dramatic, puberty rites and funeral events are always closely linked to the presence of a significant act. The methods they employ are most often ritual prayer, offerings and performances. Religion in its structure contains all the elements that gave rise to the various manifestations of collective life. Myths and legends originated from science and poetry; the ceremony became ritual practices that possessed moral qualities.

Finally, the change in the concept of religion has brought big changes in the social structure. The emergence of monotheism transformed human society in an industrial structure, a phenomenon which, in turn, acting on psychic life, has enabled the development of scientific thought. All the events of psychic life must note Profane ceremony, which consists of all the attitudes of people observed between them during social activities. The main purpose of the ceremony is to regulate Profane human actions. It includes gifts, visits, courtesy formulas to interpellate, titles, costumes, trophies and mutilation. Its essential character is symbolism and expressions are the current submission, deference and respect. Nowadays, much of this ceremonial highly developed in primitive peoples survived. This is not due to its practical use, but that largely ceremonial Profane satisfy our aesthetic instinct. However, most of these ceremonials disappeared due to loss of time. Its evolution is parallel with the evolution of ideas and depends largely on the environment.

In religion there is also the basis of another manifestation of psychic life that is based on scientific thinking. Between these two ways of manifestations there is a strong antagonism, progress finally bringing itself after the decline of the former. We find common notions of both events but clearly indicating that they have a common origin. Thus, the concept of force, the concept of cause and concept of law are common to both mental manifestations. But what characterizes scientific thinking is disinterestedness and objectivity of the scholar, freedom and individuality. The transition from religion to science was done by magic. Indeed, the magician appears as one of the first individuals who are trying to liberate religion and social groups. But magic cannot be identified by religion, since it works by methods that religion does not prescribe; nor science, that it is a mixture of free and accurate knowledge assumptions. The emergence of science is conditional on freedom of the spirit and the possible use of leisure time, factors that are closely related to the existence of a rich society where constraining forces of the primitive beliefs have lost their vigor. While primitives are very close to magic, scientifically civilized peoples are different from the first, thanks to diffusion of knowledge. Preserving knowledge through writing was possible through creation of specialists, thanks to precision instruments and because the correlations between various branches of science.

2. Ethnic manifestations - correlations with manifestations of material life

What distinguishes man from all other living creature is its ability to react and adapt to the vicissitudes of the external environment, the ups and downs of nature, effort strengthened by employing artificial instruments and using articulated language. Man responds to the external environment throughout its entire structure, so both through the psyche, as well as his physical. The manifestations of these reactions may be general for all people or different from one group to another group. The reasons underlying human activity are: a) biological factors (organic necessities); b) social factors; and c) psychological factors. Biological determinism works hand in hand with social and psychological determinism, each being a process of cooperation and convergence. Biological and psychological factors are the heritage of the individual; social factors are external factors. In the following lines, the human events shown will be analyzed through the factors which determine each particular part of human events.

Events which take a unique form to all human groups is the use of articulated language, creating and using artificial instrument and achievement through community awareness of organic connection. Progress is not possible unless, alongside creative initiative, the human group gains conservation. This property of transmission from one generation to another cannot be established unless the means of communication of thought are sufficiently developed, i.e. when language is almost definitively established. Certainly articulate language is not the only means of understanding and communication between people. Besides he also found other aids that link the individuals. These features are: gestures, facial expressions, signals, writing and fine arts. However, given that the secondary means that are insufficient to establish a perfect bond between individuals, language remains the main mode of understanding.

The tool that it is articulated language is an intermediary between the human being and the outer reality. Man does not see the real objects than covered by their verbal symbols, symbols or associated immediate. Thinking and reflective capacity thus become an inner speech, any thought process based on the image of the spoken word. Thinking, in turn, builds on the other expressing signs, symbols; they substitute things or external phenomena. With language, an individual can affect another man's conscience in such a way that the latter perception of sensations arising not only sound but also images or associations consciousness induced by these images. Such language can convey feelings or ideas; it will contain emotional or rational elements. In this way, an individual can transfer it to another person everything he possesses the experience, and conservation gain is thus ensured. Since all these signs create language only when signs have real meaning for individuals whom they are addressed, it follows that they are conventional and presuppose society; Indeed, the language appeared with the advent of society and has evolved with the latter! Vocabulary words and meaning have changed with the evolution of social conditions. The emergence of social classes, progress in invention from the material production, historical moments that brought cultural progress. Language should therefore be amended with the transformation of social life, totally corresponding to the degree of differentiation of society. Creating artificial instruments has, after Bergson, differentiated humans from animals. Intelligence is therefore the starting point of reflective abilities. Indeed, while in animals, the instrument is part of the body, there is an instinct that drives its use in humans. Social life has always revolved around the manufacture and use of instruments. Most often there is always a gap between a new facility and social reaction produced by inventing this instrument. Finally, the collective achievement of the organic connection between conscious human manifestations is the product of stark human intellectual function and produce, in turn, within the human group, the emergence of a consciousness, which distinguishes human societies from those of other animals.

In addition to these general human events, we find different human manifestations within different ethnic group, events relating to material life, mental life and social life. These human activities are the direct or indirect relationships with biological functions. Therefore, the most important activities are related to the preservation of life while at the same time, the major manifestations of biological functions. The activities necessary for the conservation of individual existence and social functions are the most visible manifestations of the body namely nutrition, reproduction, protection and innervation. They will form the substrate of the other activities in the sense of increasing complexity. The product of these activities and functions are fundamental: locomotion, aesthetic function, communicating ideas and social institutions that form the indirect means of survival.

In the events of material life, we will deal with those events concerning the nature, preparation and food preservation; livelihood; garments and ornamentation. Eating is the most important human activity related to the function of nutrition, running a dominant role in the preservation of life. Type of food preparation and preservation vary from group to group. Generally, all vegetables are considered edible. There are people that find most curious types of food, genres which often are related to factors that have no relation in nutritional function. Thus, cannibalism is practiced either out of necessity in cases where the missing food or for other reasons: pleasure, superstition or in some cases reducing litter. Scatophagy be explained by economic reasons; undigested grains and other particles are kept in dry faeces and thus consumed in times of famine.

People all over the earth eat uncooked foods. This is either due to the need to facilitate digestion or the need to conserve food. In cooking, the man uses different methods, but underlying all these methods is the use of fire. Once he discovered fire, man had the means to make edible and digestible food for his peers. Since the man has ensured the preservation and preparation of food, he made his debut in the human condition. Along with agriculture, food preparation freed man from the obligation to hunt and thus to be based on the problem of eating.

Fire made it possible for human habitation in cold regions, ensuring warmth and the light needed. Finally, the use of fire has allowed the birth and development of the industry; the myth of

Prometheus can therefore capitalize on this important enough human conquest. Around the fire, man developed intellectually and morally. The culinary evolution has two great periods, namely: one before and another after the discovery of pots. First the man was satisfied with roasting food. The second phase is going back to the time in which they could boil water.

Until the man became a farmer, cooking remained in a primitive stage. With the advent of agriculture, the power plant has a preponderance of the animal being safer. The peoples who earn their hunting territories need very large areas. But that does not show that they were nomadic. Of course, agglomerations of people in regions favorable appear impossible, for any congestion would destroy the whole game. Groups dealing with primitive people hunting exploits the most often only district that belongs to them. Man, needing a varied diet, in addition to hunting and picking berries, because by consuming the latter he could break the monotony of a carnivorous diet. Of course, all thanks to this cause, people who adopted agriculture and cattle breeding do not cease to hunt. The idea of conservation and preservation of food has led them to not touch plants before their maturation and not eat birds whose eggs are edible. The fact is the origin of agriculture and cattle farming. Of great inventions, it was the most fertile agriculture. Hunting, fishing and gathering fruit were indeed unsafe food sources, allowing frequent occurrence of famines. Thanks to agriculture, man began to foresee a period of security.

Another question which is based on the origin of agriculture is the return to nomadic tribes of the same age in the same places. Fruit picking and capturing small animals entered in the duties of women, we can consider agriculture and animal husbandry as the operated by the latter. Agriculture thus formed a first form of division of labor. So, the crucial importance of agriculture lies in the fact that it increases the chances of survival and helps to develop mental faculties. At the same time, it enables man to secure a modicum of free time, time that man has used it to indulge with crafts. True agriculture appears only once animals were domesticated. Besides the considerable number of cultivated plants, domesticated animals appear in a curiously low percent. Domestication has not been made but due to reasons of expediency, but due to reasons of ceremonial nature, sports or entertainment. Practical use is the result of domestication and not its cause. We do not know when and how we started to domesticate animals.

The protective function is, like that of nutrition, one of the fundamental functions of the body. Nutrition is the purchase of energy from the environment; protection appears once this energy has been conserved. Thus, prehistoric populations living in caves; nomadic peoples, dealing with hunting, living in tents; those dealing with fishing villages can establish standing, at least for a certain period of the year; people dealing with agriculture and industry have fixed housing. The prototype is fixed dwelling hut, which probably comes from a screen of branches, as can be seen today in certain primitive peoples. Huts form is conditioned by climate and the nature of the inhabitants have it handy. Nature of the material is dependent, in turn, the geographic location and transport. Thus, in ancient times, when the Egyptian temples were built of stone brought into the path of the Nile in Nubia, Assyrian palaces and temples were built of brick, Assyrians having handy ways and means of transport to ensure their material transportation in the mountains. Once past the primitive stages, the specific architecture of each region begins to develop. A round-conical hut primitive presenting a grave inconvenience (where they do not allow the house to take too large), replacement plane circular with a rectangular plan was a major breakthrough in the evolution of architecture, progress achieved in a period early history of civilization. May I bring great progress through the discovery Romans vault.

Geographical environment has a great influence on human ingenuity when it comes to determining land use. Such groups established in swampy regions have built houses built above the marshes by stakes; Eskimos build their homes in the snow. However, the nature and place of human settlement also depend, in addition to geographical conditions and conditions purely social. The presence of water, food, fuel and enemies determined, in large measure, the place of human settlements. The need to protect the body gave birth, on the other hand, mantle. Secondary causes underlying the mantle are modesty and aesthetic instinct. Body protection garments is determined by the body's fight against the cold, insects and road accidents. Modesty is developed in all nations, but not always expresses the shame of nudity. Often even lack of ornament such as ring nasal brownies, causing feelings of shame. What is certain is that the issue has always been conditioned mantle of applications ornamentation and even seems curious that preceded mantle ornamentation. However painting or tattooing the body should be considered as a pre ceremonial vestment or coquetry. Material they are made garments vary in relation to social life and climate. Use of material such as leather clothing belonging to hunters, cotton and flax belongs to farmers, tree bark belongs to the inhabitants of forests, and silk worms belong to farmers. Mantle varies with climate, moving from one of the parties covering sexual characteristic equatorial areas, until thick and complicated garments inhabitants from the cold. In warmer regions are used in garments manufacturing plant products, while in the cold animal products are used.

We see that among the reasons that push man to cover his body, modesty plays a relatively weak need protection and determine the place that the individual must occupy in society are the important factors. With the study of material manifestations of life in keeping with nutrition and protection, we must say a few words about industries. They aim to build artificial instrument which helps the man to fulfill its fundamental functions. Primitives, dealing with hunting cannot find enough free time to be able to deal with any trade in these populations and therefore we will not only find an extremely weak industry. The emergence of industry will be put on the presence of free time and a notable development of intelligence and inventive spirit. The company is more evolved, much more free time is dedicated to crafts and individuals who practice them come to specialize in certain industrial Professions.

Industrial progress was not a sudden jump never produced the results are the sum of a series of slow improvement. The invention of capital industry was due to the discovery of fire. The discovery of first order industries as pottery gave rise to metallurgy. Once in possession of primary inventions the state of civilization of mankind begins to be born. There are some primitive industries which have played a significant role in human history. Thus, basket weaving, leather preparation, preparation of linen, pottery and metallurgy were the starting point of a series of human events, bringing an important contribution to the history of civilization.

Social life brought transformations by industrial inventions that are considerable. These innovations have contributed to the evolution of economic and hence social life. But what you need to note is that an innovative industrial order is never immediate to social reaction, but between these two for quite a pronounced lag, after which social reaction almost always occurs. From what has been said, it appears that the evolution of material life events can assist with two major stages, which limits, if not fixed, may still be readily discerned. One of these steps is prior to the occurrence of agriculture. At this stage, winning unsafe food is done through hunting, fishing or picking fruit; food is preserved and is most often consumed raw; homes are reduced to simple partitions caverns or branches; mantle is made of crude, unprocessed. The second phase marks the beginning of civilization and parallels the development of intelligence. It begins with the discovery of fire and is characterized by the appearance of agriculture and industries. In this period, we find the regulation of feeding, housing emergence fixed and processed protective mantle. During this period, human primary functions are met and secured in this way the man can begin to fully realize his human condition. The issue of cultural anthropology in conjunction with the typology presented in Chapters put physical anthropology with poignancy but in actuality postulate Socratic "I know that I know nothing" and expressing the "cogito ergo Dubito, cogito ergo sum". It raises two issues remain unanswered:

1. Man has a social environment and a spirituality whose product is all that is conditioned thinking and talent; Biblical truth itself says that "in the beginning was the word" animal and plant world but does not have any of this? It seems the answer is firmly negative.

2. Are we matter that we know in part plus the etheric, astral, mental, spiritual and less clarified or are "shadow-fire" metaphor Plato who considered the real world as a shadow of the real world of ideas?

3. The Human Condition in The East-Asian Cultural And Anthropological Vision A Comparison Between The Buddhist And The Christianist Concept

People have always been attracted to the great mysteries of life, often asking questions about their own existence or the existence of other beings who are superior to them. Such questions are often conceptual, like the difference between the concepts "good" and "bad" (together with all the questions derived from them); How they were created, what would happen after their death, etc.?

These questions, which have stirred man since ancient times, have led him to devote his life to trying to find an answer or to open at least a path for others to follow, sharing the information he found. As we know, man is, by definition, a social being, which urges us to understand that all his achievements were not individual, but that they are the result of group ideas that, following the logical thread of human thought, have set out on a solitary journey to develop and give birth to new ideas and concepts.

Consequently, religion was created to answer these questions in an abstract way capable of satisfying the little curiosity of the human mind. *Nishida* said that "*religion is about God. God is fundamental to religion in any form. As the color is shown to the eye as color, and the sound of the ear as sound, so God also shows to the religious self as an event of his own soul.*" (*Nishida*, 1987). However, this does not prevent us from seeing man differently, but on the contrary, his uniqueness is emphasized, depending on how he was conceived.

Thus, in Buddhism, the human condition is perceived as a negative thing described in harsh words beginning with The Four Noble Truths in which we are told that the entire human existence is "suffering" and continues with the Noble Truth of Suffering: *"Birth is suffering, aging is suffering, sickness is suffering, death is suffering, sorrow and lamentation, pain, grief, and despair are suffering; association with the loathed is suffering, dissociation from the loved is suffering, not to get what one wants is suffering — in short, suffering is the five categories of clinging objects."*

The categories to which the Buddha refers are a body, sentiment, knowledge, will, and conscience. They are an ensemble of the elements that make up man, but neither together nor separately can make up the "self." The human essence lies within but can not be defined or identified. In this regard, we can see how Buddhism admits to some extent that the existence of the inner "self" is distinct and personal to each individual due to his physical and psychic attributes that can be considered and defined separately. However, this does not extend, at all, to what Christians recognize as an eternal spirit, because the metaphysical manifestation, like all the elements of this universe, is transient. Thus, the essence of human nature is trapped in an illusory reality full of desires that lead to suffering. This reality is in perpetual change and decay, an eternal cycle that does not forgive anyone. That is why the Buddha denies the existence of an eternal "self" that defines our own nature that will remain unchanged as it passes through the millions of reincarnations, and then obtain the much-desired release. That is why Buddhist doctrine preaches the existence of a "non-self.'

However, the Buddha accepts the idea of *karma* (the law of cause-effect of the material world) and *samsara* (the process of reincarnation), concepts that can not be fulfilled without the existence of an eternal "self." Thus, the nature of the rebirth of a person is conditioned by the karmic law. In other words, it is not necessary to reincarnate the same original "self," but components of the human structure, thus creating a new version of the same "self." All actions and decisions in the course of time are closely linked to the cause-effect cycle, consequences that can become a burden for the contingent "self," creating the potential for future rebirth. According to karmic laws, in samsara, the self can be rewarded or punished, so Buddha goes further in his perception of our world and the law of reincarnation. *Ernest* states that the Buddha sees karma as the only living going from life to life "*using the shadows created by candlelight, which are derived from another candle without having its own substance.*" Thus, "*there is rebirth without self-transfer from one birth to another.*" (*Ernest*). In Christianity, Hinduism, Daoism, and even in Confucianism, there is a discourse of an eternal "self," trapped in the body, but which is to rise to be "rescued" through different ethical, moral or ritualistic methods, but the way they perceive the "man" is not nearly as hard as Buddhism does. In this reality in which we are caught "*everything burns*" (Buddha, "The Feast of Fire"), and the human body is "*made of plagues, tormented by illusory desires, dying slowly, falling into the dust. Old age consumes the body, this place of rottenness, always under the threat of ruin* "(Dhammapada, v. 147-148).

According to the Bible, Christians see man as being created in the likeness of God."*Then God said, "Let us make mankind in our image, in our likeness, so that they may rule over the fish in the sea and the birds in the sky, over the livestock and all the wild animals,[a] and over all the creatures that move along the ground." So God created mankind in his own image, in the image of God he created them; male and female he created them." (Genesis 1:26-27)*

According to the Genesis, at first it was nothing, and it was God. God created everything from nothing. This creative power rests with Him, the supreme authority that constantly oversees us. The great Creator "*taking (...) dust from the earth, made man, and breathed before him a breath of life, and made man alive*" (Genesis 2: 7). Through all this, we see His power to create the physical universe. In this universe resides the man who is composed of body and spirit - the physical dimension and the spiritual dimension. Christianity through its existence promotes a multitude of dimensions with a well-defined status, compared to other religions, and God is above all. He has never been in the physical dimension of the universe because He belongs to the spiritual world, the place where the human soul goes after the separation from the flesh.

When man was created in the likeness and image of God, he received a part of the creator, but he did not receive His nature, only qualities similar to Him. Thus man was given the ability to be connected with divinity. From a biblical point of view, we will see how the human`s will and communication with the "self" within, fall on a lower plan, Christianity emphasizing the obedience and fulfillment of God's commandments and laws, but this does not in any way prevent the free will. In this way, with the "*image of God, projected into man*" as a personal example, by applying His laws in everyday life, the doctrine becomes a way of living.

In Christianity, according to *Ernest*, man has the body and soul, its attributes, as real as possible, being not completely bad or illusory."*(...) the serpent said to the woman." For God knows that when you eat from it your eyes will be opened, and you will be like God, knowing good and evil." When the woman saw that the fruit of the tree was good for food and pleasing to the eye, and also desirable for gaining wisdom, she took some and ate it. She also gave some to her husband, who was with her, and he ate it. Then the eyes of both of them were opened (...) And the* L*ORD God said, "The man has now become like one of us, knowing good and evil." (Genesis, 3:4-7,22)*

According to the Genesis, in the vision of Christianity, man is perceived as "neutral." He is neither evil nor good. As God, when Adam and Eve ate the apple, they began to know and distinguish between good and evil. Man is the being able to understand, to think and to become good or bad according to the choices made. The human body is real as it is made of "dust," and its soul is an ephemeral, intangible, but "real" element. The soul exists, and without a body, it would not make the man. Thus, together, they are not evil or illusory, they are present to "become." That is why the elements of psycho-mental life do not contain anything wrong in them, which is why Christianity demands discernment between good and evil, using free will for good purposes." *Do not conform to the pattern of this world, but be transformed by the renewing of your mind. Then you will be able to test and approve what God's will is—his good, pleasing and perfect will." (Romans 12:2)* Nowhere in the Bible does it say that desire should be annihilated to reach the supreme spiritual universe, the dimension in which God is.

Unlike Buddhism (where desire is evil, suffering is evil, need is bad, etc.) Christianity does not see desire as a bad thing in essence, but as an integral part of human nature, and acts as an impulse to reach as close as possible to God." *You, my brothers and sisters, were called to be free. But do not use your freedom to indulge the flesh; rather, serve one another humbly in love. So I say, walk by the Spirit, and you will not gratify the desires of the flesh. For the flesh desires what is contrary to the Spirit, and the Spirit what is contrary to the flesh. They are in conflict with each other, so that you are not to do whatever you want." (Galatians*, 5:13,16-17)

Taking this opposition idea further, we can make a resemblance to the *yin-yang*[6] (dark-light) theory of Chinese thought. This gives us the opportunity to explain the concepts that have built what we know today to be Chinese thinking: Confucianism and Daoism.

Confucianism began by being an ethical system to improve the Chinese society of that time. It focused on social life and principles that should govern the welfare of society, family, and personal life. According to Confucius, the human ideal could be achieved by morality and ethics, not by religious rituals. He put a great emphasis on teaching, virtue, and reciprocity.*"The Master said: Negligence in the cultivation of character, lack of thoroughness in study, incompetence to move towards recognized duty, inability to correct my imperfections - these are what cause my solicitude." (Analects* 7: 2)

All of Confucius's lectures were based on how man should behave according to his situation, implicitly transforming these teachings into a lifestyle. Having managed to follow the instructions given by the Master, the man manages to achieve the perfection of the human character, the most noble medal he can hold.

Daoism, on the other hand, complements Confucianism by the fact that man must be in harmony with nature and its energies. The instinct, the desire, the will, the imagination, the need to create, all must be allowed to manifest freely, because only so can they be an integral part of nature.*"Dao gives birth to beings and nourishes them, creates them, but does not control them, works and does not boast; He is the master of all beings and things, but leaves them to their will - this is called deepest* De *(virtue)* "(*Dao De Jing*, 10)

---

[6] The yin-yang theory refers to the duality of the material world. Yin represents the darkness, the shadow, the bottom, the rest, the interior, the water, the night, the earth, etc., and yang represents light, heat, upward, motion, exterior, fire, day, sky, and so on. This duality is, in chinese thinking, the foundation of understanding of the natural world.

In Daoism, it is very important not to interrupt the sacred energies of the universe. Here the order and the chaos have another meaning, the moral discipline of Confucianism being seen as emprisoning man." *Let go of the doctrine and keep your heart free. What is the difference between "Yes" and "Yeah" ? And what is the difference between "good" and "bad" ? What scares people can not be dreadful. A! How vain and endless is the teaching of the world!* "(Dao De Jing, 20). It is believed that Dao, even though God has the same aspect (undefined, formless, invisible to the eye), created the universe of His own substance, allowing it to be omnipresent and omnipotent." *Dao is empty, no form and shape, but we can serve him indefinitely! Deep and impenetrable, He seems to be the ancestor of the ten thousand things. Tinkering sharpening, untie the ties, putting harmony in all its shining, one with the dust, It seems like in a deep water it is, and it is not. Whose son I do not know, but it was before all the gods with a face." (Dao De Jing*, 4)

Daoism views the human condition as being reflected in nature. In the universe that hosts the man, the same laws of ascent and decay apply for all "*ten thousand things.*" Man ascends to the moment of birth when he reaches the climax, after which the period of decay begins. (*Ernest*) "*I alone sit quietly and undisturbed, innocent as a child*" (*Dao De Jing*, 20). The moment of decay, the effective life of man, the period between birth and death, is seen as the incompetence of men to keep their vital energy intact, wasting it in the mood of chaos. Thus, they die until they come to align with nature perfectly. Progress and regression are elemental concepts for the universe, but man's inability to perceive these things makes it incomplete and return to a new form until the "elementary" becomes "elementary" to the human mind, and the energies of the universe will merge with it. We must also remember that man has always felt the need for "ritual" to understand, communicate, and achieve a certain purpose in terms of the mysteries of the universe. In this sense, ritual arts exist to meet the psychological desires of man. The human mind is the ideal home for "chaos," that is why there is constant need to create "order" through the appearance of various categories, meaningful, in order to perceive both the external world and the internal world. For example, through the tea ceremony, man tries to relate to the "self," to remove the fog that envelops him and to reach "nothing." The ritual of the tea ceremony is one of physical and mental cleansing. This ritual helps the practitioner to make "order" in his soul.

Also, we must bear in mind that before the emergence of technology, man attempted to understand and control nature through various rituals. That is why religion has been seen as a constant that man can define and be able to find in it. In the great religions of the world the doctrine merged with culture and created a special concept for man and his way of being. Knowledge discovered in the search for "self" or "non-self" was a gift that could not be preserved only for the discoverer, and the man felt the need to share with his "close" the great discovery. Thus, we find him in many ways the protagonist loved or punished by his universe: the traveling man, the seeker man and the religious man, all three being connected to each other.

Man, until he becomes a seeker or a religious one, is first a traveler. The journey has an important role for people; it can be divided into two categories: moving from a point A to a point B (travel with a specific purpose: craft, goods transport, trade, having a commercial role) and the religious journey (Religious character, self-finding, pilgrimage). We will continue to talk about his pilgrimage and religious character, given that not only monks participated in such actions, although they are most popular because of trips to isolated places for their spiritual cleansing. Such journeys are found in many writings throughout history that refer to merchants, seekers of new lands, pilgrims, followers to share the teaching of the master or the teacher. However, the most important thing is that, through the journey, the monks have passed on, from one country to another, culture, religious teaching and many other invaluable values, which today we can regard as some of them Cultural jewelry. The *Dalai Lama* said that "*all religions have one message: love.*" According to his words, we are all united under one umbrella of religion, and yet we are so different. Here we can see how culture plays an important role in interpreting religious teaching and thus the concept of "man," "self." In East Asia it is important to remember that "order" plays an important role in people's thinking." Chaos" and "order" are present from the time of creation so that religion (in addition to writing, culture, and teaching), both local (Shintoism[7] - Japan) and foreign (Buddhism, Christianity) was passed through the filter of cultural thinking Can be understood. For East Asia, thought and way of life blend harmoniously so that religious influences can be detected even in scientific and literary works.

The spiritual journey has played an important role in East Asian culture. For hundreds of years, people have resorted to a journey to find spirituality. We could even say that going through long and solitary roads is a characteristic of this area. If we think of Dao principles, it is understandable why travels are closely related to the harmonization of energies, the search for "self" or the maintenance of "order" in the human universe. According to the laws of the universe, we can imagine the flow of energies in the form of the infinity sign. They are in a continuous process of transformation, moving from Ascension to decay. For example, in Buddhist writings, we will find references to real points of nature, time and space. The greatest difficulty, however, is to interpret and identify past points with those of the present. However, for the listener and a good observer, such problems can become simple and easy to solve.

The things that scare the man are usually the reason why he is moving in some directions. For travelers, it is quite possible that karmic law is precisely the main cause of the impetus to understand the great teachings and to seek answers to the last questions of the "soul" by venturing into spiritual journeys. By following some trails, they may even end up doing their "order" in the "chaos" inside. This may be a reason for people to go to pilgrimage to some places indicated by great teachers. Ackerman brought to light a new category of travel: the journey for treatment and relaxation. This category includes the famous walks on the onsen caves (thermal baths), one of Japan's pride and an integral part of the culture of this country. Because of the religion found at the base of East Asian countries, there is no exception to the application of the laws of the universe that are omnipresent in this world. Because of this, any information that has entered this cultural area has been passed through a filter of thought specific to the contact area, so all the knowledge received has undergone a transformation. In antiquity, it was believed that by traveling they could help align the energies that form a sort of "*barrier of protection.*" If this "*barrier of protection*" becomes interrupted or "holes" in it, people have to participate or create a ritual by which both the flux of the energies of the universe and the human body was "reorganized" and "repaired" until a future disturbance appeared. For the universe, such rituals were held at periods of time calculated and established by the great priests of the time.

Through such a "filter of thought," Buddhism has passed, which, like most religions, has begun a journey." In the sixth century, before Christ, India goes through a period of intense spiritual and intellectual travel." [8] Starting from this early period of Buddhism, it has undergone many essential transformations which, due to the interpretation of the doctrine, have led to the birth of many branches of which one can be considered an integral point in East Asian culture.

---

[7] Shinto, Shintō, or The Way of the Gods is the ethnic religion of Japan. It focuses on the ritual and communion of man with the gods. In Shintō's belief, man sees deity everywhere. The spirits that dwell in nature and the spirits of the ancestors must be respected and venerated, being considered "Divinities."

[8] Cited from: Focşeneanu, Anca. „Civilizație japoneză – de la origini până în epoca clasică"; Crombé Veronique 1995, Prezentarea budismului în Gaudin Phillippe – editor, p 358-407

Bodhidharma[9] (*Putidamo* in Chinese and *Daruma* in Japanese) is the first monk to bring Mahayana Buddhism to China. He is also considered to be the first Patriarch of Chinese Zen. (*Taisen, Etienne* 2013) In other words, we can say he is the founder of Zen Buddhism, but what does *Zen* mean? *Zen* is the Japanese pronunciation of the Chinese word *Chan*, which is a transcription of the Sanskrit word *dhyana*, meaning "*meditation.*" Thus "Zen School" means "School of Meditation." So Zen is not a separate branch of Buddhism, but it is the very meditation the Buddha practices under the sacred fig. Thus, Bodhidharma brought to China Buddhism that focuses on meditation. Zen Buddhism, this school of meditation, believes that each person has two personalities, one in the world we live in, the physical personality and one in Nirvana, the celestial world - virtual personality. In order to reach Nirvana, Heaven in the Christian religion, the physical personality must enter the same plane as virtual personality, that is, become identical with each other. To this end, Zen Buddhism comes with the method by which to accomplish this, namely the perfect activity of virtual activity. Thus, for example, a street-cleaning worker must do it perfectly, and a teacher who attends students must be as perfect as possible in presenting the notions he conveys to those who hear him.

In this way, Zen Buddhism comes with the solution which helps every human personality to get as close as possible to divinity. Once this point has been reached, the human personality remains in Nirvana, and no reincarnation takes place. If not too exaggerated, we could say that Zen Buddhism is a militant teaching of perfection comparable to the Catholic teaching that states the thesis that every person must be, through what he does, the appearance and the thought of God. With the spread of this religion, the Buddhist temples, places of pilgrimage, spiritual cleansing and Buddhist practices have appeared. The temples were situated in the mountains, far from the noise of people, and the roads were long and dangerous.

From this point of view, we only have to relate to the way in which travel (by extension, which is perceived as a ritual) can be integrated into the Buddhist doctrine. Although Buddhists, by definition, regard places regarded as spiritual energy points as mere illusions, that is, "evil" places, they may at the same time be regarded as "seeds of salvation." Once a man realizes his mistake, and the "wickedness" of the place, awareness of this is the first step to enlightenment. In other words, what is initially seen as "evil" can be transformed into "good" by simply realizing this. By concentrating on the journey, we can consider the path to enlightenment as a journey of transformation full of seeds of the truth that emerge to the seeker one by one, being peculiar to the situation in which they were planted. Both physical and spiritual suffering is caused by *bonnō* (worldly desires and passions), and this prevents the traveler from clearly seeing the way to enlightenment, but even under these conditions man does not have to despair because *bonnō sunawachi bodai* (worldly desires are nothing but enlightenment). Applying this expression, we can consider that man, as long as he gradually transforms the desires and illusions of this world into small truths, he can attain enlightenment. If he follows the road carefully, the careful observer will come to understand the essence and cause of the suffering of this world, but everything has a price. Like the ancient rituals that needed a periodic "renewal," and the Buddhist core ritual (meditation and sutra songs) must be repeated until the seeker reaches Nirvana. (*Ackermann*)

The journey is a process of detachment that helps to "transform" the interior, pointing the traveler towards a road meant to understand the concept of "detachment." The past does not matter. Only this is important. Therefore, the practitioner must leave behind everything that

---

[9] His name consists of *Bodhi*, *satori* and *dharma*, the cosmic order, the highest truth of this world, the cosmic truth. (*Taisen, Etienne*: 2013)

represents worldly attachment (feelings, memories, objects, people, etc.). To make this possible, we first need to understand the ephemeral nature of things, thus bringing the detachment from the karmic cycle of growth and rot. Knowing these things, we can easily admit that pilgrimage is the way to enlightenment, a road to health and good fortune.

A well-known example of the journey of transformation is the migration of the people of Israel from Egypt to the Promised Land. (*Bayley*, 2008) Egypt, a symbol of civilization and power, is perceived as the material world, a world created and developed by man away from God. If we go further with the analysis, then we could say that Egypt is a "bad" place. In order to come closer to God, to find the way and to return to the simplicity of faith and hope, the sons of Israel must go to a pure, untouched place they will care for and love because it is the Promised Land. The departure from Egypt is heavy and painful, leaving behind sacrifices. Detachment and detachment are necessary to go forward because, in order to rise, we must "cleanse" in the soul. During the journey, the "order" lies, and we learn not to look back, as happened with the people guided by Moses to Canaan when they crossed the Red Sea." *Then Moses stretched out his hand over the sea, and all that night the Lord drove the sea back with a strong east wind and turned it into dry land. The waters were divided, and the Israelites went through the sea on dry ground, with a wall of water on their right and on their left." (Exodus,* 14:21-22). This episode can be seen as a crucial moment when traveling, as travelers are about to turn.

The moment when the waters are separated is at night. In many writings, we find the night as a climax of change. The Buddha began its own change at sunset, the night "fought" to find the truth, and when it was found and touched the illumination was done in the morning. A similar episode also passes these travelers, because when their dawn approaches their transformation is complete." *Moses stretched out his hand over the sea, and at daybreak, the sea went back to its place. The Egyptians were fleeing toward it, and the Lord swept them into the sea. The water flowed back and covered the chariots and horsemen—the entire army of Pharaoh that had followed the Israelites into the sea.(…) And when the Israelites saw the mighty hand of the Lord displayed against the Egyptians, the people feared the Lord and put their trust in him…" (Exodus*, 14:27-28,31) We can consider this transcendence as a ritual of purification, in which the Egyptians are the "chaos" we take with us and enslaves us without feeling. The moment the waters flooded over this "chaos," the man freed himself and began to understand and see what he could not see and eventually to fear what could become. Thus, the transforming journey is an integral part of the spiritual journey, for as the "sons of Israel" and the pilgrim seek the truth and the change in the spiritual points that we can see as the "Promised Land" - a pure place necessary for the finding of faith. The spiritual journey, known as pilgrimage, is a centuries-old phenomenon, both in the east and in the west. The importance of the pilgrimage began to be recognized when the intercultural and inter-religious dialogue that emerged during these spiritual paths was discovered.

Pilgrimages to holy places were often made in organized groups because the roads were long and dangerous. Most of the trails were deserted, so besides those who wanted to reach the sacred places adventures and robbers or jails and freshly released were adventures. These characters were making it difficult for wildlife and other unforeseen events. That is why the leaders of these areas had to implement new laws to protect pilgrims. Armed guards were located in points considered particularly dangerous on the road to protect robbers. The pilgrim groups, when they left their towns, were seen by all the neighbors, blessed by the priest and dressed in a "uniform" specific to them: a hat, a bracelet, a water gourd and a long cane with which they could support and defend against wild animals, dogs and parasites. Jesus Gonzales Valles, in his "Pilgrimage Roads in Spain and Japan," tells us about such relationships.

One of the most famous pilgrimage trips in Europe is the road to Santiago de Compostela. The classical route traversed the traveler through seven Spanish provinces until it reached its famous location in northwestern Spain. This road is considered to be a meeting road for cultures, and this gives the spiritual journey an opening to universality, equality, brotherhood, and solidarity. Travelers from different European countries who participated in such trips have discovered an opportunity for cultural exchange and a new way of inter-human communication. Pilgrims were interacting by sharing suffering caused by natural disasters or disasters, and by exchanging material goods (food, crafts, etc.) that they had with them. With this exchange of experience, a new connection was created between the participants of this hike, namely, the spiritual understanding that each of them dwelt in their own soul.

Even if cultural and social elements are important, we can not ignore the religious foundation of the road to Santiago, embodied in Christian beliefs and beliefs. In essence, the path of *St. Apostle James* is neither a touristic route nor a playful one, although they are also found. It is imminently a religious pilgrimage in which pilgrims do not go to *Santiago de Compostela* to see museums but to affirm their own faith. (*Valles*)This road rooted in the Christian faith for ten centuries witnessed a spiritual and cultural abundance for all the European Christian peoples who followed it. In Japan an equivalent of pilgrimage to Santiago de Compostela is pilgrimage to Ise. It is distinguished by the fact that the route is visited by 88 Buddhist temples covering an area of 1374 km, hence the name *hachijūhakkasho meguri* (the pilgrimage of the 88 temples), the most famous pilgrimage in Japan around the southern island of Shikoku By Honshu - Japan's largest island. Many of the temples here are said to have been founded or restored by the famous monk *Kūkai*. Japanese pilgrims wishing to follow the traditional road have, like the Europeans, a "uniform" specific to them. They are called *henro san* and carry *byakue* (wallet white coat), *wagesa* (scarf around the neck, usually purple to indicate that you are in the pilgrimage), *sugegasa* (straw hat, cone), *kongōtsue* (the cane which is the indispensable sign that identifies you as a pilgrim). Also, most pilgrims carry a notebook called *nōkyōchō*, collecting red *shuin* stamps from each temple they visit. On the white coat, *Dōgyō Ninin* is written and means "*two traveling together*," the other being the spirit of *Kōbō Daishi* the post-mortem title of monk *Kūkai*. On long trips, usually through the woods, the pilgrims were reciting sutras to rejuvenate the atmosphere. Such trips allow man to contemplate the "self," the experience of the road, the beauty of nature, the religious aspect of the journey, and, of course, the purpose of this journey. Pilgrims not only worship those who pray but during the journey, they pay homage to cultural heritage while being enveloped by the beauties of nature that lead them to their destination, giving them time to meditate on the salvation and the teachings given by Great teachers. There are considerable differences between Christianity and Buddhism. As the Buddha taught the "way," Jesus assumed to be the "path." The Buddhist Pilgrimage in Japan is mainly circular (the pilgrim being forced to visit most of the temples on the route if he can not make the whole journey) and the Christian pilgrimage is linear (the traveler goes directly to the ultimate goal of the journey). But with all the differences, pilgrimage is always a road to a meeting with the "self" and others, a path to asceticism and enlightenment. (*Valles*)

In conclusion, human nature is closely related to the universe and its laws. The karmic law governs the human condition and the "judgment" it receives when the period of "decay" ceases. Religions militate for the existence of an "essence" that is found in the deepest layers of human nature. Man is perceived differently for each religion. Buddhism denies the existence of a "self," but Christianity accepts the "self" and its eternity. In Christianity, desires are seen as sins to be punished, and in Buddhism, these are nothing more than human ignorance that prevents man from seeing the truth. Although there are similarities between religions, the human condition is not one of them.

CHAPTER XIII.
NOTIONS OF METAPSYCHOLOGICAL ANTHROPOLOGY

In regard to parapsychology, there are two variations of such defined name, i.e., parapsychology and metapsychology.

Entering your metapsychology by Charles Richet

Charles Richet, Nobel laureate for medicine (discovery of anaphylaxis) is the one who gave the name of metapsychological anthropology, a term that is gaining more ground within the borders of anthropology. As to detail, we can say that the situation is somewhat similar to that of alternative medicine or traditional medicine, which also was raised terminological issues.

Etymological variations between parapsychology and meta-psychology, considering that the latter term is more relevant as we approach the concept of metaphor, saying, lately there is growing evidence demonstrating Aristotle's maxim, founder of materialism, who emphasize that "there is spirit over matter." At the same concept, Charles Richet, analyzing vibrations in the world around us, imperceptible usually to our senses, advocating the existence of sixth sense in communication with the divine spirit." In fact, the neperian 2.14 logarithm, which ordered the five known human senses, is a free zone between listening and visuality, which would explain the presence of this sixth sense to some people with existing metapsychological capabilities.

Religion is an emanation of human culture, in our opinion pertaining to cultural anthropology, which defines human typology. In fact, cultural anthropology provides a whole other aspect of physical anthropology. Structuralist concept fully proves that "full" does not equal "sum of the parts", which makes anthropology a very complex science that "unknown is far greater than the known" (Ashby). Pythagoras said that everything in the universe is vibration, rhythm and movement, and that all phenomena, observations with the naked eye have a "translation" ciphered and radioestesy is based on this concept.

Physical body, etheric and astral body, mental body, spiritual body

Starting from this, without detailing the issues at hand, it is extremely complex to define constitutional typologies much deeper than the visible matter, we note that the techniques find their application in maintaining the health, medicine, dietetics, of character and human psychology - these last two areas are essential components of the body's constitutionality.

Lately it grows increasingly more and in connection with investigations by scientific methods a new area of research, namely, metapsychology. Parapsychology as a science is meant by addressing phenomena that cannot be explained by our current knowledge, only partially or sometimes not at all. The body is made of matter containing atoms expressed by protons and electrons. But a new question materialized on how to present the spaces between these particles: are they form vacuum or other components that we cannot explain. Based on these questions and other unexplained phenomena began research that considers human bodies and even the animals would consist of:

- **The physical body,**
- **Etheric and astral**
- **The mental body,**
- **The spiritual body**

Astral matter exists as seven distinct states, which correspond to seven physical states of matter, i.e.: solid, liquid, gaseous, ethereal, ethereal super, sub atomic and atomic. But since there have been no created names for these astral states, it is useful to call the number under that plane, the coarser material having number one in correspondence with physical states, and the subtle, number seven. For example, we are talking about solid astral matter, to name the first condition, the coarser; ethereal astral matter about to name the fourth state in the subtle plane; and so on.

Astral matter, being more subtle than physical matter enters the latter. As a result, each physical atom floating in an ocean of astral matter, perhaps other energy that surrounds and fills all the interstices of physical matter. It is well known that even the toughest substances, there are no two atoms that can achieve space between two adjacent carbons atoms is enormous compared to the size of atoms. Therefore, a living being from the astral world can occupy space as being in the physical world, and yet each of them knows anything about the existence of the other and not to hinder in any way movements.

The astral world or astral plane is, therefore, a different state of nature and not separated. Precisely because it is imperative that the physical body is contained in physical matter located in all states of aggregation - solid, liquid, gaseous and ethereal, so it is essential that astral body to include in it particles of every seven under the planes, even if their proportions may vary greatly from case to case.

Thus, man's astral body is composed of seven sub planes belonging to matter; it has the opportunity to experience all kinds of desires, from the noble to the lowest. If a man undeveloped astral body is a hazy mass of astral matter hardly organized, vaguely outlined, having regard to the prevailing lower level in a measure: it is coarse, dark color and dense; often is so dense that barely distinguishable outline of the physical body; and it is very likely to respond to stimuli related to coarse passions and desires. It expands in all directions at a distance of 25 to 30 cm outside the body. If a man has a moral and intellectual environment, the astral body is much larger and extends to about 45 cm, one side of the physical body; it contains greater elements in top quality, pure and elevated presence of these elements give the whole a certain lightness and its outline is clearly defined. In the case of a very evolved spirit, astral body it is even higher and is composed of the purest elements of each subdivision of the astral plane. As I said, man's astral body is intertwined not only to the physical body but expands around in all directions like a cloud.

That portion of the astral body that extends beyond the physical body is called, usually with the term of astral "aura". It is said that Buddha's aura was within 5 km. Not only the physical body of man has a counter part of astral matter, but all things cannot be separated only by occult power consumption, separation ceased as soon as the power is not exercised. In other words, any physical object has an astral counterpart. But as the astral particles are constantly moving, like those of a physical liquid, there is no permanent association between particle and some amount of astral matter. The main colors emitted by the astral body and which can be highlighted with special equipment, each have a specific meaning. Powell said they can represent:

- Black gray: hate and malice;
- Red: flashes of dark red, usually on a black background: anger;
- Red scarlet cloud: irritability;
- Bright scarlet red "noble indignation"
- Blood-red and dark red: sensuality;
- Gray brown, dark gray: selfishness, one of the most common colors in the astral body;
- Red brown, dark, rusty color close: avarice, usually in the form of parallel strips on the astral body;
- Greenish brown color illuminated by flashes of dark red or scarlet: jealousy. For a man accustomed usually he has much of this color when feeling "love";

- Gray: depression; as brown and red signifies avarice is arranged in the form of parallel lines that give the impression of a cage;

- Pale gray, a shade repulsive and frightening: fear;

- Cramoisi (purple red): selfish love;

- Pink: non selfish love. When color is exceptionally bright with shades of lilac, showing spiritual love for humanity;

- Orange: pride and ambition. It is often simultaneously with irritability;

- Yellow: intelligence. Ranging from dark to bright golden color and a lemon yellow, clear and bright;

- Dark yellow ocher: shows the use of intelligence for selfish purposes;

- Yellow Cambodia: obviously indicates a more evolved person;

- Primrose-yellow: indicates an intellect devoted to spiritual purposes;

- Gold: pure intelligence used to indicate philosophy or mathematics;

- Emerald green: versatility, ingenuity used in a selfless manner;

- Pale blue and light green: deep sympathy and compassion, accompanied by a power of adaptability that only these feelings can give;

- Blue (open or closed) show a religious feeling. It can be tainted by many other qualities and therefore may vary from indigo or a beautiful violet blue to gray, through all intermediate shades;

- Bright blue or cobalt blue: show devotion to a noble spiritual ideal. A purple color indicates a mixture of affection and devotion;

- Bright lilac blue, usually accompanied by sparkling golden flashes: highest spirituality with the noblest aspirations;

- Purple: developing the highest and purest of mental faculties;

Astral body functions can be classified briefly as follows:

1. To enable sensations;

2. To play the role of intermediary between the soul and physical matter;

3. Play the role of independent vehicle for knowledge and action.

Factors that determine the quality of the astral body during physical life can be classified mainly as follows: 1) The physical life; 2) emotional life; 3) mental life.

1. Physical life

Each particle of the physical body has an astral counterpart. As a result, as solids, liquids, gases and ether making up the physical body can be coarse or subtle, so does astral body. A physical body fed with impure food will match a vehicle impure, while food and drink pure helps to purify astral vehicle. The astral body is the vehicle of emotions, passions and sensations. Coarse astral body type will be easily influenced by the grossest kinds of passions and emotions, while a more refined astral body vibrates more easily influenced by emotions and aspirations more elevated. It is impossible to have a coarse physical body and the mental and astral bodies should be targeted for elevated, as it is not possible to have a purely physical body and the mental and astral bodies to be impure. These three bodies are closely related to each other.

2. *Emotional Life*

It hardly needs to remind this - the quality of the astral body is mainly determined by the way that it expresses feelings and emotions through it constantly.

3. *Mental Life*

The third and final factor leading astral body during ordinary waking life is mental life.

Mental activities have the largest effects on the astral body for two reasons:

1. Lower mental matter: Manas (as it is also called) is so closely linked to astral matter, Karma, that is almost impossible for most people to use one without the other, few people are able to think without, at the same time, to feel something.

2. Because organizing and controlling the astral body makes the mind, this is an example for the general principle that every body is molded of active consciousness of the next higher plane. Without creative power of thought, the astral body could not be organized.

Any momentum that starts from the mental to the physical body must pass through the astral body and produce such an effect on him. Moreover, since the astral matter is more sensitive to vibrations of thought than physical matter, that mental vibration effect is greater on them than on the physical body. Conversely, if the mind has no active control on the astral body, then it is especially sensitive to the influence of currents of thought from the environment, continually receives external stimuli and reacts to them.

When we analyze and divide man principles, i.e. modes of manifestation of life, the four lower principles, sometimes called "lower quaternary" are:

1. The physical body;

2. Etheric, astral;

3. Prana, or vitality;

4. Karma or desire.

In the plant kingdom, it is obviously much better developed, thus showing a greater faculty to use the lower astral matter. Specialists in botany know affinities and dislikes (desires) are more prominently in the vegetable kingdom than in the mineral world and many plants that exhibit great ingenuity and intelligence to achieve remarkable goals Plants respond to the care of the people who love them and are noticeably affected by human feelings towards them. They are particularly sensitive to the admiration and are also capable of individual attachment and repulsion. Animals are able to obtain lower strong desires, but are more limited in terms of higher desires. And they still exist and, in exceptional cases, an animal is able to show affection or devotion, with a highly elevated character. For the student of spirituality, it is of fundamental importance to gain complete control over all its vehicles, the physical, astral and mental one. To study these three bodies, we need to acknowledge each one, so that later we can develop them; in practical life, their development can be achieved at the same time each.

The third element is the mental body composed of mental matter. Vibration emanating from the mental body whose nature has been less explored is also accompanied by a color effect. Any thought of mental well-defined, produces two effects: first a vibration that propagates and the second effect is a form called form going. Astral matter is more sensitive than physical matter to the impulses of the mental world; As a result, the human astral body also has this ease to react to thoughts and vibrates in response to any thought that it touches, whether this thought comes from outside, i.e. from the mind of another man, or mind 'owner "his.

The discontinuity of consciousness between the physical and astral life is due to either lack of development astral body or the absence of links between the astral and etheric dense physical body. The spiritual body, yet without being able to prove scientifically, is part of the spirit of divinity. A variety of elements and facts advocate for this view. The soul has to some extent the ability to predict and may sometimes know in advance the events that will occur, or rather those events that could occur if measures are not taken to be avoided and may send warnings to the physical brain. In some cases, it is possible to take account of these warnings and to take all actions required to change or avoid the event foretold.

ALBERT EINSTEIN equation - $E = MC^2$

Metapsychologically interpreted

Energy E results when mass M is accelerated to speed C^2, square of the speed of light (300000 km/sec). This equation in mechanics is written this way: $E = MV^2$. The difference between the two formulations comes from the fact that it`s applied to two different levels of the matter structure. The mechanics and physics equation, looks at the energy contained in natural bodies at an atomic maximum size, while Einstein's equation refers to the energy contained and turned to the subatomic level or atomic energy as it`s usually called. So, then we have E = energy? But what form of energy? In mechanics, forms of energy are described in the chapter on thermodynamics, one of the main forms being heat energy; with it are described, however, other forms of energy, such as electric, field, the information entropy, and the forms are presented in the other, the potential, kinetic and other three forms. Atomic energy is manifested also by heat in nuclear reactors, radiant and heat in the atomic bomb and obviously the field energy of particle components of mass M. This equation if we apply a limited amount of material it cracks. The reaction is currently widely used in nuclear reactors.

But if we apply Einstein's equation to the "Big Bang" moment? We do nothing else than to assert that the whole matter MC^2 is born from an energy form "E" whose nature we do not know, but we can simply speculate what was before gave birth to immense accumulation of energy condensed at a point and which, at some point, exploded. It can be any form of energy that preceded the birth of the universe. What form of energy was it? Is it also currently out of the limits of our universe? Science can only respond with speculation to this question. But there is a source, much blasted and declared mystical, and primitive, and untrue, in which we find a response and still a very modern and incomprehensible one, before the era of computer science. In the Gospel of John, the first verses begin with the statement, "At the beginning was the word, and the word was with God, and God was the word." What is the word, what does it stand for? The answer is clear in the light of current scientific concepts, he is the bearer of information. Words, in any language, have the meaning of spoken, written codes, more recently fixed on discs, tapes, cassettes, micro disks, sticks, etc. transmitted by bright or hertzian waves, all but when the receiver knows the code and only then the information becomes intelligible for him.

But what is the information? It is now considered to be a form of energy, a force that is accepted in science and as such must be subject to the laws of thermodynamics:

Law no. 1 of Robert Mayer is the law of energy conservation. In a closed system, the forms of energy can be transformed from one to another without any loss.

Law no. 2 is the principle of Carnot, which states that energy cannot circulate spontaneously but from higher potentials to lower ones.

Law no. 3 is Clausius' postulate that asserts that spontaneously the energy transfer is from a higher potential to a lower potential. Some processes can also reverse, but in this case it is necessary to inject energy that is able to increase potential. Likewise, information can only circulate from teacher to student, whose information potentials are different, more often than not, of teachers. Information is a special form of energy that has the capacity to turn into various other forms of energy or can intervene in the structuring of matter. Information is the initiating idea, the prelude to any action, an idea followed by a project that develops the creation of material or mental structures when it does not act upon matter and remains abstract, mental, ideological, non-material, but materializable by writing, drawing, etc. The word spoken in the Bible, in Genesis, is God's command word. All creation of six days (divine and not terrestrial) because there were not yet the benchmarks to determine the notion of day, it is made by commands: "God said" and made, for example, "Light". When there is a source that generates structured information in the form of commands with a precise objective, we can admit that the source is intelligent. In Genesis, in the Bible, the making of the universe, of the earth, the appearance of life as of man all appear to us as an act of the will of a supreme intelligence that organizes and orders the execution of what ultimately will be our focus universe on Terra. It is clear from the story that this construction was step by step, in an order that, to a great extent, hugs on what historical geology found and described. Here severe criteria come to find and point out the differences between the times and sequences of biblical creation and those found geologically. The sequence of events in the Bible is correct, the appearance of Bible light corresponds to that of the first photons in the first fractions of a second of the "Big Bang," the description of the stages is perhaps too brief, there is no Precambrian life, no bacteria, and Adam's and Eve`s creation do not appear as a corollary of evolution, having as a predecessor a long line of hominids starting with Sahealantropus Tschadensis, passing through the Homo erectus, and finally hominids that we know to have had an intelligence close to that of Homo sapiens sapiens, Homo Heidelbergensis, the man of Neanderthal, Denisovanii. That is, if the anatomical evolution can be deduced after the skeletons, found more or less complete. But if we are referring to the mental evolution, the consciousness of the individuals, the work gets complicated, and it develops in successive phases. Some philosophers, like Ken Wilber, describe eight phases, and mankind is now in the fourth. In this evolution, human consciousness goes to a level called uroboric, in which the individual confuses himself with nature and passes through successive phases in which he realizes his own personality but also the limit of his existence, death, and transcends in higher phases until he reaches to understand the duality of one's own person and the existence of a transcendent domain of which his self belongs. We know about Adam, however, that he has emerged in an already superior stage of intellectual development, mind, self-consciousness, and the ability to have an abstract, information-creating thinking capable of activating and creating tools, houses, clothes, footwear, culture, painting, music, civilization, but also to make philosophy, to think abstractly. We do not know exactly where to place Adam on this development line along with his consort. But what we know from genetic studies is that Homo sapiens, sapiens, are drawn from a pair of individuals who lived in the African rift area about 200,000 years ago. This has proven to us the DNA molecules of the Y chromosome for Adam and the mitochondrial for Eve. So it seems that Adam and Eve, however, existed and lived in the heaven represented by nature in the area at that time.

Returning to the discussion regarding the nature of primordial energy E in Einstein's equation, we can say that we have no information about its nature, but we must admit that its field contains a compulsory element, namely the one who had the initiative and then realized the "Big Bang" and I believe that this is the point where the discussion begins. Who is the initiator? Incident, hazard, or a creative intelligence with initiative, are capable of materializing this information. That is, to be the creator. The struggle between these two currents is fierce despite its theoretical aspect.

The Industrial Revolution and the progress of concrete sciences have given people arguments to speculate on the fundamental problems of the origin of the universe and of life, and apart from constructing theories and models based on the latest discoveries of science. Some vehemently combat old-fashioned concepts, considering them to be outdated. And for many, they are sometimes right. This made it bluntly reject all the facts, assumptions, and new plans. To this was added a doctrinal opposition against religious cults, churches, and especially Catholic ones who, through authoritarianism and monetary materialism, on the one hand, and by opposition to any way of thinking different from the dogmas resulting from the unilateral interpretation of the Bible, on the other hand, and the adaptability of the customs to the acquisitions of the present civilization, and highlighted the dictatorial and mercantile spirit that he exercised. However, starting from denying or overturning conceptions and explanations, expanding aversion and denial on an entire domain and assigning everything and time is incorrect and harmful. I do not want to go into the critique of the concepts of creation and evolution through hazard and time and by denying an intelligent factor, but I think the discussion is not Profitable to thinking and acting as we would like, but I say that this theory desires to impose despite the fact that the scientific arguments violate the fundamental laws of physics and computer science, a fact recognized by some technicians (De Duve, Nobel Prize for Biochemistry), which states that life was created by chance, evolved through random genetic mutations, and the appearance of life on earth and its evolution an exception to the laws of nature, statistical mathematics and probability calculations. This, apart from the fact that his entire demonstration wants to explain the appearance of the DNA molecule, which he counts as the starting point for the life's genesis. But this molecule only has the role of a letter in the genetic alphabet: where is the word, where are the phrases that constitute the text of the genetic message? The letters of the alphabet, even if they exist, are nothing in the absence of the text, we have the letter, but we do not have the poetry or the short story, there must be a writer for the existence of the text.

I ask the question: who wrote the genetic code?

The symbolism of "E" will remain a subject of debate, but I continue to argue that "E" is, or has a very large component, a large portion of intelligent energy information.

The "Big Bang" was the moment when a process in which native intelligence had the initiative to create the material universe was triggered. I want to emphasize here that "E" is not material, it has no space or time. But the same thing I want to remind is that the only element in our universe that resembles the domain of "E" is information that is equal to the idea and is non-material but needs material support to act in a material environment that has space and time. The initial headquarters of information in the human social environment are the brains of people, they have ideas, initiatives, plans, they call concrete or abstract things, some of them can turn them into written recordings, and others can turn them into the most different material objects.

And now let's talk about the "=" sign of the equation. Does he represent not only the equality tie between the two terms of the equation? So, if we apply it to a mass of "m" matter, this logic has led to the release of nuclear fission energy. First the atomic bomb and then the nuclear reactors. But if we apply it dynamically (personal hypothesis), it will have the meaning of vector, as in $E\text{-}MC^2$ and will represent the "Big Bang", the moment of the genesis of our universe that creates the "M", meaning the matter, mass and speed, which, in its turn, is composed of Space and Time, that is, of the basic components of our material universe. Primitive data on nature and its evolution come from the ancient writings of many peoples. This means that human consciousness has reached a high stage of development in some individuals in ancient societies, shamans, magi, philosophers. These were people who transcended the initial stages of the development of the self and had the revelation of the transcendental domain, of a field outside the everyday universe, the material. Around everywhere, the evolution of consciousness and intellect, theories and hypotheses on the genesis of the Universe and matter, of our universe, including life, have emerged. The emergence of concrete science based on evidence and experience has led to the answer to many questions formulated by philosophy and has been the basis for development on all levels of human society. Scientific discoveries have an experimental and material basis and constitute the instrument by which the whole material basis of mankind, from food to cosmic missiles and computers, is conceived and built. But what are these products than information placed on various media, especially paper, but also any other material support. The information itself is non-material, it is born in the brain and has no informative value but for the brains that can decode it. It is born in a non-material character, part of it remains in this area, but most of it materializes in words, which remain in all materials of material storage and processing material or turn into material objects. from silex to cyclotron CERN. This transformation was first spent in the "Big Bang" when primordial information energy or a variant of it transformed into matter, "M" in the equation. Of course, there is the argument that we basically do not know anything about the environment, the domain from which the matter was born in a sequence of phenomena whose sequence is precisely known and described by astrophysics and which largely corresponds to biblical genesis. Here is a work written by a great astrophysicist (Harvard) and theologian (Jerusalem), Gerald Schroeder, who has analyzed verse by verse the Genesis and interpreted in astrophysics all those asserted there, finding a perfect concordance between the words of the Bible and the present interpretations of astrophysicists. Many scientists are vehemently fighting the phenomenon of creation itself, but also the fact that it is intelligent, arguing with the presence of inconsistencies in the sequence of events and the inconsistency of statements. It is worth mentioning, only for this chapter I of Genesis that interests us, the following:

1. The Bible is written 3000 years ago by humans, of course intellectual peaks of the time, but probably with a level of development of the ego that exceeds the average of the population but with the culture, language and knowledge of the time. The Bible was written for their congeners with limited knowledge in the field of philosophy and less of science. The facts quoted in Genesis cannot be considered to spring from the minds of religious leaders of the time. There has also been a source of revelation that happens periodically to various scientists who make unexpected leaps and emit theories that overturn classical and immutable concepts. In Genesis, such a revelation (called the thought underlying the text) took place as it did in Newton, Plank or Einstein centuries later, who in turn explained the phenomenon both in scientific style and mathematical support as well as by popular texts, both respecting the scientific truth.

2. The whole Bible has, in addition to the narrative of land events, especially in the history of the Jewish people, and a high symbolic character, especially in Genesis, to suggest that there was an intelligent initiative that initiated the "Big Bang" which the Bible calls God.

3. All construction, of the Universe, of the Earth, of life and of man is done by verbal commands, "God said..." and after execution a verification of realization expressing the opinion "And the Lord saw that it is good..." Verbal commands are information transfers that have the ability to have the effects described, but in any case, have materialized.

God made man of clay, instilled life, and the information and the clay made man. It is worth mentioning that no living creature, plant or animal, has benefited from the divine breath, nor from the information that it has made man "in His image and likeness". How can these statements be interpreted? Simply, God gave man the ability to materialize the thought. Thinking is a human faculty that raises many problems of philosophy, so serious scientists say that "The human mind cannot be defined by the actual terms of science" (Kandel), that is, the state of consciousness of man, his mind, cannot be defined in the current terms of science. Of course, the conflict between creationists and evolutionists continues to be fierce. Creationists admit that the self, the mind, the consciousness of the self, is a creation of the Creator, and is the only link of the individual's connection with the divinity. The connection with the Creator occurs only in the mind of a believer, God exists in this material universe only in the mind of the believer. Christ has shown us where God dwells. Our Father says, "You are in the Heaven," and in a few statements before the Sanhedrin and Pilate when, at the question of being a king of the Jews, he answers at least twice "My kingdom is not of this world."

Evolutionists claim that the self is a creation of the brain and dies with him. There is no later life, there is no trial, so you have the freedom to do all the mischiefs that, if not punished on earth, by human society, will in no way count, for there is no life after the death of the body. Convenient, don`t you think so? The statements of some physicists, such as Hawking, that there is no need for God to explain how the universe works, are real and correct; but they are looking for God where he says he is not, looking for him in the Einsteinian universe, temporally material, and he is transcendent, and the only connection with him is possible only through human consciousness. Faith is the only element that certifies its existence. The domain of our universe is an area in which we cannot find God, as we do not find in a car the name of the one who conceived it, Otto, Daimler or Diesel, no matter how much we seek it. They are found only in the information about their life and work contained in historical documents, but not in their material creation, the automobile, which I have just bought. So it is with the creator of the universe, it is not found in his "Our Universe", but is found in documents, the Bible, and in the minds of the faithful people. The domain of God is transcendental, it is outside our universe, which is "E" in Einstein's equation, and the sign (=) is the moment of creation, the initial burst of super condensed energy at one point. The sign (=) can also be seen as a vector (>) as we have shown before but as a bisensual vector (<>) if we take into account the military and peaceful uses of nuclear energy. For people who do not accept the existence of the transcendent and therefore of God, they do not exist and they can do it very well. Faith is a matter of free will and in no case an element of discrimination as counted by certain religions and individuals. What you think is only for you!

And now let's move on, briefly, with the discussion to the second term of the equation. We begin with (M) the mass, the Newtonian mass, which has the capacity to produce an attraction force that attracts any mass directly proportional to its size and density and inversely proportional to the square of the distance between the two masses considered. This proves the existence of a field that Newton has embodied in the law of universal attraction, gravity, whose behavior we know all about, because it enters into all the calculations of the cosmic trajectories of space vehicles, but whose nature we do not know yet or almost nothing with the exception of assumptions. But the mass itself is composed of what? From molecules, atoms, electrons and nuclei, protons, neutrons, some with electric charge, other (neutrons), with low mass (electrons) or higher mass (protons and neutrons). The particles described have been considered elementary, but we now know that they are made up of quarks that also seem to be based on smaller particles but which have a more theoretical existence (strings), being in fact a form of oscillatory energy. If we examine the structure of an atom, we see that its mass is actually concentrated in the nucleus because electrons have a negligible mass. Looking at the dimensions of these objects, we see that if the core is the size of an orange, it would be at the center of a system of circular circles that orbits the electrons, the first circle located at a distance of about 10 km. The atom is empty in terms of material mass, the rest of the structure being formed by the field created by the forces of attraction between the nucleus and the electrons. So energy. But more energy is found in the nucleus, where the protons are bound to neutrons by gluons, which prevents the disintegration of the nucleus as a consequence of the presence of electropositive tasks that tend to reject, leading to the disintegration of the nucleus, which occurs in atomic nuclei containing a larger number of protons. These substances are radioactive, because their nuclei slowly disintegrate, eliminating the components. Generally, matter, which is the whole nature and objects around us, is nothing but "structured" energy, by understanding that all the components presented, with their specific characters, make assemblies that produce stable materials, the raw material upon which the human mind works. We have here a primary structure that started with the Big Bang and continued to generate atoms from Mendeleev's painting in successive supernova explosions. This is a first form of energy structuring to produce matter. The human mind operates on a second structure through chemistry and physic chemistry operations and creates the whole arsenal of tools for both the advancement of science and the creation of current use goods. Everything that creates the human mind is proudly described as creations of the mind, human intelligence, while for the first structure of the energy that created the matter (M) from Einstein's equation, the author is considered to exist or to be pure simple happening. What material did the conversion of E into MC^2? From nothing, many say, from (E) says Einstein. Which and what is (E) we have discussed before, so it is certain that we have only theories and speculations, but no other proof outside of Einstein's equation. And now let's discuss (V) and (C) speed and specifically the speed of light, the greatest possible speed in our Universe. What hides this term tells us any physics treaty or even school textbooks. V = S / T, the speed, the space in the unit of time. (V) Therefore, conceals the space and time genesis which, together with (M), the mass, form the definition of our universally tempo material space. This is the area in which physics and all the other sciences work, the results of which are evidenced by material evidence and repeatable experiments. But where specialists in the field do not find God and I repeat, because God is not here. He is in (E), which is transcendent. Just as Otto is not in the gasoline engines of the cars. With or without our understanding or knowledge, we must accept, unless we are in bad faith that a creator exists. If we look at (V), respectively (C) composed of the two elements (S) and (T), it involves movement, another defining element of the Universe. There is nothing in the stationary, resting position, everything moves, from quarters to quarters. But the movement implies impulse, that is, energy, but in a form other than that of (M). Another element that shows that everything is nothing but structured energy.

In conclusion, both (M) and (V) or (C) of the equation represent energy forms from which we have begun to recover something, broad chemical energy, enough atomic energy, mechanical energy of nature, wind, sunlight, atomic energy, etc. What energy is structured in the form of the energy categories described in physics cannot be said because we have no information about it and everything that was before the “Big Bang”.

But what does structure mean is to arrange certain objects according to a particular scheme or structure, which is the plane that objects are arranged for. The plan often has a purpose, the structure often has a functionality and a destination. This is precisely the process a design engineer goes through when he makes the plan of the structure he had the idea to create. It is the process of materializing an idea, essentially, of transforming non-material information, the idea, in a material structure, the object (the material structure) created in the workshop. It is consistent with the Bible statement that man was made in the likeness and likeness of God. I believe that the statement merely shows, confirming that the Divinity endowed man with the same quality that he himself has, that of transforming an intangible idea into a material object, that is, exactly what God did in the moment Big Bang, when it materialized a new, unknown, form of energy into the material universe. The question that arises and discusses is whether this structure of primary energy has been made spontaneously and randomly, as some say, or was a clever act, that is, it had a purpose and a plan conceived and executed by a creator. The first observation I have to make is that no matter how this structure was made, by spontaneous genesis or by intelligent act, what was produced was the condensation of some energy quanta that gave birth to the smallest material body known, quark. Associated quarks form atomic particles, protons, neutrons, electrons, etc. Associated atoms form the molecules that make up matter in the Universe. The Universe also contains other forms of matter, such as black matter and energy, the black energy, whose existence we detect but whose nature we do not know much about. A lot of types of radiation and fields, of which gravity is the most involved in the movement of material bodies in the Universe. There are also other particles such as photons, which were the first formations in the early stages of the "Big Bang", which is also mentioned in Genesis when the Creator split the darkness of light and many other short-lived particles that appear in cyclotrons when certain materials are bombarded with accelerated particles at MeV energy levels. All construction of the material universe can be compared to a LEGO game in which the pieces are quantum energy or materialized energy (Quark). One of the modern philosophers, Ken Wilber, even has this concept and denotes the "HOLON" particles, each of which consists of underlying holons and also being part of the superhuman holons of which they are part of. If these holons have spontaneously formed or intelligent constructions cannot be proved experimentally, so scientifically, but only logically, so at the immaterial level of ideas.

Finally, I ask: can Einstein's equation suggest an answer to the question "Spontaneous Random Genesis or Creation." My answer is that he cannot. What we can do, however, is to present the arguments of the two theses that appear in many works of the partisans of the respective theses. I will not reproduce these arguments here but ask a question: Why do we consider everything created by the human mind and materialized in the civilization that surrounds us as an intelligent creation having a purpose and a logical and functional structure, and when it comes to us ourselves and the geographic and cosmic environment in which we live, as well as life itself, in all its complexity, as being generated by chance and evolution over time?

The needle with a pile is accepted by everyone that it is an intelligent creation, and a living cell of algae or bacterium has spontaneously arisen from the interaction of the elements, without purpose and without a plan, so the problem is very simplified. Genesis is an informational process, and information is considered a form of energy, and hence obeys the laws of thermodynamics. The second law (Carnot) and the third (Clausius-Clapeyron) say: Energy can only flow from a higher potential to a lower one. A man-made intelligent construction comes from his mind, which generates the information needed for construction, which has a purpose and function. This is the builder's intelligence. A product like a cell of a living organism, a mechanism of immense complexity, did it have a project, a plan after which it was made or made alone? The universe, in all its vastness and complexity, has been intelligently conceived, with a plan and functionality, or has it done by itself and by chance? Why do we do this double judgment, all we humans have done is intelligent creation, but ourselves and the environment are we a random product from which we exclude any kind of intelligence? Do not we confuse intelligent creation with the doctrines of the various religious beliefs and churches of mankind, and leave with the very field of science, according to De Duve, that life is an exception to the laws of nature and that random mutations can be winning as there are winners and the lottery.

We point out in the conclusion of this chapter that, apart from the Vatican, there is a research institute which, scientifically demonstrating the sublimation of matter from solid to eternal state, brings clear evidence of the existence of divinity.

AFTERWORD

Acad.Prof.Dr. Mircea Ifrim, the coordinator of the paper

I will briefly open a discussion on metapsychology and, implicitly, on its metapsychological type and its normality. I will present some lived and unusual personal experiences that make the metapsychological type a component that has beneficial motives.

SAI BABA

An experience for me was that of my visit to India in 2008 at a New Delphi Congress of Morphological Sciences when I had the opportunity to meet in Bangalore with the famous Sai-Baba, a prominent exponent in the metapsychology universe. Considered a parapsychological, renowned and adulated prophet, Sai-Baba is the author of an impressive journey of miraculous acts, amazing healings, and resolving incredible situations, likened by the recipients of his "powers" with Jesus Christ. His miraculous capabilities have been recorded in highly recognized scientific works written by leading personalities from U.S.A., England, and Switzerland.

Once I arrived in Bangalore in 2007, I attended a Sai-Baba audience, facilitated by the Bangalore Hospital's head physician, a medical institution pending by the SAI-BABA Foundation, one of the most modern hospitals in the world, where any man without income is treated free of charge! About 100 people, men and women, of any age, sitting separately, men in front, women in the back are welcomed to the audience. I had Prof. Steward Johns, on the left, and Indian General Salid Mohami on the right. The Professor confessed to me that he came here three years ago, having an inoperable lung cancer, and he was cured with ash given by Sai-Baba, fact verified and confirmed radiologically and clinically. The general told me that he had a small, private audience of only 10-12 people, where Sai-Baba offered the gift of a talisman, offered him, from the so-called ash of his hand, a watch gold-talisman. Gifts are offered to all people present, while the prophet discusses with them the problems they have and which he can solve.

The collective audience has another ritual. The invitees either give Sai-Baba a detailed request in which the wishes are written - what can be received or thrown or broken - or give him a gift that can be received - in which case the prophet hands his hand and blesses him - or throw it away. When Sai-Baba entered the room, chants dedicated to God, began. He started his shift from one visitor to the next and came to my side. He embraced the Professor and the general, then blessed my gift-a painting, which meant that the gift absorbed talisman like powers, then he put a hand on my head, which meant I would benefit from a private audience next time. After talking to all the men, he went to the women's group. When he came to my wife, he spoke in English (a sign of goodwill).

- You are from where?
- From Romania.
- Very bad place! - remarks Sai-Baba and moves away.

This is often the controversial attitude of the prophet, about which his disciples and admirers state that it is in accordance with what he feels, with what influx he gets from the person, with what he conveys, mentally, his ability to synthesize, to perceive, to penetrate the person in front of him: is he a person of good or evil?

I could also clearly see how, from finger movements, he leaves an ash with curative therapeutic properties for incurable diseases.

Next year, I didn`t go.

My wife did not agree with Sai-Baba because, she said, Jesus helps all people, regardless of the social condition, makes no choices or special audiences with people of a certain rank!

KAMAKURA

I arrived in Kamakura, where I wanted to visit a temple on the outskirts of the village, in a secluded, forested area. The moment I entered that temple, characterized by a perfect silence, in which everything, the air, the lights and the penumbra seemed to be stunned in a strange stillness, I suddenly stumbled upon the place, and suddenly I felt that a supernatural force flowed over me, transmitting something that communicated to me, a force that held me in strict relation to that place where I was - the middle of the temple - above which there was a huge classical Chinese lamp, in front of it is the altar with the statue of the Buddha. I could not move, I could not leave, and gradually I had the feeling that someone was talking to me, and the words were beginning to gradually become intelligible, to get strong, the words got the resonance needed for the hearing, and "Someone" told me I had to follow in my life the moral principles that I have followed so far, putting me ahead what will happen to me in the future, telling me that life will not be easy, that I will fall, but all these attempts will not weaken my ability to be just and fair, because by giving up momentary tendencies to gaining momentary advantages I will lose everything, but if I follow these tips, these guidelines, despite the hardships, everything will eventually be bright. I could clearly hear the words spoken by a voice whose resonance seemed to come from within the deepness of it all! I could not move, I could not figure out where I am, who I am, what I do, and so it went over an hour when I started to come back, realizing that I was left in that place, all that time, after which we left the temple. I was asking myself, is it a psychological disorder? I'm a doctor! What had happened? Was I too impressed? This is the first time I ever came here to Kamakura, and I was so intrigued by everything I saw that I began to have visions, or is it really a communication with the Devine? Over time, I read the book Conversations with God by Donald Walsch, where the author, asking God why He punishes him so much, begins to hear his voice and starts to write down what the voice says to him, and in that way, with question and answer, he wrote down all three volumes of his book. I felt very frustrated, and I was wondering: is my life going to be as hard as this voice has made me more detailed? Will I have to go through all those challenges? As my voice prefigured for me in the future the fall from UNESCO, the fall from the place I had set up, the University of Medicine in Oradea, the convulsions of life that would be a trial for me, I left deeply impressed with this communication with the Divinity.

Later, meeting in Paris with Professor Suzuki Tahito, from Ohio University, he told me that when he was a young assistant after completing his studies at Sorbonne, he was given the mission to accompany JP Sartre on a visit he made to Japan. What happened to me at Kamakura, Prof. Suzuki heard from the great philosopher J. Paul Sartre: after he visited and stayed for nearly two hours at the "Golden Temple" in Kyoto. Prof. Suzuki Tahito's story showed me that I was not suffering from a mental disorder, but I had lived a revelation experience. There are no coincidences.

DORU DAVIDOVICI - A TERRESTRIAL EMISSARY OF THE GALCTIC WORLDS

In 1988, we published the “Motricity Anthropology”. This book raised some issues, as it addressed some fewer material aspects and related to the metapsychological constitutional type. They had to be removed from the work, because at that time there could not be too many ideas about immateriality, and the fact that the human being is not represented only by the psychic-physical body. Being receptive to the requests of the Scientific and Encyclopedic Publishing House, at that time, the director of the publishing house proposed me the following:

- In Anthropology, you understand that some things cannot be published and you've arranged your book for this, leaving of course some elements that are not so pregnant and disagree with what can and cannot be printed and published. But we have a problem with that way of doing things. There is the Galactic Worlds of Mr. Doru Davidovich. He does not want to accept, in any way, to get something out. Look at this one, there is a whole chapter: "The human world, a zooparc". This cannot happen! We thought that it will be a good idea to put you in this book. We will give you a copy so you can have a discussion with the author. Maybe you can convince him.

- Agree.

I had a meeting with the author of this book, and I told him what my task I was:

- Commander, I am your referent. Know that I do not want to make you any difficulty, you are making your report, I sign it, you can leave your book just like this or not, the decision is yours to make, I sign it, you send it and you have my signature. But I would like to tell you a few things. I also have my Anthropology. I had some aspects about the parapsychological type, because, please believe me, I believe in parapsychology. Parapsychology is science dealing with phenomena that we cannot explain through our knowledge system. For example, I read: *Mourir ou ne pas mourir*, *Life after Life* by Raymond Moody. At the moment of apparent death, people have some visions, the spirit comes out of the body and sees a number of things that he remembers if he returns to life. Moreover, I read a work about the miracles of life, an American psychologist, Powell, who gives only facts, does not interpret anything, and these facts are very curious: for example, at one point, a young woman enters a coma is hospitalized in a clinic in Paris. This person, in a coma, has a moment of revelation and says, "I was an Egyptian princess, I was buried in this place, on my grave the following words are written." He recovers from the coma, heals himself; having a stroke, does not remember anything.

There are archaeological excavations in the place indicated by her, and there is exactly a tomb with these inscriptions. The author gives all the data, the hospital in Paris, the person's name, the address, everything, and other such facts. And I want to tell you that by telling these facts to a great surgeon, he tells me the following: I had a patient from the countryside, to whom I did a cholecystectomy with general anaesthesia. At the time of the operation, she began to ask me, in perfect English, how the operation goes, to which I answered - the operation went well - the patient returned from general anaesthesia and did not remember anything, it was a simple person from the countryside, who didn`t speak English, and the English she spoke during the operation was a perfect English, with the perfect accent, not the English we know by learning. So, sir, I believe in these things, but cannot say, and to make a chapter in saying that the human world is a zoopard is not possible. To which, Doru Davidovici tells me:

- Professor (I was called a Professor, although I was a lecturer), remember one thing. We, the ones who go in Cosmos, know some things, some very big secrets, including UFOs - which exist, and this zoopard - which is a reality; but I cannot give you more details, I can only give you this generality: that everything is determined, that there is a fate and, you see, I have also put in there certain elements that prove this.

- Yes, Commander, I have a fate too; and I told him how I got away from the 1977 earthquake. Yeah, and I can tell you that this is reality, we're a zoo. I believe you, of course, you cannot tell me more, do what you think.

Doru Davidovich probably reflected on the conversation with me, he made the report, I signed it, got it out of the paper. So, thinking retrospectively, that all these things were consuming me, that so much is happening, and that God is determining your fate, I was saying to myself: it is a fate in the course of life.

This means you're surfing the storm. What will come next? And here I am wondering what will happen in the future, what is left of the encounter with God in Kamakura, yet have I navigated this storm? I try, navigating like this, to draw as much as I can from many past teachings. I'm trying to figure out how much I can of these things, because in fact it's a splitting of clouds and waters without onboard instruments, and in which only the intuition and the junction between your spirit and the universal spirit can make you sail more wisely. But at the same time, the awareness of the fact that there is a fate, the awareness that not everything is reduced to materiality, gives you the power to think that everything that is happening is an internship, and this stage depends on what the future will be.

It is possible for death to mean life, and this life is the result of what, in this terrestrial existence, you realize and, at the same time, there is a cycle of spirit in which you have the more chances of remaining in the spirit world and in a more elevated area, the more you understand your fate and choose what is in accord with your predestination.

*

*   *

I conclude this essay through a poetry prayer written by the brilliant poet and philosopher Mihai Eminescu, less known poetry, which was recited in Romanian by Pope John Paul II in Vatican.

Empress of our choosing
We kneel praying,
Ascend us, save us
From the wave that haunts us:
Be shielding
And the wall of salvation,
Your gaze is worshiped
Come down among us,
Oh, mother too clean,
And always virgin,
    Mary!
We, from the mercy of the saint
Make shadow upon the earth,
Praying for forgiveness,
To the star upon the Seas;
Listen to our complaints,
Queen over Angels,
From mist show thyself,
Clear sweet light,
Oh, mother too clean
And always virgin,
    Mary!

By Acad. Mircea Ifrim, the coordinator of this treatise

SELECTIVE BIOGRAPHY

*** Bible
*** Dhammapada
Ackermann, Peter; Maria Rodriguez del Alisal; Dolores P. Martinez (ed.). *Pilgrimages and Spiritual Quests in Japan*. London, New York: Routledge. 2007
Alexandrescu, Constantin, *Igiena educației fizice și sportului*, Editura Sport-Turism, București, 1980
Alvarado, C.S., *Human radiations: Concepts of force in mesmerism, spiritualism and psychical research*, Journal of the Society for Psychical Research 70, 138-162, 2006
Ardelean, Tiberiu, *Unele aspecte privind dezvoltarea calităților motricitye*. în *Revista de educație fizică și sport*, 1983-1985
Ashby, Robert H., *The Guidebook for the Study of Psychical Research*, Rider, 1972
Aubaret, D., *L'Anatomie sur le vivant*, Ed. Baillière, Paris, 1920
Avramoff, E., *Unele aspecte medico-biologice în gimnastică*, Editura Sport-Turism, București 1983
Baroga, Nicolae, *Calități motricitye combinate*, Editura Sport, București,1985
Basarab, Mihai, Broadbent, B.H., *Ontogenie development of occlusion*. Angle Orthodontist. Nr. I 1:223-241, 1941
Baskin, Diana, *Divine Memories*, SRI Sathya SAI Books & Publications Trust, India
Bayer, M.L., *The assessement of somatic androgynity*, American Journ of Phys. Anthrop, 4, p. 433-462, 1946
Bălăceanu-Stolnici, Constantin, *Cunoaştere şi ştiinţă*. Ed. Fundației Andrei Şaguna, Constanţa, 1997
Bălăceanu-Stolnici, Constantin, *Cibernetica* (în colab. cu Edmond Nicolau), 1961
Bălăceanu-Stolnici, Constantin, *Dialoguri despre cele văzute şi nevăzute*, 1995
Bălăceanu-Stolnici, Constantin, *Incursiune în lumea sufletului. O abordare antropologică*, Editura Paideia, 2003
Bălăceanu-Stolnici, Constantin, *Les fondements cybernétiques de l'activité nerveuse*, Paris, 1971
Bălăceanu-Stolnici, Constantin, *Neuropsihologia postmodernistă*, 2000
Bălăceanu-Stolnici, Constantin, *Personalitatea umană – o interpretare cibernetică* (în colab. cu Edmond Nicolau), 1972
Bălăceanu-Stolnici, Constantin, *Tratat de geriatrie practică*, 1998
Beerli, P., "Bioinformatics", 2006, *Oxford Univ. Press*
Bayley, Jonathan. *From Egypt To Canaan: Being The Divine Description Of The Regenerate Life Shown By Israel In Egypt, The Journey In The Wilderness, And The Conquest Of Canaan (1867).* Kessinger Publishing, LLC. 2008
Bielicki,T., Welon Z., *The sequence of growth velocity peaks of principal body dimensions in girls*. In *Mat. i Prace Antrop.*, nr. 86, 1973
Blaga, Lucian, *Aspecte antropologice*. Ed. Facla, Timişoara, 1970
Boca, Arsenie, *Tinerii, familia şi copii născuți în lanțuri. Din învățăturile părintelui Arsenie Boca,* Editura Credința Strămoșească, 2009
Bouchard, C., Thibault, M.C., Jobin J., *Advanced in selected areas of human work physiology*, In Yearbook Phys. Anthrop., vol. 24:1, 1981
Bouchard,C., Malina R.M., *Genetics of physiological fitness and motricity performance*, In Laval Univ. Press, 306, 1983
Bourgine, Jérôme, *Din tainele călătoriilor extracorporale*, Editura Ram, 1999
Brătescu, Gh. Neagu, *Jurnalele lui Fr. Rainer*, Ed. Eminescu, 1979
Brower, M. Brady, *Unruly Spirits: The Science of Psychic Phenomena in Modern France*, University of

Illinois Press, 2010
Brozek, J., Keys A., *The evolution of leaness-fatness in man: norms and inter-relantionships*. In Brit. J. Nutr., vol. 5:194, 1951
Buckland, Raymond, T*he Spirit Book: The Encyclopedia of Clairvoyance, Channeling, and Spirit Communication*, Visible Ink Press, p. 131, 2005
Burnet, John, *Early Greek Philosophy*, Adam&Charles Black, London, 2014
Carrel, Alexis, *L'homme cet inconnu*, versiune în limba română de Dan Oprescu. Ed. Victor-Victor, Bucureşti, 2004
Cauhepe, Jean, *Les variations de la tête,* L'orthodontie française, 1951
Charzewski, J., et al., *Zarys antropologii* (pod redakcja Haliny Milicer), Warsawa,1980
Chranowskiej Maria, Materialydo cwiczen Z antropologii
Church, George M., Edregis, *How synthetic Biology will reinvent nature and our selves*, în *Regenesis*, oct. 2, 2012
Confucius. *The Analects*. Arcturus Publishing Limited. 2010
Corander, J., Waldmann, P., Sillanpää, MJ., *Bauesian analysis of genetic differentiation between populations,* 2003
Cornford, Francis M., *Plato's Cosmology*, Hackett Publishing Co., Cambridge, 2005
Covic, Mircea, Ştefănescu, Drago, Sandovici, Ionel, *Genetica medicală*, Polirom, 2011
Cremo, Michael A., *Human Devolution – A Vedic Alternative to Darwin'sTheory*, Torchlight Publishing, 2014
Cummings, Michel, *Human Heredity: Principles and Issues*, 2013
Demeter, A., *Bazele fiziologice ale educaţiei fizice*, Editura Sport-Turism, Bucureşti, 1972
Demeter, A., *Calităţile fizice*, Editura Sport-Turism, Bucureşti, 1983
Demeter, A., *Fiziologia sporturilor*, Editura Sport-Turism, Bucureşti, 1978
Dennett, Daniel, *Tipuri mentale, o încercare de înţelegere a conştiinţei*, Ed. Humanitas, Bucureşti, 1996
Djuvara, Neagu, *O scurtă istorie a românilor povestită celor tineri (Carol I)*, Ed. Humanitas, Bucureşti, 2002
Drăgan, I., *Medicină Sportivă*, Editura Stadion, Bucureşti, 1974
Drăgan, I., *Selecţia medico-biologică în sport*, Editura Sport-Turism, Bucureşti 1979
Dumitru, Carmen, *Selecţia în gimnastică*, Com. *Daciana*, 1983
Dumitru, V., *Aspecte ale creşterii şi dezvoltării în etapa postpubertară*, în *Palestra*, nr.13, 1973
Dumitru, V., *Studiul dezvoltării fizice la şcolari printr-un sistem de proporţii corporale*. Comunicare, în vol. Acad. de Şt. Med., 1979
Eliade, Mircea, *Istoria credinţelor şi ideilor religioase* (vol. I şi III), Ed. Ştiinţifică şi enciclopedică, Bucureşti, 1981
Epuran, M., *Personalitatea*, Editura I.E.F.S., Bucureşti, 1983
Falconer, D.S., *Dziedziczenie ceh ilosciowych*, PWN, Warsawa, 1974
Feldman, D.R., Wendkos, Olds, S., Papalia, E.D., *Dezvoltarea umană*, Ed. Trei, Bucureşti, 2010
Ferembach D., Susanne C, Chamla M-C., *L'Homme, son évolution, sa diversité*. Ed. Doin, 1986
Firea, Elena, Ifrim, Mircea, *Valoarea unghiului biiliac în selecţia sportului*. Com. *Congres Anatomie Insbruck*, 1984
Firea, Elena, *Metodica Educaţiei Fizice şi Sportului*, Editura I.E.F.S., Bucureşti, 1984
Firu, P., Apostolescu, *Asistenţa şi învăţământul de medicină dentară din trecut până în prezent*, Ed. Junimea, Iaşi, 2006
Firu, P., *Introducere în studiul anomaliilor dento-maxilare*
Firu, P., Slăvescu, Dan, Apostolescu, Svetlana, *Periodontita la copii şi adolescenţi*. Ed. Romcartexim,

București, 1998
Firu, P., *Stomatologia infantilă*. Ed. Didactică şi pedagogică, Bucureşti, 1983
Firu, P.; Apostolescu, *Asistenţa şi învăţământul de medicină dentară din trecut până în prezent*. Ed. Junimea, Iaşi, 2006.
Firu, P.; Slăvescu, Dan; Apostolescu Svetlana, *Periodontita la copii şi adolescenţi*. Ed. Romcartexim, Bucureşti, 1998
Floru, Eugen, *Tractul ilio-tibial*, Ed. Imprimeriile statului, București 1946
Focșeneanu, Anca. *Civilizație japoneză – de la origini până în epoca clasică*. Cluj-Napoca: Editura Eikon. 2014
Forbes, G.B., *Toward a new dimension in human growth*, în *Pediatrics*, vol. 36: 825, 1965
Forna N., coordonator, *Actualităţi în clinica și terapia edentației parţial întinse*, Ed." Gr.T. Popa" 2009
Forna N., coordonator, *Protetica dentară,* vol. I şi II, Editura Enciclopedică, 2011
Fuller, J., Denehi, G., *Concise Dental Anatomy and morphology*. Ed. Yearbook Med. Publ. Chicago London, 1979
Gagea, A., *Selecţia sportivă în tir şi scrimă*, în vol. *Cercetări*, I.E.F.S., Bucureşti, 1982
Gane, C., *Trecute vieţi de doamne şi domniţe*, vol. I şi II, Ed. Orizonturi, Bucureşti
Gardner, Mark and Barbara, *Sai Baba and You – Practical Spirituality*, SRI Sathya SAI Books & Publications Trust, India
Gavrilă, Lucian – *Principii de ereditate umană*, Editura ALL 2004.
Gavrilă, Lucian, *Principii de ereditate umană*, Editura ALL, 2004.
Ghooi, Charanjit, Dr. (Mrs.), *Spirituality and Health*, SRI Sathya SAI Books & Publications Trust, India
Giroud, A., Lelièvre, A., *Elements d'embriologie*. Ed. Libr. François, Paris, 1965
Glavce, C., *Studiul mixt-longitudinal al copiilor de vârsta preşcolară mică (5-8 ani) provenind din localităţi cu grade diferite de urbanizare şi altitudine*, Universitatea Iaşi; 1979 (teză de doctorat)
Glavce, C. et al., *Atlasul antropologic al Banatului de Sud-Est*, Ed. Academiei Române, 2004
Glavce, C. et al., *Secolul XXI şi provocările antropologiei*, Ed. Bioedit, Ploieşti, 1999, 316 pagini
Glavce, C., Avăpăloaie, Ligia, Radu, Elena, Popa, Ion, *Atlasul antropologic al Transilvaniei*, vol. II, Ed. Academiei Române, 2005
Glavce, C., Firu. P., Vlad, V., *Curs de pedo-ortodontică*, 160 de pagini, Univ. Ecologică Bucureşti, Curtea Veche SRL, VII, *Particularităţile examenului clinic în prevenirea afecţiunilor buco-dento-maxilare*, 1993, p. 93-138
Glavce, C., Iancu, E., Rodewald, A., *Relaţii între nivelul hormonilor sexuali, parametri biochimici şi tipologia constituţională*, Ed. Bioedit 2002, 246 pagini, 2005
Glavce, C., Iancu, E.E., *Elemente de tipologie constituţională*, Ed. Bioedit 2002, 119 pagini
Glavce, C., Iancu. E., Bălteanu, C.,Stârcea-Crăciun, M., *Francisc I. Rainer – Colecţii Antropologice*, Ed. Bioedit, 50 de pagini, in print
Glavce, C., Radu, E., Dragomirescu, I., *Ghid practic de antropologie*, vol. I, *Iniţiere în antropometrie, Natura Practică 1 – colecţia biologie-ecologie, Universitatea Bucureşti*, Ed. Ars Docendi 2002, 55 pagini
Glavce, C., *Antropologia Rainer*, 2003
Glavce, C., *Antropologia Rainer*, 2003
Glavce, C., *Atlasul antropologia al Munteniei*, Ed. Academiei Române, 1999 – Premiul I.C. Parhon al Acadeiei Române, 2001
Glavce, C., *Atlasul antropologic al Munteniei*, Ed. Academiei Române, 1999 – Premiul I.C. Parhon al Academiei Române, 2001
Glavce, C., *Atlasul antropologic al Transilvaniei*, vol. I, Ed. Academiei Române, 2005
Glavce, C., *Studiul mixt-longitudinal al copiilor de vârsta preşcolară mică (5-8 ani) provenind din localităţi*

cu grade diferite de urbanizare şi altitudine, Universitatea Iaşi, 1979 (teză de doctorat)
Gray, Henri, *Gray's Anatomy. Anatomy Descriptive and surgical et. XV-e*, Ed. Pickering Pick London,1999
Griffiths, William M., Miller, Jeffrey, H., Suzuki, David T. et al., "Genetics and the Organism: Introduction". *An Introduction to Genetic Analysis* (ed. 7th), New York: W.H. Freeman, 2000
Guieu, Jean-Michel, *6 – Tensions nationalistes et efforts pacifistes. La France, l'Allemagne et l'Europe (1871-1945)* (in French), 2005, Retrieved 2015-03-11
Guja, Cornelia et al., *Caracterizarea biofizică a adultului tânăr*, Lucrare plan. Centrul de Antropologie, 1984
Guja, Cornelia şi Pavalan, Mariana, *Critères anthropologiques pour la constitution d´une typologie humaine naturelle*
Guja, Cornelia, *An Interdisciplinary Method: INTEGRONIC THINKING*, Bulletin A.O.S. *Commission D´études interdisciplinaires*, janvier-juin, p. 33-39, 1984
Guja, Cornelia, Electronographical Results, în Anthropology, Ann. Roum. Anthropol., 115, 53-55, 1978
Guja, Cornelia, *Parametrii biofizici proporţionali, variabilitatea lor*, Teză de doctorat, Conducător ştiinţific, Acad. Ştefan M. Milcu.
Guja, Cornelia, *Propriétés bioélectriques de l´enveloppe cutanée humaine. Résultats de quelques recherches expérimentales, Bull. et Mém. de la Soc. d´Antrop. de Paris*, t. 7, séries XIII, p. 205-220,1980
Gupta, Gauri Shankar, *Unraveling Mysteries of Life: Modern Science and Ancient Wisdom*, Reálszisztéma Dabasi Nyomda Zrt, 2012
Gysel, Carlos, *La naissance de la morphologie dento faciale*. Ed. Beaux arts Lyon, 1980
Hamon, Hervé, *Nos médecins*, Ed. Du Seuil, Paris, 1994
Hartl, Daniel L., *Essential Genetics*, Oct. 12, 2012
Hein, J., Schierup, M.H., y Carstein, W., *Gene Genealogies, Variation and Evolution: a primer in Coalescent Theory*, Oxford University Press, 2006
Hrişcă, Aristeia et al., *Baschetul*, Editura Sport-Turism, Bucureşti, 1984
Ifrim, M, Iliescu, Andrei, *Anatomia şi Biomecanica Educaţiei Fizice şi Sportului*, Editura Didactică şi Pedagogică, Bucureşti, 1979
Ifrim, M. et al., *Atlas de Anatomie Umană*, vol. I, II, III, Editura Ştiinţifică şi Enciclopedică, Bucureşti, 1983-1985
Ifrim, M. et al., *Contribution à l´étude du type anthropologique optimum et des critères de sélection pour les jouers de handball*, Congrès International D´Anatomie, Mexic, 1980
Ifrim, M. et al., *Recherches antropologiques concernant la corrélation entre les facteurs génétiques et la performance sportive*, în *Médecine du Sport*, 1982, nr. 4
Ifrim, M. et al., *Riscul malformativ în reproducerea umană*, Editura Medicală, Bucureşti, 1978
Ifrim, M., *Antropologie motricityă*, Editura Științifică şi Enciclopedică, 1988
Ifrim, M., *Actualităţi în antropologie cu aplicabilitate în sport*, Editura I.E.F.S., Bucureşti, 1981
Ionescu, Adrian, *Creşterea şi dezvoltarea*, Editura Stadion, Bucureşti, 1970
Izard, C., *Orthodontie,* Ed. Masson, Paris, 1950
Jakobsson, M., Rosenberg, N.A., *Bioinformatics*, Oxford Univ. Press, 2007
Kanu, Victor, *Sathya Sai Baba God Incarnate*, SRI Sathya SAI Books & Publications Trust, India
Katch, F., Ardle, W.D., *Validity of body composition prediction equations for college men and women*, în *Amer. Clin. Nutr.*, vol. 28: 105, 1975
Kenny, Anthony, *Aristotle On the Perfect Life*, Clarendon Press, Oxford, 2014
Kirk, G.S., Raven, J.E., Schofield, M., The Pre-Socratic Philosophers, Cambridge University Press, 2012
Kovar, R., *Human variation in motricity abilities and its genetic analysis*, Univ. Ivarl, Praha, 1980
Kovar, R., *Prispevekke studiu geneticke podminenosti lidske motricityiky*, Autoref. Dys. Dokt. Uniw. Karola, Praga, 1974

Krystal, Phyllis, *Sai Baba – The Ultimate Experience*, SRI Sathya SAI Books & Publications Trust, India
Kunst Ghermănescu, Ioan et al., *Handbalul*, Editura Didactică şi Pedagogică, Bucureşti, 1983
Lao Zi. *Dao De Jing.* București: Editura Herald. 2014
Larchet, Jean-Claude, *Teologia bolii.* Ed. Oastea Domnului, Sibiu, 1997
Lewis, Ricki, *Human Genetics*, Oct 7, 2011
Maliţa, M., *Aurul Cenuşiu*, Editura Politică, Bucureşti, 1975
Maliţa, M., *Orizontul fără limite al învăţăturii*, Editura Politică, Bucureşti, 1981
Marchocka, M. et al., *Specific body build of judo athletes depending out the fighting technique used*, Biology of Sport, Warszawa, vol. 1/3-4, 1984
Martin, A.O., Kurczynski, T.W., Steinberg, A.G., *Familial studies of medical and anthropometric variables in a humanisolate*, în *Amer. J. Hum. Genet.*, vol. 25: 581, 1975
Martin, R., Saller, K., Muzj, Edmondo – *Lehrbuch der Antropologie*. Ed. Gustav Fischer, Stuttgart, 1956. Antropometrie oro-facială. Ed. J. Prelat, Paris, 1967
McCabe, Joseph, *Scientific Men and Spiritualism: A Skeptic's Analysis*, The Living Age. 12 June, pp. 652-657, 1920
McMartin, Grace J., *A Recapitulation of Baba's Divine Teachings*, SRI Sathya SAI Books & Publications Trust, India
Milcu, Şt.M., Ulmeanu, Fl., *Beitrag zum Studium den endokrinen Drüsen bei den Sportlern*, Berlin II., Intern Sport Kongress, 1936 (36)
Milcu, Şt.M., Ulmeanu, Fl., *Contribution à l´étude des glandes endocrines chez les sportifs*, Buc. Soc. Med. de educaţie fizică, 1936, V/3-4 (57-60)
Milcu, Şt.M., Ulmeanu, Fl., *L'influence des exercices sportifs sur les glandes endocrines*, Anal. Educ. Fiz, 1937, VI/3 (244-248)
Milcu, Şt.M., *Examenul clinic al glandelor endocrine la 50 de atleţi participând la Balcaniadă*. Anal. Educ. Fiz. 1937, VI/4 (310-311)
Milcu, Şt.M., *Genetica*, Editura Academiei R.S.R., Bucureşti, 1974
Milcu, Şt.M., *Influenţa travaliului muscular asupra glandelor endocrine*. Educaţia Fizică la individul normal şi patologic. Metodă, tehnică, indicaţii. Conferinţe, Bucureşti, 1933 (136-144)
Milcu, Şt.M., *Introducere în antropologie*, Editura Academiei R.S.R., Bucureşti, 1978
Milcu, Şt.M., *Les Glandulas Endocrinas en Relación con la Performance y el Sobreentrenamiento*, în *Medicina de la Cultura Fisica*, Red. Dr. Fl.C. Ulmeanu, pg. 113, editorial Pax Mexico, 1969
Mogoş, I., Mitra, Gh., *Metodica educaţiei fizice*, Editura Sport-Turism, Bucureşti, 1984
Mueller, W.H., Titcomb, M., *Genetic and environmental determinants of growth of schooll aged children in a rural Colombian population*, în *Ann. Hum. Bio.*, vol. IV, nr. 1:1, 1974
Muller, F. Max (edited & translated), *The Sacred Books of the East – The Upanishads*, volume I to XV, Low Price Publications, Delhi, 2010
Nickell, Joe, *Adventures in Paranormal Investigation*, The University Press of Kentucky. p. 215, 2007
Nicu, Alexe et al., *Potenţialul biomotricity al populaţiei şcolare din R.S.R.*, Editura C.N.E.F.S., Bucureşti, 1972
Niculescu, I.D., *Anatomia dinţilor*, Ed. Cultura, Bucureşti, 1931
Nikitjuk, B.A., Kogan, B.I., *Blizneţovii metod v biologii, mediţine i sporte, Naucini sovet AN SSSR. po problemam genetike*, Mediţinschii Institut im. Pirogova Gosudarsvenii Teatralnâi, ordena Lenina, Institut fiziceschii cultura, 1984
Nishida, Kitarō. *Last Writings: Nothingness and the Religious Worldview.* SUA: University of Hawaii Press. 1987
Oprescu, L., Glavce, Cristina, *Însemnări memorialistice prezentate de Ştefan Marius Milcu*, Ed. Academiei Române, 2006

Osho, *Povestiri Zen comentate de Osho*, Editura Ram, 2003
Papilian, V., *Anatomia omului*, vol. I, II, Ed. Didactică şi pedagogică, Bucureşti, 1974
Pariskowa, J., *La masse active, la graisse deposée et la constitution corporelle chez les sportives de haut niveau*, în *Kinatropologie*, 95, 1972.
Pariskowa, J., *Siledovani zmen podilu aktivni telesne hmoty a tuku pri ruzne intensite a prepuseni pohygu*, în *CS. Fyxiol.* t. 9, 253, 1960
Păscanu, Mariana, Andreescu, Florin, Radu, D., Adumitroaiei, C., *Oltenia de Nord*, Ed. Ad. Libri, Bucureşti, 2006
Pensrose, L.S., *Wstep do genetyki czlowieka*, PWN, Warszava, 1965
Petrescu, A., *Stomatologia bucureşteană la 1878*, revista Stomatologia nr. 5:451, 452, Bucureşti
Plutschow, E. Herbert. *Chaos and Cosmos: Rituals in Early and Medieval Japanese Literature.* Netherlands: Suntory Fundation. 1990
Polidoro, Massimo, *Final Séance: The Strange Friendship Between Houdini and Conan Doyle.* Prometheus Books, pp. 171-172, 2001
Popa, Fr., Popa Florica, *Anatomia lui Gray descriptivă şi aplicată*, Ed. Jean Leon, Bucureşti, 1944
Powell, A.E., *Corpul Astral*, Editura Ram, 2009
Powell, A.E., *Corpul Cauzal*, Editura Ram, 2007
Preda, Victor, *Tratat elementar de antropologie*, Ed. Dacia Traiana, 1947
Rabacky, Raoul, *Anatomia funcţională,* vol. I, II, III, Editura Scrisul Românesc, 1986
Raczynka, B. et al., *Investigations of heredity of blood. Plasma cortisol level in human, Biology of sport*, Vol. I, Nr. 2/1984
Rainer, Fr.I., *Jurnale*, Ed. Eminescu, Bucureşti, 1979
Rainer, Fr.I., *Oeuvre scientifique*, Editura Academiei Române, Bucureşti, 1945
Răduţ, C., *Criterii de selecţie*, Editura C.N.E.F.S., Bucureşti, 1967
Răzuş, Mircea, *Un model morfofiziopsiho-cibernetic al personalităţii umane, Conferinţa Naţională de Cibernetică* – 1983
Richet, C., *Our Sixth Sense*, London: Rider (First published in French, 1928), nd, ca 1928
Richet, C., *Thirty Years of Psychical Research*, New York: Macmillan (Translated from the second French edition), 1923
Richet, C., *Traité de métapsychique*, Ed. Félix Alcan, Paris, 1922
Rossman, J., *Anatomic and body composition changes with ageing*, în *Handbook of the biology of ageing, Van Nostrand Reinhold co*, 1977
Russel, Bertrand, *Human Knowledge*, Routledge, New York, 2001
Sandweiss, Samuel H., Dr., *Sai Baba – The Holy Man and Psychiatrist*, SRI Sathya SAI Books & Publications Trust, India
Sandweiss, Samuel H., *Spirit and the Mind*, SRI Sathya SAI Books & Publications Trust, India
Saville, P.D., Heaney, R.P., *Osteoporosis, Practical geriatrics*, Karger, Basel, 1975
Săhleanu, V., *Dinamica şi problematica antropologică a vârstei adulte, Varia Antropologice*, 9/1974 Bucureşti
Săhleanu, Victor, *De la omul necunoscut la omul cognoscibil.* Ed. Ramida, Bucureşti, 1996
Sedley, David, *The Cambridge Companion to Greek and Roman Philosophy*, Cambridge University Press, 2000
Sharma, S.C., Dr., *Ayurveda – The Ultimate Medicine*, Wisdom Tree, New Delhi, 2003
Siclovan, Ion, *Teoria educaţiei fizice*, Editura Sport-Turism, Bucureşti, 1980
Silverman, S., *Oral physiology*, Ed. Mosby Co ST. Louis
Simu, Octavian. *Shintō – Calea zeilor.* București:Editura Herald. 2008
Sina, Abu Ali (Avicenna), *Poemul medicinei, canonul ştiinţei medicale*, ed. Medicală, Bucureşti 1962

Skibińska, A., Sklad, M., *Genetic determination of heath Carter somatotype*, *Biology of Sport*, Vol. I/1984 Warszawa

Skibińska, A., *Ciezar tkanki tluszczowei podskornej i ciala szczuplego*, în *Wych Fiz. i Sport*, t. 5: 57, 1961

Starosta, V. et al., *Variation of selected agility (cocrdonation) indices in young wrestlers during training*, *Biology of Sport*, vol. II, Nr. 1/1985

Starosta, W., *Mouvement coordination as an element in sport selection system*. *Biology of Sport*, Vol. I, Nr. 2/1984

Stănculescu, Victor, *Antrenamentul în fotbal*, Editura Sport-Turism, Bucureşti, 1983

Swarz, W.S., *O roli nosredstwiennych e sredowych factorow w razwitii fiziczescoj robotosposobnosti n dietej i podrostkow*, în *Issledowanije blizniecow*, Dys. Dokt., Tatra, 1972

Swarz, W.S., *Orali nosredstwiennych i sredowych factorow w razwitii fiziczeskoj robotosposobnosti w dietej i podrostkow*, în *Issledowanije blizniecow*, Dys. Doct., Tatra, 1972

Sykes, Bryan, The Seven Daughters of Eve, W.W. Norton & Company Inc., 2001

Szopa, J., Mleczko, E., Miernik, Cz., Niklinska, K. – *Wplyw selekcji i zwiekszonej oktymnosci ruchowej na poziom rozwoju fizycznego, psychomotricityycznego i sprawnosci fizycznej chlopcow i dziewxzat z krakowskich klas sportowych na tie populacii porownawczej*, în *Wych. Fiz i Sport*, Nr. 1:4, 1984

Szopa, J., *Dziedziczenie wymiarow I wskaznika glowy u czlowieka przegland, Antropologiczny*, Tom 43 z.1, Poznan, 1977, Nadbitka

Szopa, J., *Dziedziczenie wysokosci ciala u czlowieka*, în *Mat. i Prace Antrop.*, Nr. 92:53, 1976

Szopa, J., *Genetic and environmental determination of the body weight in man. Results of family studies*, în *Genet. Pol.*, vol. 23, nr. 1:257, 1982

Szopa, J., *Genetic determination of the body height man,* în *Genet. Pol.* vol. 20, nr. 2:277, 197

Szopa, J., Genetic determination of the human head measurements, în Genet. Pol. vol.19, nr. 3:345, 1978

Szopa, J., *Genetycznei srodowiskowe czynniki rozwoju niektorych cech metrycznych glovy, twarzi i nosa oraz wysokosci ciala u czlowiek*, în *Mat. i Prace Antrop.* Nr. 100:57, 1981

Szopa, J., *Inheritance of measurements of shoulder and thigh breadth and body proportion in man*, în *Genet. Pol.* vol. 18, nr. 3:275,1977

Szopa, J., Inheritance of the dimensions and facial index in man, în Genet. Pol., vol. 19, Nr. 3:401, 1976

Szopa, J., *Ksztaltowanie sie zwiazkov korelaccynych miedzy wymiarami glowy i twarzy oraz wzrostu rodzicow i dzieci w procesie biomorfozy*, Zeszyty Naucowe Uniwercytetu jagielloskiego, *Prace – Zoologiczne – Zeszyty* 2, 1978

Szopa, J., *Oblicbzanie prawdopodobienstwa ojcostwa napodztawie wybranych cech antropometrycznych*, Zessyty Naucowe Uniwersytetu Jaguellonskiego, *Prace Zoologiczne – Zeszyty* 27, 1981

Szopa, J., *Zmienosc oraz genetyczne uwarunkowania niektorych przejawow sily miesni u czlowjeka. Wyniky badan rodzinnych*", în. *Mat. i Prace Antrop.* Nr. 103:131, 1983

Şteflea, D., *Reflectări cronobiologice în medicină* Editura Medicală, Bucureşti, 1984

Taisen, Deshimaru; Etienne, Zeisler. *Satori – Mari maeștri zen.* București, Editura Herald. 2013

Tanner, J.M., Israelsohn, W.J., *Parent-child correlation for body measurements of children between ages of one months and seven years*, în *Ann. Hum. Genet.*, vol. 26:245, 1963

Tanner, J.M., *Growth and Adolescence*, Oxford, Blackwell Sci. Publ., 1955

Tanner, J.M., *Rozwoj w okresie pokwitania z uwzglednieniem wplywu czynnikow dziedzicznich i srodwiskowych na wzrastanie i dojrzewanie od urodzenia da dojrzalosci*, Pzwl, Warszawa, 1963

Tatu, Titus et al., *Atletismul*, Editura Didactică şi Pedagogică, Bucureşti, 1984

Teodorescu, Dem., Mic atlas de anatomia omului, Ed. Didactică şi pedagogică, Bucureşti, 1974

Testut, L., Latarjet, A., *Traité d'Anatomie humaine,* Ed. Gaston Doin, Paris, 1930

Valea, Ernest. *The Human Condition in World Religions.* http://www.comparativereligion.com/man.html - accessed on 17.05.2017

Viola, G., *La costituzione individuale*, Ed. Cappelli, Bologna, 1951

Walker, R., *Standards for somatotopy children, The prediction of young adult height from children´s growth data, Ann. of. Human Biology* 1; 145-159; 1974

Watson, D. James, Baker, Tania A., Bell Stephen P. and Gann, Alexander, *Molecular Biology of the Gene* (ed. 7th), 2013

Watson, D. James, Berry, Andrew, DNA: "The Secret of Life", *Knoph*, 17 august 2004

Wolanski, N., *Antropometria, inzymieryjna*, Kiw Warszawa, 1975

Wolanski, N., Parizkowa, J., *Sprawnosk fizyczna a rozwoj cztowieka*, Sit, Warszawa, 1976

https://www.scribd.com/doc/197970294/Last-Writings-Nothingness-and-the-Religious-Worldview-by-Kitaro-Nishida -accessed on 10.05.2017

http://booksandjournals.brillonline.com/content/journals/10.1163/18725473-12341299;jsessionid=OoqzjnW-h6Gpqx_tPDAVe7m9.x-brill-live-03 – accessed on 12.05.2017

http://www.accesstoinsight.org/lib/authors/nanamoli/wheel017.html#s1 – accessed on 05.05.2017

http://fromhankototokyochichibu.blogspot.ro/2016/05/day-one-of-pilgrimage-walking-walking.html - accessed on 07.05.2017

ARA Publisher, an international publishing house of the
American Romanian Academy of Arts and Sciences
University of California Davis
http://www.AmericanRomanianAcademy.org
Email: info@AmericanRomanianAcademy.org
Address: P.O. Box 2761, Citrus Heights, CA 95611-2761

Lightning Source UK Ltd.
Milton Keynes UK
UKHW051933270219
338150UK00009B/294/P

9 781935 924272